Clinical Cases in
Implant Dentistry

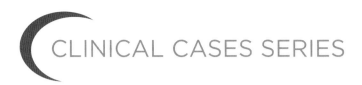

CLINICAL CASES SERIES

Clinical Cases in
Implant Dentistry

Edited by

Nadeem Karimbux, DMD, MMSc

Professor of Periodontology
Associate Dean
Academic Affairs
Tufts University School of Dental Medicine
Boston, MA
USA

and

Hans-Peter Weber, DMD, DrMedDent

Professor and Chair
Department of Prosthodontics
Tufts University School of Dental Medicine
Boston, MA
USA

WILEY Blackwell

Editorial offices: 1606 Golden Aspen Drive, Suites 103 and 104, Ames, Iowa 50010, USA
The Atrium, Southern Gate, Chichester, West Sussex, PO19 8SQ, UK
9600 Garsington Road, Oxford, OX4 2DQ, UK

For details of our global editorial offices, for customer services and for information about how to apply for permission to reuse the copyright material in this book please see our website at www.wiley.com/wiley-blackwell.

Library of Congress Cataloging-in-Publication Data

Names: Karimbux, Nadeem, editor. | Weber, Hans Peter, 1950- editor.
Title: Clinical cases in implant dentistry / edited by Nadeem Karimbux and
    Hans-Peter Weber.
Other titles: Clinical cases (Ames, Iowa)
Description: Ames, Iowa : John Wiley & Sons, Inc., 2017. | Series: Clinical
    cases | Includes bibliographical references and index.
Identifiers: LCCN 2016036137 (print) | LCCN 2016037395 (ebook) | ISBN
    9781118702147 (paper) | ISBN 9781119019930 (pdf) | ISBN 9781119019923
    (epub)
Subjects: | MESH: Dental Implantation | Dental Prosthesis Design | Case
    Reports
Classification: LCC RK667.I45 (print) | LCC RK667.I45 (ebook) | NLM WU 640 |
    DDC 617.6/93--dc23
LC record available at https://lccn.loc.gov/2016036137

A catalogue record for this book is available from the British Library.

Wiley also publishes its books in a variety of electronic formats. Some content that appears in print may not be available in electronic books.

Cover image: top middle – courtesy of Do-Gyoon Kim

Set in 10/13pt Univers Light by Aptara Inc., New Delhi, India
Printed and bound in Singapore by Markono Print Media Pte Ltd

1   2017

CONTENTS

CONTENTS

CONTRIBUTORS

Paulina Acosta
Private Practice
Tijuana, Baja, CA, USA

Mohammed N. Alasqah
Periodontist and Esthetic Dentistry
Assistant Professor
Department of Preventive Dental Sciences
College of Dentistry
Prince Sattam Bin Abdulaziz University
Al Kharj, Saudi Arabia

Abdullah Al Farraj Aldosari
Director of Dental Implant and Osseointegration
Research Chair
Associate Professor and Consultant of Prosthodontics
and Implantology
Department of Prosthetic Science
College of Dentistry
King Saud University
Riyadh, Saudi Arabia

Shatha Alharthi
Advanced Graduate Resident
Department of Periodontology
School of Dental Medicine
Tufts University
Boston, MA, USA

Emilio Arguello
Clinical Instructor
Division of Periodontology
Department of Oral Medicine, Infection, and Immunity
Harvard University School of Dental Medicine
Boston, MA, USA

Federico Ausenda
Advanced Graduate Resident
Department of Periodontology
Tufts University School of Dental Medicine
Boston, MA, USA

Gustavo Avila-Ortiz
Assistant Professor
Department of Periodontics
University of Iowa, College of Dentistry
Iowa City, IA, USA

Christopher A. Barwacz
Assistant Professor
Department of Family Dentistry
University of Iowa, College of Dentistry
Iowa City, IA, USA

Seyed Hossein Bassir
Division of Periodontology
Department of Oral Medicine, Infection and Immunity
Harvard School of Dental Medicine
Boston, MA USA

Francesca Bonino
Advanced Standing Student for Internationally Trained
Dentists
Henry M. Goldman School of Dental Medicine
Boston University
Boston, MA, USA

Suheil M. Boutros
Private practice limited to periodontics and dental implants
Grand Blanc, MI, USA;
Visiting Assistant Professor
Department of Periodontics and Oral Medicine
The University of Michigan
Ann Arbor, MI, USA

Eriberto Bressan
Professor
Department of Neuroscience
University of Padova
Padova, Italy

Minh Bui
DMD Candidate
Department of Diagnosis & Health Promotion
Tufts University School of Dental Medicine
Boston, MA, USA

Michael Butera
Prosthodontist
Private Practice
Boston, MA, USA

Jacinto Cano-Peyro
Periodontist, Private Practice
Marbella, Spain;
Visiting Professor, Department of Restorative Dentistry
Complutense University of Madrid
Madrid, Spain

Chun-Jung Chen
Instructor in Periodontics
Department of Dentistry
Chi Mei Medical Center
Tainan, Taiwan

Sung Mean Chi
Prosthodontist
Private Practice
Stow, OH, USA

Sung-Kiang Chuang
Associate Professor in Oral and Maxillofacial Surgery
Massachusetts General Hospital and Harvard School of Dental Medicine
Boston, MA, USA

Luis Del Castillo
Clinical Assistant Professor
Department of Prosthodontics
Tufts University School of Dental Medicine
Boston, MA, USA

Rustam DeVitre
Director of Alumni
Tufts University School of Dental Medicine
Boston, MA, USA;
Private Practice
Boston, MA, USA

Irina Dragan
Department of Periodontology
Tufts University School of Dental Medicine
Boston, MA, USA

Satheesh Elangovan
Associate Professor
Department of Periodontics
The University of Iowa College of Dentistry
Iowa City, IA, USA

Karim El Kholy
Advanced Graduate Resident
Division of Periodontics
Department of Oral Medicine, Infection, and Immunity
Harvard School of Dental Medicine
Boston, MA, USA

Waeil Elmisalati
Clinical Assistant Professor of Periodontology
University of New England College of Dental Medicine
Portland, ME, USA

Zameera Fida
Associate in Pediatric Dentistry
Boston Children's Hospital
Boston, MA, USA

Marcelo Freire
Advanced Graduate Resident
Division of Periodontology, Oral Medicine, Infection and Immunity
Harvard School of Dental Medicine
Boston, MA, USA

Rumpa Ganguly
Assistant Professor and Division Head
Oral and Maxillofacial Radiology
Department of Diagnostic Sciences
Tufts University School of Dental Medicine
Boston, MA, USA

Hamasat Gheddaf Dam
Adjunct Assistant Professor in Prosthodontics
Tufts University School of Dental Medicine
Private Practice
Boston, MA, USA

Hadi Gholami
Research Fellow
Department of Prosthodontics
Tufts University School of Dental Medicine
Boston, MA, USA

Mindy Sugmin Gil
Visiting Postgraduate Research Fellow
Department of Oral Medicine, Infection, and Immunity
Harvard School of Dental Medicine
Boston, MA, USA

Luca Gobbato
Clinical Instructor
Department of Oral Medicine, Infection and Immunity
Division of Periodontics
Harvard University School of Dental Medicine
Boston, MA, USA

Maria E. Gonzalez
Clinical Assistant Professor
Division of Operative Dentistry
Comprehensive Care Department
Tufts University School of Dental Medicine
Boston, MA, USA

Mitchell Gubler
Advanced Graduate Resident
Department of Periodontics
University of Iowa College of Dentistry
Iowa City, IA, USA

Sergio Herrera
Post Graduate Resident
International Academy of Dental Implantology
San Diego, CA, USA

Daniel Kuan-te Ho
Assistant Professor
Department of Periodontics
School of Dentistry
University of Texas Health Science Center at Houston
Houston, TX, USA

Hsiang-Yun Huang
Private Practice
Taipei, Taiwan;
Clinical Instructor
School of Dentistry
National Defense Medical Center
Taipei, Taiwan

Yong Hur
Assistant Professor
Department of Periodontology
Tufts University School of Dental Medicine
Boston, MA, USA

Y. Natalie Jeong
Assistant Professor
Department of Periodontology
Tufts University School of Dental Medicine
Boston, MA, USA

Nadeem Karimbux
Division of Periodontology
Department of Oral Medicine, Infection and Immunity
Harvard School of Dental Medicine
Boston, MA, USA;
Professor of Periodontology
Department of Periodontology
Tufts University School of Dental Medicine
Boston, MA, USA

Ioannis Karoussis
Assistant Professor of Periodontology
Dental School
University of Athens
Athens, Greece

David Minjoon Kim
Associate Professor
Director, Postdoctoral Periodontology
Director, Continuing Education
Division of Periodontology
Department of Oral Medicine, Infection & Immunity
Harvard School of Dental Medicine
Boston, MA, USA

Samuel Koo
Assistant Professor
Department of Periodontology
Tufts University School of Dental Medicine
Boston, MA, USA

Chun-Teh Lee
Post-Doctoral Fellow in Periodontology
Harvard School of Dental Medicine
Boston, MA, USA

Samuel Lee
Director of International Academy of Dental
Implantology
San Diego, CA, USA

Paul A. Levi, Jr.
Associate Clinical Professor
Department of Periodontology
Tufts University School of Dental Medicine
Boston, MA, USA

Diego Lops
Assistant Professor in Periodontology and Implant
Dentistry
University of Milan
Milan, Italy

Lauren Manning
Assistant Professor
Oregon Health & Science University
Portland, OR, USA

Sonja Mansour
Assistant Professor
Department of Prosthodontics
Institute for Dental and Craniofacial Sciences
Charité
Berlin, Germany

Mariam Margvelashvili
Postdoctoral Fellow
Department of Prosthodontics
Tufts University School of Dental Medicine
Boston, MA, USA

Fabio Mazzocco
Visiting Professor
Department of Implantology at Padova
University of Dental Medicine
Padova, Italy

Luigi Minenna
Research Centre for the Study of Periodontal and Peri-
Implant Diseases
Department of Periodontology
School of Dentistry
University of Ferrara
Ferrara, Italy

Adrian Mora
Post Graduate Resident
International Academy of Dental Implantology
San Diego, CA, USA

Lorenzo Mordini
Advanced Graduate Resident
Department of Periodontology
Tufts University School of Dental Medicine
Boston, MA, USA

Hidetada Moroi
Assistant Clinical Professor
Department of Periodontology
Tufts University School of Dental Medicine
Boston, MA, USA

Zuhair S. Natto
Visiting Assistant Professor
Department of Periodontology
Tufts University School of Dental Medicine
Boston, MA, USA;
Assistant Professor
Department of Dental Public Health
School of Dentistry, King Abdulaziz University
Jeddah, Saudi Arabia

Christina Nicholas
Department of Anthropology and Dows Institute for
Dental Research
The University of Iowa College of Dentistry
Iowa City, IA, USA

Yumi Ogata
Board Diplomate
American Board of Periodontology
Assistant Professor
Department of Periodontology
Tufts University School of Dental Medicine
Boston, MA, USA

Rory O'Neill
Associate Clinical Professor
Department of Periodontology
Tufts University School of Dental Medicine
Boston, MA, USA;
Clinical Professor of Dentistry
Roseman University
College of Dental Medicine
Henderson, NV, USA

Pinelopi Pani
Advanced Graduate Resident
Department of Periodontology
Tufts University School of Dental Medicine
Boston, MA, USA

Gianluca Paniz
Visiting Professor
Department of Implantology at Padova
University of Dental Medicine
Padova, Italy

Panos Papaspyridakos
Assistant Professor of Postgraduate Prosthodontics
Department of Prosthodontics
Tufts University School of Dental Medicine
Boston, MA, USA

Kwang Bum Park
Director
MIR Dental Hospital
Daegu, South Korea

Carlos Parra
Department of Periodontics
Texas A & M University College of Dentistry
Dallas, TX, USA

Lucrezia Paterno Holtzman
Department of Periodontology
Tufts University School of Dental Medicine
Boston, MA, USA

Aruna Ramesh
Diplomate, ABOMR
Associate Professor and Interim Chair
Department of Diagnostic Sciences
Division of Oral and Maxillofacial Radiology
Tufts University School of Dental Medicine
Boston, MA, USA

Tannaz Shapurian
Associate Clinical Professor
Department of Periodontology
Tufts University School of Dental Medicine
Boston, MA, USA

Teresa Chanting Sun
Department of Periodontology
Tufts University School of Dental Medicine
Boston, MA, USA

Rainier A. Urdaneta
Prosthodontist
Private Practice
Implant Dentistry Centre
Jamaica Plain, MA, USA

Jeff Chin-Wei Wang
Clinical Assistant Professor
Department of Periodontics and Oral Medicine
University of Michigan School of Dentistry
Ann Arbor, MI, USA

Hans-Peter Weber
Professor
Department of Prosthodontics
Tufts University School of Dental Medicine
Boston, MA, USA

Wichaya Wisitrasameewong
Post-Doctoral Fellow
Division of Periodontology
Department of Oral Medicine, Infection and Immunity
Harvard School of Dental Medicine
Boston, MA, USA

PREFACE

We are excited to present 49 Clinical Cases in Implant Dentistry. The cases have been authored by invited clinicians and residents that have diverse training and different backgrounds. Each case presents a real patient scenario with the appropriate clinical and radiographic information. The cases convey the steps involved with diagnosis, treatment planning and treatment covering both the surgical and restorative aspects.

Although each chapter is presented under certain thematic headings, we realize that many aspects of each case and each discussion cross over to areas covered in other chapters/cases. There is also redundancy in topics discussed/presented since each author was presenting their own cases with self-generated study questions/discussions. It is this diversity of clinical viewpoints and reviews of the literature that we believe will give our readers the best overview of the multiple challenges, topics and reviews of the literature presented by the cases.

Each case and the discussions and literature presented should be treated and appreciated with this in mind. We hope that you use the cases and information supplied to add to your clinical expertise in the areas presented, and as a review for potential clinical and board exams!

Hans-Peter Weber
Nadeem Karimbux

ACKNOWLEDGMENTS

A special thanks to my spouse and children (Hema Ramachandran and Naavin and Tarin Karimbux) for putting up with all my "lap-top" time processing chapters and manuscripts as a part of my academic pursuits.

NK

My gratitude goes to my spouse Cheryl for supporting me throughout my career and generously accepting the fact that projects like this book are not possible without spending personal time at home on them.

HPW

An acknowledgment is extended to all the residents at Harvard and Tufts University Schools of Dental Medicine. We learn from you every day as you grow in your pursuit of clinical knowledge and skills. A special thanks to the faculty for their commitment to our students and for contributing to the chapters in this book.

NK, HPW

1

Examination and Diagnosis

Case 1

Clinical Examination

CASE STORY

A 39-year-old Caucasian male who had just moved in from another city presented to our clinic with a chief complaint of "I lost my lower molar tooth and I need a fixed replacement." Five months before this visit the patient had acute pain on mastication in tooth #30. Periodontal examination revealed a localized 7 mm pocket depth on the distal of tooth #30. The Slooth test was positive and there was severe pain on percussion of the lingual cusps. This led his previous dentist to suspect vertical root fracture of tooth #30. Exploratory flap surgery was performed, which revealed a fracture extending all the way to the middle of the root. The tooth was extracted in the same visit and the socket was grafted with bone allografts and covered with resorbable collagen membrane. When he presented to our clinic, it was 5 months since the time of extraction and ridge preservation. The patient reported that he was getting regular dental care, including periodontal maintenance, from his previous dentist.

LEARNING GOALS AND OBJECTIVES

- ■ To be able to understand the necessary elements in the examination and documentation portion of dental implant therapy
- ■ To be able to understand the several diagnostic tools available for comprehensive evaluation and implant treatment planning
- ■ To understand the importance of systemic, periodontal, and esthetic evaluation in dental implant therapy

Medical History

The patient when presented was a well-controlled type II diabetic. His last glycated hemoglobin was 6.2, measured a month before his initial visit. He was taking metformin 1000 mg per day. Other than diabetes, the patient did not present with any other relevant medication condition, allergies, or any untoward incidents during his previous dental visits.

Review of Systems

- Vital signs
  - ○ Blood pressure: 120/77 mmHg
  - ○ Pulse rate: 76 beats/min (regular)
  - ○ Respiration: 14 breaths/min

Social History

The patient did not smoke but he reported that he was a social consumer of alcohol.

Extraoral Examination

No significant findings were noted. The patient had no masses or swelling, and the temporomandibular joint was within normal limits. No facial asymmetry was noted, and lymph nodes assessment yielded normal results.

Intraoral Examination

- Oral cancer screening was negative.
- Soft tissue exam, including his buccal mucosa, tongue, and floor of the mouth, was within normal limits.
- Periodontal examination revealed pocket depths in the range 2–3 mm (Figure 1).
- Color, contour, and consistency of gingiva was within normal limits, with localized erythema of marginal gingiva in the lingual of mandibular anterior areas.

Buccal	323	323	333	212	212	212	222	212	212	323	213	323	323	323	333	323
Palatal	333	323	333	222	323	213	212	212	212	212	223	212	313	323	333	323

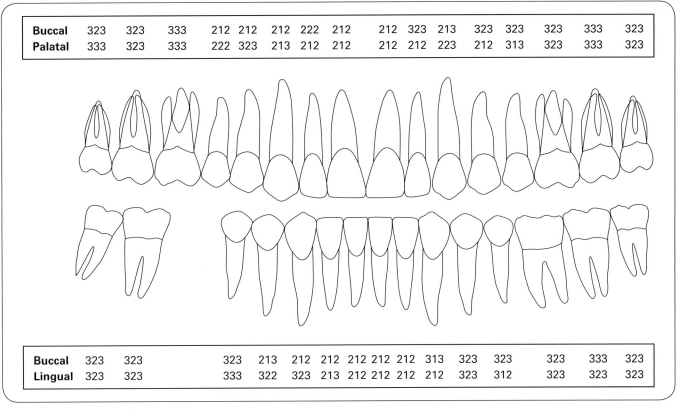

Buccal	323	323		323	213	212	212	212	212	212	313	323	323	323	333	323
Lingual	323	323		333	322	323	213	212	212	212	212	323	312	323	323	323

Figure 1: Probing pocket depth measurements during the initial visit.

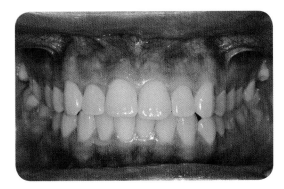

Figure 2: Initial presentation (facial view).

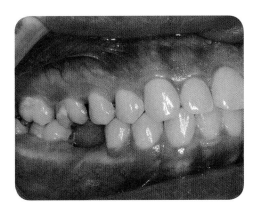

Figure 3: Initial presentation (right lateral view).

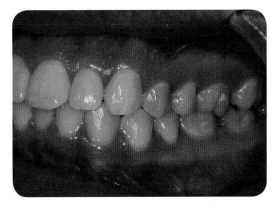

Figure 4: Initial presentation (left lateral view).

- Oral hygiene was good when he presented to the clinic (Figures 2, 3, and 4).
- Localized areas of dental plaque-induced gingival inflammation were noted.
- Slight supragingival calculus was noted in the mandibular lingual areas.
- Dental caries, both primary and recurrent, was noted in a few teeth.
- The ridge in the site #30 healed adequately, which revealed a slight buccal deficiency (Figure 5).

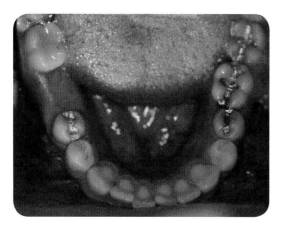

Figure 5: Initial presentation (occlusal view).

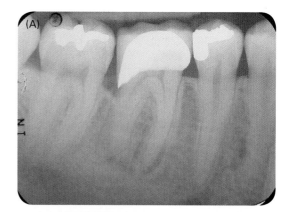

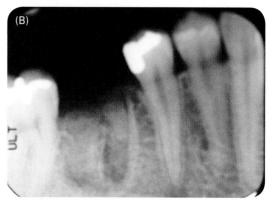

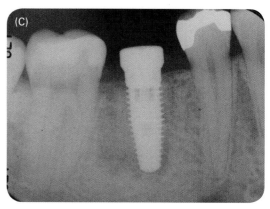

Figure 6: Periapical radiographs: (A) pre-extraction; (B) postextraction; (C) postimplant placement.

- On palpation, the ridge width was found to be adequate to place a standard diameter implant (to replace the molar tooth), without the need for additional bone grafting.
- No exaggerated lingual concavity was noted in the area.
- Normal thickness and width of keratinized mucosa was noted (Figure 3).
- No occlusal disharmony was noted, and there was adequate mesio-distal and apico-coronal space for the future implant crown (Figure 3).

Occlusion

There were no occlusal discrepancies or interferences noted (Figures 2, 3, and 4).

Radiographic Examination

A full mouth radiographic series was ordered. (See Figure 6 for patient's periapical radiograph of the area of interest before extraction of #30 and after extraction and ridge preservation.) The postextraction radiograph revealed radiographic bone fill of the #30 socket. The crestal bone level was well maintained. Normal bone levels in the adjacent teeth were noted. The inferior alveolar canal was not visible in any of the three radiographs.

Diagnosis

American Academy of Periodontology diagnosis of plaque-induced gingivitis with acquired mucogingival deformities and conditions on edentulous ridges was made.

Treatment Plan

The treatment plan for this patient consisted of disease control therapy that included oral prophylaxis and oral hygiene instructions to address gingival inflammation. This was followed by implant placement. After an

adequate time for osseointegration (4 months), the implant was restored.

Examination and Documental Visit

The patient when presented to our clinic had already lost tooth #30, which had been extracted 5 months previously. The healing at the extraction site was found to be satisfactory. Systemically, the patient was a diabetic but with good glycemic control and was a nonsmoker. Periodontal examination revealed healthy periodontium with localized areas of mild gingivitis. His part dental history revealed that he was a compliant patient and was on a regular dental maintenance schedule. Occlusal analysis revealed no occlusal disharmonies. These factors together made him a good candidate for dental implant therapy.

The site-specific clinical and radiographic evaluation revealed enough bucco-lingual width and mesiodistal and apico-coronal space for both the placement and the restoration of the implant. The inferior alveolar canal was not in the vicinity of the planned implant site. For these reasons, additional imaging analysis such as cone beam computed tomography (CBCT) was not planned. Impressions were taken during this initial visit

that were utilized for doing diagnostic wax-up and for making a surgical guide. Extraoral and intraoral clinical photographs were taken during this visit for patient education and communication with the restoring dentist. Once the treatment plan was finalized, the patient was educated about the dental implant and the treatment sequence. This was followed by implant placement on a separate day using a surgical guide and a drilling sequence recommended by the implant manufacturer.

Self-Study Questions

(Answers located at the end of the case)

A. Why is systemic evaluation important in a dental implant patient?

B. Is the success rate of dental implants different in smoker versus nonsmoker?

C. How important is periodontal evaluation before planning for dental implants?

D. What are the site-specific assessments that need to be done prior to placing implants?

E. What are the components of esthetic evaluation for planning implants in the esthetic zone?

F. What are the anatomical landmarks that have to be examined carefully that may influence treatment execution?

G. What are the presurgical adjunctive evaluations required on a case-by-case basis?

H. How are ridge deformities classified?

References

1. Chen H, Liu N, Xu X, et al. Smoking, radiotherapy, diabetes and osteoporosis as risk factors for dental implant failure: a meta-analysis. PLoS One 2013;8(8):e71955.
2. Oates TW, Huynh-Ba G, Vargas A, et al. A critical review of diabetes, glycemic control, and dental implant therapy. Clin Oral Implants Res 2013;24(2):117–127.
3. Johnson GK, Hill M. Cigarette smoking and the periodontal patient. J Periodontol 2004;75(2):196–209.
4. Heitz-Mayfield LJ, Huynh-Ba G. History of treated periodontitis and smoking as risks for implant therapy. Int J Oral Maxillofac Implants 2009;24(Suppl):39–68.
5. Safii SH, Palmer RM, Wilson RF. Risk of implant failure and marginal bone loss in subjects with a history of periodontitis: a systematic review and meta-analysis. Clin Implant Dent Relat Res 2010;12(3):165–174.
6. Heitz-Mayfield LJ. Peri-implant diseases: diagnosis and risk indicators. J Clin Periodontol 2008;35(8 Suppl):292–304.
7. Lin GH, Chan HL, Wang HL. The significance of keratinized mucosa on implant health: a systematic review. J Periodontol 2013;84:1755–1767.
8. Weber HP, Buser D, Belser UC. Examination of the candidate for implant therapy. In: Lindhe J, Lang NP, Karring T (eds), Clinical Periodontology and Implant Dentistry, 5th edn. Oxford: Wiley-Blackwell; 2008, pp 587–599.
9. Benavides E, Rios HF, Ganz SD, et al. Use of cone beam computed tomography in implant dentistry: the International Congress of Oral Implantologists consensus report. Implant Dent 2012;21(2):78–86.
10. Handelsman M. Surgical guidelines for dental implant placement. Br Dent J 2006;201(3):139–152.
11. Seibert JS. Reconstruction of deformed partially edentulous ridges using full thickness onlay grafts: part I – technique and wound healing. Compend Contin Educ Dent 1983;4:437–453.

Answers to Self-Study Questions

A. There are several factors that influence the success rate of dental implants. Systemic factors are one among them and have a strong influence in the outcome of dental implants. Any systemic condition that has the influence to alter the bone turnover or wound healing process has to be carefully considered. It is clear from a well-conducted recent systematic review that smoking and radiotherapy (before or after implant placement) are associated with a higher (35% and 70% respectively) risk of implant failure [1]. With regard to other medical conditions, such as diabetes, it is becoming clearer that poor glycemic control is not an absolute contraindication for implant therapy provided that appropriate accommodation for delays in implant integration are considered [2]. Other commonly encountered systemic conditions that may modify the treatment plan include uncontrolled hypertension, intake of anticoagulants, patients on bisphosphonate therapy, or patients with psychiatric conditions. In select cases, getting clearance from the patient's physician is required. Therefore, it is extremely important that a thorough systemic evaluation be completed prior to planning for dental implants.

B. It has been shown that smoking affects periodontium by more than one mechanism [3]. Smoking was shown to negatively influence the oral microbial profile, suppress the immune system, and alter the microvascular environment, leading to disrupted healing [3]. Smokers have a two times higher risk for dental implant failure than nonsmokers do [1]. Apart from the lower success rate of implants in smokers, the incidence of peri-implantitis (a condition synonymous with periodontitis around natural tooth) is also shown to be high in smokers compared with nonsmokers [3,4]. Though smoking is not an absolute contraindication for dental implant therapy, explaining the higher risk for implant failure to the patients who are current smokers is the responsibility of the clinician.

C. Doing a thorough periodontal examination prior to implant therapy is as important as doing a systemic evaluation of the patient as this allows the clinician to obtain information on the patient's current periodontal disease status, oral hygiene status, and mucogingival parameters, such as the level of frenal attachments, width of keratinized mucosa, and vestibular depth. A moderate level of evidence suggests that patients with a history of periodontitis (especially the aggressive form of the disease) are at a higher risk for implant failure and marginal bone loss [5]. Poor oral hygiene is considered to be another important risk factor for dental implant failure [6]. Certain mucogingival conditions, such as low vestibule or high frenal attachments, may necessitate a soft tissue procedure in addition to implant placement. There is emerging evidence that lack of keratinized mucosa around dental implants is associated with more plaque buildup, inflammation, and mucosal recession [7]. Therefore, a thorough periodontal examination will guide the clinician to modify the treatment approach based on the periodontal findings.

D. For placing implants of standard diameter and length, having adequate bone volume both buccopalatally/-lingually and apico-coronally is a prerequisite. Therefore, site-specific examination, including evaluating for height and width of the bone, should be performed. This is accomplished by digital palpation of the area and by imaging techniques (described in question G). As a general rule, for a 4 mm diameter implant, at the level of the bone crest there should be at least 7 mm of mesiodistal space and buccolingual bone thickness to safely place the implant without encroaching on adjacent anatomical structures or without encountering bony dehiscence. It is a general guideline that there should be at least 1.5 mm distance between the implant and the adjacent tooth and 3 mm space between two implants placed adjacently. It is also important to make sure that there is sufficient distance from the proposed implant platform to the opposing teeth for restoring the implant with proper sized abutment and crown.

E. The esthetic analysis of an implant patient should include the following elements [8]:
- patient's smile line (high, medium, and low) and course of gingival line assessment;
- gingival phenotype (thick or thin) assessment;
- examination of tooth size and space distribution;
- examination of the shape of anatomical tooth crowns;
- examination of the length to width ratio of clinical crowns;
- examination of the hard and soft tissue anatomy of the site;
- interproximal bone heights (from radiographs);
- occlusal assessment (overjet and overbite).

F. In the maxilla, if the proposed implant site is in close vicinity to maxillary sinuses, nasal cavities, and the nasopalatine canal, those sites should be carefully evaluated to avoid encroaching on these structures while placing the implant. In the mandible, knowing the buccolingual and apico-coronal location of the inferior alveolar canal within the bony housing and the extent of lingual concavity of the mandible are important. This is usually accomplished by taking a CBCT of the area of interest. It is a general rule to maintain a safety distance of at least 2 mm between the implant and inferior alveolar canal (to account for radiographic distortions). In some instances, neurovascular bundles can be seen exiting lingual of the anterior mandible near the midline. Any trauma to these vessels may lead to severe hemorrhage in the sublingual area that can be life threatening.

G. Apart from a clinical oral examination that includes periodontal evaluation, in select cases adjunctive diagnostic assessments such as imaging, diagnostic wax-up, and clinical photographs are required to aid in diagnosis and/or treatment planning. Imaging typically includes periapical radiographs, bitewing radiographs, panoramic radiographs, or CBCT. CBCT is more advantageous than radiographs as it gives three-dimensional information of the proposed treatment site. It also allows the clinician to accurately determine the proximity of vital anatomic structures [9]. Doing a diagnostic wax-up allows the clinician to determine the need for additional implant site preparation, help with patient education, and for making surgical guides [10]. Clinical photographs are useful diagnostic aids, especially in anterior esthetic cases to document the patient's smile and also to discuss the case with peers.

H. There are several classifications that exist to categorize ridge deformities, but the most commonly used one is the classification proposed by Seibert in 1983 [11]. This classification was originally proposed in the context of soft tissue augmentation, but it has been adapted and is widely used in the context of implant site preparation.

The three classes of ridge deformities according to Seibert are:

class I – buccolingual/-palatal resorption;
class II – apico-coronal resorption;
class III – combination of buccolingual/-palatal and apico-coronal resorption.

Case 2

Medical Considerations

A 70-year-old Caucasian male presented with a chief complaint of "I am missing my back teeth and I have difficulty in eating normally." The patient lost teeth #2–#5, #12–#15, #18, #19, #26, and #28–#31 several years ago due to severe periodontal disease. The third molars were impacted and removed at a very young age. The patient had a maxillary and mandibular interim partial denture fabricated before proceeding with a fixed solution, which he was wearing irregularly (Figures 1 and 2). The patient visited his dentist regularly for uninterrupted dental care to maintain the remaining teeth and reported that he brushed twice per day and flossed at least once a day. He had two class V composite restorations in teeth #20 and #21 buccally and a composite restoration in the incisal edge of #8.

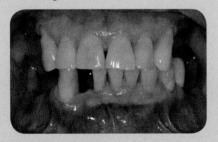

Figure 1: Pre-op presentation (facial view).

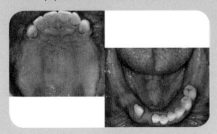

Figure 2: Pre-op presentation (occlusal view).

Medical History

At the time of treatment the patient presented with type II diabetes, controlled with medications (metformin). His last glycated hemoglobin (HbA1c) level was 6.7%, measured a few weeks before his initial exam. His fasting blood sugar was 120 mg/dL in the last physical exam. The patient was also hypertensive, controlled with medications (hydrochlorothiazide, doxazosin methylate, benazepril). In addition, he had hypercholesterolemia that was controlled with medication (simvastatin). Last, he suffered from a knee injury 4 years prior to his initial visit, which resulted in a blood clot formation that traveled to the lungs. The patient had surgery on his knee and has been taking Coumadin since then. The patient's last international normalized ratio (INR) was 2.3. The patient's body mass index was 33.9, which put him in the obese category. The patient denied having any known drug allergies.

Review of Systems
• Vital signs
  ○ Blood pressure: 135/70 mmHg
  ○ Pulse rate: 85 beats/min (regular)
  ○ Respiration: 16 breaths/min

Social History

The patient had no history of smoking or alcohol consumption at the time of treatment.

Extraoral Examination

There was no clinical pathology noted on extraoral examination. The patient had no masses or swelling. The temporomandibular joints were stable, functional, and comfortable. There was no facial asymmetry noted, and his lymph nodes were normal on palpation.

Intraoral Examination

- Oral cancer screening was negative.
- Soft tissue exam, including his tongue and floor of the mouth and fauces, showed no clinical pathology.
- Periodontal examination revealed pocket depths in the range 1–3 mm (Figure 3).
- Localized areas of slight gingival inflammation were noted.
- The color, size, shape, and consistency of the gingiva were normal. The keratinized tissue was firm and stippled.
- Generalized moderate with localized severe attachment loss and generalized recession were noted.
- An aberrant maxillary and mandibular bilateral labial frenum was also noted, which was extending also to the edentulous posterior areas.

- Localized plaque was found around the teeth, resulting in a plaque-free index of 90%.
- Evaluation of the alveolar ridge in the edentulous areas revealed both horizontal and vertical resorption of bone (Seibert class III).
- Class V composite restorations in teeth #20 and #21 buccally and a composite restoration in the incisal edge of #8 were also noted.

Occlusion

An overjet of 3.5 mm and overbite of 4 mm were noted. Angle's molar classification could not be determined due to loss of these teeth. Canine classification could only be determined on the left side, which was class II. Signs of secondary occlusal trauma (worn dentition, mobility, fremitus) were also noted. Functional analysis of the occlusion revealed anterior guidance during protrusion and canine guidance during lateral extrusion movements.

Radiographic Examination

A panoramic and a full mouth radiographic series was ordered (Figure 4). Radiographic examination revealed generalized moderate horizontal bone loss. There was also vertical loss of bone noted in the edentulous areas. A cone beam computed tomography scan was also ordered for better evaluation of the edentulous areas. The height of bone between the crestal bone and maxillary right sinus, in the position of the future implant, as indicated by the radiographic stent, was 4.95 mm and the height of bone between the crestal bone and maxillary left sinus was 8 mm. The height of bone between the

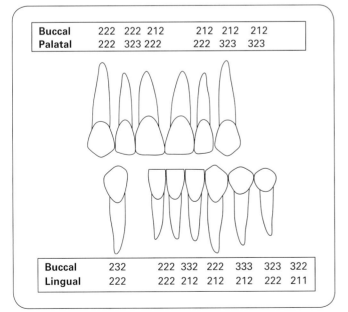

| Buccal | 222 | 222 | 212 | | 212 | 212 | 212 |
| Palatal | 222 | 323 | 222 | | 222 | 323 | 323 |

| Buccal | 232 | | 222 | 332 | 222 | 333 | 323 | 322 |
| Lingual | 222 | | 222 | 212 | 212 | 212 | 222 | 211 |

Figure 3: Periodontal chart. Probing pocket depth measurements during the initial visit.

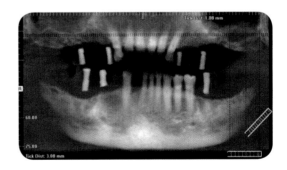

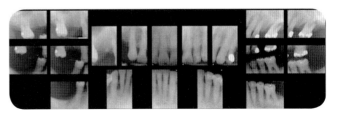

Figure 4: Panoramic and full mouth radiograph.

crestal bone and the inferior alveolar nerve canal was 12 mm bilaterally. The distance from the right mental foramen was 10 mm (Figure 5). The buccal–lingual width seemed adequate in all indicated positions for placement of dental implants.

A round, well-circumscribed radiopacity with well-defined borders was noted in the maxillary right sinus. The lesion occupied a big area of the right maxillary sinus space. Slight sinus membrane thickening was noted in the maxillary left sinus (Figure 5).

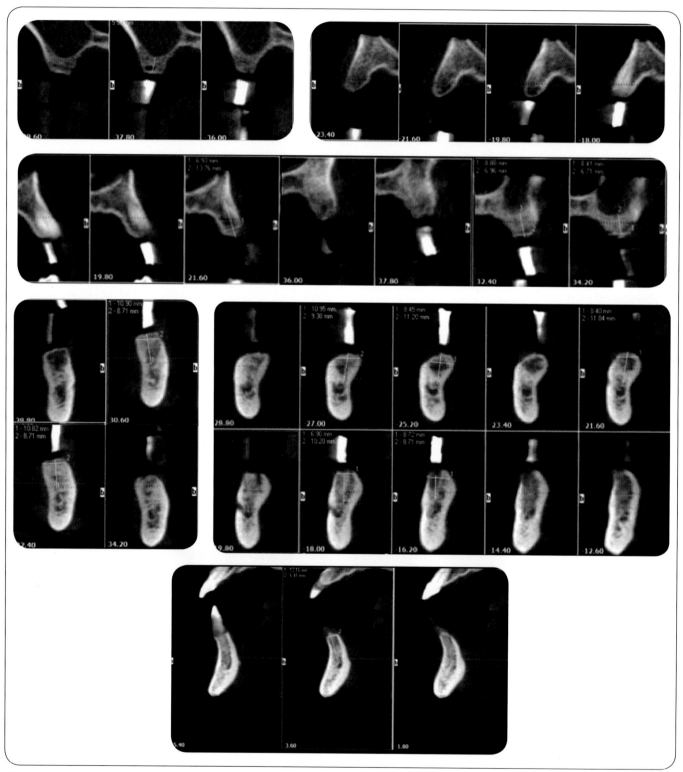

Figure 5: Cone beam computed tomography scan.

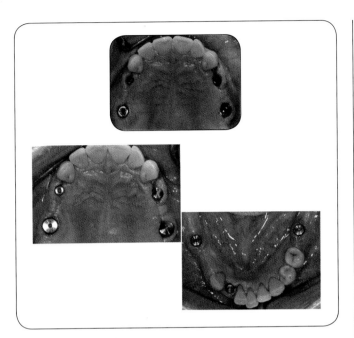

Figure 6: Implant placement.

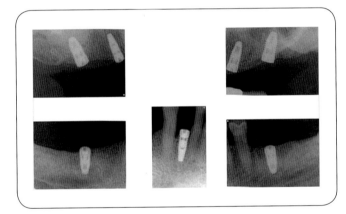

Figure 7: Implants placed.

Diagnosis

A diagnosis of generalized moderate and localized severe chronic periodontitis with mucogingival deformities and conditions around teeth (facial, lingual, and interproximal recession and aberrant frenum), mucogingival deformities and conditions on the edentulous ridges (horizontal and vertical ridge deficiency in all edentulous areas and aberrant frenum), and occlusal trauma (secondary) was made. Additional diagnosis of partial edentulism with Kennedy class I in the maxilla and Kennedy class I (mod 2) in the mandible was made.

Treatment Plan

Interdisciplinary consultation along with diagnostic casts and wax-up led to different treatment plan

options. Financial limitations also played a role in the final decision. The treatment plan for this patient consisted of an initial phase therapy that included oral prophylaxis and oral hygiene instructions to address gingival inflammation. This was followed by implant placements #3 and #5 with external sinus elevation, implants #12 and #14 with internal sinus elevation, and implants in locations #19, #26, and #30 (Figures 6 and 7). After adequate time for osseointegration (6–8 months in the maxilla, 4 months in the mandible), the implants were restored.

Treatment

Prior to any treatment, primary care physician and ear, nose, and throat (ENT) consultations were obtained. The primary care physician recommended that the patient should stop warfarin treatment 5 days prior to surgery and start using Lovenox (low molecular weight heparin) until 24 h prior to surgery. The patient should restart warfarin and Lovenox 24 h after surgery until his INR ≥2.0, when Lovenox should be discontinued.

The ENT report stated that patient had a benign asymptomatic mucous retention cyst in the maxillary right sinus and a slight membrane thickening in the maxillary left sinus. Neither condition would interfere with the implant surgery or sinus elevation procedure. In the case of membrane perforation, though, the procedure should be stopped, no implants or bone grafts should be placed, and the patient should be referred to the ENT doctor for cyst removal and sinus treatment.

After the initial phase therapy, the patient presented for implant placement. Implant placement took place in three visits (Figures 6 and 7).

Implant placement and restoration will not be described in this chapter, since these topics will be addressed in later chapters.

Discussion

In this case, the primary concern was the patient's past and current medical history. The patient was being treated for several systemic diseased that he controlled with specific medication. These factors should be taken into consideration prior to any surgical implant treatment to minimize any possible complications and optimize implant therapy outcome.

In medically healthy patients, the success rates of some dental implant systems are reported to be between 90 and 95% at 10 years. Dental implants may fail, however, due to a lack of osseointegration during early healing, or when in function due to breakage, or infection of the peri-implant tissues leading to loss of implant support. The long-term outcome of implant therapy can be affected by local factors or systemic diseases or other compromising factors. In fact, it has been suggested that some local and systemic factors could represent contraindications to dental implants treatment [1,2].

The impact of health risks on the outcome of implant therapy is unclear, since there are few if any randomized controlled trials evaluating health status as a risk indicator [1]. Certain conditions, such as uncontrolled diabetes, bleeding disorders, a weakened/suppressed immune system, or cognitive problems, which interfere with postoperative care, increase the risk of implant failure. There is still, however, a lack of high-quality substantiated evidence to confirm all the associations [1,2]. Therefore, proper patient selection is important to increase the likelihood of implant therapy success.

It is important to realize that the degree of disease control may be far more important than the nature of the systemic disorder itself, and individualized medical management should be obtained prior to implant therapy, since in many of these patients the quality of life and functional benefits of dental implants may outweigh any risks [1]. In patients with systemic conditions, it is critical to outweigh the cost–benefit considerations with the patient's quality of life and life expectancy, and it is very important to undertake the implant surgical procedures with strict asepsis, minimal trauma, and avoiding stress and excessive hemorrhage. Equally essential in these patients is to ensure proper maintenance therapy with optimal standards of oral hygiene, without smoking, and with avoidance of any other risk factors that may affect the outcome of dental implants [1,2].

Self-Study Questions

(Answers located at the end of the case)

A. What is the impact of systemic diseases and/or medications used to treat systemic diseases on the success of implant therapy?

B. What are the contraindications of dental implants in medically compromised patients?

C. Which medical/systemic diseases have a *high* risk associated with implant success and what is the level of association with lack of osseointegration, peri-implant bone loss, and/or implant failure?

D. Which medical/systemic diseases have a *significant* risk associated with implant success and what is the level of association with lack of osseointegration, peri-implant bone loss, and/or implant failure?

E. Which medical/systemic diseases have a *relative* risk associated with implant success and what is the level of association with lack of osseointegration, peri-implant bone loss, and/or implant failure?

F. Which other medical/systemic diseases have an *increased* risk associated with implant success and what is the level of association with lack of osseointegration, peri-implant bone loss, and/or implant failure?

G. Which medical/systemic conditions are considered to be absolute contraindications for implant therapy?

H. Which medication may affect osseointegration?

References

1. Diz P, Scully C, Sanz M. Dental implants in the medically compromised patient. J Dent 2013;41:195–206.
2. Gómez-de Diego R, Mang-de la Rosa M, Romero-Pérez MJ, et al. Indications and contraindications of dental implants in medically compromised patients: update. Med Oral Patol Oral Cir Bucal 2014;19(5):e483–e489.
3. Bornstein MM, Cionca N, Mombelli A. Systemic conditions and treatments as risks for implant therapy. Int J Oral Maxillofac Implants 2009;24(Suppl):12–27.
4. Clementini M, Rossetti PHO, Penarrocha D, et al. Systemic risk factors for peri-implant bone loss: a systematic review and meta-analysis. Int J Oral Maxillofac Surg 2014;43:323–334.

5. Berglundh T, Lindhe J, Ericsson I, et al. The soft tissue barrier at implants and teeth. Clin Oral Implants Res 1991;2:81–90.

6. Sanz M, Alendaz J, Lazaro P, et al. Histopathologic characteristics of peri-implant soft tissues in Brånemark implants with 2 distinct clinical and radiographic patterns. Clin Oral Implants Res 1991;2:128–134.

7. Quirynen M, Van Steenberghe D. Bacterial colonization of the internal part of two stage implants: an in vivo study. Clin Oral Implants Res 1993;4:158–161.

8. Hermann JS, Cochran DL, Nummicoski PV, et al. Crestal bone changes around titanium implants: a radiographic evaluation of unloaded nonsubmerged and submerged implants in the canine mandible. J Periodontol 1997;68:1117–1130.

9. Jansen VK, Conrads G, Richter EJ. Microbial leakage and marginal fit of the implant abutment interface. Int J Oral Maxillofac Implants 1997;12:527–540.

10. De Souza JGO, Pereira Neto ARL, et al. Impact of local and systemic factors on additional peri-implant bone loss. Quintessence Int 2013;44:415–424.

11. Albrektsson T, Isidor F. Consensus report of session IV. In: Lang NP, Karring, T (eds), Proceedings of the 1st European Workshop on Periodontology. London: Quintessence; 1994, pp 365–369.

12. Wennström J, Palmer R. Consensus report session 3: clinical trials. In: Lang NP, Karring T, Lindhe J (eds), Proceedings of the 3rd European Workshop on Periodontology. Implant Dentistry. Berlin: Quintessence; 1999, pp 255–259.

13. Fransson C, Lekholm U, Jemt T, Berglundh T. Prevalence of subjects with progressive bone loss at implants. Clin Oral Implants Res 2005;16:440–446.

14. Meijer GJ, Cune MS. Surgical dilemmas. Medical restrictions and risk factors. Ned Tijdschr Tandheelkd 2008;115:643–651 (in Dutch).

15. Bornstein MM, Cionca N, Mombelli A. Systemic conditions and treatments as risks for implant therapy. Int J Oral Maxillofac Implants 2009;24(Suppl):12–27.

16. American Society of Anesthesiologists. New classification of physical status. Anesthesiology 1963;24:111.

17. Maloney WJ Weinberg MA. Implementation of the American Society of Anesthesiologists physical status classification system in periodontal practice. J Periodontol 2008;79:1124–1126.

18. Smith RA, Berger R, Dodson TB. Risk factors associated with dental implants in healthy and medically compromised patients. Int J Oral Maxillofac Implants 1992;7:367–372.

19. Van Steenberghe D, Quirinen M, Molly L, Jacobs R. Impact of systemic diseases and medication on osseointegration. Periodontol 2000 2003;33:163–171.

20. Blanchaert RH. Implants in the medically challenged patient. Dent Clin North Am 1998;42:35–45.

21. Sugerman PB, Barber MT. Patient selection for endosseous dental implants: oral and systemic considerations. Int J Oral Maxillofac Implants 2002;17:191–201.

22. Hwang D, Wang HL. Medical contraindications to implant therapy: part I: absolute contraindications. Implant Dent 2006;15:353–360.

23. Hwang D, Wang HL. Medical contraindications to implant therapy: part II: relative contraindications. Implant Dent 2007;16:13–23.

24. Buser D, von Arx T, ten Bruggenkate CM, Weingart D. Basic surgical principles with ITI implants. Clin Oral Implants Res 2000;11(Suppl):59–68.

25. Sugerman PB, Barber MT. Patient selection for endosseous dental implants: oral and systemic considerations. Int J Oral Maxillofac Implants 2002;17:191–201.

26. Mombelli A, Cionca N. Systemic diseases affecting osseointegration therapy. Clin Oral Implants Res 2006;17(Suppl):97–103.

27. Krennmair G, Seemann R, Piehslinger E. Dental implants in patients with rheumatoid arthritis: clinical outcome and peri-implant findings. J Clin Periodontol 2010;37:928–936.

28. Weinlander M, Krennmair G, Piehslinger E. Implant prosthodontic rehabilitation of patients with rheumatic disorders: a case series report. Int J Prosthodont 2010;23:22–28.

29. Friberg B, Sennerby L, Roos J, Lekholm U. Identification of bone quality in conjunction with insertion of titanium implants: a pilot study in jaw autopsy specimens. Clin Oral Implants Res 1995;6:213–219.

30. Jaffin RA, Berman CL. The excessive loss of Branemark fixtures in type IV bone: a 5-year analysis. J Periodontol 1991;62:2–4.

31. Sakakura CE, Marcantonio Jr E, Wenzel A, Scaf G. Influence of cyclosporin A on quality of bone around integrated dental implants: a radiographic study in rabbits. Clin Oral Implants Res 2007;18:34–39.

32. Heckmann SM, Heckmann JG, Linke JJ, et al. Implant therapy following liver transplantation: clinical and microbiological results after 10 years. J Periodontol 2004;75:909–913.

33. Gu L, Yu YC. Clinical outcome of dental implants placed in liver transplant recipients after 3 years: a case series. Transplant Proc 2011;43:2678–2682.

34. Gu L, Wang Q, Yu YC. Eleven dental implants placed in a liver transplantation patient: a case report and 5-year clinical evaluation. Chin Med J (Engl) 2011;124:472–475.

35. Dijakiewicz M, Wojtowicz A, Dijakiewicz J, et al. Is implanto-prosthodontic treatment available for haemodialysis patients? Nephrol Dial Transplant 2007;22:2722–2724.

36. Porter SR, Scully C, Luker J. Complications of dental surgery in persons with HIV disease. Oral Surg Oral Med Oral Pathol 1993;75:165–167.

37. Scully C, Watt-Smith P, Dios P, Giangrande PLF. Complications in HIV-infected and non-HIV-infected hemophiliacs and other patients after oral surgery. Int J Oral Maxillofac Surg 2002;31:634–640.

38. Oliveira MA, Gallottini M, Pallos D, et al. The success of endosseous implants in human immunodeficiency virus-positive patients receiving antiretroviral therapy: a pilot study. J Am Dent Assoc 2011;142:1010–1016.

39. Koo S, König Jr B, Mizusaki CI, et al. Effects of alcohol consumption on osseointegration of titanium implants in rabbits. Implant Dent 2004;13:232–237.
40. Marchini L, de Deco CP, Marchini AP, et al. Negative effects of alcohol intake and estrogen deficiency combination on osseointegration in a rat model. J Oral Implantol 2011;37(6):633–639.
41. Galindo-Moreno P, Fauri M, Avila-Ortiz G, et al. Influence of alcohol and tobacco habits on peri-implant marginal bone loss: a prospective study. Clin Oral Implants Res 2005;16:579–586.
42. Alissa R, Oliver R. Influence of prognostic risk indicators on osseointegrated dental implant failure: a matched case–control analysis. J Oral Implantol 2011;38:51–61.
43. Linsen SS, Martini M, Stark H. Long-term results of endosteal implants following radical oral cancer surgery with and without adjuvant radiation therapy. Clin Implant Dent Relat Res 2012;14:250–258.
44. Harrison JS, Stratemann S, Redding SW. Dental implants for patients who have had radiation treatment for head and neck cancer. Special Care Dent 2003;23:223–229.
45. Javed F, Al-Hezaimi K, Al-Rasheed A, et al. Implant survival rate after oral cancer therapy: a review. Oral Oncol 2010;46:854–859.
46. Landes CA, Kovacs AF. Comparison of early telescope loading of non-submerged ITI implants in irradiated and non-irradiated oral cancer patients. Clin Oral Implants Res 2006;17:367–374.
47. Granström G. Radiotherapy, osseointegration and hyperbaric oxygen therapy. Periodontology 2000 2003;33:145–162.
48. Coulthard P, Patel S, Grusovin GM, et al. Hyperbaric oxygen therapy for irradiated patients who require dental implants: a Cochrane review of randomised clinical trials. Eur J Oral Implantol 2008;1:105–110.
49. Esposito M, Grusovin MG, Patel S, et al. Interventions for replacing missing teeth: hyperbaric oxygen therapy for irradiated patients who require dental implants. Cochrane Database Syst Rev 2008;(1):CD003603.
50. Verdonck HW, Meijer GJ, Laurin T, et al. Implant stability during osseointegration in irradiated and non-irradiated minipig alveolar bone: an experimental study. Clin Oral Implants Res. 2008;19:201–206.
51. Michaeli E, Weinberg I, Nahlieli O. Dental implants in the diabetic patient: systemic and rehabilitative considerations. Quintessence Int 2009;40:639–645.
52. McCracken M, Lemons JE, Rahemtulla F, et al. Bone response to titanium alloy implants placed in diabetic rats. Int J Oral Maxillofac Implants 2000;15:345–354.
53. Fiorellini JP, Nevins ML, Norkin A, et al. The effect of insulin therapy on osseointegration in a diabetic rat model. Clin Oral Implants Res 1999;10:362–368.
54. Morris HF, Ochi S, Winkler S. Implant survival in patients with type 2 diabetes: placement to 36 months. Ann Periodontol 2000;5:157–165.
55. Alsaadi G, Quirynen M, Komárek A, van Steenberghe D. Impact of local and systemic factors on the incidence of late oral implant loss. Clin Oral Implants Res 2008;19:670–676.
56. Dowell S, Oates TW, Robinson M. Implant success in people with type 2 diabetes mellitus with varying glycemic control: a pilot study. J Am Dent Assoc 2007;138:355–361.
57. Anner R, Grossmann Y, Anner Y, Levin L. Smoking, diabetes mellitus, periodontitis, and supportive periodontal treatment as factors associated with dental implant survival: a long-term retrospective evaluation of patients followed for up to 10 years. Implant Dent 2010;19:57–64.
58. Turkyilmaz I. One-year clinical outcome of dental implants placed in patients with type 2 diabetes mellitus: a case series. Implant Dent 2010;19:323–329.
59. Oates TW, Dowell S, Robinson M, McMahan CA. Glycemic control and implant stabilization in type 2 diabetes mellitus. J Dent Res 2009;88:367–371.
60. Javed F, Romanos GE. Impact of diabetes mellitus and glycemic control on the osseointegration of dental implants: a systematic literature review. J Periodontol 2009;80:1719–1730.
61. Tawil G, Younan R, Azar P, Sleilati G. Conventional and advanced implant treatment in the type II diabetic patient: surgical protocol and long-term clinical results. Int J Oral Maxillofac Implants 2008;23:744–752.
62. Beikler T, Flemmig TF. Implants in the medically compromised patient. Crit Rev Oral Biol Med 2003;14:305–316.
63. Gornitsky M, Hammouda W, Rosen H. Rehabilitation of a hemophiliac with implants: a medical perspective and case report. J Oral Maxillofac Surg 2005;63:592–597.
64. Scully C. Medical Problems in Dentistry, 6th edn. London: Elsevier; 2010.
65. Madrid C, Sanz M. What influence do anticoagulants have on oral implant therapy? A systematic review. Clin Oral Implants Res 2009;20:96–106.
66. Bacci C, Berengo M, Favero L, Zanon E. Safety of dental implant surgery in patients undergoing anticoagulation therapy: a prospective case–control study. Clin Oral Implants Res 2011;22:151–156.
67. Hong CH, Napeñas JJ, Brennan MT, et al. Frequency of bleeding following invasive dental procedures in patients on low-molecular-weight heparin therapy. J Oral Maxillofac Surg 2010;68:975–979.
68. Napeñas JJ, Hong CH, Brennan MT, et al. The frequency of bleeding complications after invasive dental treatment in patients receiving single and dual antiplatelet therapy. J Am Dent Assoc 2009;140:690–695.
69. Glaser DL, Kaplan FS. Osteporosis. Definition and clinical presentation. Spine 1997;22(24, Suppl):12S–16S.
70. Glösel B, Kuchler U, Watzek G, Gruber R. Review of dental implant rat research models simulating osteoporosis or diabetes. Int J Oral Maxillofac Implants 2010;25:516–524.
71. Blomqvist JE, Alberius P, Isaksson S, et al. Factors in implant integration failure after bone grafting: an osteometric and endocrinologic matched analysis. Int J Oral Maxillofac Surg 1996;25:63–68.
72. Alsaadi G, Quirynen M, Komarek A, van Steenberghe D. Impact of local and systemic factors on the incidence of oral implant failures, up to abutment connection. J Clin Periodontol 2007;34:610–617.

73. Slagter KW, Raghoebar GM, Vissink A. Osteoporosis and edentulous jaws. Int J Prosthodont 2008;21:19–26.

74. Dvorak G, Arnhart C, Heuberer S, et al. Peri-implantitis and late implant failures in postmenopausal women: a cross-sectional study. J Clin Periodontol 2011;38:950–955.

75. Friberg B, Ekestubbe A, Mellström D, Sennerby L. Brånemark implants and osteoporosis: a clinical exploratory study. Clin Implant Dent Relat Res 2001;3:50–56.

76. Sheper HJ, Brand HS. Oral aspects of Crohn's disease. Int Dent J 2002;52:163–172.

77. Alsaadi G, Quirynen M, Michilis K, et al. Impact of local and systemic factors on the incidence of failures up to abutment connection with modified surface oral implants. J Clin Periodontol 2008;35:51–57.

78. Alsaadi G, Quirynen M, Komarek A, van Steenberghe D. Impact of local and systemic factors on the incidence of late oral implant loss. Clin Oral Implants Res 2008;19:670–676.

79. Khadivi V, Anderson J, Zarb GA. Cardiovascular disease and treatment outcomes with osseointegration surgery. J Prosthet Dent 1999;81:533–536.

80. Van Steenberghe D, Jacobs R, Desnyder M, et al. The relative impact of local and endogenous patient-related factors on implant failure up to the abutment stage. Clin Oral Implants Res 2002;13:617–622.

81. Bayes J. Asymptomatic smokers: ASA I or II? Anesthesiology 1982;56(1):76.

82. Wilson Jr TG, Nunn M. The relationship between the interleukin-1 periodontal genotype and implant loss. Initial data. J Periodontol 1999;70:724–729.

83. Bain CA, Moy PK. The association between the failure of dental implants and cigarette smoking. Int J Oral Maxillofac Implants 1993;8:609–615.

84. De Bruyn H, Collaert B. The effect of smoking on early implant failure. Clin Oral Implants Res 1994;5:260–264.

85. Lambert PM, Morris HF, Ochi S. The influence of smoking on 3-year clinical success of osseointegrated dental implants. Ann Periodontol 2000;5:79–89.

86. Weyant RJ. Characteristics associated with the loss and peri-implant tissue health of endosseous dental implants. Int J Oral Maxillofac Implants 1994;9:95–102.

87. Minsk L, Polson AM, Weisgold A, et al. Outcome failures of endosseous implants from a clinical training center. Compend Contin Educ Dent 1996;17:848–850.

88. Kumar A, Jaffin RA, Berman C. The effect of smoking on achieving osseointegration of surface-modified implants: a clinical report. Int J Oral Maxillofac Implants 2002;17:816–819.

89. Sverzut AT, Stabile GA, de Moraes M, et al. The influence of tobacco on early dental implant failure. J Oral Maxillofac Surg 2008;66:1004–1009.

90. Bain CA, Weng D, Meltzer A, et al. A meta-analysis evaluating the risk for implant failure in patients who smoke. Compend Contin Educ Dent 2002;23:695–699.

91. Itthagarun A, King NM. Ectodermal dysplasia: a review and case report. Quintessence Int 1997;28:595–602.

92. Candel-Marti ME, Ata-Ali J, Peñarrocha-Oltra D, et al. Dental implants in patients with oral mucosal alterations: an update. Med Oral Patol Oral Cir Bucal 2011;16:e787–e793.

93. Sweeney IP, Ferguson JW, Heggie AA, Lucas JO. Treatment outcomes for adolescent ectodermal dysplasia patients treated with dental implants. Int J Paediatr Dent 2005;15:241–248.

94. Bergendal B, Ekman A, Nilsson P. Implant failure in young children with ectodermal dysplasia: a retrospective evaluation of use and outcome of dental implant treatment in children in Sweden. Int J Oral Maxillofac Implants 2008;23:520–524.

95. Guckes AD, Scurria MS, King TS, et al. Prospective clinical trial of dental implants in persons with ectodermal dysplasia. J Prosthet Dent 2002;88:21–29.

96. Percinoto C, Vieira AE, Barbieri CM, et al. Use of dental implants in children: a literature review. Quintessence Int 2001;32:381–383.

97. Scully C, Carrozzo M. Oral mucosal disease: lichen planus. Br J Oral Maxillofac Surg 2008;46:15–21.

98. Hernandez G, Lopez-Pintor RM, Arriba L, et al. Implant treatment in patients with oral lichen planus: a prospective-controlled study. Clin Oral Implants Res 2012;23:726–732.

99. Czerninski R, Eliezer M, Wilensky A, Soskolne A. Oral lichen planus and dental implants – a retrospective study. Clin Implant Dent Relat Res 2013;15(2):234–242.

100. Wolff K, Johnson RA, Suurmond D. Fitzpatrick's Color Atlas & Synopsis of Clinical Dermatology, 5th edn. New York: McGraw Hill; 2006, pp 398–402.

101. Jensen J, Sindet-Pedersen S. Osseointegrated implants for prosthetic reconstruction in a patient with scleroderma: report of a case. J Oral Maxillofac Surg 1990:48:739–741.

102. Langer Y, Cradash HS, Tal H. Use of dental implants in the treatment of patients with scleroderma: a clinical report. J Prosthet Dent 1992:68(6):873–875.

103. Patel K, Welfare R, Coonae HS. The provision of dental implants and a fixed prosthesis in the treatment of a patient with scleroderma: a clinical report. J Prosthet Dent 1998;79:611–612.

104. Haas SE. Implant supported, long span fixed partial denture for a scleroderma patient: a clinical report. J Prosthet Dent 2002;87:136–139.

105. Öczakir CS, Balmer S, Mericske-Stern R. Implant prosthodontic treatment for special care patients: a case series study. Int J Prosthodont 2005;18:383–389.

106. Ekfeldt A. Early experience of implant-supported prostheses in patients with neurologic disabilities. Int J Prosthodont 2005;18:132–138.

107. Addy L, Korszun A, Jagger RG. Dental implant treatment for patients with psychiatric disorders. Eur J Prosthodont Restor Dent 2006;14:90–92.

108. Cune MS, Strooker H, Van der Reijden WA, et al. Dental implants in persons with severe epilepsy and multiple disabilities: a long-term retrospective study. Int J Oral Maxillofac Implants 2009;24:534–540.

109. Delaleu N, Jonsson R, Koller MM. Sjögren's syndrome. Eur J Oral Sci 2005;113:101–113.

110. Mathews SA, Kuien BT, Scofield RG. Oral manifestations of Sjögren's syndrome. J Dent Res 2008;87:308–318.

111. Isidor F, Brondum K, Hansen HJ, et al. Outcome of treatment with implant-retained dental prosthesis in patients with Sjögren syndrome. Int J Oral Maxillofac Implants 1999;14:736–743.

112. Attard NJ, Zarb GA. A study of dental implants in medically treated hypothyroid patients. Clin Implant Dent Relat Res 2002;4:220–231.

113. Carabello B. Valvular heart disease. In: Goldman L, Ausiello D (eds), Cecil Textbook of Medicine, 22nd edn. St. Louis, MO: Saunders; 2004, pp 439–442.

114. Chambers H. Infective endocarditis. In: Goldman L, Ausiello D (eds), Cecil Textbook of Medicine, 22nd edn. St. Louis, MO: Saunders; 2004, pp 1795–1796.

115. Proceedings of the Seventh ACCP Conference on Antithrombotic and Thrombolytic Therapy: evidence-based guidelines. Chest 2004;126:172S–696S.

116. Drews RE. Critical issues in hematology: anemia, thrombocytopenia, coagulopathy, and blood product transfusions in critically ill patients. Clin Chest Med 2003;24:607–622.

117. Jolly DE. Interpreting the clinical laboratory. J Calif Dent Assoc 1995;23:32–40.

118. Mealey BL. Periodontal implications: medically compromised patients. Ann Periodontol 1996;1:256–321

119. Karr RA, Kramer DC, Toth BB. Dental implants and chemotherapy complications. J Prosthet Dent 1992;67:683–687.

120. Steiner M, Windchy A, Gould AR, et al. Effects of chemotherapy in patients with dental implants. J Oral Implantol 1995;21:142–147.

121. Kennedy J. Alcohol use disorders. In: Jacobson J (ed.), Psychiatric Secrets, 2nd edn. Philadelphia, PA: Hanley & Belfus; 2001, p 103.

122. Fu E, Hsieh YD, Nieh S, et al. Effects of cyclosporin A on alveolar bone: an experimental study in the rat. J Periodontol 1999;70:189–194.

123. Wu X, Al-Abedalla K, Rastikerdar E, et al. Selective serotonin reuptake inhibitors and the risk of osseointegrated implant failure: a cohort study. J Dent Res 2014;93(11):1054–1061.

124. Ferlito S, Liardo C, Puzzo S. Bisphosphonates and dental implants: a case report and a brief review of literature. Minerva Stomatol 2011;60:75–81.

125. Flichy-Fernández AJ, Balaguer-Martínez J, Peñarrocha-Diago M, Bagán JV. Bisphosphonates and dental implants: current problems. Med Oral Patol Oral Cir Bucal 2009;14:E355–E360.

126. Wang HL, Weber D, McCauley LK. Effect of long-term oral bisphosphonates on implant wound healing: literature review and a case report. J Periodontol 2007;78:584–594.

127. Lazarovici TS, Yahalom R, Taicher S, et al. Bisphosphonate-related osteonecrosis of the jaw associated with dental implants. J Oral Maxillofac Surg 2010;68:790–796.

128. Jacobsen C, Metzler P, Rössle M, et al. Osteopathology induced by bisphosphonates and dental implants: clinical observations. Clin Oral Investig 2013;17(1):167–175.

129. Memon S, Weltman RL, Katancik JA. Oral bisphosphonates: early endosseous dental implant success and crestal bone changes. A retrospective study. Int J Oral Maxillofac Implants 2012;27:1216–1222.

130. Advisory Task Force on Bisphosphonate-Related Ostenonecrosis of the Jaws, American Association of Oral and Maxillofacial Surgeons. American Association of Oral and Maxillofacial Surgeons position paper on bisphosphonate-related osteonecrosis of the jaws. J Oral Maxillofac Surg 2007;65:369–376.

131. Madrid C, Sanz M. What impact do systemically administered bisphosphonates have on oral implant therapy? A systematic review. Clin Oral Implants Res 2009;20:87–95.

132. Javed F, Almas K. Osseointegration of dental implants in patients undergoing bisphosphonate treatment: a literature review. J Periodontol 2010;81:479–484.

Answers to Self-Study Questions

A. The achievement of osseointegration is a biological concept already adopted in implant dentistry [3]. The long-term maintenance of bone around an osseointegrated implant is paramount to clinical success, and peri-implant bone remodeling is important to long-term survival rates [4]. It is believed that several factors may affect peri-implant bone resorption: local, surgical, implant, post-restorative, and patient-related risk factors, which include systemic diseases, medications used to treat systemic diseases, genetic traits, chronic drug or alcohol consumption, and smoking status [4]. The widely accepted theory for physiologic bone loss is related to the formation of a peri-implant biologic distance and should be understood as a physiologic phenomenon. This is shaped by bone resorption that occurs to accommodate soft tissue structures, with a vertical extension measuring from 1.5 to 2 mm in the apical direction [5–9]. Later or additional bone loss is characterized by gradual loss of marginal bone after osseointegration. Different levels of bone loss have been reported as acceptable [10]. One study reported that a gradual bone loss of 0.2 mm after the first year in function and ≤0.2 mm per year in subsequent years can be considered successful [11]. Another study tolerated 2 mm bone loss between the installation time and 5 years later [12]. However, another more recent study reported about 3 mm loss of bone apical to the abutment–implant interface after 5–20 years in function [13]. Although these studies [11–13] consider as acceptable bone loss up to 2 mm over the years, there is no consensus regarding this statement. Moreover, the relative importance of local and systemic factors to the development of alveolar bone loss around osseointegrated dental implants remains controversial [10].

The impact of health risks on the outcome of implant therapy is unclear, since there are a few randomized controlled trials evaluating health status as a risk indicator. In principle, only patients with an American Society of Anesthesiologists (ASA) physical status grade I (P1: a normal healthy patient) or II (P2: a patient with mild systemic disease) should qualify for an elective surgical procedure, such as dental implant placement, and the patient's surgical risks should be weighed against the potential benefits offered by the dental implants [1,14–16]. For very severe and acute medical problems (ASA physical status categories P3 to P6) calculating the risk of failure in affected subjects seems impossible because patients with such conditions hardly ever receive dental implants. A recent publication stated that elective dental treatment of patients classified as P4 or higher should ideally be postponed until the patient's medical condition has stabilized and improved to at least P3 [17].

Systemic diseases may affect oral tissues by increasing their susceptibility to other diseases or by interfering with healing. In addition, systemic conditions may be treated with medications or other therapies that potentially affect dental implants and the tissues carrying them [3]. There are different studies, mainly retrospective ones, that deal with the impact of medical/systemic factors and/or medications on the outcome osseointegrated implants, but the extrapolation of their results should be cautious, since it is not possible to collect

much information from such studies if not much insight into the occurrence and nature of systemic disease is given [18,19]. Several authors have also identified diseases for which dental implants are not recommended, or are at least questionable, but it often remains unclear what type of evidence these statements are based on [20–23]. Therefore, it still remains a debated question whether some systemic factors/medications compromise the achievement of an intimate bone to implant interface and what their role is during the healing time [18,19].

B. A medically compromised patient can be described as one who has a distinctive physical or mental feature regarding people of the same age. In these sorts of patients there is a higher risk of interactions between their disease and the implant surgery, implying a higher medical risk [2]. A thorough and exhaustive medical examination will help not only to determine the specific measures that must be adopted for a medically compromised patient but also to carry out the estimation of the patient's risk. The system proposed by the ASA [16] to the dental patient is commonly used to define the patient's risk [23]. These classifications and the medical history allow the dentist to identify the systemic disease and the success rate expected in the medically compromised patient that is going to be rehabilitated with dental implants [2]. It seems like the medical control of the disease is more important than the disease itself. This evidence proves the need for carrying out personalized medical examinations [1].

To achieve and maintain successful osseointegration over time, which is the goal and outcome of successful implant treatment, indications and contraindications must be carefully balanced. Therefore, proper patient selection is the key issue in treatment planning [20]. Contraindications can be divided into local and systemic/medical. In a recent Consensus Conference [24] it was proposed to subdivide the general/medical risk factors into two groups:
- *Group 1 (very high risk).* Patient with serious systemic diseases (rheumatoid arthritis, osteomalacia, osteogenesis imperfecta), immunocompromised patients (HIV, immunosuppressive medications), drug

abusers (alcohol), and noncompliant patients (psychological and mental disorders).

- *Group 2 (significant risk)*. Patients with irradiated bone (radiotherapy), severe diabetes (especially type 1), bleeding disorders/severe bleeding tendency (hemorrhagic diathesis, drug-induced anticoagulation), and heavy smoking habit.

Other authors have recommended certain patient groups or conditions as relative contraindications for dental implants [25]:

- children and adolescents
- epileptic patients
- severe bleeding tendency
- endocarditis risk
- osteoradionecrosis risk
- myocardial infarction risk.

Other reported relative contraindications include adolescence, ageing, osteoporosis, smoking, diabetes, positive interleukin-1 genotype, HIV positivity, cardiovascular disease, hypothyroidism, and Crohn's disease [22].

In more recent studies, the following diseases and conditions were examined for their increased risk for dental implant treatment failure: scleroderma, Sjögren syndrome, neuropsychiatric disorders/Parkinson disease, lichen ruber planus/oral lichen planus, HIV infection, ectodermal dysplasia, long-term immunosuppression after organ transplantation, cardiovascular disease, Crohn's disease, diabetes, osteoporosis, oral bisphosphonate medication, and use of radiotherapy for the treatment of oral squamous cell carcinoma [3,26].

Suggested absolute contraindications for implant placement (severe and acute medical conditions for which implant therapy has always been considered a contraindication) include the following: acute infections, severe bronchitis, emphysema, severe anemia, uncontrolled diabetes, uncontrolled hypertension, abnormal liver function, nephritis, severe psychiatric disease, conditions with severe risk of hemorrhage, endocarditis, recent myocardial infarction and cerebrovascular accident, transplant or valvular prosthesis surgery, profound immunosuppression, active treatment of malignancy, drug abuse, and intravenous bisphosphonate use [1,15,23]. There is, however, little or no evidence to support most of these conditions [1].

Generally, though, the evidence level of implant failures in the medically compromised patient is limited due to the low number of controlled randomized studies [2]. Therefore, different reviews have tried to evaluate certain disease categories as possible contraindications to implant therapy and their evidence on implant treatment complications/failures. The existing evidence has been generally drawn from a wide range of sources, ranging from case reports to controlled cohort investigations, including both human and animal studies [1].

The implant outcome assessment has varied from histological and radiographic outcomes, to objective and subjective determinations of implant and treatment failure [1].

Contraindications are mainly based on both the risk of medical complications related to implant surgery (e.g., hemorrhage risk in patients with bleeding disorders) and the rate of dental implant success in medically compromised patients (e.g., in patients with head and neck cancer receiving radiotherapy) [1].

The medical risk factors will be analyzed according to the different classification systems (high risk, significant risk, relative risk, and other medical conditions) described earlier.

C.

- *Rheumatoid arthritis.* There are some retrospective series on dental implants outcomes involving females suffering from autoimmune rheumatoid arthritis with or without concomitant connective tissue diseases, and the authors conclude that a high implant and prosthodontic success rate can be anticipated in rheumatoid arthritis patients, but peri-implant marginal bone resorption and bleeding are more pronounced in those with concomitant connective tissue diseases [27,28].
- *Osteomalacia.* This is a defective mineralization of the organic bone matrix (i.e., collagen). The disorder is usually associated with vitamin D deficiency and alimentary deficiencies. The vitamin D deficiency reduces the intestinal uptake and the mobilization of calcium from the bone and thus results in hypocalcemia. This leads to an increased parathyroid hormone secretion, which in turn increases the clearance of phosphorus by the kidneys. The decrease in the concentration

of phosphorus in the bone fluids prevents a normal mineralization process. The radiologic characteristics of bone in osteomalacia are a thinning of the cortices and a decreased density of the trabecular part [19]. No reports could be found on the clinical relevance of osteomalacia for the outcome of oral implants. It could be that some osteomalacia patients have been categorized as patients with "poor bone quality," category IV bone, which has been clearly associated with a higher failure rate [29,30].

- *Immunocompromised patients (HIV, immunosuppressive medication).* There have been some studies (mainly animal models) that have shown that cyclosporin impairs peri-implant bone healing and implant osseointegration [31]. However, many patients receiving organ transplantation (mainly liver and kidney) with long-term cyclosporin therapy have had successful dental implant therapy [32–35]. Similarly, no significant problems after dento-alveolar surgery have been reported in HIV-positive patients [36,37]. In a recently published case–control series of HIV-positive patients receiving different regimens of highly active antiretroviral therapy, after assessing peri-implant health, the authors concluded that dental implants may represent a reasonable treatment option in HIV-positive patients, regardless of CD4 cell count, viral load levels, and type of antiretroviral therapy [38]. It seems that dental implants are well tolerated and have predictable short-term outcomes for HIV-infected individuals, but published evidence is limited and the predictability of the long-term success remains unknown. It would seem wise though to proceed with implant therapy when CD4 rates are high and the patient is on antiretroviral therapy. In general, there is no evidence that immune incompetence is a contraindication to dental implant therapy, but medical advice should be obtained before considering dental implant therapy, and strict anti-infective measures should be enforced when treating these patients [1,3].
- *Drug abusers (alcohol).* There is no reliable evidence that alcoholism is a contraindication to implants, but patients that consume alcohol may be at increased risk of complications. Negative effects of alcohol intake on bone density and

osseointegration have been demonstrated in animal models [39,40]. In humans, there is evidence of increased peri-implant marginal bone loss and dental failures in patients with high levels of alcohol consumption [41,42]. Generally, it is worth considering before placing implants to alcohol consumers that alcoholism (a) is often associated with tobacco smoking (which itself may be considered as contraindication to implant therapy), (b) impairs liver function and may cause bleeding problems, (c) may cause osteoporosis (another relative contraindication to implant placement), (d) may impair the immune response, and (e) may impair nutrition, especially folate (vitamin B9) and vitamin B in general [1].

D.

- *Radiotherapy.* This can significantly affect dental implant outcomes mainly during the healing period [43]. Radiotherapy may induce obliterating endarteritis, and hence can predispose to osteoradionecrosis of the jaw [1]. Some studies involving implants placed in adult patients who have received radiotherapy reported lower success rates [44], but there are also several clinical studies demonstrating that dental implants can osseointegrate and remain functionally stable in patients who had received radiotherapy [45]. Other authors have reported successful dental implant outcomes but occurrence of late complications, such as bone loss and mucosal recession, possibly due to altered saliva flow and increased bacterial colonization [46]. Several case–control studies have shown evidence of improved outcomes in patients with history of radiotherapy and dental implants with the addition of hyperbaric oxygen therapy mainly through reduction in the occurrence of osteoradionecrosis and failing implants [47]. However, in a recent systematic review the authors were unable to find any strong evidence to either support or contradict the use of hyperbaric oxygen therapy for improving implant outcome, concluding that the use of hyperbaric treatment in patients undergoing implant treatment does not seem to provide significant benefits [48,49]. Radiotherapy could be responsible for the reduction in the success rate of dental implants when it is administered in doses exceeding 50 Gy, as has already been proven for extraoral implants [23]. An animal case–control study with irradiated maxilla and mandible (24–120 Gy) showed a decrease of implant stability quotient values long term in irradiated bone when compared with nonirradiated bone [50].

To increase implant success in irradiated head and neck cancer patients, the following precautions should be considered [47]:

1. Implant surgery is best carried out >21 days before radiotherapy.
2. Total radiation dose should be <66 Gy if the risks of osteoradionecrosis are to be minimized or <50 Gy to reduce osseointegration failure – avoiding implant site/portals.
3. Hyperbaric oxygen should be given if >50 Gy radiation is used.
4. No implant surgery should be carried out during radiotherapy.
5. No implant surgery should be carried out during mucositis.
6. Deferral of implant placement for 9 months after radiotherapy.
7. Use implant-supported prostheses without any mucosal contact and avoidance of immediate loading.
8. Ensure strict asepsis during surgical procedure.
9. Consideration of antimicrobial prophylaxis.

• *Diabetes mellitus.* This is a metabolic disorder resulting in hyperglycemia caused by a defect in insulin secretion, impaired glucose tolerance, or both. Diabetes is the most prevalent endocrine disease, comprising the third highest cause of disability and morbidity in the Western world [51]. HbA1c is a measure of long-term glucose control. Normal level is 4.0–6.0%; good balance is 6.0–7.5%, fair is 7.6–8.9%, and poor balance is 9.0–20.0% [51].

It is well established that diabetic patients are more prone to healing complications, with usually delayed wound healing [2]. There are two major types of diabetes. Type 1 (previously termed "insulin dependent") is caused by an autoimmune reaction destroying the beta cells of the pancreas, leading to insufficient production of insulin. Type 2 (previously termed "noninsulin dependent") is viewed as a resistance to insulin in combination

with an incapability to produce additional compensatory insulin [3].

Metabolic changes produced by diabetes are associated with the synthesis of the osteoblastic matrix induced by insulin. Variation in the differentiation of osteoblastic cells and hormones that regulate calcium metabolism produce homeostasis in the mineral bone tissue, an alteration in the level of bone matrix required to produce mature osteocytes that enhance the osseointegration of dental implants [2]. Epidemiological case–control studies carried out in animals show a variation in the bone density surrounding the implant in samples of noncontrolled diabetic patients [52,53]. Most studies reviewed confirm these experimental results. In a 3-year retrospective study, a higher frequency of implant failure was shown in diabetic patients (7.8%) than in healthy patients (6.8%) [54].

These data are also confirmed in recent thorough reviews [3,26]. Some other recent publications produce different results in spite of insisting on the higher risk of failure in diabetic patients [51,55]. Most case series, cohort studies, and systematic reviews support that dental implants in diabetics with good metabolic control have similar success rates when compared with matched healthy controls [51,56–58]. However, impaired implant integration has been reported in relation to hyperglycemic conditions in diabetic patients [59]. In a recent systematic review the authors concluded that poorly controlled diabetes negatively affects implant osseointegration [60]. This fact is consistent with the known effects of hyperglycemic states on impaired immunity, microvascular complications, and/or osteoporosis [1]. Generally, there is no evidence that diabetes is a contraindication to dental implant therapy, but as HbA1c may represent an independent factor correlated with postoperative complications and due to the known effects of hyperglycemic states on healing, medical advice and strict glycemic control before and after dental therapy are recommended [61]. Antimicrobial cover using penicillin, amoxicillin, clindamycin, or metronidazole should be provided during the implant surgery [62]. These patients should also quit smoking, optimize oral hygiene measures, and use antiseptic mouth rinses to prevent the occurrence of periodontal and peri-implant infections [1].

In the light of the results, the total contraindication to placing dental implants in diabetic patients because of their higher frequency of failure due to the risk of infection [51] has been modified. If controlled diabetics receive an antibiotic prophylaxis protocol and aseptic techniques with chlorhexidine gluconate 0.12% during implant placement the failure rates are similar to those of healthy patients [54,62].

- *Bleeding disorders/severe bleeding tendency (hemorrhagic diathesis, drug-induced anticoagulation).* Even though hemorrhage can be a relatively common complication in dental placement there is no reliable evidence to suggest that bleeding disorders are a contraindication to the placement of implants: even hemophiliacs have successfully been treated with dental implants [63]. Any oral surgical procedure may lead to hemorrhage and blood loss, and if this bleeding reaches the facial spaces of the neck it can endanger the airway [1]. In patients with bleeding disorders, hemorrhage associated with implant surgeries is more common and can be prolonged particularly with warfarin or acenocoumarol [64]. In these patients, the current recommendation is to undertake the implant surgical procedure without modifying the anticoagulation, provided the INR is less than 3 or 3.5 [64]. There is evidence that anticoagulated patients (INR 2–4) that have not discontinued their anticoagulant medication do not have a significantly higher risk of postoperative bleeding, and topical hemostatic agents are effective in preventing postoperative bleeding [65]. Oral anticoagulant discontinuation is therefore not recommended for dentoalveolar surgery, such as implant placement, provided that this does not involve autogenous bone grafts, extensive flaps, or osteotomy preparations extending outside the bony envelope [1,66]. The bleeding risk is also low in patients treated with heparin [67]. Generally, there is no evidence that any bleeding disorders are an absolute contraindication to dental implant surgery, although these patients may be at risk of prolonged hemorrhage and blood loss, and medical advice should be taken first, especially in

congenital bleeding disorders [1]. The primary care physician may decide any medication alteration or "bridging" the patient with low molecular weight heparin prior to implant placement in order to keep the INR at levels suitable for surgical treatment. The practitioner should take into consideration that the risks of altering or discontinuing use of the antiplatelet medications – increased risk of thromboembolism – far outweigh the low risk of hemorrhage, and medical advice is necessary prior to any treatment [68].

E.

- *Osteoporosis.* This is a common metabolic condition characterized by generalized reduction in bone mass and density with no other bone abnormality and an increased risk and/or incidence of fracture [3]. The World Health Organization has established diagnostic criteria for osteoporosis based on bone density measurements determined by peripheral dual-energy radiographic absorptiometry. A diagnosis of osteoporosis is made when the bone mineral density level T is at least 2.5 standard deviations below that in the mean young population ($T \leq 2.5$) [69]. The major concern about osteoporosis with respect to implant placement is the possibility that the disease modifies bone quality, formation, or healing to an extent that osseointegration is compromised [23]. When evaluating whether dental implants in osteoporotic patients have a different long-term outcome, even though failure rates have been reportedly higher in animal models [70] and patients [71,72], a systematic review revealed no association between systemic bone mineral density (BMD) status, mandibular BMD status, bone quality, and implant loss, concluding that the use of dental implants in osteoporosis patients is not contraindicated [73]. Another study found no relation between osteoporosis and peri-implantitis [74], and even patients with severe osteoporosis have been successfully rehabilitated with dental implant-supported prostheses [22,75]. The authors in a recent study concluded that taking into consideration the existing evidence, osteoporosis alone does not affect implant success [23]. A recent review, though, showed a weak association between osteoporosis and the risk of implant failure [3]. It is recommended, therefore, to thoroughly evaluate and accurately analyze the bone quality prior to implant placement. A further potential complication in osteoporotic patients is the possible effect on bone turnover at the dental implants interface of systemic antiresorptive medication and the risk of developing bisphosphonate-related osteonecrosis of the jaw (BRONJ) [1].

- *Crohn's disease.* This is an idiopathic chronic inflammatory disorder of the gastrointestinal tract that may also involve the oral cavity. The disease process is characterized by recurrent exacerbations and remissions [76]. Crohn's disease has also been suggested as a relative contraindication for dental implants. It is associated with nutritional and immune defects, and hence it may impair dental success [72]. However, the literature regarding the performance of dental implants in patients with Crohn's disease is scarce and with a very low level of evidence [3]. In different prospective and retrospective studies it was shown that implants placed in Crohn's disease patients integrated successfully, with limited early implant failures in patients with Crohn's disease [72,77,78]. Owing to limited evidence, a final conclusion cannot be drawn, but caution is indicated when implants are planned in such patients. The circulating antigen–antibody complexes in Crohn's disease may lead to autoimmune inflammatory processes in several parts of the body, including the bone-to-implant interface during the healing phase. Factors associated with the disease, such as medication or malnutrition, may also play a role in regard to implant placement [2].
- *Cardiovascular disease.* Five forms of cardiovascular disease (hypertension, atherosclerosis, vascular stenosis, coronary artery disease, and congestive heart failure) may impair the healing process, which depends on oxygen supply delivered by a normal blood flow [23]. The cardiac systemic disease can endanger and reduce the amount of oxygen and nutrients in the osseous tissue, which may affect the osseointegration process of dental implants. Some authors even point out the relative contraindication of placing dental implants in patients with certain cardiac systemic disease due to their higher risk of

developing infective endocarditis [3,23]. On the contrary, no correlation seems to exist between the lack of osseointegration of dental implants and patients with certain cardiac systemic disease, as concluded in a retrospective case study: similar implant failure rates were found in both the cardiovascular disease and control groups [79]. Despite causing physiological alterations, cardiovascular disease seems not to affect clinical implant success. Additionally, in two retrospective studies and one prospective study from the same center, the investigators also found no relation between early implant failure and cardiovascular disease, though patients with possibly noncontributory cardiovascular disease (such as angina, heart valve anomalies, and arrhythmia) were included [72,77,80]. The literature addressing dental implants and their success and failure rates in patients with cardiovascular disease is scarce. Further studies with implants in function are needed, but it appears that cardiovascular disease does not diminish initial implant survival. It is important, though, to understand that patients with cardiovascular disease often take medications for the disease control that may have an impact on implant treatment.

- *Smoking.* Smokers are categorized in ASA II physical status classification (mild systemic disease) [81]. Cigarette byproducts such as nicotine, carbon monoxide, and hydrogen cyanide incite toxic biological responses. Nicotine attenuates red blood cell, fibroblast, and macrophage proliferation, increases platelet adhesion, and induces vasoconstriction via the release of epinephrine; this leads to a lack of perfusion and compromised healing. Carbon monoxide competitively binds to hemoglobin and, thus, reduces tissue oxygenation. Hydrogen cyanide inhibits enzyme systems necessary for oxidative metabolism and cell transport. In addition, smoking promotes expression of inflammatory mediators (e.g., tumor necrosis factor and prostaglandin E2), and impairs polymorphonuclear neutrophil chemotaxis, phagocytosis, and oxidative burst mechanisms. It also increases matrix metalloproteinase production (e.g., collagenase and elastase) by polymorphonuclear neutrophils [23]. Several investigations implicate tobacco use in implant failure. Several retrospective studies showed that smokers have a higher failure rate, which sometimes was as high as 2.5 times greater, compared with nonsmokers [82]. Significantly more implants in the maxilla failed in smokers than in current nonsmokers, leading to the maxilla having greater failure disparity between smokers and nonsmokers [83,84]. In an 8-year long, randomized, prospective clinical trial the researchers concluded that persistent tobacco use following implantation lessened the ability of bone or other periodontal tissues to adapt over time, thus compromising all stages of treatment after fixture uncovering. They suggested smoking cessation for all implant candidates [85]. Only a few studies conclude that smoking status does not influence implant success [86–88]. Two retrospective studies concluded that the consumption of tobacco is not a decisive factor in the loss of dental implants [72,89]. In another study it was observed that surface-modified implants may resist effects of smoking [90]. On the whole, smoking appears to reduce implant success in the maxilla, but smoking cessation prior to implant rehabilitation appears to improve results. Generally, many authors have associated the consumption of tobacco with the implant loss significantly [23,72,77]. The use of surface-modified fixtures may decrease the risk of failure in smokers, though evidence is preliminary [23].

F.
• *Ectodermal dysplasia.* This is a hereditary disease characterized by congenital dysplasia of one or more ectodermal structures. Common extra- and intraoral manifestations include defective hair follicles and eyebrows, frontal bossing, nasal bridge depression, protuberant lips, hypo- or anodontia, conical teeth, and generalized spacing [91]. There have been several case reports and case series for patients with ectodermal dysplasia treated with dental implants. Most series demonstrate an excellent implant success rate in adults with ectodermal dysplasia [92], although results reported in children and adolescents mainly when implants were placed in the maxilla or the symphyseal region of the anterior mandible

have been less encouraging [93,94]. The most appropriate age for dental implant treatment in growing children remains controversial [95,96]. There are no controlled studies, though, to demonstrate any positive or negative effect of the disease on the implant treatment [3].
• *Lichen planus.* Oral lichen planus is a common T-cell-mediated autoimmune disease of unknown cause that affects stratified squamous epithelium virtually exclusively [97]. It has been suggested that dental implants are not ideal for patients with oral lichen planus because of the limited capacity of the epithelium involved to adhere to the titanium surface [20]. Case control and case reports have showed successful outcomes of implants placed in patients with oral lichen planus. Peri-implant mucositis and peri-implantitis seem to be slightly more frequent in patients with oral lichen planus than in controls, and desquamative gingivitis was associated with a higher rate of peri-implant mucositis [98]. Implant placement does not influence the disease manifestations, though [99]. Careful long-term monitoring of both lesions and dental implants is recommended [92]. With the available literature at present, oral lichen planus as a risk factor for implant surgery and long-term success cannot be properly assessed.
• *Scleroderma.* This is defined as a multisystem disorder characterized by inflammatory, vascular, and sclerotic changes of the skin and various internal organs, especially the lungs, the heart, and the gastrointestinal tract. Typical clinical features in the facial region include a masklike appearance, thinning of the lips, microstomia, radial perioral furrowing, sclerosis of the sublingual ligament, and indurations of the tongue [100]. The skin of the face and lips as well as the intraoral mucosa is tense, thereby hindering or complicating dental treatment. There are only case reports and case series with up to two patients with scleroderma and treated with dental implants in the literature [101–105]. According to a recent review, no further controlled studies for scleroderma were found and, therefore, the level of evidence for the efficacy of dental implants in such patients is low [3].
• *Neuropsychiatric disorders.* The literature with respect to implant placement in patients

with neuropsychiatric disorders is scarce and contradictory. Some case reports and case series have shown implant treatment to be successful in some patients with various degrees of both intellectual and physical disability, including cases of cerebral palsy, Down syndrome, psychiatric disorders, dementia, bulimia, Parkinson disease, and severe epilepsy [105–108]. However, poor oral hygiene, oral parafunctions such as bruxism, harmful habits such as repeated introduction of the fingers into the mouth, and behavioral problems are not uncommon in patients with neuropsychiatric diseases, and dental implants in such patients may lead to complications. Therefore, the success of oral rehabilitation depends fundamentally on appropriate patient selection, and adequate medical advice should be taken prior to implant therapy. It is important to keep in mind, though, that patients with diseases affecting motor skills can benefit from implant-retained overdentures. In contrast, full fixed prosthetic restorations over implants should be avoided because of the difficulty of effective cleaning [3].

- *Sjögren syndrome.* This is a chronic autoimmune disease affecting the exocrine glands, primarily the salivary and lacrimal glands. The most common symptoms are extreme tiredness, along with dry eyes (keratoconjunctivitis sicca) and dry mouth (xerostomia). Xerostomia can eventually lead to difficulty in swallowing, severe and progressive tooth decay, or oral infections. Currently, there is no cure for Sjögren syndrome, and treatment is mainly palliative [109,110]. Literature on implant treatment in patients with Sjögren syndrome is scarce. There are no controlled studies available; but there is one case series study, which showed an implant-based failure rate of 16.7% and patient-based failure rate of 50% [111].

- *Hypothyroidism.* Thyroid disorders affect bone metabolism. Thyroxine and, to a lesser extent, triiodothyronine regulate several homeostatic processes. In soft tissue and bone fractures, these hormones manage wound healing. Hypothyroidism decreases recruitment, maturation, and activity of bone cells, possibly by reducing circulating levels of insulin-like growth factor-1; this suppresses bone formation

as well as resorption [23]. Fracture healing is therefore inhibited. It can be assumed, therefore, that hypothyroid states lead to greater failures in implant osseointegration. There are a few studies, though, on thyroid status and implant success rates where no correlation was found [80,112]. Thus, in a controlled patient, hypothyroidism fails to influence implant survival [23].

G.

- *Recent myocardial infarction or cerebrovascular accident or ischemic stroke.* When ischemia to the heart or the brain occurs, it generates necrosis and functional deficits. With intervention and a healing period of roughly 6–12 months after preliminary care, patient stability occurs. In the interim period and for 3–6 months after initial stability, it is necessary to avoid any stress, including surgical, that could trigger post-ischemia complications. Owing to the high risk of complications following a myocardial infarction or cerebrovascular accident, the dental provider must wait until preliminary stabilization. The patient may pursue elective dental care only if at least 6 months have passed since the ischemic incident and they obtain medical clearance. Additionally, the health-care professional must be aware of any anticoagulant or thrombolytic therapy administered and understand that the desire for oral implants does not necessarily justify interruption of a therapeutic INR [22].

- *Transplant or valvular prosthesis placement.* Repair of cardiac or vascular defects with autografts or particular materials often becomes completely encased in endocardium or endothelium within the first month, rendering them relatively impervious to bacterial seeding, increasing possible risks from exposure such as endocarditis or endarteritis. Especially prone to microbial infection, prosthetic valves restore function to those with progressive congestive heart failure, systemic emboli, or endocarditis [22,113]. Three forms of prosthetic valve exist: bioprostheses (porcine), mechanical valves, and homografts or autografts. All but the autograft fall subject to endocarditis, as well as regurgitation, stenosis, and degeneration. The prevalence of prosthetic valve endocarditis lingers around

1–3%, and the greatest risk occurs within the first 3 months [114]. By 6 months the prosthetic valve endocarditis rate drops to 0.4%. With prosthetic valve replacement, stability occurs at least 6 months to 1 year after cardiac surgery [113,114]. Avoidance of invasive periodontal procedures is mandatory in order to prevent bacteremia and possible subsequent valve loss. Depending on the type of valve used (mechanical or bioprosthesis), the patient requires different drug regimens (anticoagulants or plasma volume elevators, respectively) [113]. Additionally, premedication with antibiotics prior to any invasive surgical procedure may be required. Practitioners must take such medications into consideration prior to any implant treatment.

- *Conditions with severe risk of hemorrhage.* If proper hemostasis cannot occur, elective surgery must not take place. Uncontrolled hemorrhage stems from a multitude of conditions, including platelet and clotting factor disorders, but often originates from drug therapy. Patients taking oral anticoagulants (e.g., aspirin, warfarin, clopidogrel) for cardiovascular diseases must receive careful supervision of bleeding time and INR. Little risk of significant bleeding following dental surgical procedures in patients with a prothrombin time of 1.5–2 times is normal. The medical literature, however, proposes that a patient with an INR of 3 or less tolerates invasive oral therapies, including extractions or implant therapy [115]. If, for some reason, the INR must be kept higher, elective implant treatment is inappropriate [22]. A lack of platelets due to infection, idiopathic thrombocytopenia purpura, radiation therapy, myelosuppression, and leukemia may lead to bleeding issues during or after surgery as well. Mild thrombocytopenia, or platelet count 50,000–100,000/mm^3, may produce abnormal postoperative bleeding. Levels below 50,000/mm^3 lead to major postsurgical bleeding; spontaneous bleeding of mucous membranes occurs below 20,000 cells/mm^3 [116]. Such patients often require transfusion before surgery. For most dental patients, the hematocrit is crucial to outpatient care only when values drop to roughly 60% of low normal range. Patients who are to undergo sedation or general anesthesia require hemoglobin and hematocrit values within about 75–80% of normal [117].

- *Profound immunosuppression.* The ability to obtain an adequate immune response is crucial to wound healing. Oral surgery is typically contraindicated when the total white blood count falls below 1500–3000 cells/mm^3, as the patient becomes susceptible to infection and compromised repair or regeneration [118]. A normal absolute neutrophil count level lies between 3500 and 7000 cells/mm^3. A person with levels between 1000 and 2000 cells/mm^3 requires broad-spectrum antibiotic coverage [117]. Those with less than 1000 cells/mm^3 require immediate medical consultation and cannot receive dental implantation [22].

- *Active treatment of malignancy.* While needed to destroy rapidly dividing malignant cells, both ionizing radiation and chemotherapy disrupt host defense mechanisms and hematopoiesis. Because the patient on such regimens cannot mount an appropriate response to wounding from surgery, implantation is prohibited [22]. The total dose of ionizing radiation for cancer treatment ranges from 50 to 80 Gy. This is given in fractions of 1–10 Gy per week in order to maximize death of neoplastic cells and minimize injury to host cells. Four stages of biological interactions occur with radiation. Overall, the tissues and systems of the periodontium have intermediate radiosensitivity compared with those with more rapid turnover (marrow, skin, gastrointestinal cells). Typical head and neck radiation, however, makes the periodontal apparatus prone to injury. Osteocytes of outer lamellar and haversian bone in the direct path of ionizing radiation die, and blood vessels of the haversian canals may be obliterated. Mucositis and xerostomia, resulting from radiation damage to mucosa and salivary glands respectively, also contribute to a poor oral environment. Patency and hemopoietic potential of bone decrease. The posterior mandible in particular experiences osteoradionecrosis simply because it often lies adjacent to the radiation source. Additionally, it is less vascular, and contains less and larger trabeculae. Most studies that involve implant placement in irradiated bone reflect this. Additionally, active use of cytotoxic anticancer drugs, which induce rapid granulocytopenia, followed by thrombocytopenia, may contraindicate implant rehabilitation [22]. There are, though, a very limited number of investigations on chemotherapeutic effects on implant survival. Case reports on subjects with dental implants who then undergo cancer chemotherapy show conflicting, though mostly adverse, results [119,120].

- *Severe psychiatric disorders.* In a patient unable to comprehend and anticipate dental treatment logically, it is best not to proceed with implant therapy. Several conditions have been identified as incompatible with implant placement. These include psychotic disorders (e.g., schizophrenia), severe character disorders (hysteroid and borderline personalities), dysmorphophobia, cerebral lesions, and presenile dementia, as well as alcohol and drug abuse [22]. There are no biological reasons for patients with most of the above disorders to lose implants (at least none that have been determined), but various case reports blame removal of osseointegrated fixtures on psychiatric factors [22].

- *Drug abuse.* Addictions to alcohol and other drugs lower resistance to disease, increase possibility of infection, retard healing aggravated by malnutrition, cause incoherence, and result in poor oral hygiene [121]. Alcohol abuse in particular induces hepatic disease and subsequent platelet disorders, hypertension, distress infarction, aneurysm, and insidious hemorrhage. A patient who abuses alcohol or drugs may suffer from an inability not only to recognize or accept realistic treatment outcomes but also to heal [22].

H. Some medications may cause complications during or after implant therapy or may have an impact on healing, early or late osseointegration, and possibly on implant failure.
- *Medications that cause gingival overgrowth.*
  ○ Antiepileptics (phenytoin). Phenytoin is an antiepileptic drug that is known to provoke gingival enlargement in the presence of plaque. Gingival overgrowth may also happen around transgingival/mucosal abutments in the presence of plaque accumulation. Resection of the enlarged soft tissue can be performed by

gingivectomy (for limited overgrowths) or flap surgery (when larger volumes are involved). No data are available for oral implants in patients receiving phenytoin [19].
  ○ Antihypertensives (calcium channel blockers). Dihydropyridine calcium channel blockers for hypertension have gingival overgrowth as a common side effect. Data concerning the risk of gingival overgrowth in patients rehabilitated by means of implants are lacking [19].
  ○ Immunosuppressives (cyclosporin). Cyclosporin, and immunosuppressive medication usually given to patients with transplants, also has gingival enlargement as a common side effect. The gingival overgrowth does not appear to be plaque related. Cyclosporin has a more challenging effect on osseointegrated implants, namely its well-documented effect on accelerating bone turnover and provoking a negative bone balance [19,122].
- *Selective serotonin reuptake inhibitors (SSRIs).* These are the most widely used drugs for the treatment of depression and have been reported to interfere with bone metabolism, having a direct negative effect in bone formation by increasing osteoclast differentiation. As a result they reduce bone mass and bone mineral density and increase the risk of osteoporosis and bone fracture. In a recent cohort study, the authors' findings indicated that treatment with SSRIs is associated with an increased failure risk of osseointegrated implants, which might suggest a careful surgical treatment planning for SSRI users [123].
- *Bisphosphonates.* The bisphosphonates are drugs indicated in the prevention and treatment of illnesses associated with bony resorption (osteoporosis or Paget disease), bony metastasis of cancer, paraneoplastic syndromes, and multiple myeloma. They can be used orally or intravenously [2]. The risk in patients using bisphosphonates is well recognized, in terms of BRONJ [124–126]. The largest series of patients developing BRONJ following dental implants published to date involved 27 patients on bisphosphonates, taken either orally or intravenously (alendronate, zoledronic acid, and pamidronate). There was a mean duration of 16 months from implants placement until the

appearance of BRONJ [127]. In another series of BRONJ following dental implants, again involving patients on bisphosphonates either orally or intravenously, it has been suggested that posteriorly placed implants seem to be at higher risk of BRONJ development [128]. BRONJ is a real issue for patients treated with intravenous bisphosphonates, but the occurrence of BRONJ in patients receiving oral bisphosphonates medication is minimal [1]. The use of oral bisphosphonates at the time of implant placement and during healing does not seem to affect early implant success [129]. In 2007, the American Association of Oral and Maxillofacial Surgeons [130] produced guidelines for patients treated with oral bisphosphonates, based on the clinical situation of the patient and the length of treatment with the drug, indicating that greater caution prior and subsequent to surgery should be taken during 3 years after discontinuing bisphosphonate treatment. Two systematic reviews showed that the placement of dental implants in patients with chronic intake of oral bisphosphonates did not lead to BRONJ and did not influence short-term implant survival rates. The authors concluded that dental implants might be considered a safe procedure in patients taking oral bisphosphonates for <5 years [131] and that dental implants can osseointegrate and remain functionally stable in patients treated with bisphosphonates [132]. In summary, there is a consensus on contraindicating implants in cancer patients treated with intravenous bisphosphonates [131]. In patients with osteoporosis treated with bisphosphonates, they should be informed of the risk of possible implant loss as well as of the risk of suffering bony necrosis and a poor outcome from sinus lifts, and, therefore, adequate informed consent prior to dental implant surgery should be obtained [1].

• *Corticosteroid therapy.* Corticosteroid adverse effects include reduced bone density, increased epithelial fragility, and immunosuppression [64]. In consequence, the use of systemic glucocorticoids might compromise dental implant osseointegration and peri-implant healing. There is no evidence that corticosteroid therapy is a contraindication to dental implants, but it is important to consider that systemic corticosteroids can cause suppression of the hypothalamo–pituitary–adrenal axis and, therefore, standard recommendations for any oral surgery in patients on steroid therapy should be implemented [64]. The Medicines Control Agency still advises that patients who have finished a course of systemic corticosteroids of less than 3 weeks' duration and might be under stresses, such as trauma, surgery, or infection, and who are at risk of adrenal insufficiency receive systemic corticosteroid cover during these periods.

Conclusions

Patient selection is the critical factor for implant survival. In most cases an appropriate healing response allows for, if not ensures, success. Not all of those who desire implant rehabilitation, however, are candidates for surgery. Absolute medical contraindications exist and must be adhered to, lest the clinician contend with infection, implant failure, or even patient death. There are conditions that, if stabilized, do not seem to interfere perceptibly with repair. The careful practitioner understands the nature of a number of diseases, evaluates evidence regarding implant therapy in such patients, and picks their cases based on this knowledge. It is an informed choice that we make, and if we choose properly, then predictability results. A number of these relative contraindications to elective implant therapy exist. If controlled or isolated, the vast majority of diseases fail to affect conspicuously implant survival [22,23]. Not every patient who requires implant therapy initially qualifies for it; the good clinician possesses the ability to discriminate between candidates, make appropriate decisions, and instigate medical treatment as necessary.

Case 3

Implant Stability

Past Dental History

The patient had a history of root canal therapy on teeth #9 and #10. These teeth were splinted by porcelain fused to a metal prosthesis. There was an uneven incisal alignment seen on tooth #9 with a maxillary anterior open bite (Figure 1).

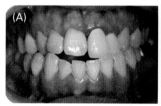 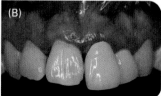

Figure 1: (A) Intraoral presentation and (B) close-up of tooth #9 (facial view).

Medical History

There were no significant medical problems reported. However, the patient is a heavy smoker (10 per day). The patient's family is healthy without any reported medical problems.

Review of Systems

- Vital signs
  - ○ Blood pressure: 110/72 mmHg
  - ○ Pulse rate: 73 beats/min (regular)
  - ○ Respiration: 15 breaths/min

Social History

The patient smokes and is a social consumer of alcohol. The patient was placed in a smoking cessation program.

Extraoral Examination

No significant findings were noted on extraoral examination. The patient had no masses or swellings and the temporomandibular joint was within normal limits. There was no facial asymmetry.

Intraoral Examination

- Soft tissue examination, including buccal mucosa, tongue, and floor of the mouth, was within normal limits.
- Oral hygiene was considered good, with an O'Leary plaque score of 22%.
- Slight calculus accumulation of lower anterior was found.
- Tooth #9 presented with crowding, uneven incisal alignment, and labioversion (Figure 1).
- Periodontal examination revealed probing depths in the range 2–3 mm (Figure 2).
- Loss of attachment and black triangle between teeth #7, #8, and #9 (Figure 1).

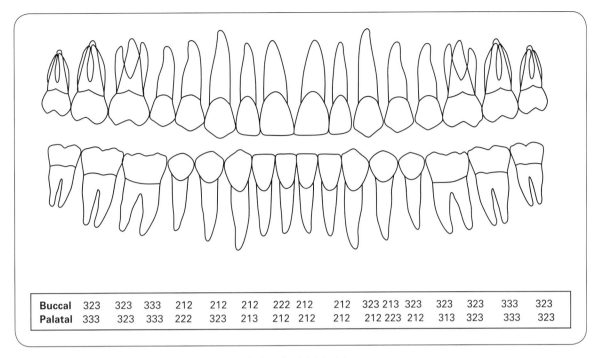

Buccal	323	323	333	212	212	212	222	212	212	323	213	323	323	323	333	323
Palatal	333	323	333	222	323	213	212	212	212	212	223	212	313	323	333	323

Figure 2: Maxillary probing pocket depth measurements during the initial visit.

- There was no primary or recurrent dental caries, and gingival inflammation was minimal.
- Localized erythema was noted on the margin of tooth #9.
- Normal thickness and width of keratinized mucosa noted.

Occlusion

The patient presented with a maxillary anterior open bite and group function.

Radiographic Examination

An initial panoramic radiograph (Figure 3) was ordered and subsequently a full mouth radiographic series was exposed. A cone beam computed tomography (CBCT) scan of the maxilla was also ordered. Buccal bone level and bone crestal height on the anterior maxilla were evaluated for proper diagnosis using CBCT scan selected images. Thin buccal bone was observed in the CBCT scan by three-dimensional reconstruction (Figures 4 and 5).

Diagnosis

An American Academy of Periodontology diagnosis of plaque-induced gingivitis with traumatic, accidental, physical injury [1].

Treatment Plan

The treatment plan for this case included disease control therapy to effectively reduce gingival inflammation and surgical and prosthetic reconstruction of tooth #9.

Examination and Treatment Visits

The patient presented to our clinic with the chief complaint of tooth mobility. The medical and dental

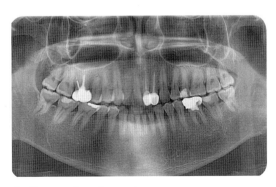

Figure 3: Panoramic radiograph.

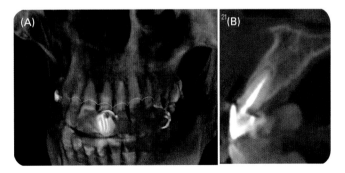

Figure 4: (A) CBCT reconstruction. (B) Sagittal view of the alveolar bone.

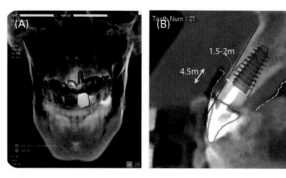

Figure 5: Virtual implant position plan: (A) facial view; (B) sagittal view.

histories were obtained. Systemically, the patient was healthy with the exception of being a smoker. The patient had a history of root canal therapy on tooth #9 and #10 and splinting by porcelain fused to a metal prosthesis. Periodontal examination revealed healthy periodontium with localized areas of mild gingivitis. Occlusal analysis revealed uneven incisal level alignment on tooth #9 with maxillary anterior open bite. These factors together made her a good candidate for dental implant therapy.

The patient had periodontal phase I treatment to resolve periodontal tissue inflammation. After a CBCT scan of the maxilla, a surgical stent was fabricated. The site-specific clinical and radiographic evaluation revealed enough buccolingual width and mesiodistal and apico-coronal space for both the placement and the restoration of the implant. Impressions were taken during this initial visit that were utilized for doing a diagnostic wax-up and creating a surgical guide. Immediately after the extraction of tooth #9 the implant was placed by using flapless surgery using the prefabricated surgical stent (Figure 6). Implant stability buccolingually and mesiodistally was measured using an Osstell device

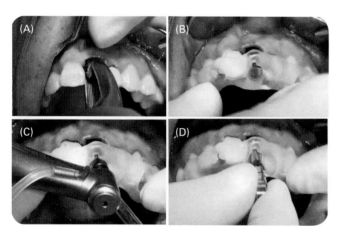

Figure 6: (A) Tooth #9 extraction. (B) Surgical stent placed. (C) Osteotomy. (D) Implant placement.

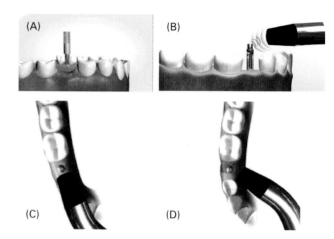

Figure 7: Schematic demonstration of implant stability measurement by Osstell device. (A) Attaching SmartPeg to implant; (B) transmission of magnetic pulses; (C) buccal and lingual measurements; (D) mesial and distal measurements.

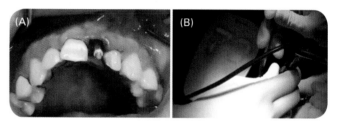

Figure 8: Clinical implant stability: (A) after SmartPeg placement; (B) Osstell measurements.

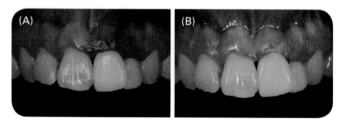

Figure 9: (A) Temporary crown postimplant placement. (B) At 2 weeks postimplant placement.

(Figures 7 and 8). A provisional crown was placed immediately after surgery without any occlusal contact. When the patient presented to the clinic, 2 weeks after extraction and implant placement, the peri-implant tissue was healthy (Figure 9). CBCT evaluation of the implant placement and its relationship with the buccal bone demonstrate optimal angulation (Figure 10). The final porcelain fused to zirconia restoration was delivered 8 weeks after implant placement (Figures 11 and 12).

Discussion

Dental implants have been widely used since the first development [2]. Implant placement has been advocated to be in sites that the bone is completely

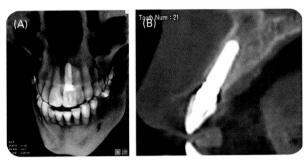

Figure 10: CBCT scan of new implant position: (A) facial view; (B) sagittal view.

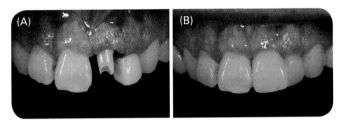

Figure 11: (A) Zirconia abutment. (B) Final crown.

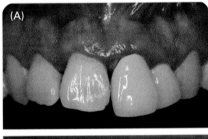

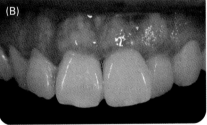

Figure 12: (A) Pre-extraction. (B) Postimplant placement (8 weeks).

healed and after placement there should be at least 3–6 months without any forces [3]. During implant–bone wound healing, forces may interfere with osteoprogenitor cells and proper bone formation. In fact, covering the implant was a strategy developed to prevent both infection and epithelial invasion, favoring osseointegration. The high clinical success rates of implant therapy have led to the indications of more demanding clinical situations, including immediate placement [4]. For both biologically and clinically

successful implants, proper diagnosis is crucial to the final treatment outcome. Here, we describe proper techniques to diagnose the presurgical site and implant stability.

Site evaluation is a critical factor for the success of the short- and long-term success of the implant [5–7]. There are many factors that influence the surgical site, including soft tissue biotype and quantity, bone quality and shape, socket healing status, adjacent teeth periodontal tissue, presence of pathology, and esthetic considerations. In this patient, immediate placement was feasible because she presented with most of the key factors that favor a good outcome. It is important to point out that a thin gingival biotype can be a risk factor for future esthetics (Figure 13) of the implant because of buccal plate resorption and tissue recession [8–10]. If the buccal plate is lost and one tries to place an implant without grafting, the risks of recession and esthetic concerns after restoration are even higher. Thus, when the biotype is not thick and is highly scalloped, concomitant augmentation therapy is recommended. In addition, minimally invasive techniques are recommended to prevent trauma in both hard and soft tissues. In addition to surgical techniques, the surgical site requires optimal tissue quality and a quantity of soft and hard tissues without pathological lesions for implant placement [11].

Among all surgical factors that influence implant success, the most relevant and determining factor in the immediate implant scenario is primary stability. And this is imperative for immediate loading treatment options [7,12–14]. As reported in this clinical case, primary stability was achieved and evaluated by additional diagnostic techniques, including an Osstell device [15]. The concern for implant movement comes

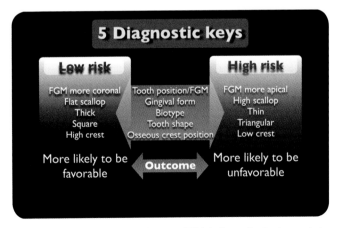

Figure 13: Diagnostic key factors (FGM: free gingival margin).

from the notion that micromovement has been shown to interfere with bone healing [16]. Connective tissue encapsulation was found in implants placed with poor initial stability. This has been illustrated by many studies demonstrating that micromotions of more

than 100–150 µm influence the healing and even promote fibrous encapsulation [17,18]. Therefore, site-specific diagnosis and pre- and postimplant placement evaluation are tools predictive of osseointegration and implant success.

Self-Study Questions

(Answers located at the end of the case)

A. What are the key factors that contribute to immediate implant success?

B. How does immediate implant placement influence esthetic outcomes of the case?

C. What are the clinical methods to evaluate implant stability?

References

1. Armitage GC. Development of a classification system for periodontal diseases and conditions. Ann Periodontol 1999;4(1):1–6.
2. Brånemark PI, Adell R, Breine U, et al. Intra-osseous anchorage of dental prostheses. I. Experimental studies. Scand J Plast Reconstr Surg 1969;3(2):81–100.
3. Albrektsson T, Zarb G, Worthington P, Eriksson AR. The long-term efficacy of currently used dental implants: a review and proposed criteria of success. Int J Oral Maxillofac Implants 1986;1(1):11–25.
4. Schulte W, Kleineikenscheidt H, Lindner K, Schareyka R. The Tübingen immediate implant in clinical studies. Dtsch Zahnarztl Z 1978;33(5):348–359 (in German).
5. Schwartz-Arad D, Chaushu G. Placement of implants into fresh extraction sites: 4 to 7 years retrospective evaluation of 95 immediate implants. J Periodontol 1997;68(11):1110–1116.
6. Becker W, Dahlin C, Lekholm U, et al. Five-year evaluation of implants placed at extraction and with dehiscences and fenestration defects augmented with ePTFE membranes: results from a prospective multicenter study. Clin Implant Dent Relat Res 1999;1(1):27–32.
7. Polizzi G, Grunder U, Goene R, et al. Immediate and delayed implant placement into extraction sockets: a 5-year report. Clin Implant Dent Relat Res 2000;2(2):93–99.
8. Zigdon H, Machtei EE. The dimensions of keratinized mucosa around implants affect clinical and immunological parameters. Clin Oral Implants Res 2008;19(4):387–392.
9. Kim BS, Kim YK, Yun PY, et al. Evaluation of peri-implant tissue response according to the presence of keratinized mucosa. Oral Surg Oral Med Oral Pathol Oral Radiol Endod 2009;107(3):e24–e28.
10. Gobbato L, Avila-Ortiz G, Sohrabi K, et al. The effect of keratinized mucosa width on peri-implant health:

a systematic review. Int J Oral Maxillofac Implants 2013;28(6):1536–1545.
11. Barone A, Orlando B, Cingano L, et al. A randomized clinical trial to evaluate and compare implants placed in augmented versus non-augmented extraction sockets: 3-year results. J Periodontol 2012;83(7):836–846.
12. Becker W, Sennerby L, Bedrossian E, et al. Implant stability measurements for implants placed at the time of extraction: a cohort, prospective clinical trial. J Periodontol 2005;76(3):391–397.
13. Artzi Z, Beitlitum I, Kolerman R. From an immediate implant placement in the post-extraction phase towards immediate loading application: current status. Refuat Hapeh Vehashinayim (1993) 2011;28(1):36–45,78 (in Hebrew).
14. Schrott A, Riggi-Heiniger M, Maruo K, Gallucci GO. Implant loading protocols for partially edentulous patients with extended edentulous sites – a systematic review and meta-analysis. Int J Oral Maxillofac Implants 2014;29(Suppl):239–255.
15. Meredith N, Alleyne D, Cawley P. Quantitative determination of the stability of the implant–tissue interface using resonance frequency analysis. Clin Oral Implants Res 1996;7(3):261–267.
16. Brunski JB. Avoid pitfalls of overloading and micromotion of intraosseous implants. Dent Implantol Update 1993;4(10):77–81.
17. Prendergast PJ, Huiskes R, Soballe K. ESB Research Award 1996. Biophysical stimuli on cells during tissue differentiation at implant interfaces. J Biomech 1997;30(6):539–548.
18. Szmukler-Moncler S, Salama H, Reingewirtz Y, Dubruille JH. Timing of loading and effect of micromotion on bone–dental implant interface: review of experimental literature. J Biomed Mater Res 1998;43(2):192–203.

Answers to Self-Study Questions

A. Several risk factors influence implant survival. Systemic and local factors influence the outcome of the therapy directly and indirectly. Immunocompromised patients and patients with uncontrolled diabetes and other systemic conditions can have poorer outcomes. Failures of endosseous implants were subdivided into early and late stages. In early failures there is an inability to establish implant-to-bone contact. Late failures are associated with plaque-induced inflammation and occlusal overloading. Early failures have been highly associated with hypertension, gastric problems, osteoporosis, diabetes type I and II, chemotherapy, and intake of medications. Heavy smoking should be considered a relative contraindication for immediate placement due to reduced peripheral blood circulation and proper tissue healing activation.

Local factors of the bone and soft tissue are important factors for implant success. Single tooth implants have high survival and low complications when compared with multiple implants. Bone quality and degree of resorption influences early and late outcomes. In addition, presence of buccal plate, thick soft tissue biotype, optimal implant position and sites influence a successful therapy.

B. Immediate implant placement introduces a high risk of esthetic complications. Because of this, proper diagnosis and augmentation for soft and hard tissues is frequently necessary. Several clinical studies have shown that the facial mucosa is the main complication observed with immediate implants. To achieve a correct mucosal level on the facial aspect the implant needs to be positioned in a coronal–apical direction and the mucosa must be supported by a buccal plate that has sufficient height and thickness. Papilla height is also another important factor, and this can be affected by many factors, including tooth extraction technique, incision placement, the timing of implant placement, and adjacent hard tissue, soft tissue, and tooth relationships. Thus, an array of biological and surgical concepts influence treatment outcomes.

C. Implant stability can now be evaluated by many tests, such as reverse torque, bone implant contact, micromobility, and resonance frequency analysis (i.e., implant stability quotient or ISQ). Ostell devices were developed in 1999 by Integration Diagnostics Ltd (Sweden). This method allows the assessment of implant stability by measuring implant oscillation frequency on the bone. The ISQ ranges from 0 to 100. Implants with an ISQ of 70–85 are considered very stable (loading is acceptable), 65–70 as moderately stable (one-stage approach), and 60–65 as minimally stable (two-stage approach). Osstell devices can be used to assess primary stability, follow-up stability after surgery, and diagnosing detrimental actions of overloading in the early stages. The ISQ has been to shown to provide a standard and predictable method to assess biological changes in the bone–implant relationship.

Torque is the rotational friction between the implant and the bone and is normally measured in newton centimeters. Insertion torque describes the cutting friction of the tip of the implant in the bone as well as the friction between the implant surface in the bone. Seating torque is measured when the implant is fully inserted, while reverse torque is used to test the friction between the implant and the surrounding bone, but it has the risk of negatively influencing osseointegration.

Case 4

Oclussal/Anatomical Considerations

CASE STORY

A 60-year-old female presented for dental implant therapy in the maxillary left quadrant (sites #11–#14) and mandibular right quadrant (sites #29–#31). She was also missing tooth #18. The patient had lost her teeth in those areas due to failed restorations more than 5 years ago. She did not wish to restore the edentulous site #18 for the time being. She reported episodes of grinding and currently had a night guard, which according to her was worn down and needed to be replaced. The patient presented with a recent panoramic radiograph (Figure 1).

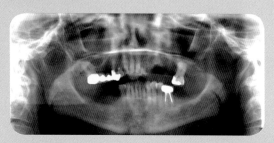

Figure 1: Initial panoramic radiograph.

LEARNING GOALS AND OBJECTIVES

- To determine the importance of a prosthetically driven implant placement and how it relates to the different anatomical landmarks
- To categorize and systematically analyze and evaluate the different anatomical landmarks
- To elucidate the pathologic conditions that may restrict implant placement
- To appreciate the importance of a team approach

Medical History

Not significant.

Social History

The patient did not smoke or drink alcohol at the time of treatment.

Extraoral Examination

No significant findings were noted. The patient did not have any masses, swellings, facial asymmetry, or lymphadenopathy. The temporomandibular joints (TMJs) were within normal limits.

Intraoral Clinical and Radiographic Examinations

See Figures 1, 2, 3, and 4.

- Class I maxillo-mandibular occlusal relationship, with normal vertical and horizontal bites.
- General assessment of TMJs within normal limits.
- Edentulous areas: #18, #11–#14, #29–#31.
- Residual alveolar ridge in the edentulous areas appeared atrophic.

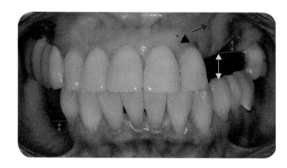

Figure 2: Frontal intraoral picture illustrating the reduced interocclusal distance for the maxillary left edentulous area (yellow double-headed arrow); buccal recession #10 (blue arrow); buccal frenum (red arrow); vertical bone loss (pink double-headed arrow). *Source*: image courtesy of Dr. Francesca Bonino.

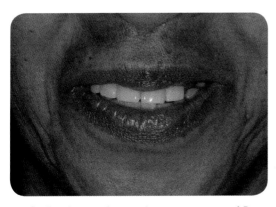

Figure 3: Smile picture. *Source*: image courtesy of Dr. Francesca Bonino.

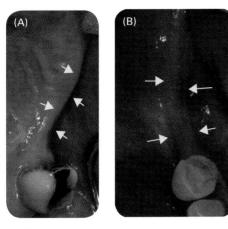

Figure 4: (A) Occlusal view of maxillary edentulous area illustrating atrophic residual alveolar ridge (arrows). (B) Occlusal view of mandibular site illustrating atrophic residual alveolar ridge (arrows). *Source*: images courtesy of Dr. Francesca Bonino.

- Soft tissue exam within normal limits.
- Low smile line.
- Periodontal examination revealed pocket depths in the range of 3–4 mm.
- Localized areas of gingivitis and a moderate oral hygiene were noted.
- The anterior teeth were triangular in form with a thin surrounding tissue biotype.
- A 2 mm buccal area of recession was noted on tooth #10.
- A 2.5 mm area of buccal recession was noted on tooth #28.
- Multiple restorations on existing teeth and periapical rarefying osteitis on tooth #19.
- Supra-eruption of tooth #15.
- The available mesiodistal space between #10 and #15 was 30 mm.
- The available space from distal of tooth #29 to the ascending mandibular ramus was 37 mm.

Implant Diagnosis and Treatment Plan

Upon evaluation of the patient's clinical and radiographic findings it was decided that the maxillary treatment plan should include placement of a single-unit implant retained crown in site #11 and an implant retained fixed partial denture (FPD) in sites #12–#14. The mandibular treatment plan should include placement of a three-unit FPD on implants #29–#31. A diagnostic wax-up of the desired size, anatomy, three-dimensional placement, and occlusion of the future restorations was done on the patient's mounted casts. A cone beam computed tomography (CBCT) scan was then performed with a radiographic stent in place (Figure 5) and the following detailed site analysis was completed. The radiographic stent was later converted into a stereolithographic surgical guide.

Detailed Site Analysis

Implant site analysis was performed intraorally, on mounted casts, and in CBCT images. Linear measurements were made using the CBCT measurement tool (Figure 6).

Site #11

- In the CBCT cross-sectional images, the density of trabeculae within cortical plates appeared within the range of normal. The density of trabeculae in cancellous bone appeared within the range of normal.
- In the CBCT cross-sectional images, the height of available alveolar ridge measured 19.68 mm and the width of the available ridge measured 4.08 mm.
- The apical area of tooth #10 was tipped distally, causing encroachment into the available space for dental implant #11 (red arrow, Figure 6A).
- The available bone height was limited by the floor of the nasal fossa or hard palate superiorly (Figure 6B).
- There was a pronounced labial concavity that would require careful angulation of the long axis of the implant to prevent perforation of the buccal cortical plate (yellow arrow, Figure 6A).

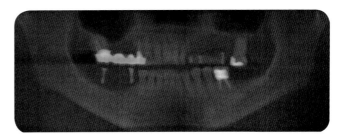

Figure 5: Reconstructed panoramic radiograph from CBCT with radiographic stent in place.

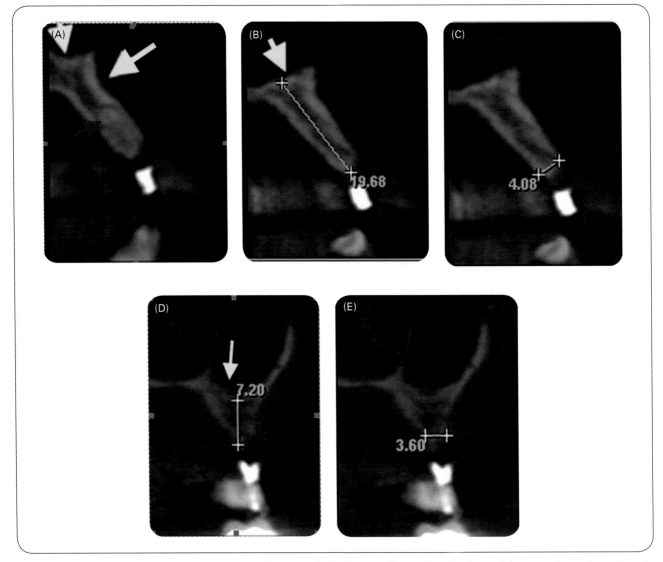

Figure 6: (A) Cross-sectional CBCT image showing the area of missing #11 illustrating the floor of the nasal fossa (arrowhead) and the labial concavity (yellow arrow) and the root of #10 (red arrow). (B) Cross-sectional CBCT image illustrating the height of available bone in area #11 limited superiorly by the floor of the nasal fossa (arrow). (C) Cross-sectional CBCT image illustrating the width of available bone in area #11. (D) Cross-sectional CBCT image illustrating the height of available bone in area #14 limited superiorly by the floor of left maxillary sinus (arrow). (E) Cross-sectional CBCT image illustrating the width of available bone in area #14.

- The available buccal keratinized soft tissue width was 4 mm.
- The available interocclusal space was 8.5 mm.

Site #12
- In CBCT cross-sectional images, the density of trabeculae within cortical plates appeared within the range of normal. The density of trabeculae in cancellous bone appeared within the range of normal.
- In CBCT cross-sectional images, the height of available alveolar ridge measured 18.01 mm and the width of the available ridge measured 2.34 mm; the ridge appeared narrow buccolingually due to atrophy.
- There was a low lateral frenulum attachment.
- Clinically, the available buccal keratinized soft tissue width measured 6 mm.
- Clinically, the available interocclusal space measured 8.0 mm.

Site #14
- In CBCT cross-sectional images, the density of trabeculae within cortical plates appeared reduced.

The density of trabeculae in cancellous bone appeared within the range of normal.
- The available bone height was limited by the floor of maxillary sinus superiorly (Figure 6D).
- In CBCT cross-sectional images, the height of available alveolar ridge measured 7.20 mm and the width of the available ridge measured 3.60 mm (Figure 6D and E).
- Mild soft tissue thickening was noted in the left maxillary sinus consistent with mucositis superior to the site of implant placement (Figure 6D and E).
- Clinically, the available buccal keratinized soft tissue width measured 4 mm.
- Clinically, the available Inter-occlusal space was 15 mm.

Site #29

- In CBCT cross-sectional images, the mental foramen was located approximately 6.50 mm distal and inferior to the marker.
- In CBCT cross-sectional images, the available bone height was limited inferiorly by the anterior extension of the inferior alveolar nerve (IAN) canal (Figure 7).
- In CBCT cross-sectional images, the available height of alveolar ridge measured 15.79 mm and the width of the available ridge measured 5.03 mm (Figure 7).
- Clinically, the available buccal keratinized soft tissue width measured 3.5 mm.
- Clinically, the available interocclusal space measured 10 mm.

Site #31

- The available bone height was limited inferiorly by the IAN (Figure 8).

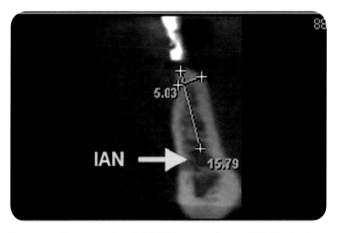

Figure 7: Cross-sectional CBCT image of area #29 illustrating the height of available bone above the IAN (red dot) and the width of available bone at the crest.

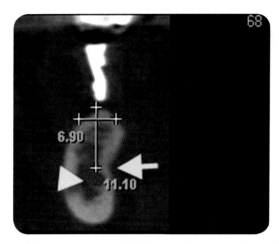

Figure 8: Cross-sectional CBCT image of area #31 illustrating the height of available bone above the IAN (red dot, arrowhead) and the width of available bone at the crest. The arrow indicates the submandibular salivary gland fossa.

- In CBCT cross-sectional images, the available height of alveolar ridge measured 11.10 mm and the width of the available ridge measured 6.90 mm.
- Clinically, the available buccal keratinized soft tissue width measured 3 mm.
- Clinically, the available interocclusal space measured 11.50 mm.

Treatment

The treatment for this patient was initiated with oral prophylaxis and oral hygiene instructions to reduce existing gingivitis.

Maxillary Arch

Owing to the limited buccolingual width in the edentulous area, it was decided to perform a hard tissue augmentation prior to implant placement (Figure 9). After the healing phase, one narrow and one regular-size implant was placed in sites #11 and #13 respectively, and a large-size implant was placed in site #14 with the guidance of the surgical stent (Figure 10). All implants were placed with a slight lingual orientation in order to allow for screw-retained restorations. Care was taken during the placement of implant #11 to avoid the distally tilted root of tooth #10. Owing to the patient's thin tissue biotype, the existing recession on tooth #10, and the low frenulum attachment in the area of #11 and #12, special care was taken to place the implants more lingually in order to maximize the amount of residual buccal plate and keratinized tissue. Both implants were also placed slightly deeper (approximately 3 mm apical to the CEJ of tooth #10) in order to avoid exposing the metal

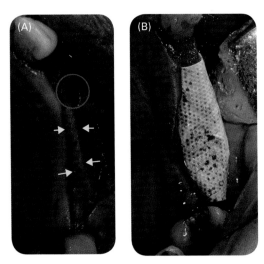

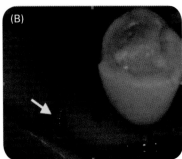

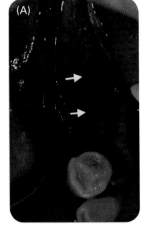

Figure 9: Intraoperative photographs illustrating (A) the maxillary residual ridge (arrows) and the labial concavity in the area of missing #11 (green circle) and (B) the ridge augmentation procedure for the maxillary site. *Source:* images courtesy of Dr. Francesca Bonino.

Figure 11: (A) Intraoperative view of the atrophic mandibular residual alveolar ridge (arrows). (B) Reflection of flap and exposure of mental foramen (arrow). *Source:* images courtesy of Dr. Francesca Bonino.

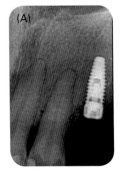

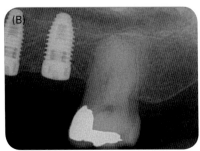

Figure 10: Periapical radiograph illustrating (A) the narrow-sized implant placed in area #11 and (B) the regular-sized implant placed in area #13 and large-sized implant placed in area #14.

occlusal surfaces of the restorations on #12–#14 were made in metal without porcelain coverage due to the patient's bruxing habit.

Mandibular Arch

A hard tissue augmentation was performed prior to implant placement of #29 and #30 (Figure 11), due to the reduced buccolingual width in the edentulous area of #29 and #30 (Figure 12). The flap was reflected to expose the mental foramen surgically, permitting its visualization (Figure 11B). After healing was established, with the guidance of the surgical stent a regular-size implant was placed in site #29 and a wide-size implant was placed in site #30 (Figure 13). Care was taken to place implants #19 and #30 in a parallel orientation to one another, to support the future FPD.

Both implants were placed so as to allow a screw-retained restoration. Following osseointegration, a temporary implant-retained FPD was fabricated to shape the peri-implant and pontic soft tissues to the desired level. After a couple of weeks of the temporary bridge in function, a three-unit FPD was delivered. Again, a metal occlusal surface of the FPD was suggested due to the patient's bruxing habit.

A new hard acrylic night guard was delivered to the patient at the end of the treatment.

Discussion

Placement of a short implant (<10 mm) instead of a standard-length implant would have eliminated the need

abutment margin during the final restoration. The patient's thin biotype makes her prone to that risk. An internal sinus lift was performed concomitantly with the implant placement of #14 in order to overcome the issue of limited bone height in that area. Care was taken to place implants #12 and #14 in a parallel orientation to one another, to support the future FPD.

Following osseointegration, temporary implant retained restorations were recommended in order to shape the peri-implant and pontic soft tissues to the desired level. After a couple of weeks of the temporaries in function, a single-unit porcelain-fused-to-metal crown was placed on #11, and a screw-retained three-unit FPD was placed on implants #12–#14. The

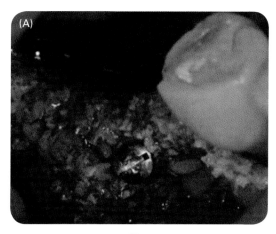

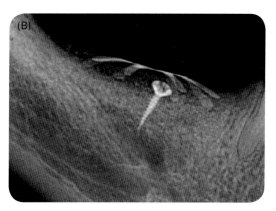

Figure 12: (A) Clinical photograph illustrating ridge augmentation procedure for mandibular site. *Source:* image courtesy of Dr. Francesca Bonino. (B) Postsurgical periapical radiograph illustrating the graft in place.

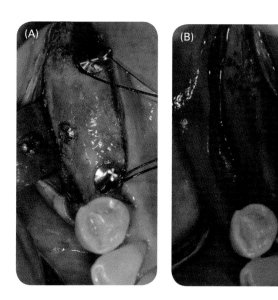

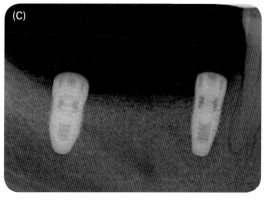

Figure 13: Clinical photographs illustrating (A) mandibular implants placements and (B) mandibular implant site healing. *Source:* images courtesy of Dr. Francesca Bonino. (C) Periapical radiograph illustrating mandibular implants in place.

for the internal sinus lift procedure. Research supports the use of short implants if prosthetic and occlusal considerations are respected [1].

Even though this patient had a low smile line, the thin tissue biotype placed her in a high-risk category for esthetic concerns [2,3]. Careful planning and placement of the anterior maxillary teeth (including the premolars) was crucial. If a soft tissue graft was necessary, the ideal timing would be during the temporary restorations stage. The temporary crowns would then be relined and reshaped to follow the new soft tissue contour and allow its maturation prior to the placement of the final restorations. To help categorize the difficulty level of a given treatment, in 1999 the Swiss Society of Oral Implantology proposed a system for classifying implant patients from a surgical and prosthetic standpoint. In the SAC classification system, S represents simple, A advanced, and C complex treatment procedures. In the surgical classification, all esthetic indications have been placed in either the A or C category, acknowledging the clinical challenges faced in the anterior maxilla and the frequent need for bone augmentation procedures [4].

Adjacent implant placement, such as areas 13 and 14 in the case presented herein, challenges the treatment team's ability to place dental implants in a position that allows for subgingival shoulder location and an ideal emergence profile while maximizing the osseous crest height and consequently papillary appearance [2].

Effective communication between the clinician and the patient is very important. After the evaluation of the clinical and radiographic findings, a separate consultation appointment is arranged to present the different treatment options to the patient along with the predictable treatment alternatives. This will help the patients understand the extent of the limitations and present them with the available options to reconstruct their mouth. In this way, treatment plans may be formulated to the patient's best advantage and will allow for treatment outcomes to be more predictable and successful [5].

Self-Study Questions

(Answers located at the end of the case)

A. What is the importance of a prosthetically driven implant placement and how does it relate to the different anatomical landmarks?

B. How can we categorize and systematically analyze and evaluate the different anatomical landmarks?

C. What pathologic conditions may restrict implant placement?

D. How important is a team approach?

References

1. Sun HL, Huang C, Wu YR, Shi B. Failure rates of short (≤10 mm) dental implants and factors influencing their failure: a systematic review. Int J Oral Maxillofac Implants 2011;26(4):816–25.
2. Buser D, Martin W, Belser UC. Optimizing esthetics for implant restorations in the anterior maxilla: anatomic and surgical considerations. Int J Oral Maxillofac Implants 2004;19:43–61.
3. Belser UC, Buser D, Higginbottom F. Consensus statements and recommended clinical procedures regarding esthetics in implant dentistry. Int J Oral Maxillofac Implants 2004;19:73–74.
4. Dawson, A., Stephen, C. The SAC Classification in Implant Dentistry. Quintessence; 2009.
5. Tatum Jr OH, Lebowitz MS. Anatomic considerations for dental implants. J Oral Implantol 1991;17(1):16–21.
6. Garber GA, Belser UC. Restoration driven implant placement with restoration generated site development. Compend Contin Educ Dent 1995;16:796–804.
7. Floyd P, Richard P, Barrett V. Treatment planning for implant restorations. Br Dent J 1999;187:297–305.
8. Lekholm U, Zarb GA. Patient selection and preparation. In: Brånemark PI, Zarb GA, Albrektsson T (eds), Tissue Integrated Prostheses: Osseointegration in Clinical Dentistry. Chicago, IL: Quintessence; 1985, pp 199–209.
9. Prasad DK, Shetty M, Mehra DR. Anatomical considerations in implant selection and positioning. Int J Oral Implantol Clin Res 2013;4(1):24–29.
10. Shah KC, Lum MG. Treatment planning for single tooth implant restoration: general considerations and the pretreatment evaluation. J Calif Dent Assoc 2008;36:827–834.
11. Blum IR, Smith GA. A quick and simple method to obtain a radiographic evaluation of remaining alveolar bone height before implant placement. Aust Dent J 2002;47:266–268.
12. Kois JC. Predictable single tooth peri-implant esthetics: five diagnostic keys. Compend Contin Educ Dent 2001;22:199–206.
13. Jung RE, Zembic A, Pjetursson BE, et al. Systematic review of the survival rate and the incidence of biological, technical, and aesthetic complications of single crowns on implants reported in longitudinal studies with a mean follow-up of 5 years. Clin Oral Implants Res 2012;23:2–21.
14. Misch CE. Contemporary Implant Dentistry, 3rd edn. St Louis: Mosby; 2010, pp 40, 130–146, 245–250, 280.
15. Isidor F. Influence of forces on peri-implant bone. Clin Oral Implants Res 2006;17:8–18.
16. Reiser GM, Bruno JF, Mahan PE, Larkin LH. The subepithelial connective tissue graft palatal donor site: anatomic considerations for surgeons. Int J Periodontics Restorative Dent 1996;16(2):130–137.
17. Sonick M, Abrahams J, Faiella R. A comparison of the accuracy of periapical, panoramic and computerized tomographic radiographs in locating the mandibular canal. Int J Oral Maxillofac Implants 1994;9:455–460.
18. Angelopoulos C, Thomas SL, Hechler S, et al. Comparison between digital panoramic radiography and cone-beam computed tomography for the identification of the mandibular canal as part of presurgical dental implant assessment. Int J Oral Maxillofac Implants 2008;66:2130–2135.
19. Tyndall DA, Price JB, Tetradis S, et al. Position statement of the American Academy of Oral and Maxillofacial Radiology on selection criteria for the use of radiology in dental implantology with emphasis on cone beam computed tomography. Oral Surg Oral Med Oral Pathol Oral Radiol 2012;113:817–826.

Answers to Self-Study Questions

A. The overall success of implant placement and restoration depends on careful patient selection and a comprehensive treatment plan. If the patient is indeed a candidate for implant therapy, a systematic protocol should be followed to assess the site-specific considerations. This chapter goes over some of the most frequently encountered anatomic structures that clinicians need to be attentive to when treatment planning an implant procedure.

Proper anatomic site evaluation along with restorative-driven planning will optimize final results. This involves a visualization of the emergence and position of the definitive implant-supported restoration. This is not only important for the planning of the ideal placement of the future implant, but can also aid in the diagnosis of hard and soft tissue deficiencies prior to implant placement

Articulated diagnostic casts will allow for the evaluation of the residual ridge, remaining dentition, existing occlusion, and available space in the edentulous site to receive the implant. The use of diagnostic wax-ups and templates for determination of anatomic comfort and danger zones is crucial in the initial planning process. This diagnostic wax-up will help with the determination of the number and position of the teeth to be replaced, implant location, angulation, relation to the remaining teeth, and the occlusal relationship with the opposing dentition. A resin template can be prepared from the finished diagnostic wax-up to serve as a radiographic and surgical template [6,7].

B. Identification and keeping clear of critical anatomical structures are key factors in the successful outcome and longevity of dental implants.

Anatomic structures to be taken into consideration with respect to implant placement can be classified into general and site-specific categories (Table 1).

Table 1: Classification of Anatomical Landmarks into General and Specific Categories

General	Site specific
Bone density	*Maxilla*
Mesiodistal interdental space	• Maxillary sinus/floor of maxillary sinus
Width of residual alveolar ridge	• Premaxilla–labial concavity
Height of residual alveolar ridge	• Floor of nasal fossa
Angulation of adjacent teeth	• Nasopalatine canal
Interocclusal space	• Palatine foramen and vessels
Occlusal forces	*Mandible*
Soft tissue biotype and smile analysis	• Inferior alveolar canal and mental foramen
	• Anterior extension of the inferior alveolar canal
	• Interforaminal area
	• Lingual canal
	• Submandibular salivary gland fossa
	• Sublingual fossa

General
• *Bone density.* This is a prime determinant in treatment planning, from implant design, to surgical approach, healing time, temporization, and loading protocol for the finalized restoration. Four types of mineralized bone have been described by Lekholm and Zarb based on its radiographic appearance and the resistance to drilling: type 1 bone, in which almost the entire bone is composed of homogenous compact bone; type 2 bone, in which a thick layer of compact bone surrounds a core of dense trabecular bone; type 3 bone, in which a thin layer of cortical bone surrounds a core of dense trabecular bone; and type 4 bone, characterized as a thin layer of cortical

bone surrounding a core of low-density trabecular bone of poor strength [8]. These differences in bone quality can be associated with different areas of anatomy in the upper and lower jaw. Mandible is generally more densely corticated than maxilla, and both jaws tend to decrease in their cortical thickness and increase in their trabecular porosity posteriorly.

A balance between the cortical and trabecular bone is desired. Too much cortical bone can delay osseointegration, while an excess of trabecular bone may limit the primary stability of the implants as well as its early stability in the bone [9].

- *Mesiodistal interdental space.* Adequate mesiodistal space must be present to provide a restoration that mimics natural tooth contours. It gives an indication of the number of implants that can be ideally placed. This has to be correlated with the buccolingual width of the bone, diagnostic wax-up of the future restoration, and the angulation of the crowns and ro ots of adjacent teeth (see later). Excesses or deficiencies in these areas must be previously addressed through the use of orthodontics, enameloplasty, or restorative materials prior to implant placement [5].

The following recommendations should be used when selecting implant size and evaluating mesiodistal space for implant placement [10]:
  ○ the implant should be at least 1.5 mm away from the adjacent teeth;
  ○ the implant should be at least 3 mm away from an adjacent implant.

Placement of the implant too close to the adjacent tooth can cause resorption of the interproximal alveolar crest to the level of that on the implant. With this loss of the interproximal crest height comes a reduction in the papillary height. This will also result in poor embrasure form and emergence profile, both of which will result in a restoration with a long contact zone and nonideal clinical results.

- *Width of residual alveolar ridge.* One of the first things to be assessed is buccolingual ridge anatomy, including whether there is sufficient crest width and the presence or absence of facial bone atrophy, and/or lingual undercuts. Deficient alveolar crest width and/or buccal

bone resorption require a bone augmentation procedure so that the implant can be positioned in an accurate buccolingual orientation. Presence of bony undercuts may cause perforation of the bone. Clinical bone mapping and different three-dimensional radiographic techniques, such as computed tomography and CBCT, can assist in diagnosing deficiencies in this dimension [11].

The minimum required residual bone width for stability of soft tissues following osteotomy and implant placement should be ≥1 mm. This is critical on the facial side since any bone resorption and ensuing change in the position of the gingival margin will be extremely unesthetic [3].

- *Height of residual alveolar ridge.* The apico-coronal dimension or height of the available bone is measured from the crest of the edentulous ridge to the anatomical landmarks that limit the placement of the implant. The assessment of implant length should allow adequate safety and distance from vital anatomic structures, particularly as many drills are designed to prepare the implant site slightly longer than the chosen implant. There should be at least 2 mm of bone between the apical end of the implant and neurovascular structures [5].

Patients with excess tissue height require attention as well. Bone present in excessive amounts is not a conducive clinical situation to place implants as it could create occlusal plane interferences in the completed restoration. In some cases, bone or soft tissue scalloping procedures will be required to allow placement of the implant shoulder in a position that ensures a harmonious gingival contour along with the adjacent teeth/ implants and result in a favorable crown/root ratio and appropriate occlusal scheme [9,12].

These landmarks can be outlined accurately in cross-sectional slices of CBCT to indicate the amount of available height of bone. Clinical situations with reduced vertical bone on adjacent teeth are challenging, because there are currently no surgical techniques available to predictably regain lost crest height. In an attempt to regain this lost tissue, orthodontic tooth extrusion techniques have been proposed [13,14]. In addition, short dental implants have shown predictable results when placed in a reduced ridge height, as long as occlusal forces are evenly distributed and lateral forces and parafunctions are controlled [1].

- *Angulation of adjacent teeth.* The inclination of the adjacent crown or root is a key parameter to avoid interference from a convergent structure during surgical placement. A panoramic or periapical radiograph can offer a basic clue to interroot space. Migration and tipping of teeth adjacent to an edentulous space will often compromise mesiodistal distance available for implant placement.

- *Interocclusal space.* This is the distance from the occlusal plane (posterior) or incisal edge (anterior) to the crest of the alveolar ridge of the arch in question This space will influence the type of prosthesis (cement or screw retained), material choices, and surgical technique that will be used.

  A satisfactory restorative outcome is obtained only if adequate crown height space is available. The ideal vertical dimensions of each region are 3 mm for the soft tissue, 5 mm for the abutment height, and 2 mm for the occlusal metal or porcelain. Screw-retained restorations generally require less crown height space compared with cement-retained prostheses, since they can screw directly onto the implant body [13].

  The consequences of inadequate crown height space include a decrease in abutment height, inadequate bulk of restorative material for strength, and esthetics, leading to prosthetic complications and poor hygiene conditions due to inadequate emergence profiles.

- *Occlusal forces.* Masticatory forces developed by a patient restored with implant-supported restorations are equivalent to those of natural dentition. Implants can tolerate much better axial loads as opposed to lateral forces [15]. Also, owing to the lack of proprioception that is found in the periodontal ligament surrounding natural teeth, implant-supported restorations are more susceptible to occlusal overloading than natural teeth are. Consequently, it is important to understand the factors contributing to the anticipated load on the implant. Patients with occlusal wear or abfraction-type defects due to clenching or bruxism should be identified since

the parafunctional habits will affect the long-term predictability of the implant [13].

- *Soft tissue analysis.* An evaluation of the soft tissue at the future implant site should determine the amount of attached keratinized tissue, thickness of the fibrous connective tissue, and the harmony or disharmony of the gingival scallop.

  Tissue biotypes are classified as thick and thin. Thick and keratinized tissue is more favorable, easier to manipulate, and provides a more predictable esthetic outcome, compared with thin tissue, which is more likely to go through recession [2]. A thin biotype with a highly scalloped gingival architecture is often linked with triangular teeth when compared with a thick biotype featuring blunted contours of the papillae, and is often associated with square and bold teeth [3].

  Characteristics of the soft tissue biotype will play a vital role in planning for final shoulder position of the implant.

  A patient with the combination of a high lip line and a thin biotype is extremely difficult to treat and should be considered an anatomic risk. Tissue deficiencies often require bone augmentation procedures such as the guided bone regeneration technique, which uses a simultaneous or staged approach to regenerate adequate volumes of bone to allow for implant placement.

Site specific
Maxilla

- *Maxillary sinus.* The amount of residual ridge available in the posterior maxilla for implant placement is limited by the floor of the maxillary sinus. Accurate identification of this structure and its extent on radiographs, including the locations of septae, is important in estimating the available bone volume to prevent iatrogenic perforation of the sinus floor. This has been found to be a potential cause for implant failure in the posterior maxilla [9]. When performing a sinus lift procedure one should also try to anticipate the location of the posterior superior alveolar artery, which can be visualized in a CBCT scan, to prevent unnecessary bleeding during implant placement.

- *Premaxilla.* This zone is also known as the traumatic zone/esthetic zone. It consists of the alveolar ridge of the premaxilla and eight anterior teeth: four incisors, two canines, and two first premolars. Implant therapy in the anterior maxilla is challenging for the clinician because of the esthetic demands of patients and difficult preexisting anatomy, such as development of labial concavity subsequent to tooth loss. This may lead to difficulty in implant placement in a prosthetically favorable position and may necessitate bone augmentation [5].

- *Floor of nasal fossa.* The amount of residual ridge available in the anterior maxilla for implant placement is limited by the floor of the nasal fossa. Accurate identification of this structure and its extent on radiographs is important in estimating the available bone volume to prevent iatrogenic perforation of the nasal floor. This has been found to be a potential cause for implant failure in the anterior maxilla.

- *Nasopalatine canal.* The location of the nasopalatine canal dictates the placement of a dental implant in the area of the maxillary central incisors. The nasopalatine canal contains the nasopalatine nerve, the descending branch of the nasopalatine artery, and fibrous connective tissue and is located in the middle of the palate, with the inferior end of the canal opening posterior to the maxillary central incisors. The knowledge and identification of the location of this canal is crucial to avoid perforating it. Any contact of dental implant with neural tissue could result in failure of osseointegration and may lead to prolonged neurological clinical signs and symptoms [10]. Limited volume CBCT imaging has been proposed to be of benefit to determine the location and morphology of the nasopalatine canal in all three planes before dental implant surgery.

- *Palatine foramen and vessels.* The area of greater and lesser palatine foramen is often a donor site for harvesting soft tissue grafts as this is the area where the thickest tissue may be found [16]. When harvesting the graft it is necessary to avoid the neurovascular bundle that enters the palate through these foramina. The location of the greater and lesser palatine foramen should be evaluated with respect to the proposed surgical site in CBCT images to avoid injury to the neurovascular bundle.

Mandible
- *Inferior alveolar (mandibular) canal (IAN) and mental foramen.* The most important anatomical consideration while placing an implant in the posterior is the location of the inferior alveolar canal, which contains the neurovascular bundles. Iatrogenic injury of the vital structures like the IAN and inferior alveolar artery can result in loss or alteration of sensation, pain, or excessive bleeding following implant placement.

  The IAN leaves the mandibular canal through the mental foramen in the buccal cortical plate as the mental nerve. Within the canal, the nerve is about 3 mm in diameter, and its course varies. It can run with a gentle curve toward the mental foramen, or it can have an ascending or descending pathway.

  Buccolingual location of the IAN can be classified into three types: type 1 canal (70% cases), located close to the lingual cortical plate of the mandibular ramus and body; type 2 canal (15%), located in the middle of the mandibular ramus posterior to the second molar; type 3 canal (15%), located near the middle of the ramus and body. The apico-coronal location of the mandibular canal has also been classified radiographically into high – within 2 mm of the apices of the first and second molars – intermediate, and low [5].

  Several methods are used to localize the IAN during treatment planning. These include traditional panoramic radiography, three-dimensional computed tomography or CBCT, and direct surgical exposure. The limitations and deficiencies of panoramic and periapical radiography for accurate location of the inferior alveolar canal and its variations are well documented in the literature [17,18].

  A *bifid IAN canal* has been reported to occur very infrequently. Despite the rare occurrence of the bifid IAN canal, the clinician must be on the lookout for these cases when planning for dental implants.

- *The anterior loop/extension of inferior alveolar canal.* The anterior loop refers to the anterior extension of the inferior alveolar nerve anterior to the mental foramen. Care must be taken to avoid this injury by careful identification in available images. If the anterior loop is not easily discernible on available images, then it is best to surgically visualize the area prior to placing a dental implant.

- *The lingual canal.* Located in the middle of the mandible, it carries neurovascular channels. This structure can be readily visualized in cross-sectional CBCT images of the midline area of mandible. Care must be taken to avoid perforation of the canal during implant placement, which may lead to neuropathic pain.
- *Interforaminal zone.* This zone comprises of the area of the anterior mandibular alveolar ridge between mental foramen on each side.
- *Submandibular salivary gland fossa.* Also known as the lingual concavity, the submandibular gland fossa is located below the mylohyoid ridge of the posterior mandible. The extent and morphology of the fossa may have variations that may restrict placement of dental implants with desired angulations. Assessment of this anatomy in three dimensions is crucial to avoid perforation of the dental implant through the gland leading to complications [19].
- *Sulingual fossa.* The sublingual fossa located on the lingual aspect of the anterior mandible also complicates instrumentation for implant placement by presenting as an extreme concavity. The concavity could result in lingual perforation during implant placement. Although undercuts can be palpated during an intraoral examination, the thickness of the soft tissue can mask the severity of the undercut. A CBCT scan can provide an accurate view of the lingual osseous architecture and help avoid dangerous hemorrhage in the presence of extreme sublingual undercuts [19].

C. In addition to assessment of restricting anatomical structures, the potential implant sites need to be assessed to rule out any disease that may compromise and complicate the outcome of the dental implant therapy. Commonly occurring local diseases, such as chronic odontogenic inflammatory lesions, may complicate healing of the surgical site. Local changes in normal bone architecture (as seen in fibro-osseous conditions like periapical cemento-osseous dysplasia, enostosis, or idiopathic osteosclerosis) and systemic conditions (such as osteoporosis) should be taken into consideration prior to implant placement. Thorough clinical assessment as well as assessment of all available radiographic images is necessary to rule out pathology. In the event of surgical removal of a pathologic lesion in a given implant site, care must be taken to initiate the process of implant placement after healing and remodeling of the surgical defect to ensure the availability of sufficient healthy bone for osseointegration with implants. Hard and/or soft tissue grafts may be required prior to successful implant placement in some of those cases.

D. In order to successfully meet the challenges of esthetic implant dentistry in daily practice, a team approach is beneficial and highly recommended. The team includes an implant surgeon, a restorative clinician, an oral and maxillofacial radiologist, and a dental technician. In special situations, an orthodontist can also supplement the team [13,14].

There is a learning curve associated with placing and restoring dental implants. The implant should be placed in an optimal position to effectively support its overlying prosthesis and surrounding soft and hard tissues, but also in a position that does not violate neighboring anatomic structures.

Case 5

Radiographic Interpretation and Diagnosis

Medical History

History of myocardial infarction 6 years ago with subsequent placement of stents, hypertension, hypothyroidism, and macrocytic anemia. The patient reported to be on metoprolol, aspirin, Lipitor, Diovan, Levoxyl, and B12 injections.

Review of Systems

• Vital signs
  ○ Blood pressure: 107/65 mmHg
  ○ Pulse rate: 53 beats/min
  ○ Respiration: 14 breaths/min

Social History

The patient did not drink alcohol and did not smoke.

Extraoral and Intraoral Examination

No significant findings, no swellings, lymphadenopathy, assymetries, ulcerations, or exophytic lesions were present.

Occlusion

No occlusal discrepancies or interferences present.

Radiographic Examination

A panoramic radiograph (Figure 1) was obtained for initial screening. The endodontically treated tooth #5 presented with radiographic signs indicating chronic periapical inflammation.

A preoperative cone beam computed tomography (CBCT) scan with a radiographic stent was prescribed after extraction and healing to assess the edentulous areas for prospective dental implants. The radiographic stent had markers in the regions corresponding to teeth #3 and #5. The findings in the CBCT scan included disuse alveolar atrophy in the edentulous

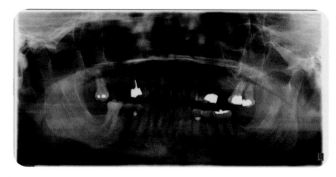

Figure 1: A panoramic radiograph for initial assessment of overall dentition and specifically edentulous areas in the right posterior maxilla.

region corresponding to the first molar. Figures 2, 3 and 4 present approximate height and width of available alveolar bone along with the edentulous saddle length for implant treatment planning. The floor of the maxillary sinus was intact. However, there was mucosal thickening, consistent with maxillary sinus mucositis. The morphology and quality of residual alveolar ridge (RAR) in area #3 could be described as Seibert class I and Lekholm and Zarb type IV. The morphology of the RAR in the edentulous region corresponding to the first premolar was within normal limits, and quality could be described as type II with a thick cortical outline surrounding a core of dense cancellous bone.

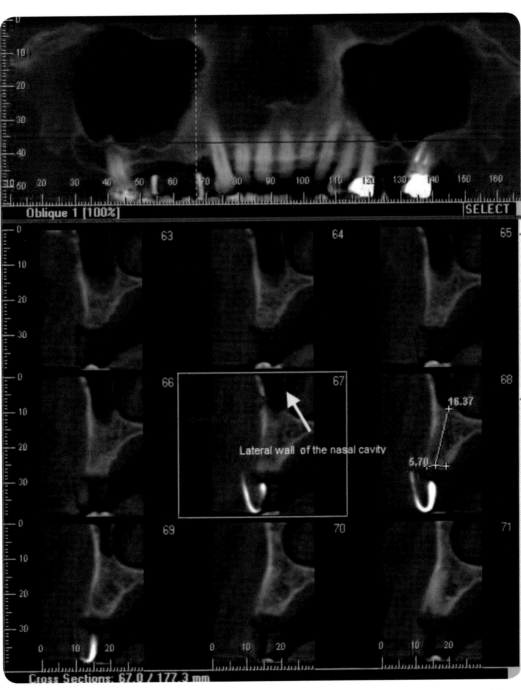

Figure 2: Cross-sectional and panoramic views from the preoperative CBCT scan of the maxilla with radiographic stent with a marker in edentulous area #5, showing cross-sectional morphology of the alveolar process, including width, height, and location of anatomic structures such as floor of the maxillary sinus and lateral wall of the nasal cavity.

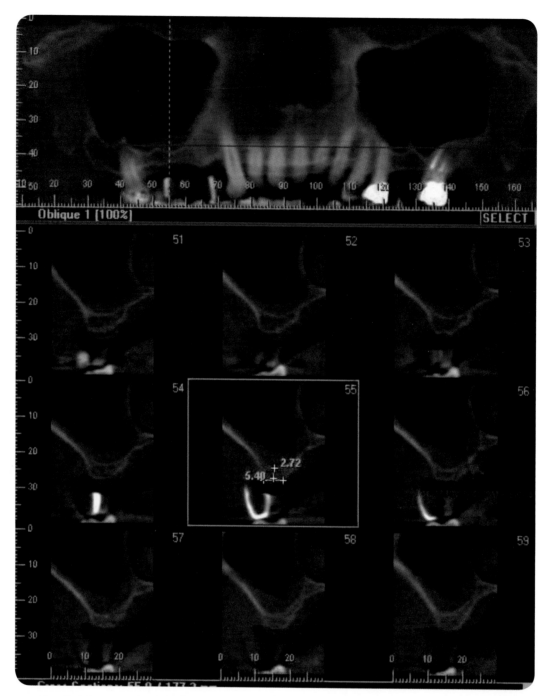

Figure 3: Cross-sectional and panoramic views from the preoperative CBCT scan of the maxilla with radiographic stent with a marker in edentulous area #3, showing cross-sectional morphology of the alveolar process, including width, height, and location of the floor of the maxillary sinus, along with maxillary sinus mucositis.

An external sinus lift procedure was done. A CBCT scan was obtained 2 months after the sinus lift procedure, for evaluation of the osseous graft in the region (Figure 5). This was followed by surgical placement of endosteal implant eight weeks later. A post-operative periapical radiograph (Figure 6) was taken after implant placement, that shows the location and oreintation of the implants in 2-dimension.

Radiographic Diagnosis

Diagnostic radiography is a critical aspect of implant therapy and can impact the outcomes of treatment. Today's sophisticated advanced imaging modalities make it possible to visualize and predict the final outcome of treatment in three dimensions. The aim of this case is to provide information on the imaging modalities for implant dentistry as it relates to the

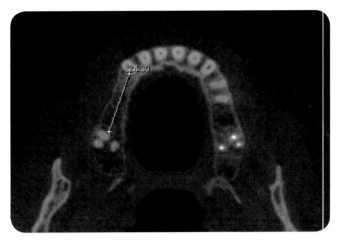

Figure 4: Axial image from the preoperative CBCT scan of the maxilla showing edentulous saddle length in the axial view.

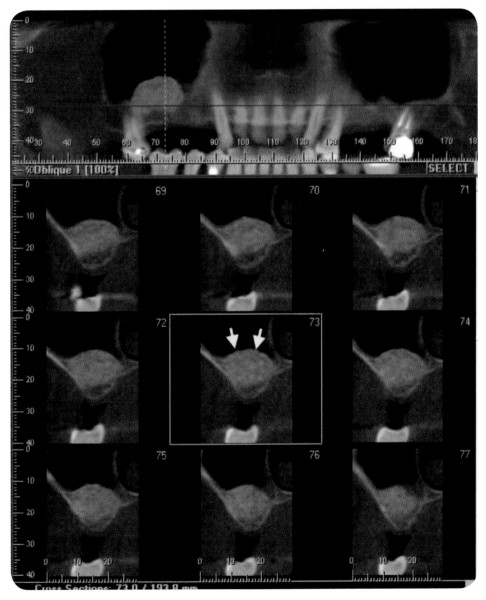

Figure 5: Cross-sectional and panoramic view from the CBCT scan taken after external sinus lift procedure showing the osseointegration of the osseous graft in the right posterior maxilla in edentulous area #3.

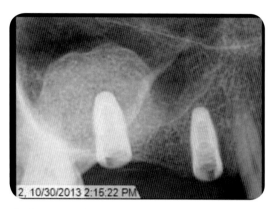

2, 10/30/2013 2:15:22 PM

Figure 6: Postoperative periapical radiograph showing the two endosseous implants in the right posterior maxilla.

presurgical, surgical, and restorative components of implant therapy. Basic principles of radiography, which also apply to imaging for implant evaluation, include:

- Appropriate training in imaging technique, including patient positioning, radiograph beam alignment, and receptor position to minimize distortion and improve precision and anatomic accuracy.
- The use of a radiographic stent with radiographic markers for implant sites during imaging.
- Imaging of the proposed implant site, including those areas that could be affected by implant placement.
- Diagnostic quality images with optimum density and contrast, free of artifacts.
- Competence in interpretation of the acquired images.

Imaging Modalities for Implant Diagnosis and Evaluation

1. Intraoral periapical radiography
2. Panoramic radiography
3. CBCT.

A good imaging protocol is critical to produce diagnostic quality images with the least amount of patient radiation dose. This is in alignment with the as low as reasonably achievable (ALARA) principle of radiation protection as per the recommendations of the National Council on Radiation Protection [1,2]. The main advantage of CBCT imaging over intraoral and panoramic radiography is that it provides three-dimensional data of the imaged volume. The range of effective doses for different CBCT devices is published to be between 52 and 1025 μSv depending on the CBCT equipment and the imaging protocol used. This range is equivalent to 4–77 digital panoramic

radiographs or 5–103 days of per capita background radiation dose in the USA. In comparison, conventional head computed tomography imparts a much larger radiation dose, with a dose range of 1400–2100 μSv [3]. When choosing a particular imaging protocol, the clinician must be aware of the effect of the technical parameters on image quality and patient dose. Reduction in patient radiation dose in CBCT imaging can be achieved by collimating the beam and using thyroid and cervical spine shielding.

Technical Parameters of Cone Beam Computed Tomography Imaging Protocol

Field of View

The ability to collimate the radiographic beam to fit the size of the region of interest (ROI) results in patient dose reduction along with improved image quality as a result of reduced scatter radiation. The dimensions of the scan volume are primarily dictated by the detector size, shape, beam projection geometry, and the ability to collimate the beam. The ROI should be the primary consideration when selecting the field of view (FOV). The beam may be collimated based on individual diagnostic needs and extend beyond the implant site and include the maxillary sinus or apposing arch. The smaller the FOV, the better the spatial resolution. A scout image taken prior to the acquisition of CBCT helps establish the accuracy of patient positioning within the FOV. This prevents unnecessary reexposure due to faulty positioning [4].

Voxel Size

The CBCT scan data is recorded and displayed as a matrix of individual blocks called voxels (volume elements). The smaller the FOV, the better the spatial resolution and smaller the voxel size. The factors controlling the voxel size in CBCT are radiographic tube focal spot size, radiographic beam projection geometry, and matrix/pixel size of the solid-state image detector [4].

Scan Time

It is desirable to reduce CBCT scan times to as short as possible to reduce motion artifacts due to patient movement. Metallic and beam hardening artifacts can result due to interaction of the radiographic beam with metallic hardware in the mouth, including dental restorations and implants. These artifacts are inherent to the technique and may obscure fine detail in the images [4].

Recommendations for Radiography for Implant Diagnosis and Management

Initial Examination

The purpose of the initial examination is the overall assessment of dentition and osseous structures, planning of location and type of proposed implant, and chronology of different treatment phases. Conventional imaging, such as periapical, bitewing, and panoramic radiographs, would be appropriate for initial examination.

Preoperative Site-Specific Imaging

CBCT is the imaging modality of choice for preoperative site specific assessment. Cross-sectional imaging is a critical component of implant site development especially when sinus augmentation or bone grafting is necessary [5]. The clinical advantage of utilizing CBCT for presurgical imaging can be enhanced by the use of a radiographic stent that will help relate the anatomic location of the proposed implant to surrounding anatomic structures. During imaging, the patient wears a radiographic stent, which is a clear acrylic stent with embedded radiopaque reference markers that indicate the proposed implant sites. This technique provides a precise reference of the location of the proposed implants. The best radiographic markers are nonmetallic, typically made of gutta-percha or composite resin to prevent metallic streaking artifacts. This radiographic stent could further serve as a surgical guide for the angulation of the implant placement. The preoperative site-specific imaging would aid in assessment of RAR characteristics, anatomic and pathologic considerations, and prosthetic considerations.

Residual Alveolar Ridge Characteristics

CBCT imaging allows the assessment of both quality and quantity of the RAR. These characteristics can be determined by vertical height, horizontal width, edentulous saddle length, and thickness and density of the cancellous and cortical bone. There are various methods that classify the quantity and quality of RAR. According to Seibert's classification [6,7], deficiency of RAR can be divided into three categories:
- class I, describing buccolingual loss of contour with normal apico-coronal ridge height;
- class II, describing apico-coronal loss of contour with normal bucco-lingual ridge width;
- class III, a combined loss in apico-coronal and buccolingual dimensions.

Lekholm and Zarb [8] described the quality of RAR as
- type I, homogenous cortical bone;
- type II, a thick layer of cortical bone surrounding a core of dense cancellous bone;
- type III, a thin layer of cortical bone surrounding a core of dense cancellous bone;
- type IV, a thin layer of cortical bone surrounding a core of low density cancellous bone.

A thorough assessment of all of these quality and quantity characteristics requires the use of cross-sectional images.

Anatomic and Pathologic Considerations

- Anatomic considerations in maxillary implant placement:
  - *Floor of the maxillary sinus and nasal cavity.* The available height of RAR for implant placement in the maxilla extends between the crest of the alveolar ridge and the floor of the maxillary sinus or nasal fossa. Assessment of the sinus and nasal cavity floor is necessary to prevent violation of these structures during implant placement or bone augmentation procedures.
  - *Nasopalatine canal and foramen.* This anatomic landmark is located in the maxillary midline. The morphology and course of the nasopalatine canal should be taken into consideration before placement of anterior maxillary implants. Violation of this structure may result in neurosensory loss, postoperative hemorrhage, or lack of osseointegration, leading to implant failure.
- Anatomic considerations in mandibular implant placement:
  - *Inferior alveolar nerve (IAN) canal and mental foramen.* The location and the course of the inferior alveolar canal are very critical for implant placement. There may be normal anatomic variations in the course of the nerve buccolingually, varying caliber or absence of distinct cortical boundaries that may negatively impact the outcome of implant therapy. Other common variations include extension of the nerve anteriorly, such as anterior loop, bifid IAN, or accessory foramen. The mental foramen is the opening of the IAN on the buccal mandibular cortical plate in the premolar region. Anatomic structures to avoid in the anterior mandible are the lingual foramen and lingual canal, in addition to larger caliber neurovascular channels.
  - *Submandibular and sublingual depressions.* These are concavities on the lingual aspect of the

mandible in the posterior and anterior mandible respectively. Improper angulation of the long axes of the implant may lead to perforation of the lingual cortical plate and result in injury to the salivary gland and vasculature.

○ *Labial concavity.* The anterior maxillary region, also known as the esthetic zone, may present with a labial concavity due to alveolar atrophy due to prolonged edentulism. This may require bone augmentation for successful treatment outcome with regard to esthetics and function. Improper vertical angulation of an implant may result in perforation of the buccal cortical plate.

Prosthetic Considerations

A prosthetically driven treatment plan in addition to anatomic and surgical considerations is essential to optimize final results of dental implant therapy. Articulated diagnostic casts are used to assess the residual ridge, remaining dentition, existing occlusion, and visualization of the ideal implant-supported restoration. A radiographic template prepared from this information is crucial for necessary modification of angulation of the proposed endosseous implant in order to allow subsequent functional loading of the prosthesis. Thus, cross-sectional imaging in the form of CBCT is vital in correlating the anatomical limitations and the desired angulation of an implant to the desired prosthetic outcome.

Intraoperative Imaging

Some instances may warrant imaging during the implant placement procedure, to either confirm correct placement of implant or to locate a lost implant. This can be achieved through intraoral or panoramic or CBCT imaging.

Postoperative Imaging

Postoperative imaging may be used to assess the bone–implant interface and the alveolar height around the implant. However, periodic imaging in asymptomatic patients is unnecessary. This may be achieved through periapical, panoramic, or CBCT imaging. One of the drawbacks of CBCT is the beam hardening and streaking artifacts due to metallic implant fixtures that may obscure subtle changes in the peri-implant bone. Panoramic and periapical radiography may prove beneficial in this regard. In case of clinically symptomatic implants, peri-implant radiographic changes, such as a radiolucency along the implant outline and crestal bone loss, may implicate a failing implant [9]. Clinical correlation would substantiate this diagnosis. Cross-sectional imaging may be necessary for planning retrieval of a failing implant.

Self-Study Questions

(Answers located at the end of the case)

A. What is the imaging modality of choice for evaluation of a single implant site in the region of tooth #25, prior to extraction of the tooth?

B. After extraction of tooth #25, a CBCT scan is prescribed for pre-implant site assessment. What are the technical considerations while planning the CBCT procedure?

C. What is the imaging modality of choice for evaluation of a complex implant case with multiple potential implant sites?

References

1. National Council on Radiation Protection and Measurements. Radiation protection in dentistry, NCRP report 145. Bethesda, MD: National Council on Radiation Protection and Measurements; 2003.
2. American Dental Association Council on Scientific Affairs. The use of dental radiographs: update and recommnedations. J Am Dent Assoc 2006;137:1304–1312.
3. Ludlow JB, Davies-Ludlow LE, Brooks SL, Howerton WB. Dosimetry of 3 CBCT devices for oral and maxillofacial radiology: CB Mercuray, New Tom 3G and i-CAT. Dentomaxillofac Radiol 2006;35:219–226.
4. Scarfe WC, Farman AG. Cone-beam computed tomography. In: White SC, Pharoah MJ (eds), Oral Radiology: Principles and Interpretation, 6th edn. Oxford: Mosby Elsevier; 2009, pp 225–243.
5. Tyndall DA, Price JB, Tetradis S, et al. Position statement of the American Academy of Oral and Maxillofacial Radiology on selection criteria for the use of radiology in dental implantology with emphasis on cone beam

computed tomography. Oral Surg Oral Med Oral Pathol Oral Radiol 2012;113:817–826.

6. Seibert J, Nyman S. Localized ridge augmentation in dogs; a pilot study using membranes and hydroxyapatite. J Periodontol 1990;61:157–165.

7. Seibert JS. Reconstruction of deformed, partially edentulous ridges, using full thickness onlay grafts. Part I. Technique and wound healing. Compend Contin Educ Dent 1983;4:437–453.

8. Lekholm U, Zarb GA. Patient selection and preparation. In: Brånemark P-I, Zarb GA, Albrektsson T (eds), Tissue-Integrated Prosthesis: Osseointegration in Clinical Dentistry. Chicago, IL: Quintessence; 1985, pp 199–209.

9. Benson BW, Shetty V. Dental implants. In: White SC, Pharoah MJ (eds), Oral Radiology: Principles and Interpretation, 6th edn. Oxford: Mosby Elsevier; 2009, pp 597–612.

Answers to Self-Study Questions

A. The best imaging modality for evaluating a single potential implant site, prior to extraction of the tooth is with a periapical or panoramic radiograph.

B. The best imaging modality of choice for pre-implant site assessment is CBCT with radiographic stent. For a single-site cross-sectional evaluation a smaller FOV and a smaller voxel size must be chosen that includes the ROI with regions just adjacent to the implant site and opposing tooth. This limited FOV scan is in compliance with the ALARA principle.

C. If imaging is required for evaluation of multiple potential implant sites, CBCT would be the imaging modality of choice. The vertical height of the FOV can be adjusted to include one jaw, both jaws, or a larger area including the temporomandibular joints.

2

Implant Design

Case 1

Regular Platform Implant Case

CASE STORY

A 33-year-old Caucasian male presented with a chief complaint of "I have an infection in my tooth, and I want a definitive solution. I don't want to be indented" (Figures 1, 2, and 3). Tooth #5 had a defective porcelain-fused-to-metal crown with an open margin (Figure 2). Radiographs showed extensive root caries lesion and periapical radiolucency (Figure 4). The patient visited his dentist regularly for uninterrupted dental care and reported that he brushed twice a day and flossed once a day.

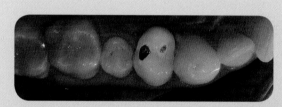

Figure 3: Pre-op presentation (occlusal view).

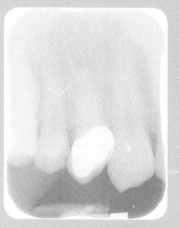

Figure 4: Pre-op presentation radiograph.

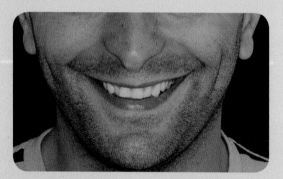

Figure 1: Pre-op presentation (extraoral view).

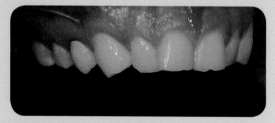

Figure 2: Pre-op presentation (intraoral view).

LEARNING GOALS AND OBJECTIVES

- To understand the concept of regular platform implants
- To understand when the use regular platform implants is recommended
- To understand the prosthodontic options for regular platform implants
- To understand loading protocols options for regular platform implants
- To understand the advantages of guided surgery

Medical History

At the time of treatment the patient presented no medical condition or known drug allergies.

Review of Systems

- Vital signs
  - Blood pressure: 115/75 mmHg
  - Pulse rate: 75 beats/min
  - Respiration: 16 breaths/min

Social History

The patient did not smoke or drink alcohol at the time of treatment.

Extraoral Examination

No significant findings were noted. The patient had no masses or swelling. The temporomandibular joint was within normal limits. There was no facial asymmetry noted and his lymph nodes were normal on palpation.

Intraoral Examination

- Oral cancer screening was negative.
- Soft tissue exam, including his tongue and floor of the mouth, were within normal limits.
- Periodontal examination revealed good plaque control (<20%) with no deep probing depths.
- Gingival biotype was thick [1].
- Mucogingival defect classified as Seibert class I [2] was noted at tooth #12.
- Minor mucogingival recession was noted at tooth #5.
- Medium smile line was displaying tooth #5 at smile.

Occlusion

There were no occlusal discrepancies or interferences noted.

Radiographic Examination

Radiographic examination revealed normal bone levels. Radiographs showed extensive root caries lesion and periapical radiolucency (Figure 4).

Diagnosis

The patient was diagnosed with extensive root caries lesion and chronic periapical periodontitis on tooth #5.

The presence of buccal cortical bone was radiographically assessed prior to the extraction of tooth #5 (FDI #14).

Treatment Plan

The treatment plan consisted of extraction and immediate implant placement with immediate loading if the primary stability was achieved.

Pretreatment

As an initial step, a radiological stent was fabricated on the master model from the plate provided by SICAT (SIRONA, Long Island City, NY, USA) (Figure 5). After obtaining the cone beam computed tomography (CBCT) scan, SICAT was further used for virtual analyses, assessment of implant position, and fabrication of the surgical stent (Figures 6 and 7). In order to fabricate an immediate screw-retained provisional crown, the implant analog was placed in the master model using the surgical stent (Figure 8).

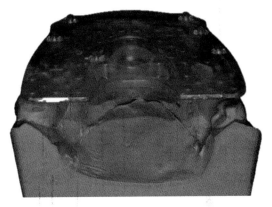

Figure 5: Plate for the fabrication of the surgical guide.

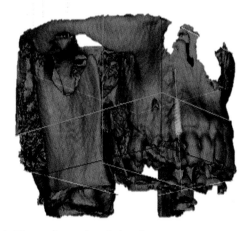

Figure 6: Three-dimensional planning.

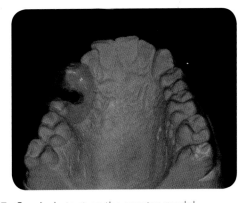

Figure 7: Surgical stent on the master model.

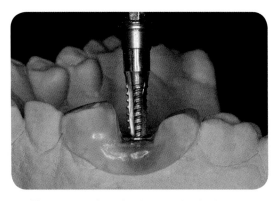

Figure 8: Placement of the implant analog in the master model using the surgical guide.

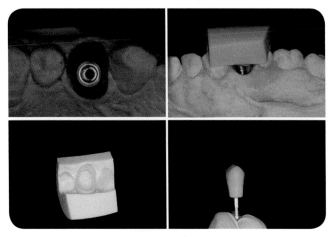

Figure 9: Fabrication of the provisional on the master model using the pick-up technique.

A provisional crown was fabricated using the conventional pick-up technique of the provisional abutment with an acrylic shell (Figure 9).

Treatment

After obtaining adequate anesthesia at the surgical site using local anesthetic, tooth #5 was extracted and the granulation tissue was removed (Figures 10 and 11). The flap was not raised, and the integrity of the buccal bone was verified. This was followed by the placement of the surgical stent. Drilling was done with increasing sequence of 2.35, 2.8, and 3.6 mm drills. The latest coincided with the implant body diameter (Figures 12 and 13). After completing the osteotomy the site was ready for implant placement. A 4.0 mm by 12 mm implant was placed (Figure 14) (Klockner Implant System, Andorra, Spain). Fully guided implant placement allowed the control of depth and direction of drilling as well as implant placement.

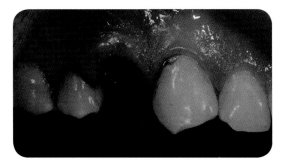

Figure 10: After extraction (vestibular view).

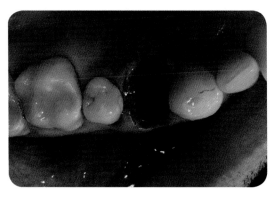

Figure 11: After extraction (occlusal view).

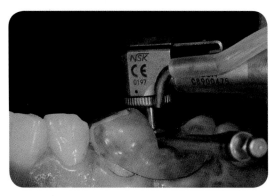

Figure 12: Preparation of implant site using surgical guide (vestibular view).

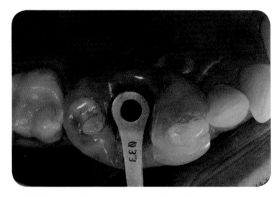

Figure 13: Preparation of implant site using surgical guide (occlusal view).

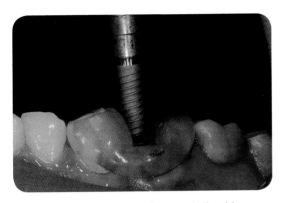

Figure 14: Implant placement using surgical guide.

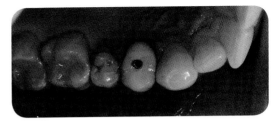

Figure 17: After surgery with implant and provisional crown in place (occlusal view).

Torque of insertion and implant stability quotient (ISQ) were measured as 45 N cm and 71 respectively. The measures are similar to the required minimum primary stability of 20–45 N cm torque of insertion and 60–65 ISQ [3].

A xenograft was carefully packed (Bio-Oss, Geistlich Biomaterials, Wolhusen, Switzerland) in the gap between the buccal plate of the bone and the implant (Figure 15). It was then that the screw-retained provisional crown was delivered and left out of occlusion (Figures 16, 17, and 18).

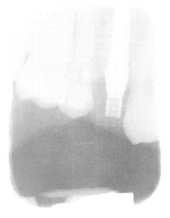

Figure 18: Periapical radiograph (PA) after the implant placement.

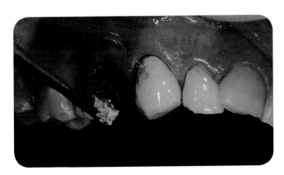

Figure 15: Application of the xenograft in the gap between the buccal bone and the implant.

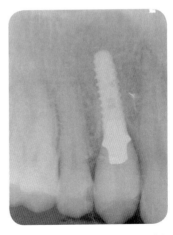

Figure 19: Periapical radiograph at 2 years of follow-up.

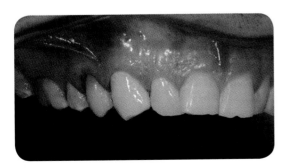

Figure 16: After surgery with implant and provisional crown in place (vestibular view).

Antibiotics (amoxicillin 1000 mg) were prescribed three times a day for 5 days.

The temporary restoration was further replaced with the permanent all-ceramic crown 12 weeks after the implant placement.

The clinical as well as radiographic two-year follow-up showed healthy soft tissue and excellent aesthetic outcome (Figures 19, 20, 21, and 22).

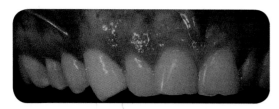

Figure 20: Intraoral view after 2 years of follow-up.

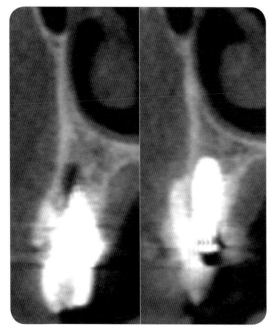

Figure 21: CBCT after 2 years displaying maintenance of buccal and palatal plates.

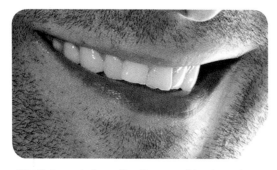

Figure 22: Extraoral view after 2 years of implant placement.

Discussion

In this clinical case, the etiology of insufficient biological width was open margin restoration. The treatment options were orthodontic extrusion or crown lengthening for achieving the desirable biological width. Biological width is defined as the natural seal that develops around teeth and/or dental implants and protects alveolar bone from bacterial invasion. It is the dimension of the soft tissue attached to the portion of the tooth coronal to the crest of the alveolar bone and is considered crucial in maintenance of periodontal health [4,5].

Alternatively, the tooth has to be extracted with two restorable options. The first option was a three-unit fixed partial denture with abutments on teeth #4 and #6 and pontic #5. The second option was an implant placement with single crown restoration.

Considering factors like treatment timeframe and preservation of healthy teeth, the patient selected the treatment option of implant placement with immediate provisionalization.

Restoring partial and/or complete edentulism using dental implants is a reliable treatment method and has become standard of care in the past couple of decades. Nevertheless, variations exist among implant types as well as loading protocols [3,6]. In general, the clinical situation dictates the technique of choice. Placement of a regular platform implant with immediate loading protocol was selected considering the existing bone volume, location of the defect, and esthetic demands. However, the protocol of immediate loading is not a standard of care in all cases, and it should be addressed cautiously even by experienced clinicians. Proper patient and site selection are important in order to increase the likelihood of the successful outcome [3,7]. Oral hygiene of the specific patient was optimal throughout the treatment, which was another well-thought-out factor.

In order to ensure precision of the implant, three-dimensional positioning surgery was conducted using a surgical guide.

Also, the ITI Consensus recommendation of simultaneous bone augmentation for immediate loading protocol was considered and a xenograft was carefully packed in the gap between the buccal plate of the bone and the implant [7].

Self-Study Questions

(Answers located at the end of the case)

A. What is a regular platform implant and when should it be used?

B. What is the minimum bone volume required around regular platform implants?

C. What is the recommended loading protocol for regular platform implants?

D. What is the platform switching technique?

E. What are the prosthetic possibilities for regular platform implants?

F. What is the advantage of using guided surgery?

References

1. De Rouck T, Eghbali R, Collys K, et al. The gingival biotype revisited: transparency of the periodontal probe through the gingival margin as a method to discriminate thin from thick gingiva. J Clin Periodontol 2009;36:428–433.
2. Seibert JS. Reconstruction of deformed, partially edentulous ridges, using full thickness onlay grafts. Part II. Prosthetic/periodontal interrelationships. Compend Contin Educ Dent 1983;4:549–562.
3. Gallucci GO, Benic GI, Eckert SE, et al. Consensus statements and clinical recommendations for implant loading protocols. Group 4 consensus statement. Int J Oral Maxillofac Implants 2014;29(Suppl):287–290.
4. Gargiulo AW, Wentz FM, Orban B. Dimensions and relations of the dentogingival junction in humans. J Periodontol 1961;32:261–267.
5. Nugala B, Kumar BS, Sahitya S, Krishna PM. Biologic width and its importance in periodontal and restorative dentistry. J Conserv Dent 2012;15:12–17.
6. Borie E, Orsi IA, De Araujo CP. The influence of the connection, length and diameter of an implant on bone biomechanics. Acta Odontol Scand 2015;73(5):321–329.
7. Weber HP, Morton D, Gallucci GO, et al. Consensus statements and recommended clinical procedures regarding loading protocols. Int J Oral Maxillofac Implants 2009;24(Suppl):180–183.
8. Pjetursson BE, Thoma D, Jung R, et al. A systematic review of the survival and complication rates of implant-supported fixed dental prostheses (FDPs) after a mean observation period of at least 5 years. Clin Oral Implants Res 2012;23(Suppl 6):22–38.
9. Schrott A, Riggi-Heiniger M, Maruo K, Gallucci, GO. Implant loading protocols for partially edentulous patients with extended edentulous sites – a systematic review and meta-analysis. Int J Oral Maxillofac Implants 2014;29(Suppl):239–255.
10. Degidi M, Piattelli A, Carinci F. Clinical outcome of narrow diameter implants: a retrospective study of 510 implants. J Periodontol 2008;79:49–54.
11. Coelho Goiato M, Pesqueira AA, Santos DM, et al. Photoelastic stress analysis in prosthetic implants of different diameters: mini, narrow, standard or wide. J Clin Diagn Res 2014;8:ZC86–ZC90.
12. Klein MO, Schiegnitz E, Al-Nawas B. Systematic review on success of narrow-diameter dental implants. Int J Oral Maxillofac Implants 2014;29(Suppl):43–54.
13. Sánchez-Pérez A, Moya-Villaescusa MJ, Jornet-Garcia A, Gomez S. Etiology, risk factors and management of implant fractures. Med Oral Patol Oral Cir Bucal 2010;15:e504–e508.
14. Ding X, Zhu XH, Liao SH, et al. Implant–bone interface stress distribution in immediately loaded implants of different diameters: a three-dimensional finite element analysis. J Prosthodont 2009;18:393–402.
15. Tarnow DP. Commentary: replacing missing teeth with dental implants: a century of progress. J Periodontol 2014;85:1475–1477.
16. Tarnow DP, Cho SC, Wallace SS. The effect of inter-implant distance on the height of inter-implant bone crest. J Periodontol 2000;71:546–549.
17. Schneider D, Grunder U, Ender A, et al. Volume gain and stability of peri-implant tissue following bone and soft tissue augmentation: 1-year results from a prospective cohort study. Clin Oral Implants Res 2011;22:28–37.
18. Schropp L, Wenzel A, Kostopoulos L, Karring T. Bone healing and soft tissue contour changes following single-tooth extraction: a clinical and radiographic 12-month prospective study. Int J Periodontics Restorative Dent 2003;23:313–323.
19. Romanos GE, Javed F. Platform switching minimises crestal bone loss around dental implants: truth or myth? J Oral Rehabil 2014;41:700–708.
20. Sailer I, Muhlemann S, Zwahlen M, et al. Cemented and screw-retained implant reconstructions: a systematic review of the survival and complication rates. Clin Oral Implants Res 2012;23(Suppl 6):163–201.
21. Wöhrle PS. Predictably replacing maxillary incisors with implants using 3-D planning and guided implant surgery. Compend Contin Educ Dent 2014;35:758–768.
22. Vercruyssen M, Hultin M, Van Assche N, et al. Guided surgery: accuracy and efficacy. Periodontol 2000;66:228–246.

Answers to Self-Study Questions

A. Implant dentistry is an expanding field that has been a subject of distinguished research interest for several decades and its achievements have greatly influenced modern techniques for restoring complete and/or partial edentulism. Currently, implant restorations are an accepted and well-documented treatment option [8,9]. Nevertheless, variations exist in shape, surface, connection, diameter, platform, and design of dental implants [6].

Implant diameter was pointed out as one of the implant-related factors influencing long-term clinical, radiological, and esthetic outcome [10], ensuring sufficient implant-to-bone contact. Based on the diameter, implants can be classified as narrow, regular and wide: <3.75 mm, <4 mm, and >4 mm respectively [11,12].

Regular-diameter implants have excellent long-term clinical results and scientifically supported treatment protocols. In other words, before the introduction of narrow- and wide-diameter implants, it was regular platform implants that were most commonly used [12]. The fracture of such implants is approximated to be as rare as 0.2% [13]. Another potential advantage of standard-diameter implants is more favorable stress distribution at the implant–bone interface. Specifically, it was shown that stress values rise significantly at the implant–bone interface when diameter is reduced from 4.1 mm to 3.3 mm. Nevertheless, the same trend could not be seen when the diameter was reduced from 4.8 mm to 4.1 mm [14].

The case presented featured restoration of a single tooth, with placement of an implant with two natural adjacent teeth. Regular implants should also be considered in the cases when multiple implants are to be placed in the posterior area. This allows keeping the minimum of 3 mm of bone between them at the implant–abutment level, the dimension that cannot always be achieved by the wide implants. Otherwise, if the two implants are not placed more than 3 mm apart the increased amount of interimplant crestal bone loss is expected [15]. Additionally, this can also influence the existence of the interimplant papilla, as there is positive correlation between the preservation of the crestal bone and existence of the papilla [16].

B. The choice of implant diameter depends on clinical variables, among which type of edentulism and available bone volume should be considered [10]. As a general guideline, at least 1 mm of bone is required around dental implants. Thus, while placing a regular platform implant, a minimum of 6–7 mm bone is required. Additionally, extra bone of 2 mm and 3 mm is necessary when an implant is placed next to a tooth or an implant respectively. This can be considered as one of the limitations of regular-diameter implants, as tooth extraction is frequently followed by bone resorption and loss of buccal bone, not leaving sufficient bone volume for placement of regular implants [15,17,18].

C. Loading protocols were defined as conventional, early, and immediate loading, when implants are loaded in 2 months after the placement, in the period between 1 week and 2 months, and earlier than 1 week respectively. There is good evidence to support all three loading protocols; however, conventional loading is still considered the only recommended protocol for all clinical situations. Nevertheless, there is a high level of comparative evidence to support the use of immediate loading of single-implant crowns. However, a minimal insertion torque in the range 20–45 N cm and a minimal ISQ of 60–65 are the prerequisites. Additionally, simultaneous bone augmentation is a recommended step for an immediate loading protocol. Overall, for the anterior region and premolars, immediate loading was assessed to be a predictable and reliable procedure. And still, owing to the inconclusive data regarding soft tissue aspects in immediately loaded implants, this protocol should be addressed cautiously even by experienced clinicians when restoring high esthetically demanding regions [3].

D. The concept of platform switching is based on the placement of a narrow-diameter abutment on a wider-diameter implant, which causes horizontal mismatch. The platform-switch technique was speculated to cause reduced peri-implant bone loss when compared with regular nonplatform-switched implants. However, controversial results have also been reported. Therefore, in the excellent review by Romanos and Javed, it was concluded that peri-implant bone loss is influenced by various factors, like cervical features of the implant design, implant positioning, prosthetic concept, bone volume, and micromotion of the implant–abutment interface. And thus, the solely platform-switching concept may not be considered as a factor defining peri-implant bone status [19].

E. In order to improve the clinical outcome of implant-supported restorations, research is ongoing to define better materials and techniques [8]. One of the actual research subjects is the fixation method between the implant and the reconstruction. Among the two major methods of fixation, screw retained or cemented, screw retained was mostly used for full-arch edentulous fixed restorations, while single-unit restorations were cemented. Cemented restorations might be easier to manipulate; however, they are surrounded with concerns like excess cement causing peri-implantitis and difficulty to remove in case of technical complications. Conversely, screw-retained reconstructions provide retrievability and better biological fit [20]. Nevertheless, three-dimensional implant positioning is more sensitive when dealing with screw-retained restorations, considering the suggestion of oral (nonvisible) positioning of the opening of the screw. Overall, cement-retained reconstructions are associated with biological complications like implant failure or marginal bone loss. In contrast, screw-retained restorations exhibit a higher rate of technical problems.

In single crown restorations both types of fixation could be applied. However, we selected screw-retained restoration, as this method offers retrievability and a better biological perspective that is crucial in the esthetic area.

F. Treatment planning can be achieved with the use of CBCT and three-dimensional software to achieve precision in implant positioning. Placement of implants using guided surgical templates is of high importance to follow the defined virtual implant position. Use of the surgical template is even more important when dealing with the limited space between adjacent teeth. Deviations in implant positioning can cause changes to bone stability and soft tissue outcome. Moreover, when a screw-retained restoration is planned, precision in implant placement is even more important. Use of guided surgery enables the surgeon to consider all the factors and take maximum advantage of available bone volume and space [20,21]. With guided surgery, not only the bone volume but also restorative parameters can be considered, allowing achievement of high esthetic and functional outcomes.

Overall, guided surgery transfers virtual digital planning to the surgical field [22]. The surgical guides can be prepared by computer-aided design and computer-aided manufacturing technologies as well as manually, using mechanical positioning devices and/or drilling machines.

Case 2

Wide-Diameter Implants

A 73-year-old male Caucasian patient presented for a consultation in regard to restorative options for replacing three missing posterior teeth in his lower right jaw. His chief complaint was: "I cannot chew well on the right side." He had lost an extended fixed dental prosthesis (FDP) in that quadrant after the distal abutment tooth (lower right second molar) had incurred a root fracture that required its extraction. The extraction of tooth #31 (FDI #47), which had included the removal of pontics #29 and #30 (FDI #45 and #46) from the fixed dental prosthesis, had been completed about 3 months prior to this consult. The patient followed a regular maintenance and recare schedule with his dentist and hygienist every 6 months.

LEARNING GOALS AND OBJECTIVES
- Understand what constitutes a wide-diameter implant
- Acknowledge the difference between the terms wide-diameter and wide-platform/wide-neck implant
- Recognize the advantages and disadvantages of wide-platform/wide-neck implants for molar replacement
- Review important criteria for implant selection in regard to diameter and platform

Medical History

The patient revealed a medical history of coronary bypass and aortal valve replacement surgery 5 years ago following a heart attack. He has recovered extremely well from these events, looks fit, and is not overweight. His blood pressure is controlled with ramipril (5 mg per day), an angiotensin-converting enzyme. He also takes 20 mg of Crestor daily to control hyperlipidemia, 50 mg of metoprolol (a beta blocker) daily, and two baby aspirins per day (162 mg). He is required to premedicate prior to any dental procedures (2 g of amoxicillin 1 h prior to each appointment).

Review of Systems

- Vital statistics
  - Average blood pressure: 128/80 mmHg
  - Average respiration rate: 17 breaths/min
  - Average pulse rate: 72 beats/min

Social History

The patient is a semi-retired academic and hospital physician, who has some dental insurance coverage. He has no history of smoking or use of tobacco-containing products. He drinks alcohol socially on occasion. He undertakes walks every day as part of his personal wellness program.

Extraoral Examination

The extraoral examination did not reveal any significant findings. No masses or lesions were noted, and his facial symmetry was normal, as were his lymph nodes of the head and neck. No discomfort, clicking, or crepitus were detected during temporomandibular joint function. Range of motion was not limited, and the palpation of the muscles of the head and neck showed no signs of soreness or tenderness.

Intraoral Examination

Inspection and, where applicable, palpation of the floor of the mouth, tongue, cheek, palate, and oropharynx were within normal limits, and no masses or lesions were noted. Salivary flow was normal as well.

Except for tooth #12 (FDI #24), which had been replaced with a four-unit FDP supported by teeth #11 (FDI #23), #13 (FDI #25), and #14 (FDI #26) many years ago, all maxillary teeth were present, including the third molars. The four incisors had intact proximal and/or labial composite restorations. All other maxillary teeth were restored either with porcelain-fused-to-metal, full-gold crowns, or gold onlays. Except for tooth #14 (FDI #26), maxillary teeth were all vital.

In the mandible, missing teeth #18 (FDI #37), #29 (FDI #45), and #30 (FDI #46) had been replaced with FDPs over 15 years ago. Owing to the fracture of tooth #31 (FDI #47), which had required its extraction and, consequently, the removal of pontics #29 (FDI #45) and #30 (FDI #46), the patient presented to our office with an edentulous space from #29 to #31 (FDI #45 to #47). The extraction site #31 (FDI #47) was well healed, and the edentulous ridge in the area #29–#31 presented itself with an excellent bone volume covered with a healthy and wide band of keratinized mucosa. Tooth vitality testing was negative for teeth #17, #20, #21, #22, #27, and #28 (FDI #38, #35, #34, #33, #43, and #44).

Periodontal Examination

The patient practiced fair oral hygiene. Localized plaque was present on the lower incisors lingually as well as in the posterior areas along crown margins and interproximally, with localized supragingival calculus in the lower front (lingual) and the upper first molar regions (buccal). Full mouth periodontal charting revealed stable conditions for the age of the patient. None of the teeth exhibited probing depths greater than 3 mm, and only localized mild bleeding on probing was noted.

Occlusal Analysis

The molar and canine occlusal relationships were consistent with an Angle class 1. No occlusal discrepancies or interferences were noted. Lateral and anterior excursions occurred in group function with the posterior antagonists out of contact as the respective movements progressed.

Radiographic Examination

The patient brought copies of recent radiographs taken by his dentist with him, a panoramic image (Figure 1) and periapical radiographs of the lower right posterior area (Figure 2). Although the panoramic radiograph was of limited quality, it was considered sufficiently diagnostic for the purpose of the envisioned treatment. No pathologic changes or lesions were noted, and

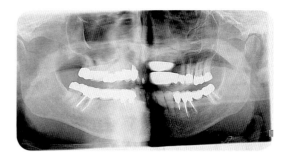

Figure 1: Pretreatment panoramic radiograph (provided by the patient).

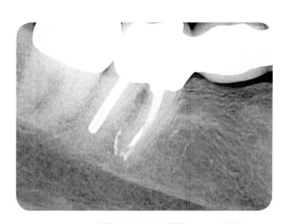

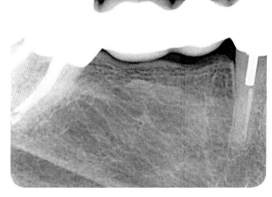

Figure 2: Periapical radiographs of area #29–#31 (FDI #45–#47) prior to the extraction of tooth #31 (radiographs provided by patient).

normal trabeculation of the jaws was present. Pneumatization of both maxillary sinuses was normal as well. Periodontal bone levels were at unreduced heights. The nonvital teeth #14, #17, #20, #21, #22, #27, and #28 (FDI #26, #38, #35, #34, #33, #43, and #44) showed successful root canal treatments and intact posts. No carious lesions were detected along the crown margins or elsewhere. Intact composite restorations were present on teeth #7 distal, #8 distal, and #10 mesial and buccal (FDI #12, #11, and #22). Radiographic views of the edentulous area of the lower right showed sufficient bone height for dental implants (Figure 2). The clinical examination of this area included bone sounding and palpation for lingual undercuts in the posterior mandible. Since the clinical examination of this area revealed excellent bone volume with a mucosal thickness of ~2 mm, as well as the absence of severe lingual undercuts, further radiographic studies, such as cone-beam tomograms, were not ordered.

Diagnosis

Partial edentulism in the mandibular right quadrant due to loss of an FDP abutment tooth after root fracture; localized mild to moderate gingivitis.

Treatment Plan

The treatment plan for this patient consisted of initial therapy that included oral prophylaxis and oral hygiene instructions to establish optimal oral conditions prior to implant treatment. The prosthodontic plan consisted of three cemented, single-unit implant restorations on tissue-level implants to replace the missing teeth. In site #29 (FDI #45), a regular neck implant was planned, and in sites #30 and #31 (FDI #46 and #47) two wide-neck implants were to be placed. The feasibility of the prosthodontic proposal was then assessed from the surgical point of view. The clinical and radiographic information confirmed the surgical feasibility of the plan. Implant length was determined from the periapical and panoramic radiographs. The distance from the top of the alveolar crest to the coronal border of the infra-alveolar nerve canal on the radiographs was 12 mm or greater. A 20% radiographic distortion factor was used to establish the safe implant lengths, which was 10 mm for each. The following implants were planned and ordered: for site #29 (FDI #45): one Straumann Standard Plus Regular Neck Implant, SLActive, diameter 4.1 mm, length 10 mm; for sites #30 and #31 (FDI #46 and #47): two Straumann Standard Plus Wide Neck Implants, SLActive, diameter 4.8 mm, length 10 mm (Straumann USA, Andover, MA).

Treatment

Surgical Treatment

Upon completion of initial phase therapy, presurgical treatment planning, and surgical stent fabrication, the patient presented for implant surgery. A course of antibiotics (2 g amoxicillin per os) was administered 1 h prior to implant surgery. Prior to administration of local anesthesia, the patient was instructed to perform an oral rinse with chlorhexidine gluconate 0.12% for 30 s. Anesthesia of the site was achieved via local infiltration

with 3.6 mL xylocaine 2%, 1:100,000 epinephrine. A mid-crestal incision was made extending from the distal surface of the first premolar to the mesial of the second molar with intrasulcular extensions to the mesiobuccal/mesiolingual aspects of the first premolar and the distobuccal/distolingual aspect of the second molar. A full-thickness flap was reflected and the three implants placed as planned and according to the manufacturer's specifications, leaving the smooth surface necks of the implants in a supracrestal position. Excellent primary stability was measured (≥35 N cm) for all three implants using the insertion torque device. Healing screws of 2 mm height were then placed on each implant and the flap closed around them using four interrupted silk 4-0 sutures leaving the implant healing screws in a nonsubmerged position. A postoperative panoramic radiograph was obtained to ensure that the implants were properly placed (Figure 3).

Postoperative Treatment

The patient was prescribed a 3-day regimen of amoxicillin 875 mg bid, ibuprofen 600 mg for pain as needed, and 0.12% chlorhexidine gluconate for twice-a-day mouth rinses for 30 s each time over a period of 1 week. The patient was scheduled for suture removal 1 week after implant placement. At that time, wound healing had progressed nicely and sutures were removed.

Prosthodontic Treatment

Eight weeks after implant placement, peri-implant tissue healing was excellent (Figure 4) and impressions for the final implant restorations were obtained. For that purpose, the healing screws were removed (Figure 5), and the closed-tray impression posts placed (synOcta RN for implant #29 and synOcta WN for implants #30 and #31; Straumann USA, Andover, MA). Shade selection was completed at this time as well (Figure 6).

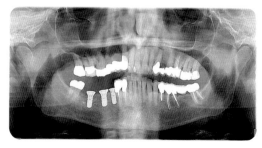

Figure 3: Postoperative panoramic radiograph after implant placement.

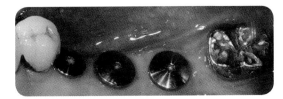

Figure 4: Healed peri-implant soft tissues 6 weeks after implant placement.

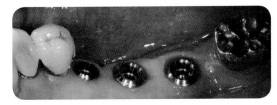

Figure 5: Implants after removal of healing screws: Regular-neck implant in site #29 (FDI #45), Wide-neck implants in sites #30 and #31 (FDI #46, and #47) (Straumann USA, Andover MA).

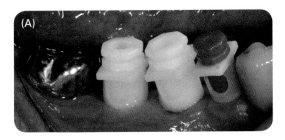

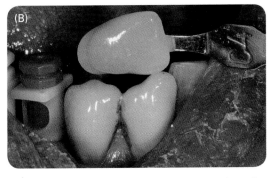

Figure 6: (A) Closed-tray impression copings and synOcta positioning cylinders for regular-neck implant #29 (FDI #45) and wide-neck implants #30 and #31 (FDI #46 and #47) (Straumann USA, Andover, MA) placed onto the implants. (B) Shade selection with Vita shade tab (Vita, Stein-Säckingen, Germany).

SynOcta cementable abutments were placed on the analogs in the master cast and slightly reduced in height to allow for sufficient interocclusal space to accommodate the necessary thickness of the restorative material (at least 1.5 mm) (Figure 7). Pressed lithium disilicate crowns (e.max pressed, Ivoclar

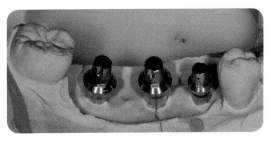

Figure 7: SynOcta abutments for cemented restorations placed onto the implant analogs on the master cast: regular neck type for implant #29 (FDI #45); wide neck types for implants #30 and #31 (FDI #46 and #47) (Straumann USA, Andover, MA).

Vivadent, Schaan, Liechtenstein) were then fabricated (Figure 8). Abutments were first tried in (Figure 9), followed by the crowns (Figure 10). Adjustments to proximal and occlusal contacts were made as necessary and the adjusted areas polished chair side using ceramic polishers. All three abutments were then tightened to 35 N cm each using a manual torque driver (Straumann USA, Andover, MA). The abutment screw heads were covered with Teflon tape and the rest of the access holes closed with a soft composite (Fermit®, 3M Espe, St. Paul, MN). The e.max crowns were subsequently cemented with Temp-Bond NE (Kerr Corporation, Orange, CA) (Figure 11). A periapical radiograph after crown insertion confirmed proper seating of the crowns on the implants as well as the complete removal of excess cement (Figure 12).

Oral hygiene instructions were given to the patient, including regular brushing with a soft toothbrush and flossing. The patient was given a follow-up appointment 4 weeks after crown delivery and encouraged to continue his regular recall visits with his hygienist/dentist every 6 months.

While he canceled the 1-month follow-up visit because everything felt fine according to him, he subsequently followed annual follow-up visits in our office, at which clinical and radiographic findings were found to be within normal limits (Figure 13).

Discussion

A patient's dentition exhibiting unilateral posterior partial edentulism involving one premolar and two molars was restored with three implant-supported crowns. Implant selection was determined first on the basis of the prosthodontic plan. Two equally predictable options for the replacement of three adjacent teeth exist: single-unit restorations requiring the placement of three implants, or a fixed partial denture supported

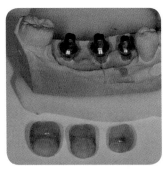
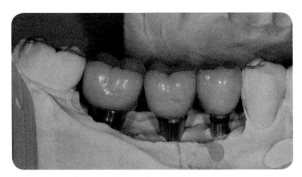
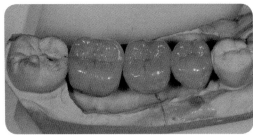
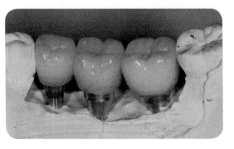

Figure 8: Cementable lithium disilicate crowns (e.max pressed; Ivoclar Vivadent, Schaan, Liechtenstein) on minimally customized synOcta titanium abutments for cemented restorations in various views; regular neck type for implant #29 (FDI #45); wide neck types for implants #30 and #31 (FDI #46 and #47) (Straumann USA, Andover, MA). Crowns made by Brendon Cornell, CDT, Boston, MA.

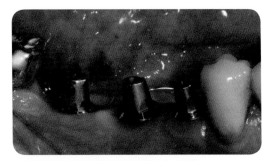

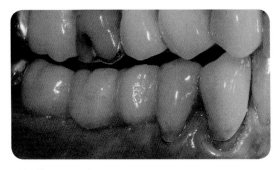

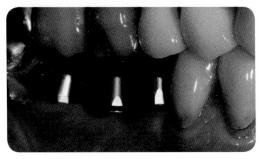

Figure 11: Cemented e.max crowns.

Figure 9: Intraoral abutment try-in.

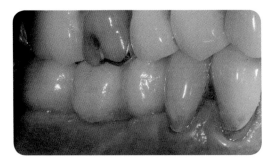

Figure 10: Crown try-in.

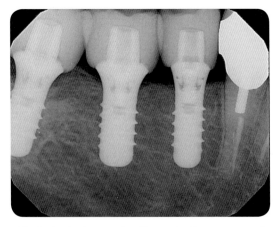

Figure 12: Periapical control radiograph after cementation.

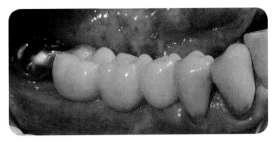 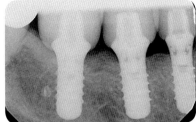

Figure 13: Clinical and radiographic documentation of 2-year follow-up condition.

by two implants [1]. The initial cost for the single-tooth alternative is higher. However, it tends to reduce the complexity and cost of managing a potential complication – biological, technical, or mechanical – later. The patient was informed about the advantages and disadvantages of both options and consented to the single-unit approach.

From a prosthodontic point of view, wide restorative platforms (wide necks) are desirable in molar areas to facilitate the design of favorable contours of molar restorations, while a regular platform is the usual choice for premolar replacements.

Tissue-level implants were chosen owing to their favorable biological and mechanical characteristics [2]. Tissue-level implants in the posterior region are usually placed in a one-stage surgical protocol, which reduces the number of surgical interventions, overall treatment time, and patient discomfort. The fact that wide-platform (wide-neck) implants were chosen meant that the endosseous portion of the implants had a diameter of 4.8 mm (wide diameter). Feasibility of placing wide diameter implants in sites #30 and #31 (FDI #46 and #47), and a standard-diameter implant in site #29 (FDI #45) was assured via conventional radiographs in combination with careful local clinical examination that included bone sounding of the area and palpation of possible lingual undercuts in that portion of the mandible.

An early loading protocol was chosen, which allowed the restorative phase to start 6 weeks after implant surgery, at which time bone and soft tissue healing had reached sufficient maturity for long-term predictable restoration. The safety and efficacy of an early loading protocol 6–8 weeks after implant placement compared with the conventional loading times after 3–6 months has been well documented in the literature [3,4].

Finally, prefabricated abutments for cemented restorations were used. The abutments were slightly customized at their coronal aspect by the dental technician to accommodate sufficient interocclusal space allowing for sufficient material thickness of the restoration. Whereas traditionally porcelain-fused-to-metal restorations would have been the primary choice, full ceramic restorations made of lithium disilicate or zirconia are being used more and more. Lithium disilicate has the advantage that it can be cemented with materials other than resin-based ones, including provisional cements such as zinc oxide non-eugenol as used in this case. Advantages are that cement excess can be easily removed, therefore minimizing the risk for biological complications. In the presence of sufficient accuracy of fit and retention of the crowns on the supporting abutments, restorations usually maintain their stability over time but can be removed by the dentist with relative ease to enhance retrievability.

Self-Study Questions

(Answers located at the end of the case)

A. What constitutes a wide-diameter implant and what is the difference between the terms wide diameter and wide platform/wide neck?

B. What are the indications or contraindications for using wide-platform/-neck implants?

C. What are the advantages of a one-stage, tissue-level implant design for posterior implant restorations?

D. What are advantages of single-unit versus splinted-implant prostheses?

References

1. Weber HP, Sukotjo C. Does the type of implant prosthesis affect outcomes in the partially edentulous patient? Int J Oral Maxillofac Implants 2007;22(Suppl):140–172.

2. Hermann JS, Buser D, Schenk RK, et al. Biologic width around titanium implants. A physiologically formed and stable dimension over time. Clin Oral Implants Res 2000;11(1):1–11.

3. Buser D, Janner SF, Wittneben JG, et al. 10-year survival and success rates of 511 titanium implants with a sandblasted and acid-etched surface: a retrospective study in 303 partially edentulous patients. Clin Implant Dent Relat Res 2012;14(6):839–851.

4. Gallucci GO, Benic GI, Eckert SE, et al. Consensus statements and clinical recommendations for implant loading protocols. Int J Oral Maxillofac Implants 2014;29(Suppl):287–290.

5. Brånemark PI, Zarb GA, Albrektsson T (eds). Tissue Integrated Prostheses. Chicago, IL: Quintessence Publishing; 1985.

6. Misch CE. Implant body size: a biological and esthetic rationale. In: Contemporary Implant Dentistry, 3rd edn. St Louis, MO: Mosby; 2007, pp 160–178.

7. Langer B, Langer L, Herrmann I, Jorneus L. The wide fixture: a solution for special bone and a rescue for the compromised implant. Part 1. Int J Oral Maxillofac Implants 1993;8:400–408.

8. Van Steenberghe D, Lekholm U, Bolender C, et al. Applicability of osseointegrated oral implants in the rehabilitation of partial edentulism: a prospective multicenter study on 558 fixtures. Int J Oral Maxillofac Implants 1990;5:272–282.

9. Davarpanah M, Martines H, Kebir M, et al. Wide-diameter implants: new concepts. Int J Periodontics Restorative Dent 2001;21:149–159.

10. Ivanoff CJ, Sennerby L, Lekholm G. Influence of mono- and bicortical anchorage on the integration of titanium implants. A study in the rabbit tibia. Int J Oral Maxillofac Surg 1996;25:229–235.

11. Ivanoff CJ, Sennerby L, Johansson C, et al. Influence of implant diameters on the integration of screw implants. An experimental study in rabbits. Int J Oral Maxillofac Surg 1997;26:141–148.

12. Balshi TJ, Wolfinger GJ. Two-implant supported single molar replacement: interdental space requirements and comparison to alternative options. Int J Periodontics Restorative Dent 1997;17:427–435.

13. Davarpanah M, Martinez H, Tecucianu JF, et al. Les implants de large diamètre. Résultats chirurgicaux à 2 ans. Implant 1995;1:289–300.

14. Anner R, Better H, Chaushu G. The clinical effectiveness of 6 mm diameter implants. J Periodontol 2005;76:1013–1015.

15. Ivanoff CJ, Grondahl K, Sennerby L, et al. Influence of variations in implant diameters: a 3- to 5-year retrospective clinical report. Int J Oral Maxillofac Implants 1999;14:173–180.

16. Attard NJ, Zarb GA. Implant prosthodontics management of partially edentulous patients missing posterior teeth: the Toronto experience. J Prosthet Dent 2003;89:352–359.

17. The Academy of Prosthodontics. The glossary of prosthodontic terms. J Prosthet Dent 2005;94(1):10–92.

18. Faucher RR, Bryant RA. Bilateral fixed splints. Int J Periodontics Restorative Dent 1983;3(5):8–37.

19. Grossmann Y, Sadan A. The prosthodontic concept of crown-to-root ratio: a review of the literature. J Prosthet Dent 2005;93:559–562.

20. Gross M, Laufer BZ. Splinting osseointegrated implants and natural teeth in rehabilitation of partially edentulous patients. Part I: laboratory and clinical studies. J Oral Rehabil 1997;24:863–870.

21. Grossmann Y, Finger IM, Block MS. Indications for splinting implant restorations. J Oral Maxillofac Surg 2005;63(11):1642–1652.

22. Weinberg LA. Reduction of implant loading using a modified centric occlusal anatomy. Int J Prosthodont 1998;11:55–69.

23. Brunski JB, Puleo DA, Nanci A. Biomaterials and biomechanics of oral and maxillofacial implants: current status and future developments. Int J Oral Maxillofac Implants 2000;15(1):15–46.

24. Isidor F. Loss of osseointegration caused by occlusal load of oral implants. A clinical and radiographic study in monkeys. Clin Oral Implants Res 1996;7:143–152.

25. Isidor F. Influence of forces on peri-implant bone. Clin Oral Implants Res 2006;17:8–18.

26. Leung KCM, Chow TW, Wat YP. Peri-implant bone loss: management of a patient. Int J Oral Maxillofac Implants 2001;16:273–277.

27. Guichet DL, Yoshinobu D, Caputo AA. Effect of splinting and interproximal contact tightness on load transfer by implant restorations. J Prosthet Dent 2002;87:528–535.

28. Wang TM, Leu LJ, Wang J, Lin LD. Effects of prosthesis materials and prosthesis splinting on peri-implant bone stress around implants in poor-quality bone: a numeric analysis. Int J Oral Maxillofac Implants 2002;17:231–237.

29. Huang HL, Huang JS, Ko CC, et al. Effects of splinted prosthesis supported a wide implant or two implants: a three-dimensional finite element analysis. Clin Oral Implants Res 2005;16(4):466–472.

Answers to Self-Study Questions

A. Over several decades, implants have gradually increased in width, from being less than 2 mm, such as those of Scialom in the 1960s, to being 3.75 mm when first introduced by Brånemark [5]. Implants of 4 mm diameter were also introduced as "back-up" implants at that time. In the late 1990s, implants with diameters of 5 mm and greater started to be produced, primarily with the intent to increase bony anchorage and mechanical strength for the support of molar restorations. The consensus today is to consider implants of 3.75–4.1 mm as the regular (standard) implant diameter, and implants with ≥5 mm width as wide-diameter implants. This refers to the diameter of the intraosseous portion of the implant [6].

The terms "wide-platform" or "wide-neck" implant refer to the restorative platform, which in one-stage (tissue-level) implants is an integral part of the implant body and is not supposed to be modified, whereas in two-part (bone-level-type) implants the restorative platform is created by the implant abutment, which can be customized.

B. Wide-diameter implants were developed based on the basic concepts of osseous integration, since anchorage surface is essential for better primary stabilization, the indication for the use of wide-diameter implants is as follows: (1) poor bone quality, (2) inadequate bone height, and (3) immediate replacement of non-osseointegrated fixtures or fractured fixtures [7]. Another indication for using wide-diameter implants is for the immediate placement of an implant after the extraction of a tooth. Because the diameters of many teeth or roots are larger than 4 mm, a wide-diameter implant will engage the extraction socket walls better and, therefore, increase primary stability. In the case of one-piece tissue-level implants, they can also enhance the design of a desirable emergence profile of the crown because of having a cervical diameter that is closer to that of the molar to be replaced and subsequently being more esthetic.

Widening the diameter of implant has been suggested to improve the biomechanical performance of implant-supported molar restorations. Studies reported that using wider implants could decrease the percentage of failures [8,9] and increase primary stability in the presence of low-density bone. Also, the diameter of the body of the implant more easily permits bicortical (buccal/lingual) stabilization in the molar region, especially above the inferior alveolar nerve, where bicortical anchorage cannot be accomplished [10,11].

It has been stipulated that using implants with larger diameters will not only increase implant stiffness, but also bone-to-implant contact surfaces, and lead to better engagement of the cortical bone [7,12]. Use of wide-diameter implants can also improve the ability of posterior implants to better tolerate the occlusal forces and create a wider platform for proper prosthesis design.

Nevertheless, the use of wide-diameter implants should be limited to situations with sufficient buccolingual dimension [9]. In fact, too large an implant may reduce the cortical support, especially around the neck of the implant, and consequently jeopardize the primary stability of the implant. The use of a wide implant may be considered if the width of the alveolar crest is equal to or greater than 8 mm [13]. A biological impediment to the use of wide-diameter implants can be a lower blood supply because of minimum existing cancellous bone [14]. Higher failure rates for wide implants were found in clinical reports [15,16] that were mainly associated with operators' learning curves, poor bone density, implant designs and site preparation, and the use of this diameter as a "rescue' implant" [15].

C. The design of a tissue-level implant includes a transmucosal, machined (smooth) supracrestal portion as an integral part of the implant. This means that any connection of a suprastructure unit (crown, custom abutment) is located coronal to the bone level unless the implant is sunk deeper into the crestal bone (e.g., for esthetic reasons). Therefore, potentially negative mechanical or biological factors causing inflammatory tissue responses due to a submucosal connection or microgap between implant and suprastructure are kept close to the soft tissue margin and are thus minimized. It has been clearly shown that a one-piece implant design without any interfering gaps in the transmucosal region facilitates the formation of a soft tissue interface that is as similar to a natural tooth as can be expected around a dental implant [2]. This type of implant design is ideal for one-stage implant placement. The fluted design of the neck portion with an internal abutment connection enhances the mechanical properties of the implant–abutment complex. Combined with the use of prefabricated abutments for cemented restorations, it represents the most straightforward and most cost-effective way of replacing a missing tooth with an implant restoration.

D. According to "The glossary of prosthodontic terms," splinting is defined as "the joining of two or more teeth into a rigid unit by means of fixed or removable restorations or devices" [17]. Splinting has long been considered as a crucial component of occlusal therapy to control the amount of forces delivered to teeth and to reduced periodontia by providing an increased positional and functional stability for the entire unit [18]. One classical clinical indication for splinting was increased crown-to-root ratio [19]. However, evidence-based data to support such an indication are largely missing for teeth, and even more so for implants [20,21], and the parameters in specific clinical situations that lead to biomechanically advantageous conditions after splinting implants are unclear [21].

Implant restorations have been splinted with fixed prostheses for reasons other than those for splinting teeth. Splinting provides stability to mobile teeth, whereas implants are nonmobile. Therefore, when nonaxial or horizontal forces are applied on an implant, the implant is unable to move immediately away from the force as it does not pivot as a tooth; instead, the forces are concentrated at the implant–abutment junction and the crest of the supporting bone [22,23]. Overload leads to stress that may cause mechanical failure of the prosthetic components and bone microfractures that could ultimately lead to implant loss [24–26]. Hence, the purposes of splinting implant crowns

are to favorably distribute the applied forces between the implants involved, to minimize the forces on the implant–abutment interfaces, and to minimize the risk of excessive horizontal loads to the bone–implant interface.

A photoelastic study showed that splinted restorations shared the occlusal loads and distributed the stresses more evenly between the implants when eccentric force was applied [27]. A three-dimensional finite-element model study – in which the effect of prosthesis splinting on peri-implant bone stress around implants in poor-quality bone was evaluated – conveyed that splinting the crowns of adjacent implants with relatively rigid restorative materials reduced the peri-implant bone stress under horizontal load, leading to the recommendation to splint implants surrounded by poor-quality bone [28]. The advantage of load sharing by the splinted prosthetic crowns is not absolute. This is notable when the supporting implants of the two crowns have a significant difference in biomechanics, such as using the standard implant in the premolar region and the wide or two implants in the molar region [29]. In addition, in cases where there is steep anterior guidance – such as in cases with a deep overbite, a reduced number of natural occlusal stops, implant restorations including canines or in patients with parafunctional habits – splinting of anterior implants will be advantageous. Moreover, the resistance and retention forms of the definitive implant-supported fixed prosthesis are other parameters to consider when evaluating the need for splinting.

It is imperative to remember that splinted restorations must not jeopardize the patient's ability to maintain proper oral hygiene. When fabricating a splinted restoration, the laboratory technician needs to design interproximal spaces and embrasures that allow easy access to these areas with hygiene devices such as superfloss, floss threaders, or interproximal brushes. In this context, nonsplinted restorations offer a major advantage in that they allow the patient to maintain optimal oral hygiene with a simple flossing technique, as on natural teeth. Recommended conditions for splinting implant restorations are listed in Table 1.

Table 1: Guidelines for Splinting Implant Restorations

Implants should be splinted	Splinting not required
Reduced number of natural occlusal stops	Multiple natural occlusal stops
Steep anterior guidance	Shallow anterior guidance
Parafunctional oral habits	Normal occlusal forces
Off-axis, angled implants	Well-oriented implants
Implants arranged around an arch	Implants arranged in a line
Implant restoration includes the canine	Implant restoration does not include the canine
Edentulous maxilla	Edentulous mandible with implants in bilateral posterior regions
Compromised retention and resistance forms of prosthetic components	Adequate retention and retention and resistance forms of prosthetic components

Source: [21].

Case 3

Special Surfaces

CASE STORY
A 60-year-old Caucasian female presented with a chief complaint of "My front tooth is infected." The patient noticed a draining fistula on the buccal fold of the maxillary right central incisor (tooth #8). There was no evidence of caries or unresolved restorative problems. She claimed to brush twice daily but only floss occasionally.

LEARNING GOALS AND OBJECTIVES
- To understand the characteristics of the bone–implant interface
- To understand how implant surface modifications impact healing and osseointegration
- To understand the use of porous Trabecular Metal™ dental implants and the evidence for their success
- To understand the structure of Trabecular Metal material (TM) and the process of osseoincorporation

Medical History
There were no significant medical problems, and the patient had no known allergies. On questioning, the patient stated that she was taking nonsteroidal anti-inflammatory drugs and antibiotics (clindamycin) for treatment of the chronic infection on tooth #8.

Review of Systems
- Vital signs
  - Blood pressure: 115/75 mmHg
  - Pulse rate: 75 beats/min
  - Respiration: 20 breaths/min

Social History
The patient reported that she drank alcohol socially but did not smoke.

Extraoral Examination
There were no significant findings. Facial symmetry and lymph nodes appeared normal and the patient had no swelling or masses. The patient reported slight bilateral temporomandibular joint clicking while chewing, but denied any physical discomfort.

Intraoral Examination
- The soft tissues of the mouth, including the tongue, appeared to be normal.
- Gingival examination revealed a localized mild marginal erythema with rolled margins around tooth #8 (Figure 1).
- The dental exam revealed a restored dentition with an anterior open bite.

Radiographic Examination
A periapical radiograph of tooth #8 revealed severe bone loss secondary to failed root canal therapy. A cone

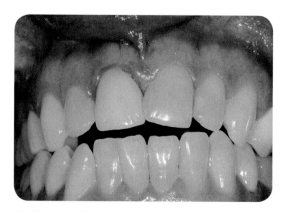

Figure 1: Preoperative presentation (facial view).

beam computed tomography (CBCT) scan confirmed the findings of severe bone loss, including the destruction of the buccal plate of tooth #8 (Figure 2).

Diagnosis

After reviewing the patient's health and dental histories, and data from the clinical and radiographic examinations, the clinical diagnosis was failed endodontic therapy on tooth #8 due to root fracture.

Treatment Plan

Based on the patient's medical and dental histories and present clinical situation, different treatment options were discussed. Since tooth #8 was nonrestorable and unresponsive to antibiotic therapy because of its fractured root, it would have to be extracted. The first treatment option was to attempt to preserve the existing ridge and soft tissue architecture by grafting the extraction socket and restoring the case with a fixed partial denture supported by the adjacent dentition (teeth #7 and #9). The second treatment option was to extract tooth #8 and immediately place a dental implant into the extraction socket. Because the implant would be placed in a prominent location within the esthetic zone of the anterior maxilla, an immediate, nonoccluding provisional restoration was planned if the implant achieved good primary stability at the time of placement. The patient did not want bone grafting or to compromise her adjacent healthy teeth to serve as abutment teeth with a pontic in the edentulous space, so she requested the second treatment option.

Because of inherent limitations in the volume and density of available bone in the anterior maxilla [1],

selection of an implant designed to augment bone fixation was indicated. A hybrid dental implant design (Trabecular Metal dental implant, Zimmer Dental Inc., Carlsbad, CA) consisting of a multithreaded titanium body with an unthreaded, highly porous, tantalum-based midsection was selected for the case. The TM (Zimmer TMT, Parsippany, NJ) in the midsection of the implant is a biomimetic scaffold that simulates the porous structure and elastic characteristics of trabecular bone [2]. The material has 75–80% interconnected porosity that is capable of achieving the development of new bone and vascular tissues inside the material [3], and the structure itself is textured at both the nanometer and micrometer levels to facilitate bone attachment [4]. TM has been extensively used since 1997 in orthopedic hip, knee, and spine implants, and more recently in the selected hybrid dental implant design [2,3,5,6].

Treatment

Phase 1: Surgery

The patient was orally sedated (Halicon 0.5 mg) and anesthesia was induced via local infiltration (lidocaine 2%, 1:100,000 epinephrine a total of 72 mg). Tooth #8 was gently extracted using an atraumatic technique to help preserve the bony walls of the alveolus (Figure 3). The socket was debrided to remove granulation tissues and infection from the socket. To preserve the architecture of the keratinzed gingiva, vestibular incisions were made and a mucoperiosteal flap was elevated to access and remove the periapical lesion (Figure 4). The extraction socket was prepared by sequential cutting with internally irrigated drills in graduated diameters and under copious external irrigation (Figures 5 and 6).

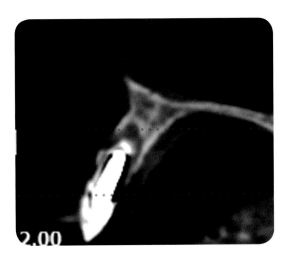

Figure 2: Preoperative CBCT scan.

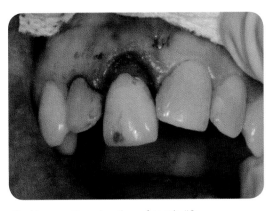

Figure 3: Atraumatic extraction of tooth #8.

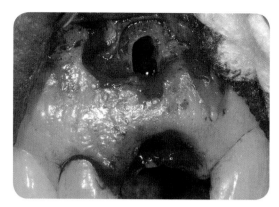

Figure 4: Elevation of a mucosal flap to access the periapical lesion.

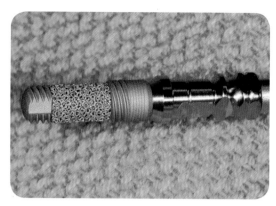

Figure 7: Trabecular Metal dental implant (4.1 mm × 13 mm).

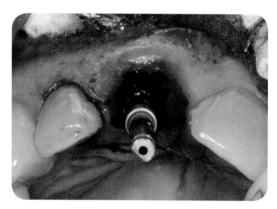

Figure 5: Palatal position of the osteotomy prepared in the extraction socket.

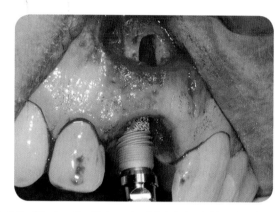

Figure 8: Placing the Trabecular Metal dental implant into the prepared extraction socket (#8).

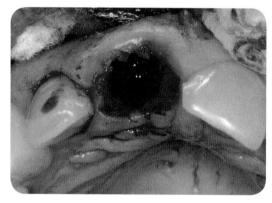

Figure 6: Completed osteotomy.

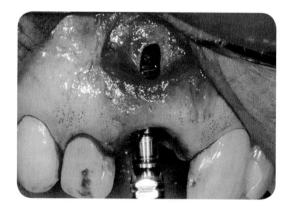

Figure 9: The fixture mount indicates the coronal–apical position of the Trabecular Metal dental implant after placement.

A Trabecular Metal dental implant (4.1 mm × 13 mm) was placed in a palatal position (Figures 7, 8 and 9). The implant achieved greater than 35 N cm of insertion torque, which indicated adequate primary stability for immediate loading based on a previous study [5] of this implant design. The fixture mount was removed and prepared for use as a temporary abutment (Figures 10 and 11). Voids created by the periapical lesion and the remaining portion of the extraction socket around the top of the implant were grafted with a mixture of mineralized allograft (Puros Cancellous Allograft, Zimmer Dental Inc.) and demineralized bone matrix (Puros DBM, Zimmer Dental Inc.) (Figures 12 and 13).

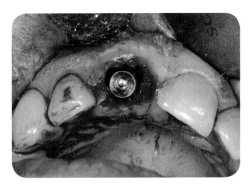

Figure 10: The buccolingual position of the implant is visible after removing the fixture mount.

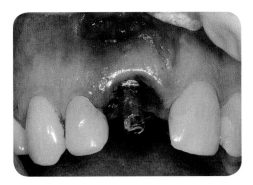

Figure 11: After preparations, the fixture mount is reattached to the implant for use as a provisional abutment.

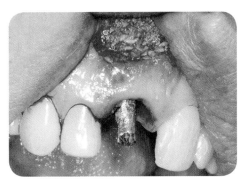

Figure 12: Periapical defect grafted with a combination of Puros mineralized bone allograft and Puros demineralized bone matrix.

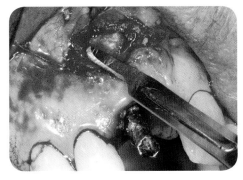

Figure 13: A collagen membrane was placed over the graft materials for guided bone regeneration.

The soft tissues of the mucosal flap were approximated and sutured using an Ethicon chromic gut 4-0 reverse cutting needle (Figure 14). A nonoccluding, acrylic provisional crown was fabricated with a screw access hole through the cingulum and cemented to the abutment with temporary cement (Figure 15). The screw access hole was occluded with a cotton pellet and sealed with autopolymerizing dental acrylic to prevent the ingress of oral bacteria. The patient was reappointed at 4 weeks. Sutures were removed and healing was proceeding without complications.

Phase 2: Definitive Restoration

Six weeks after the implant placement the patient saw the restorative dentist, who removed the provisional restoration and made a final implant-level impression (Figure 16). The provisional restoration was reattached to the implant and the patient was scheduled for delivery of the final restoration. A definitive, titanium patient-specific abutment (Zimmer Zfx® CAD/CAM abutment, Zimmer Dental Inc.) was digitally designed

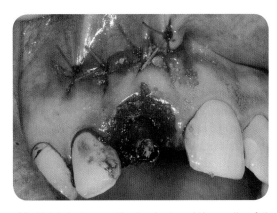

Figure 14: Voids between the implant and the walls of the socket were grafted with the same Puros allograft mixture.

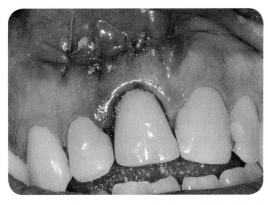

Figure 15: The implant was immediately provisionalized with a nonfunctional transitional prosthesis.

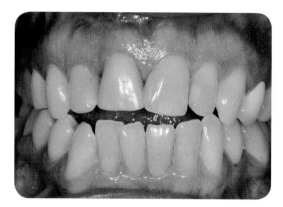

Figure 16: Postoperative presentation after 6 weeks of provisionalized healing.

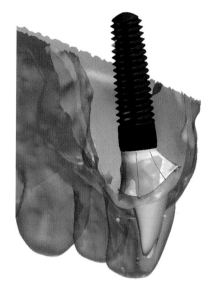

Figure 19: Digital abutment design: Zfx CAD planning to establish the optimal emergence profile.

and milled, and a definitive e.max crown was fabricated in a local dental laboratory (Figures 17, 18, 19, and 20). Twelve weeks after implant placement, the patient was reappointed by the restoring dentist. After removing the provisional restoration, the definitive abutment was attached to the implant and tightened to 32 N cm of applied torque. The definitive crown was cemented

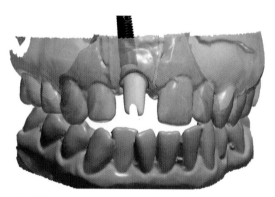

Figure 17: Digital abutment design: computer-aided design (CAD) with the Zfx system.

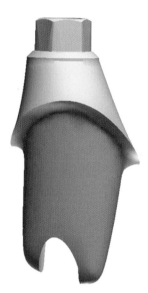

Figure 20: Digital abutment design: Zfx CAD planning of the final abutment design.

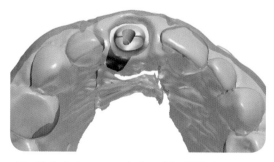

Figure 18: Digital abutment design: Zfx CAD planning of the abutment's buccolingual position.

to the custom abutment, final occlusal contacts were verified, and the patient was dismissed with oral hygiene instructions. The patient was reappointed for evaluation of oral function after 6 months of function, (Figures 21 and 22) and for evaluation and for routine oral hygiene prophylaxis 12 months after definitive restoration (Figures 23, 24, and 25).

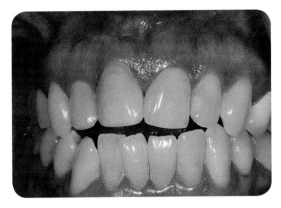

Figure 21: Presentation 6 months after final restoration.

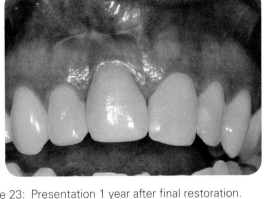

Figure 23: Presentation 1 year after final restoration.

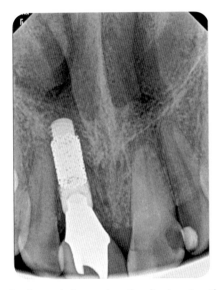

Figure 22: Radiograph 6 months after final restoration.

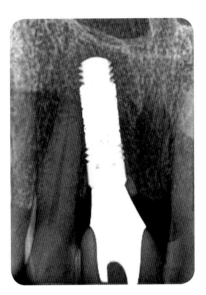

Figure 24: Periapical radiograph 1 year after final restoration.

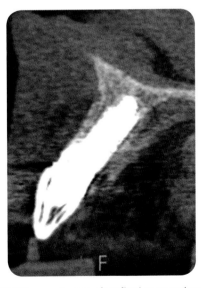

Figure 25: CBCT scan 1 year after final restoration shows
optimal implant trajectory and stable marginal bone levels.

Self-Study Questions

(Answers located at the end of the case)

A. What are the characteristic of the bone–implant surface?

B. What factors influence osseointegration?

C. What surface modifications can impact healing/osseointegration?

D. What new material was been used in this report and what is the evidence for its success?

E. What is the structure of TM and what is it designed to provide?

F. What is the current research and clinical data on TM?

References

1. Truhlar RS, Orenstein IH, Morris HF, Ochi S. Distribution of bone quality in patients receiving endosseous dental implants. J Oral Maxillofac Surg 1997;55(12 Suppl 5):38–45.
2. Bencharit S, Byrd WC, Altarawneh S, et al. (2013) Development and applications of porous tantalum Trabecular Metal-enhanced titanium dental implants. Clin Implant Dent Relat Res 2014;16(6):817–826.
3. Kim D-G, Huja SS, Tee BC, et al. Bone ingrowth and initial stability of titanium and porous tantalum dental implants: a pilot canine study. Implant Dent 2013;22(4):399–405.
4. Bobyn JD, Stackpool GJ, Hacking SA, et al. Characteristics of bone ingrowth and interface mechanics of a new porous tantalum biomaterial. J Bone Joint Surg Br 1999;81(5):907–914.
5. Schlee M, van der Schoor WP, van der Schoor ARM. Immediate loading of Trabecular Metal-enhanced titanium dental implants: interim results from an international proof-of-principle study. Clin Implant Dent Relat Res 2015;17(Suppl 1):e308–e320.
6. Schlee M, Pradies G, Mehmke W-U, et al. Prospective, multicenter evaluation of Trabecular Metal-enhanced titanium dental implants placed in routing dental practices: 1-year interim report from the development period (2010–2011). Clin Implant Dent Relat Res 2015;17(6):1141–1153.
7. Albrektsson T. Hard tissue implant interface. Aust Dent J 2008;53(Suppl 1):S34–S38.
8. Lian Z, Guan H, Ivanovski S, et al. Effect of bone to implant contact percentage on bone remodeling surrounding a dental implant. Int J Oral Maxillofac Surg 2010;39(7):690–698.
9. Brånemark P-I. Introduction to osseointegration. In: BrånemarkP-I, ZarbGA, AlbrektssonT (eds), Tissue-Integrated Prostheses, Osseointegration in Clinical Dentistry, 1st reprinting. Chicago, IL: Quintessence; 1985, pp 11–76.
10. Albrektsson T. Bone tissue response. In: BrånemarkP-I, ZarbGA, AlbrektssonT (eds), Tissue-Integrated Prostheses, Osseointegration in Clinical Dentistry, 1st reprinting. Chicago, IL: Quintessence; 1985, pp 129–143.
11. Vandamme K, Naert I, Sloten JV, et al. Effect of implant surface roughness and loading on peri-implant bone formation. J Periodontol 2008;79(1):150–157.
12. Hujoel P, Becker W, Becker B. Monitoring failure rates of commercial implant brands; substantial equivalence in question? Clin Oral Implants Res 2013;24(7):725–729.
13. Spector M. Historical review of porous-coated implants. J Arthroplasty 1987;2(2):163–177.
14. Lüthy H, Strub JR, Schärer P. Analysis of plasma flame-sprayed coatings on endosseous oral titanium implants exfoliated in man: preliminary results. Int J Oral Maxillofac Implants 1987;2(4):197–202.
15. Weiss MB, Rostoker W. Development of an endosseous dental implant (I). Quintessence Int Dent Dig 1977;8(9):87–91.
16. Weiss MB, Rostoker W. Development of a new endosseous dental implant. Part I: animal studies. J Prosthet Dent 1981;46(6):646–651.
17. Weiss MB, Rostoker W. Development of a new endosseous dental implant. Part II: human studies. J Prosthet Dent 1982;47(6):633–645.
18. Weiss MB. Titanium fiber-mesh metal implant. J Oral Implantol 1986;12(3):498–507.
19. Hacking SA, Bobyn JD, Toh KK, et al. Fibrous tissue ingrowth and attachment to porous tantalum. J Biomed Mater Res 2000;52(4):631–638.
20. Zardiackas LD, Parsell DE, Dillion LD, et al. Structure, metallurgy, and mechanical properties of a porous tantalum foam. J Biomed Mater Res 2001;58(2):180–187.
21. Wigfield C, Robertson J, Gill S, et al. Clinical experience with porous tantalum cervical interbody implants in a prospective randomized controlled trial. Br J Neurosurg 2003;17(5):418–425.
22. Nasser S, Poggie RA. Revision and salvage patellar arthroplasty using a porous tantalum implant. J Arthroplasty 2004;19(5):562–572.
23. Bobyn JD, Poggie RA, Krygier JJ, et al. Clinical validation of a structural porous tantalum biomaterial for adult reconstruction. J Bone Joint Surg Am 2004;86-A(Suppl 2):123–129.
24. Shimko DA, Shimko VF, Sander EA, et al. Effect of porosity on the fluid flow characteristics and mechanical properties of tantalum scaffolds. J Biomed Mater Res B Appl Biomater 2005;73(2):315–325.

25. Tsao AK, Roberson JR, Christie MJ, et al. Biomechanical and clinical evaluations of a porous tantalum implant for the treatment of early-stage osteonecrosis. J Bone Joint Surg Am 2005;87-A(Suppl 2):22–27.

26. Unger AS, Lewis RJ, Gruen T. Evaluation of a porous tantalum uncemented acetabular cup in revision total hip arthroplasty. Clinical and radiological results of 60 hips. J Arthroplasty 2005;20(8):100–1009.

27. Levine BR, Sporer S, Poggie RA, et al. Experimental and clinical performance of porous tantalum in orthopedic surgery. Biomaterials 2006;27(27):4671–4681.

28. Gruen TA, Poggie RA, Lewallen DF, et al. Radiographic evaluation of a monoblock acetabular component: a multicenter study with 2- to 5-year results. J Arthroplasty 2005;20(3):369–378.

29. Black J. Biological performance of tantalum. Clin Mater 1994;16(3):167–173.

30. Ring ME. A thousand years of dental implants: a definitive history – part 2. Compend Contin Educ Dent 1995;16(11):1132, 1134, 1136 passim.

31. Grenoble DE, Voss R. Analysis of five years of study of vitreous carbon endosseous implants in humans. Oral Implantol 1977;6(4):509–525.

32. Ulm C, Kneissel M, Schedle A, et al. Characteristic features of trabecular bone in edentulous maxillae. Clin Oral Implants Res 1999;10(6):459–467.

33. Ulm C, Tepper G, Blahout R, et al. Characteristic features of trabecular bone in edentulous mandibles. Clin Oral Implants Res 2009;20(6):594–600.

34. Froum SJ, Wallace SS, Cho S-C, et al. Histomorphometric comparison of a biphasic bone ceramic to anorganic bovine bone for sinus augmentation: 6- to 8-month postsurgical assessment of vital bone formation. A pilot study. Int J Periodontics Restorative Dent 2008;28(3):273–281.

35. Spinato S, Zaffe D, Felice P, et al. A Trabecular Metal implant 4 months after placement: clinical–histologic case report. Implant Dent 2014;23(1):3–7.

36. Frost HM. Bone's mechanostat: a 2003 update. Anat Rec A Discov Mol Cell Evol Biol 2003;275(2):1081–1101.

37. Misch CE, Suzuki JB, Misch-Dietsh FM, et al. A positive correlation between occlusal trauma and peri-implant bone loss: literature support. Implant Dent 2005;14(2):108–116.

38. Ormianer Z, Ben Amar Z, Duda M, et al. Stress and strain patterns of 1-piece and 2-piece implant systems in bone: a 3-dimensional finite element analysis. Implant Dent 2012;21(1):39–45.

39. Tagger Green N, Machtei EE, Horwitz J, et al. Fracture of dental implants: literature review and report of a case. Implant Dent 2002;11(2):137–143.

Answers to Self-Study Questions

A. Dental implant success is predicated on achieving mechanical stability at implant placement, followed by biologic stability over time through osseointegration. Direct bone to implant attachment is typically 50–80% of the surface, depending on the placement location, and soft tissue has been reported to always be present at the interface [7,8]. It is still unclear, however, if implants with greater bone-to-implant contact offer any greater stability [7]. At the ultrastructural level, mineralized bone has not been found to be in direct contact with the implant surface, but is linked by an interposing layer of dense, amorphous substance ranging from 20 to 500 nm in thickness, regardless of how long the implant has been in place [7]. Because the interposing layer is not present when there is a fibrous tissue interface with the implant, researchers theorized that the substance originates from organic bone matrix [7]. At the closest layer, proteoglycans with calcium deposits, occasionally in direct contact with the titanium, have been observed [7].

B. Implant surface characteristics and many other factors – such as the biocompatibility of the implant material, quality and quantity of available bone, loading conditions, and implant design – can influence the percentage and quality of achievable osseointegration [8–10]. Significant research over the last four decades has focused on increasing implant surface topography and chemistry with the goal of enhancing bone-to-implant contact [11]. While some surface modifications have shown promising results during short-term studies, there remains no clear evidence that they can provide any advantages for long-term implant survival or crestal bone maintenance compared with nontreated implant surfaces [12]. Consequently, porous surface coatings were first developed in orthopedics and later adopted by dentistry to strengthen implant fixation through bone growth into the pores of the coating [13] (Figure 26). However, all applied porous surface coatings offer limited porosity and irregular pore sizes for bone ingrowth [12], and are often

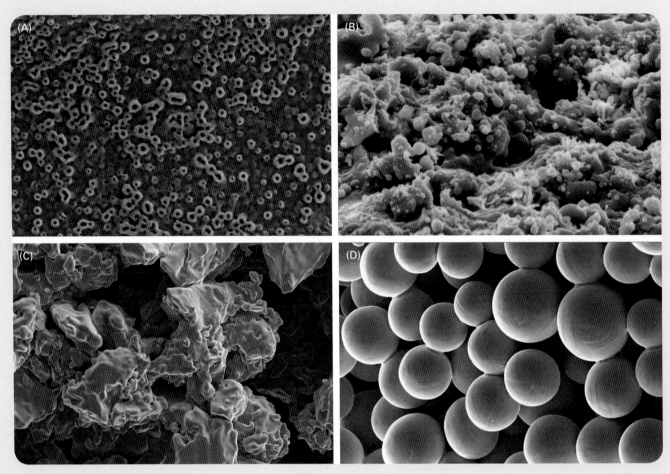

Figure 26: Examples of porous surface treatments include (A) anodization, (B) hydroxyapatite coating, (C) cancellous structured titanium coating, and (D) sintered bead coating.

prone to cracking, lamination, or dissolution in the biologic environment [14].

C. Several highly porous biomaterials were also developed for use in orthopedic and dental applications to overcome the shortcomings of porous coatings [15–18]. During the 1970s, researchers [15–18] introduced a titanium fiber mesh dental implant made of sintered, bent titanium wires. The material had at least 50% interconnected porosity and most pore channels were reportedly large enough for bone ingrowth [18]. Although the design achieved bone ingrowth between the wires and bone formation around the body of the implant, there was always a fibrous tissue interface between the bone and the metal of the implant [18]. This may have been attributable to the fact that the cylindrical implant design lacked external threads for stabilization and an adequate barrier to prevent epithelial downgrowth [18].

D. TM (Zimmer TMT), a biomimetic matrix that simulates the porous structure and elastic characteristics of trabecular bone, was developed by orthopedic researchers [19–28].

E. TM (Zimmer TMT) is fabricated by coating a vitreous carbon skeleton with elemental tantalum through a chemical vapor deposition process [2] (Figures 27, 28 and 29). Since the early 1940s, tantalum, which makes up approximately 98% of TM, has been widely used as an implantable metal in medicine, and was first introduced as a dental

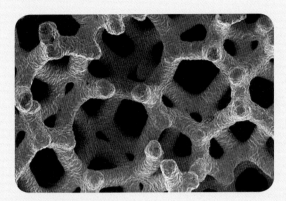

Figure 27: TM structure.

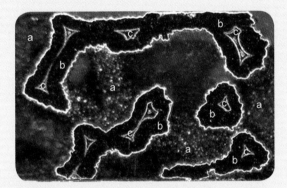

Figure 28: Cross-section of TM shows a thick tantalum layer (a) covering a vitreous carbon core (b).

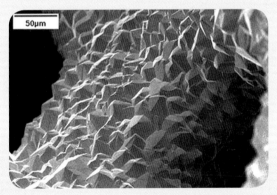

Figure 29: The microtextured and nanotextured surface of TM.

implant material in 1947 [29,30]. The vitreous carbon core, which makes up approximately 2% of TM, is also biocompatible and was used as a dental implant material during the 1970s [31]. The extensive clinical use of TM with titanium alloy in orthopedic and dental implants has affirmed

the biocompatibility and corrosion resistance of tantalum, vitreous carbon, and titanium alloy used in a single-implant design.

In addition to conventional osseointegration, TM implant fixation is augmented by bone ingrowth into the porous material, the combination of which has been termed *osseoincorporation* (Figures 30, 31, 32, 33, and 34). Despite nearly two decades of osseoincorporation with orthopedic implants, Trabecular Metal dental implants (Zimmer Dental Inc.) are still relatively new to implant dentistry. Consequently, clinical documentation of the design in peer-reviewed publications is still pending, and several clinical studies are still in process.

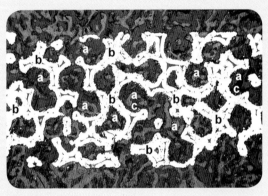

Figure 30: New bone formation (a) on the internal and external surfaces of TM (b) can be distinguished from the potting mix (c) (backscattered electron/energy dispersive radiographic, canine model). *Source:* photograph courtesy of Do-Gyoon Kim, PhD.

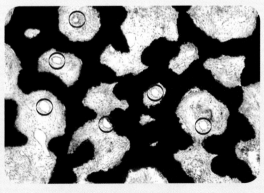

Figure 31: Human bone ingrowth, week 2: TM material pores are infused with tissue, cells and newly formed blood vessels (circles) (toluidine blue). *Source:* photograph courtesy of Celia Clemente de Arriba, MD.

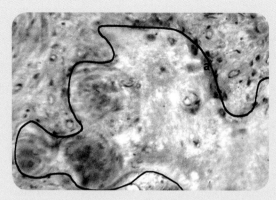

Figure 32: Human bone ingrowth, week 3: new bone formation (purple line) with a front of osteoblasts (a) in a TM pore (H & E). *Source:* photograph courtesy of Celia Clemente de Arriba, MD.

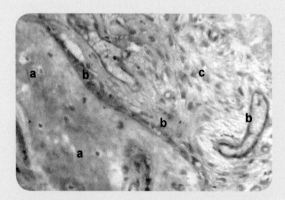

Figure 33: Human bone ingrowth, week 6: woven bone (a), a line of osteoblasts (b), pluripotent tissue (c) and a longitudinally cut blood vessel (d) inside a peripheral TM pore (hematoxylin and eosin). *Source:* photograph courtesy of Celia Clemente de Arriba, MD.

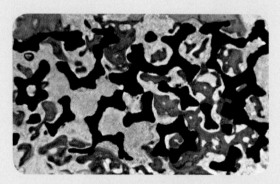

Figure 34: Human bone ingrowth, week 12: newly formed bone trabeculae (blue) penetrate the width of a TM cylinder (black) (toluidine blue). *Source:* photograph courtesy of Celia Clemente de Arriba, MD.

F. In the canine model, Kim et al. (2013) compared the hybrid tantalum–titanium Trabecular Metal dental implants with the implant's predicate Tapered Screw-Vent® implants (Zimmer Dental Inc) after 0, 2, 4, 8, and 12 weeks of healing. There were no intraoperative or postoperative complications. Implant stability, as measured by resonance frequency analysis, did not significantly differ between test and control implant designs at any time interval. Cortical bone-to-implant contact ratios exceeded 65% with no statistical difference between the two implant designs at all time periods. Histologic and backscattered scanning electron microscopic analyses revealed progressive osseointegration (bone ongrowth) with the implant surfaces and bone ingrowth and maturation inside the porous tantalum material throughout the assessment periods. Bone-to-implant contact ratio and bone inside TM had a significant positive correlation.

Schlee et al. [5] reported 1-year interim results from a 3-year, prospective, proof-of-principle clinical study on immediate loading of Trabecular Metal dental implants. The interim report consisted of the first 22 Trabecular Metal dental implants consecutively placed in 17 subjects (10 women, 7 men). Implants were provisionalized out of occlusion within 48 h of implant placement, and then definitively loaded in occlusion within 14 days. There were no implant failures or adverse events in the interim group, and mean crestal bone loss was 0.43 ± 0.41 mm.

In a second clinical study, Schlee et al. [6] reported 1-year interim results from an international, nonrandomized, prospective, multicenter clinical evaluation of Trabecular Metal dental implants placed during the implant development period (2010–2011). The objective of this 5-year study was to evaluate the functioning of TM dental implants in a cross-section of patients that clinicians would routinely treat in their practices. Noninterventional studies are designed to help avoid manufacturer bias by allowing products to be used as they would be in normal dental practices. Results are systematically documented and analyzed to determine statistically significant outcomes. For this study, a longitudinal data collection program was established to monitor the study data and provide investigators with a secure method of data collection through digital case report forms housed in a password-protected database. Patient selection and case planning were left to the professional judgments of the experienced investigators, and oversight of the 22 study sites was provided by local institutional review boards in five countries of the European Union. A total of 268 subjects have been enrolled in the longitudinal data collection program to date and treated per protocol with 377 TM dental implants (reference group). Schlee et al. [6] published an interim report on a subgroup of all subjects whose implants were placed during the implant development period from October 2010 to June 2011, and who completed 1 year of clinical follow-up after implant placement (focus group). A total of 105 subjects were selected and treated with 57 maxillary and 88 mandibular implants by the investigators. Local institutional review boards provided study oversight. Within the study group, 26.7% ($n = 28/105$) of the subjects had concomitant health conditions that could potentially elevate risks for long-term crestal bone loss and/or implant failure: smoking ($n = 17/105$), history of periodontitis ($n = 11/105$), history of osteoporosis ($n = 2/105$), history of bruxism or tooth clenching ($n = 4/105$), history of myocardial infarction or cardiac disease ($n = 4/105$), and intraoral infection that affected the implant site ($n = 1/105$). Eight (28.6%) of these subjects had two or more concomitant health conditions. A total of seven implants were lost: four failed to integrate and three failed as a result of infections. After 1 year in function, mean marginal bone loss was 0.43 ± 0.57 mm and cumulative implant survival was 95.2% ($n = 138/145$). Trabecular Metal dental implants were clinically effective under various clinical conditions in uncontrolled subjects with and without concomitant health conditions.

In another study currently (2014) pending publication, Clemente de Arriba et al. evaluated tissue response to cylinders of TM placed into human jaws. Twenty-three healthy, partially edentulous volunteers were randomly selected and scheduled for placement of one or two 3 mm × 5 mm cylinders of TM in edentulous areas of their mandibular and/or maxillary jaws. In each selected edentulous area, the alveolar bone was surgically exposed and osteotomies were prepared by sequential cutting with internally irrigated drills in graduated diameters. Each cylinder was placed slightly above the crest of the ridge without a barrier membrane. Soft tissues were approximated and sutured to obtain primary closure. Most (58%) of the cylinders were placed in molar regions. Subjects were scheduled for cylinder explantation after 2, 3, 6, or 12 weeks of healing. Each explantation interval consisted of six retrieved cylinders. Samples were prepared, sliced into sections, and analyzed histologically and histomorphometrically. Tissue infiltration and blood vessels were observed inside the internal pores and cells of the TM cylinders after 2 weeks of healing. Bone neoformation and several old bone chips were observed inside the peripheral pores of several samples after 3 weeks of healing. Progressive bone and blood vessel development inside the interconnected pores and new bone attachment to the internal and external surfaces of the TM cylinders were observed from 3 to 12 weeks of healing. After 12 weeks of healing, the mean percentage of calcified bone versus marrow was 22.74% at a depth of 0.5 mm, 16.77% at a depth of 1 mm, and 14.95% for the entire TM cylinder. Bone was still developing and maturing inside the cylinders.

The actual depth of the porous tantalum material on Trabecular Metal dental implants ranges from approximately 0.65 to 0.76 mm, depending on the implant diameter. Based on these dimensions, the mean percentage of bone tissue inside the TM cylinders at depths of 0.5 and 1.0 mm in addition to the entire sample was evaluated (Clemente de Arriba et al., unpublished results 2014). The results suggested that Trabecular Metal dental implants may be capable of achieving approximately 23% bone ingrowth after 12 weeks of healing in partially edentulous human jaws, depending on the implant diameter and the location of placement in the human jaw. The finding of approximately 23% bone ingrowth was not unexpected, since the majority of cylinders ($n = 14/24$) were placed in posterior jaws where mean trabecular bone volume in the first molar region has been reported to range from approximately 24% for males to approximately

18% for females in edentulous jaws [32,33]. Similarly, sinus lifts typically have approximately 25% vital bone in histologies taken from the same region at 6–8 months [34].

Very little peer-reviewed data have been published to date on clinician experiences with Trabecular Metal dental implants in routine dental practices. Spinato et al. [35] reported on the failure of one Trabecular Metal dental implant 4 months after placement in a maxillary right second premolar location of a 54-year-old woman with a history of moderate, chronic periodontitis. The patient was treated for her periodontal disease and the implant was reportedly placed under favorable conditions. At the surgical uncovering 4 months later, peri-implant inflammation involved the coronal one-third of the implant. With the patient's consent, the implant was surgically removed and submitted for histologic analysis, which showed greater bone formation around the TM material in the center of the implant than around the nonporous implant neck. The TM was surrounded by short, thick bone trabeculae, consisting of composite bone with both woven and lamellar structures that were growing into the peripheral pores of the implant.

To date, I have placed 75 Trabecular Metal dental implants (Zimmer Dental Inc.) in 35 cases with encouraging outcomes and no significant complications (Table 1). Over time, it will be interesting to see if TM (Zimmer TMT) will offer any long-term benefits for marginal bone preservation and esthetics based on its well-documented mechanical characteristics [19–26].

The modulus of elasticity refers to the ability of a substance to deform under applied stress. For example, both the implant and supporting bone elongate under the applied stress of chewing. Because a titanium dental implant's modulus of elasticity (~110 GPa) is significantly higher than either cortical (~15 GPa) or trabecular bone (~0.1 GPa) [20–26], the disparity creates microstrains ($\mu\varepsilon$) at the bone–implant interface during function [36–38]. These microstrains at the bone-implant interface can influence cellular remodeling in different ways, ranging from bone atrophy (disuse atrophy) (<200 $\mu\varepsilon$), to balanced

Table 1: Other Cases Treated with Trabecular Metal Dental Implants by the Author

Patients	
Number	35
Men	12
Women	23
Age (years)	
mean	56.6
range	21–74
Comorbid conditions	
none	26
smoker	4
diabetes	1
osteoporosis	1
osteopenia	3
Implants	
Number	72
Crestal options	
TMT	30
TMM	42
Lengths	
8 mm	1
10 mm	10
11.5 mm	25
13 mm	36
Diameters	
4.1 mm	45
4.7 mm	21
6.0 mm	6
Outcomes	
Follow-up[b] (months)	
mean	14.81
range	5–23
Complications	
surgical phase	0
provisional prosthesis	1[a]
follow-up	0
definitive prosthesis	0
Implant survival	
placed	72
failed	0
surviving	72
survival (%)	100

TMM: implant neck with microgrooves and a textured surface below a 0.5 mm band of machined titanium; TMT: implant neck with microgrooves and a textured surface that extends to the top of the implant.
[a]Excess temporary cement causes bone loss to the second implant thread; resolved with bone grafting before final restoration.
[b]Calculated from date of implant placement.

bone remodeling (steady state) (~200–2500 µε), bone growth (hypertrophy) (~2500–4000 µε) or bone resorption (pathological overload) (≥4000 µε), depending on the intensity of the microstrains [36–38]. Elevated microstrains (≥4000 µε) can also cause microfractures in the interfacial crestal bone, stress shielding of the subcrestal bone, and stimulate bone cells to trigger osteoclastic cytokines, all of which can result in crestal bone resorption [37]. With unresolved bone resorption, stresses can intensify to the point that osseointegration is lost or the implant fractures [39]. It is currently unknown, however, if TM's low modulus of elasticity (~3 GPa) will help to preserve crestal bone levels since it more closely approximates the elastic modulus of cortical (~15 GPa) and trabecular bone (~0.1 GPa) than titanium (~110 GPa) [20–26]. Further research is needed to fully understand the long-term benefits of Trabecular Metal dental implants.

Case 4

Narrow-Diameter Implant

CASE STORY

A 28-year-old African American female presented with an internal referral from Tufts University School of Dental Medicine Department of Orthodontics, with a chief complaint of: "I have had braces for a while and they told me that they can't make any more space. I hope there is enough space to have a tooth placed in this area." The patient was congenitally missing tooth #10. Prior to orthodontic treatment, the patient indicated she had a diastema between #9 and #11 (Figure 1). Following 1.5 years of orthodontic therapy, she presented to the department of postgraduate prosthodontics with a full set of brackets and an arch wire of the maxilla, with a tooth-colored-bracketed pontic currently occupying the #10 partially edentulous space (Figure 2). The patient indicates regular and uninterrupted 6-month visits to her hygienist and general dentist. She also reports she brushes and flosses daily. Existing restorations were limited to an occlusal composite restoration on #19 and an occlusal amalgam restoration on #31.

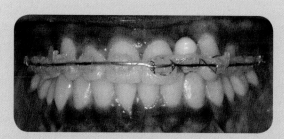

Figure 2: Orthodontic brackets and temporary.

LEARNING GOALS AND OBJECTIVES
- Recognize the specific clinical indications and applications of reduced-diameter implants
- Identify the limitations and benefits of utilizing reduced-diameter implants
- Understand the role of reduced-diameter implants in implant dentistry

Medical History

At onset and duration of treatment, the patient did not have any significant medical condition, history, and/or complications, which were contraindications for treatment. Further, she was not taking any medications and had no known drug, food, and/or material allergies.

Review of Systems
- Vital statistics
  - Average blood pressure: 118/76 mmHg
  - Average respiration rate: 17 breaths/min
  - Average pulse rate: 68 beats/min

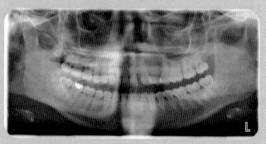

Figure 1: Pretreatment panoramic radiograph.

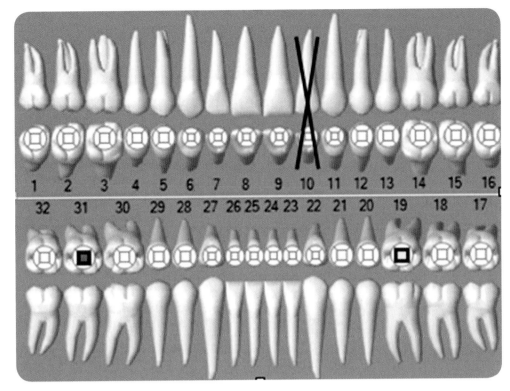

Figure 3: Periodontal charting.

Social History

The patient has no history of smoking or use of tobacco-containing products. She does indicate, however, infrequent use of alcohol, limited to less than two times per month and less than two drinks per session.

Extraoral Examination

No significant findings were noted. The lymph nodes of the head and neck were within normal limits. No clicking or crepitus noted at the level of the temporomandibular joint. Palpation of the muscles of the head and neck showed no signs of soreness, tenderness, or bruising.

Intraoral Examination

The floor of the mouth, tongue, cheek, palate, and oropharynx were within normal limits. Salivary flow was monitored to be normal. The maxilla was large and U-shaped; the mandible was also large and U-shaped.

In the maxilla, all teeth were present (including the third molars) except tooth #10. The partially edentulous site of tooth #10 had a Seibert class III ridge deformity [1].

In the mandible, all teeth were present (including the third molars), with a composite restoration on the occlusal surfaces of tooth #19 and an amalgam restoration on the occlusal surface of tooth #31.

Periodontal charting was completed with unremarkable findings, except for the absence of tooth #10 (Figure 3).

The lip line at smile was moderate, and the gingival biotype was found to be moderately thick [2,3].

Occlusal Analysis

The molar and canine occlusal relationship was class 1. No pain or tenderness was noted on loading of the joints. No occlusal discrepancies or interferences were noted.

Radiographic Examination

The patient exhibited normal trabecular bone patterns with no pathologic lesions. No history of root canal therapy or exodontia. Sinus pneumatization noted on both maxillary left and right quadrants. Generalized mild bone loss is evident. Composite occlusal restoration of tooth #19 and an amalgam occlusal restoration on #31.

Cone beam computed tomograms (CBCTs) reveal both horizontal and vertical bone loss in the partially edentulous maxilla (#10) (Figures 4 and 5). Skeletal class III.

Diagnosis

Partial edentulism due to congenitally missing left maxillary lateral incisor (#10).

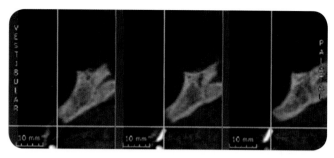

Figure 4: CBCT, sagittal cross-section.

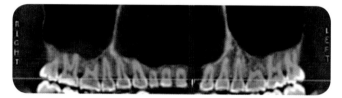

Figure 5: CBCT, panoramic view.

Treatment Plan

The treatment plan for this patient consisted of initial-phase therapy that included oral prophylaxis and oral hygiene instructions to establish a baseline prior to treatment. Both a surgical and restorative assessment were performed using the straightforward, advanced, or complex (SAC) classification, developed by the International Team of Implantology in 2007. The surgical and restorative risk assessment for the implant-based restoration of this single-tooth gap was determined as being advanced. The risk assessment was followed by presurgical treatment planning for the placement of a 3.0 mm × 10.5 mm narrow-diameter implant (BioHorizon Implant System, Birmingham, AL), hereafter referred to as a reduced-platform-diameter implant, with immediate provisionalization. An implant with a diameter of 3.0 mm was selected in order to respect the recommended intrabony implant-to-tooth distance, as the space was approximated to be 5.8 mm.

Treatment

Surgical

Upon completion of initial-phase therapy, presurgical treatment planning, and surgical stent fabrication, the patient presented for implant surgery. A course of antibiotics (2 g amoxicillin) was administered 1 h prior to implant surgery. Prior to administration of a local anesthetic, the patient was instructed to perform an oral rise with chlorhexidine gluconate 0.12% for 1 min. Anesthesia of the site was achieved via local infiltration with 2% xylocaine 1:100,000 epinephrine; a midcrestal

incision was made in site #10, followed by an intrasulcular incision that extended one tooth distal and mesial to the implant site; a vertical releasing incision was made only for the distal segment of the incision. The full-thickness flap was then reflected and one implant was placed (3.0 mm diameter × 10.5 mm height) according to the manufacturer's specifications (initial osteotomy performed with a 2.0 mm diameter drill, followed by enlargement with a 2.5 mm diameter finishing drill to length and finalized by implant placement). Confirmation of primary stability was assessed when a force of greater than 30 N cm was necessary to finalize the implant placement. The site was then sutured with interrupted 5-0 vicryl resorbable sutures until tension-free site closure was obtained. Radiography was used to determine the final implant position (Figure 6).

Provisionalization

The implant was immediately provisionalized with an indexed titanium temporary abutment. The provisional was fabricated using Quikset Jet Acrylic, finished and polished extraorally, confirmed intraorally, and then hand tightened. Teflon tape was placed above the screw to protect the screw connection, upon retrieval, and composite was placed to blend the facial access with adjacent brackets. No contacts in centric and excursive movements were allowed on the provisional (Figure 7).

Postoperative

The patient was prescribed a 5-day regimen of amoxicillin, ibuprofen for pain as needed, and a 7-day routine of 0.12% chlorhexidine gluconate. The patient was seen 1 week after surgery, at 2 weeks for suture removal, and at 8 weeks for final impressions.

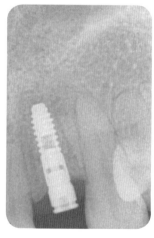

Figure 6: Periapical radiograph immediately following implant placement.

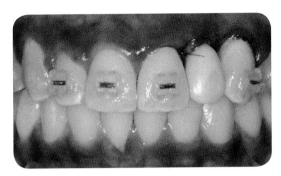

Figure 7: Immediate provisionalization.

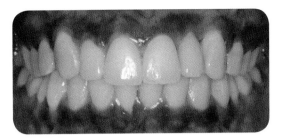

Figure 9: Final restoration.

Prosthetic Restoration

The site was allowed to heal for 8 weeks, at which time a final impression was captured using an open-tray impression technique with a customized impression coping to accurately record the emergence profile previously created by the provisional (Figure 8). The implant was then definitively restored with a gold custom abutment and a cement-retained porcelain-fused-to-metal restoration (Figure 9). Occlusion was adjusted until the shim stock pulled between the restoration and opposing tooth with light resistance in centric contact.

Discussion

This case entailed the restoration of a congenitally missing lateral maxillary incisor with a reduced-platform-diameter implant. It was further complicated by inadequate space that was partially relieved through orthodontic movements. Given the location, bone volume present, prominent upper lip, interdental position (both clinical crown and roots of adjacent teeth), and esthetic demand, it was determined that a two-piece 3.0 mm diameter bone-level implant diameter with a custom abutment and cement-retained restoration would result in the best esthetic outcome. In doing so, it allowed approximately 1.4 mm of space to be respected between the implant and adjacent tooth, placement in native bone, and met the restorative criteria of a small emergence profile [4–12].

By utilizing tools such as the SAC classification, the factors that were initially present and the factors that were necessary in order to obtain predictable surgical and restorative results were reviewed prior to treatment. This not only allows one to determine the complexity and potential risk prior to the start of the case, but also permits a case-specific assessment of the necessary capabilities of the surgeon and restorative doctor who will be performing the procedures.

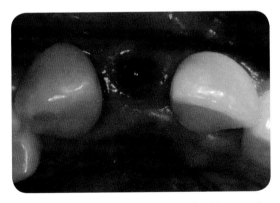

Figure 8: Contoured soft tissues prior to final impression.

Self-Study Questions

(Answers located at the end of the case)

A. What constitutes a reduced-platform-diameter implant?

B. What are the indications for placing a reduced-platform-diameter implant?

C. What are the contraindications for placing a reduced-platform-diameter implant?

D. What are the potential benefits of placing a reduced-platform-diameter implant over a standard-sized implant?

E. Are different materials utilized in fabrication of reduced-platform-diameter implants?

F. Are reduced-platform-diameter implants predictable?

References

1. Allum SR, Tomlinson RA, Joshi R. The impact of loads on standard diameter, small diameter, and mini implants: a comparative laboratory study. Clin Oral Implants Res 2008;19(6):553–559.
2. Tarnow DP, Cho SC, Wallace SS. The effect of inter-implant distance on the height of inter-implant bone crest. J Periodontol 2000;71:546–549.
3. Tarnow DP, Elian N, Fletcher P, et al. Vertical distance from the crest of bone to the height of the interproximal papilla between adjacent implants. J Periodontol 2003;74:1785–1788.
4. Seibert JS. Reconstruction of deformed, partially edentulous ridges, using full thickness onlay grafts. Part II. Prosthetic/periodontal interrelationships. Compend Contin Educ Dent 1983;4(6):549–5-62.
5. Tarnow DP, Magner AW, Fletcher P. The effect of the distance from the contact point to the crest of bone on the presence or absence of the interproximal dental papilla. J Periodontol 1992;63:995–996.
6. Davarpanah M, Martinez H, Tecucianu JF, et al. Small-diameter implants: indications and contraindications. J Esthet Dent 2000;12(4):186–194.
7. Buser D, Martin W, Belser UC. Optimizing esthetics for implant restorations in the anterior maxilla: anatomic and surgical considerations. Int J Oral Maxillofac Implants 2004;19(Suppl):43–61.
8. Zinsli B, Sagesser T, Mericske E, Mericske-Stern R. Clinical evaluation of small-diameter ITI implants: a prospective study. Int J Oral Maxillofac Implants 2004;19:92–99.
9. Reddy MS, O'Neal SJ, Haigh S, et al. Initial clinical efficacy of 3-mm implants immediately placed into function in conditions of limited spacing. Int J Oral Maxillofac Implants 2008;23(2):281–288.
10. De Rouck T, Eghbali R, Collys K, et al. The gingival biotype revisited: transparency of the periodontal probe through the gingival margin as a method to discriminate thin from thick gingiva. J Clin Periodontol 2009;36(5):428–433.
11. Kan JYK, Morimoto T, Rungcharassaeng K, et al. Gingival biotype assessment in the esthetic zone: visual versus direct measurement. Int J Periodontics Restorative Dent 2009;30(3):237–243.
12. Sohn DS, Bae MS, Heo JU, et al. Retrospective multicenter analysis of immediate provisionalization using one-piece narrow-diameter (3.0mm) implants. Int J Oral Maxillofac Implants 2011;26(1):163–168.
13. Klein MO, Schiegnitz E, Al-Nawas B. Systematic review on success of narrow-diameter dental implants. Int J Oral Maxillofac Implants 2014;29(Suppl):43–54.

Answers to Self-Study Questions

A. Classically, implants in the range of 3.75 to 4.1 mm were considered the standard regular-diameter implants [4–6]. Therefore, implants greater than or equal to 3.0 mm, but less than 3.7 mm, are given the denomination of a reduced-platform-diameter implant. However, it should be noted that subclassifications can be found in the literature that break down small-diameter implants into implants that range from 3.0 to 3.25 mm and 3.3 to 3.5 mm [4]. Lastly, implants under 3.0 mm are considered mini-implants and are often of the one-piece type, though 3.0 mm two-piece implants are also available [4,8,9]. Mini-implants are recommended for temporary use only.

B. The following are indications for reduced-platform-diameter implants [5–7,13]:
• narrow alveolar crest/limited bone volume
• limited supracrestal/mesiodistal space
• limited interradicular space
• restoration necessitating small emergence profile.

C. The main biomechanical complication is potential risk of implant fracture [6].

D.
• Placement of implant in native bone.
• Reduced potential for postoperative complications, morbidity, and failure.
• Avoid bone augmentation procedures.
• Avoid orthodontic procedures.

E. Historically, the same materials utilized for standard-sized implants are used to fabricate reduced-platform-diameter implants: grade 1 titanium [6]. Today, newer materials with improved mechanical properties, such as titanium grades IV and V (Ti6Al4V), as well as TiZr, are available and preferrably used for reduced-diameter implants.

F. According to the literature, reduced-platform-diameter implants are a reliable treatment modality in treating partially edentulous areas with three-dimensional space limitations [5–8,13].

Case 5

Short Implants

Medical History

The patient did not smoke or drink alcohol at the time of treatment and had no history of smoking. Patient reported no allergies to medications. She reported taking ursidiol (ursodeoxycholic acid) for the nonsurgical treatment of gallstones.

Review of Systems

- Vital signs
  - Blood pressure: 126/75 mmHg
  - Pulse rate: 72 beats/min
  - Respiration: 16 breaths/min

Dental History

There was no history of periodontal, orthodontic, or endodontic treatment. The maxillary right first molar was extracted due to a fracture within the last 6 months. The patient reported having cleanings and checkups every 6 months.

Extraoral Examination

No significant findings were noted. The patient had no masses or swelling, and the temporomandibular joint was within normal limits. There was no facial asymmetry noted, and her lymph nodes were normal on palpation.

Intraoral Examination

- Oral cancer screening demonstrated no pathologies present.
- Soft tissue exam, including her tongue and floor of the mouth, was within normal limits.
- Periodontal examination revealed probing depths of less than 4 mm.
- Fair oral hygiene.
- Localized gingival inflammation was noted.
- Examination of area of maxillary right first molar (#3) revealed missing tooth. Clinical and radiographic examination revealed alveolar width of more than 10 mm. The remaining ridge was significantly wider toward the distal side close to the second molar area when compared with the ridge close to the second premolar (Figure 1A). Proximity of maxillary sinus cavity and limited bone height (approximately 7 mm) were observed on the periapical radiograph, which also showed the presence of a septum on the mesial side of the edentulous area (Figure 1B).

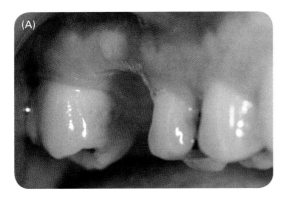

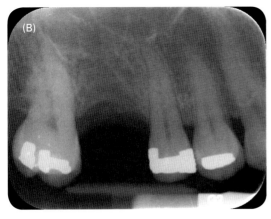

Figure 1: Preoperation evaluation showed insufficient bone height. (A) Intraoral examination revealed complete epithelialization of the socket. (B) Periapical radiograph showed about 7 mm bone height below the sinus.

- Examination of mandibular left first molar (#19) revealed subgingival fracture of both lingual cusps (deeper than 2 mm subgingivally) and no clinical crown remaining on the lingual side. Sufficient bone width more than 9 mm was noted. The distance from the crest of the ridge to the inferior alveolar nerve was approximately 17 mm.
- Sufficient keratinized gingival tissue was observed on facial side of both #3 and #19.

Occlusion

The patient had an Angle class I occlusion. Adequate posterior occlusal support was present with a total of 15 posterior teeth in contact during maximal intercuspation. On lateral excursions, canine guidance was documented on the left side and group function between three maxillary and three mandibular right posterior teeth (teeth #2, #5, #6, #27, #28 and #31) was noted. Protrusive contacts (anterior guidance) between teeth #6, #7, #9, #10, #11, #22, #23, #24, #26, #27, and #28 were noted.

Radiographic Examination

The patient brought a copy of a full-mouth radiographic series from her dentist, and a panoramic radiograph was made. Both sets of radiographs were reviewed.

Diagnosis

According to the American Academy of Periodontology, the diagnosis was plaque-induced gingivitis. The restorative diagnosis was a missing maxillary right first molar (#3) and nonrestorable mandibular left first molar (#19).

Treatment Plan

The treatment plan for this patient consisted of oral hygiene instruction and 6-month maintenance recalls at her dentist's office. Her mandibular left first molar was extracted, and implants were placed to restore the maxillary right and mandibular left first molars (#3, #19).

Treatment

This patient received oral hygiene instruction to address gingival inflammation and was educated about the importance of regular daily maintenance procedures for the better prognosis of both teeth and dental implants.

Replacement of Maxillary Right First Molar

In the maxillary right area, tooth #3 had been extracted 6 months previously with normal hard and soft tissue healing. The site appeared to be completely healed and healthy prior to implant placement (Figure 1). The timing of implant placement was classified as type IV (see Box 1) [1].

Box 1 Classification of Implant Placement in the Extraction Socket by Surgical Timing [1]

Type I: immediate placement after extraction
Type II: complete soft tissue closure of the socket (typically 6–8 weeks)
Type III: substantial clinical and/or radiographic bone fill of the socket (typically 12–16 weeks)
Type IV: healed site (typically more than 16 weeks)

A crestal incision was done and a full-thickness flap elevated. A 5 mm × 6 mm (Bicon®) implant was placed (Figure 2A).

After 4 months of healing, the implant was uncovered and a 5.0 mm × 5.0 mm titanium nonshouldered abutment was inserted and seated with the use of a seating tip and a mallet. A periapical radiograph was made to verify the proper seating of the abutment (Figure 2B). The patient was referred to her general dentist, who restored the implant with a metal ceramic crown. A periapical radiograph made 2 years postimplant placement is shown in Figure 3A.

Peri-implant bone stability was observed after 6 years of follow-up. Bone mineralization surrounding the implant–abutment interface, particularly on the mesial side, is evident when compared with the radiographs at abutment insertion and the last recall appointment (Figure 3B).

At the recall appointment (Figure 4) the following were found:

Plaque index	0, no plaque evident
Bleeding index	0, no bleeding upon probing was evident
Soft tissue inflammation	0, no inflammation observed
Probing depths MP, P, DP, MB, B, DB (mm)	3, 1, 2, 1, 1, 1
Width of keratinized peri-im plant mucosa (mm)	3
Implant stability as measured with Periotest®	−3, indicating no mobility

B: buccal; DB: distobuccal; DP: distopalatal; MB: mesiobuccal; MP: mesiopalatal; P: palatal.

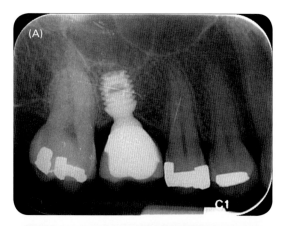

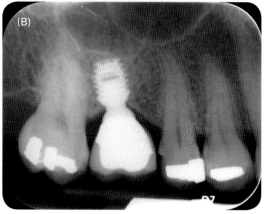

Figure 3: The radiographic film illustrated stable alveolar bone level at (A) 2 years and (B) 6 years after implant placement. Significant bone gain could be observed surrounding the mesial side of the implant–abutment interface.

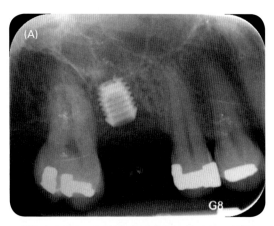

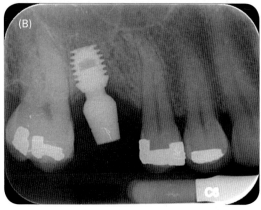

Figure 2: Implant was placed at #3 edentulous ridge (A) and the abutment was seated after 4 months of healing (B).

Replacement of Mandibular Left First Molar

Tooth #19 was extracted and an implant was placed in the same appointment (Bicon®, 5 mm × 6 mm;

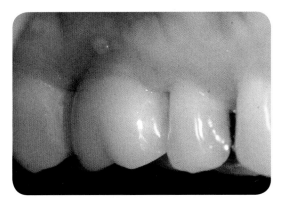

Figure 4: Clinical examination after 3 years of implant placement showed healthy peri-implant soft tissue.

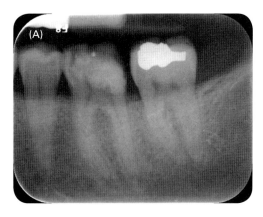

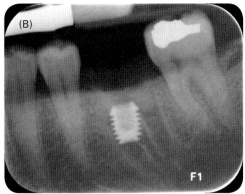

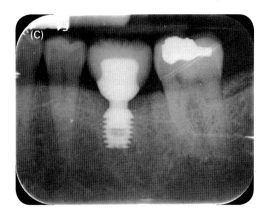

Figure 5A and B). The timing of implant placement was classified as type I. The pilot drill osteotomy was done in the intraradicular bone with the objective of expanding distally the cavity left by the mesial root. Since a 6 mm length implant was planned, the distance to the inferior alveolar nerve was a very safe 9 mm.

Beta tricalcium phosphate (Synthograft, Bicon, LLC) was placed coronal to the implant, and the area was covered with a resorbable collagen plug. The area was then sutured. The implant was submerged for a two-stage surgical approach. The implant was uncovered 3 months later after placement. A permanent crown was delivered 1 month later (Figure 5C).

Recall appointment (Figure 5D) demonstrated the following:

Plaque index	1, plaque evident with a probe
Bleeding index	0, no bleeding upon probing
Soft tissue inflammation	0, no inflammation observed.
Probing depths ML, L, DL, MB, B, DB (mm)	2, 1, 3, 3, 1, 1
Keratinized peri-implant mucosa (mm)	1.5
Implant stability as measured with a Periotest	−0.3, indicating no mobility

B: buccal; DB:distobuccal; DL: distolingual; L: lingual; MB: mesiobuccal; ML: mesiolingual.

After 4 years of follow-up, heathy peri-implant mucosa with a band of keratinized, attached tissue was noted clinically (Figure 6A), and peri-implant bone stability was shown on the radiograph (Figure 6B).

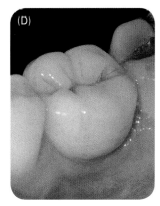

Figure 5: (A) Unrestorable mandibular left first molar before extraction. (B) Implant was placed immediately after extraction. (C) A permanent crown was delivered 4 months later. (D) At recall appointment.

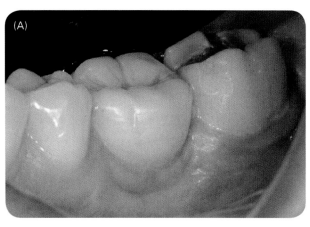
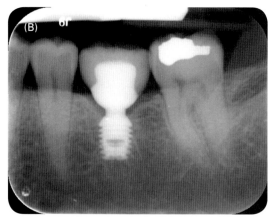

Figure 6: (A) Final restoration showed clinical success with healthy soft tissue. (B) Four years after placement, the periapical radiographic film demonstrated stable alveolar bone level.

CASE STORY 2
A 55-year-old Caucasian female presented with a failing mandibular right fixed partial denture. She complained of pain when chewing and a bad smell in the area.

LEARNING GOALS AND OBJECTIVES
■ To be able to understand the clinical applications of short/ultrashort dental implants
■ To understand the indications, contraindications, and the rationale for the use of short and ultrashort dental implants by reviewing clinical cases and literature
■ To identify differences in the surgical protocol of short implant placement when compared with conventional-size implants

Medical History
The patient reported no systemic diseases and did not take any medication. She reported no allergies to medications.

Review of Systems
• Vital signs
  ○ Blood pressure: 118/68 mmHg
  ○ Pulse rate: 66 beats/min (regular)
  ○ Respiration: 18 breaths/min

Social and Dental History
The patient stopped smoking more than 10 years ago. She did not smoke at the time of treatment. She is a social drinker. Past dental history includes fixed partial dentures in both mandibular posterior areas more than 10 years ago, implant-supported restorations in the maxillary anterior area, and endodontic treatment. The patient reported no history of periodontal disease or treatment.

Extraoral Examination
No significant findings were noted. The patient had no masses or swelling, and the temporomandibular joint was within normal limits. There was no facial asymmetry noted, and her lymph nodes were normal on palpation.

Intraoral Examination
• Oral cancer screening was negative.
• Soft tissue exam, including her tongue and floor of the mouth, was within normal limits.
• Periodontal examination revealed generalized probing depths within 4 mm and localized 3–5 mm in maxillary posterior areas. General recession and moderate plaque accumulation were presented with bleeding on probing. Calculus accumulation in mandibular anterior area was also noted.
• The oral hygiene is fair.
• Mandibular right posterior area:
  ○ Recurrent caries was detected on mandibular right second premolar (#29). This tooth with previous endodontic treatment served as an abutment for a four-unit fixed partial denture replacing missing first and second mandibular molars (#29–x–x–#32). The extent of caries rendered the tooth nonrestorable.

○ Clinical examination demonstrated sufficient bone width; more than 9 mm was noted with a periodontal probe. The distance from the crest of the ridge to the inferior alveolar nerve was approximately 11 mm when measured in the area of the mandibular right second premolar on the radiograph. Clinical examination of lingual areas demonstrated a reduction of ridge width toward the apical areas approximately 10 mm from the lingual crest corresponding to a moderately prominent mandibular fossa.

Occlusion

Angle class II occlusion with proper posterior support.

Radiographic Examination

A full-mouth radiographic series was made and reviewed.

Diagnosis

- Periodontal diagnosis: generalized mild to moderate chronic periodontitis (1999, the International Workshop for a Classification of Periodontal Diseases).
- Restorative diagnosis: #29, #30, #31 edentulous ridge.

Treatment

After initial periodontal therapy was finished, probing depths in maxillary posterior areas were reevaluated and recorded within 4 mm.

The fixed partial denture was sectioned mesial of #32. Tooth #29 was extracted. Three ultrashort implants (5 mm × 5 mm, Bicon®) were placed; this allowed for a safe distance to the inferior alveolar nerve. Quality of bone was documented as type III (see Box 2) [2]. Bone collected during the osteotomy was placed in area #29 to close the coronal space left by the extraction of the tooth and then the area was covered with a resorbable collagen membrane and sutured.

The postoperative evaluation performed 1 month after surgery revealed proper healing and no signs of infection, and the patient reported no pain. The implants were uncovered 3 months after implant placement and osseointegration was verified. Then, an implant-level impression was made. Three Integrated Abutment Crowns™ [3] were delivered 4 months after implant placement (Figure 7). Peri-implant bone stability was observed after a 3.5-year follow-up (Figure 8). No probing depth more than 4 mm was detected at all sites of implant #29, #30, #31 (Figure 9).

| Box 2 | Bone Density Classification [2] |

Type I: dense cortical bone
Type II: thick dense to porous cortical bone on crest and coarse trabecular bone within
Type III: thin porous cortical bone on crest and fine trabecular bone within
Type IV: fine trabecular bone
Type V: immature, nonmineralized bone

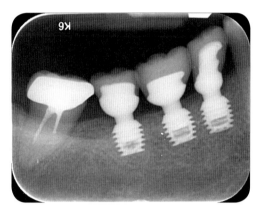

Figure 7: Three implants (#29, #30, #31) were placed and restored with nonsplinted crowns.

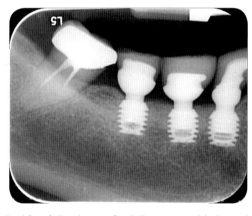

Figure 8: After following up for 3.5 years, stable bone level was noted.

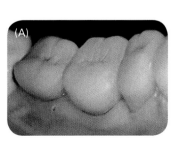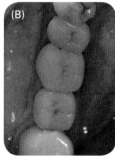

Figure 9: Intraoral examination showed healthy peri-implant soft tissue: (A) buccal view and (B) occlusal view.

A clinical examination performed on a recall appointment (Figure 9) revealed the following:

Plaque index	0, no plaque accumulation observed on the facial sides
Bleeding index	1, slight bleeding was elicited upon probing on facial side of all three implants
Soft tissue inflammation	0, no inflammation observed
Probing depths ML, L, DL, MB, B, DB (mm)	
#29	3, 3, 3, 4, 3, 2
#30	1, 1, 2, 4, 3, 2
#31	2, 1, 2, 4, 3, 3
Keratinized gingiva (mm)	2
Implant stability as measured with a Periotest:	
#29	−3, indicating no mobility
#30	−5, indicating no mobility
#31	−4, indicating no mobility

B: buccal; DB: distobuccal; DL: distolingual; L: lingual; MB: mesiobuccal; ML: mesiolingual.

Occlusal and interproximal contacts were present.

Discussion

Short implants (refer to self-study question A) are generally placed at sites with anatomic limitations, such as insufficient bone height and proximity of vital structures (refer to self-study question B). In case 1, the edentulous ridge in area #3 had limited vertical bone height (approximate 7 mm below maxillary sinus). An implant longer that 7 mm would have required sinus augmentation prior to or at implant placement. Although a sinus augmentation procedure (transalveolar or lateral approach) is a predictable treatment alternative [4], it is technically sensitive. Patients need to have multiple surgical procedures, which result in increased costs. According to a systematic review of transalveolar sinus lift, sinus membrane perforation was the most frequent surgical complication (prevalence varied between 0 and 21.4%, with a mean of 3.8%), and sinus infection was the most frequent postoperative complication (prevalence varied between 0 and 2.5%, with a mean of 0.8%) [5]. For a lateral approach, the mean prevalence of membrane perforation was 19.5% (range 0–58.3%), and the mean incidence of sinus infection was 2.9% (range 0–7.4%) [6]. Moreover, hemorrhage, nasal bleeding, blocked nose and hematomas are all possible postoperative complications. Patients who had sinus augmentation procedures lost an average of 3 days of work and needed 5 days to recover from pain, swelling and other complications [7]. Therefore, the use of short implants, which have shown similar survival rates to longer implants (refer to self-study question C), could reduce the number of appointments, the number of morbidities, and cost (refer to self-study questions B and E).

In the first case reported, the implant in the area of #19 was placed immediately after the extraction of the tooth. Immediate placement can shorten procedure time compared with delayed implant placement. The immediate placement of a 6 mm long implant restored with a molar-sized tooth demonstrated successful clinical outcome after several years.

The implant in the area of #3 was placed 6 months after extraction. The postextraction site had completely healed soft and hard tissues. It could be argued that limited primary stability will be achieved when placing 6 mm long implants in posterior maxilla. However, the implants used in the present report were a plateau design and had a hydroxyapatite (HA) coating. Several studies have reported HA-coated implants have increased bone-to-implant contact [8], increased interfacial strength with bone, and greater torque removal values when compared with an untreated titanium surface [9,10], and higher bone mineral apposition rate and higher biomechanical fixation when compared with alumina-blasted/acid-etched titanium [11,12]. Therefore, HA-coated short implants can have successful osseointegration even with low primary stability. However, the HA-coated implants could have a high peri-implantitis rate, which causes failure in the long-term follow-up [13]. The patients who have HA-coated implants placed need to have good oral hygiene and be cooperative with all maintenance appointments.

The use of short implants has been questioned in the past because of the unfavorable mechanical force distribution caused by high crown-to-implant ratio (CIR; refer to self-study questions C and D). In case 1, the short implants restoring the maxillary and mandibular first molars demonstrated healthy peri-implant soft tissues and stable marginal alveolar bone levels without complications over time. In case 2, the three unsplinted short implants demonstrated successful clinical outcomes after a 3.5-year follow-up. This supported the hypothesis that it may not be necessary to splint multiple, consecutive short implants (refer to self-study question D). According to the literature and the authors' clinical experiences, short implants have comparable clinical outcomes to long implants as long as proper surgical procedures are performed (refer to self-study question F). Short implant placement could become a routine treatment if future studies demonstrate that long-term survival and peri-implant bone stability turn out to be similar to longer implants.

Self-Study Questions

(Answers located at the end of the case)

A. What is a short dental implant?

B. What are the clinical situations where short implant placement is applicable?

C. What is the clinical evidence supporting short dental implant placement?

D. Is the high CIR a clinical concern for a short implant? Should multiple short implants be splinted?

E. What are the possible complications following short implant placement?

F. What should a clinician pay attention to while performing a short implant placement procedure or prosthetic restoration of a short implant?

References

1. Hammerle CH, Chen ST, Wilson Jr TG. Consensus statements and recommended clinical procedures regarding the placement of implants in extraction sockets. Int J Oral Maxillofac Implants 2004;19(Suppl):26–28.
2. Misch CE. Contemporary Implant Dentistry. St Louis: MO: Mosby; 1999.
3. Urdaneta RA, Marincola M. The Integrated Abutment Crown™, a screwless and cementless restoration for single-tooth implants: a report on a new technique. J Prosthodont 2007;16:311–318.
4. Wallace SS, Froum SJ. Effect of maxillary sinus augmentation on the survival of endosseous dental implants. A systematic review. Ann Periodontol 2003;8:328–343.
5. Tan WC, Lang NP, Zwahlen M, Pjetursson BE. A systematic review of the success of sinus floor elevation and survival of implants inserted in combination with sinus floor elevation. Part II: transalveolar technique. J Clin Periodontol 2008;35:241–254.
6. Pjetursson BE, Tan WC, Zwahlen M, Lang NP. A systematic review of the success of sinus floor elevation and survival of implants inserted in combination with sinus floor elevation. J Clin Periodontol 2008;35:216–240.
7. Mardinger O, Poliakov H, Beitlitum I, et al. The patient's perception of recovery after maxillary sinus augmentation: a prospective study. J Periodontol 2009;80:572–576.
8. Gottlander M, Albrektsson T. Histomorphometric studies of hydroxylapatite-coated and uncoated CP titanium threaded implants in bone. Int J Oral Maxillofac Implants 1991;6:399–404.
9. Bell R, Beirne OR. Effect of hydroxylapatite, tricalcium phosphate, and collagen on the healing of defects in the rat mandible. J Oral Maxillofac Surg 1988;46:589–594.
10. Carr AB, Larsen PE, Papazoglou E, McGlumphy E. Reverse torque failure of screw-shaped implants in baboons: baseline data for abutment torque application. Int J Oral Maxillofac Implants 1995;10:167–174.
11. Coelho PG, Lemons JE. Physico/chemical characterization and in vivo evaluation of nanothickness bioceramic depositions on alumina-blasted/acid-etched Ti–6Al–4V implant surfaces. J Biomed Mater Res A 2009;90:351–361.
12. Coelho PG, Bonfante EA, Pessoa RS, et al. Characterization of five different implant surfaces and their effect on osseointegration: a study in dogs. J Periodontol 2011;82:742–750.
13. Wheeler SL. Eight-year clinical retrospective study of titanium plasma-sprayed and hydroxyapatite-coated cylinder implants. Int J Oral Maxillofac Implants 1996;11:340–350.
14. Kotsovilis S, Fourmousis I, Karoussis IK, Bamia C. A systematic review and meta-analysis on the effect of implant length on the survival of rough-surface dental implants. J Periodontol 2009;80:1700–1718.
15. Friberg B, Jemt T, Lekholm U. Early failures in 4,641 consecutively placed Brånemark dental implants: a study from stage 1 surgery to the connection of completed prostheses. Int J Oral Maxillofac Implants 1991;6:142–146.
16. Jemt T, Lekholm U. Oral implant treatment in posterior partially edentulous jaws: a 5-year follow-up report. Int J Oral Maxillofac Implants 1993;8:635–640.
17. Lekholm U, Gunne J, Henry P, et al. Survival of the Brånemark implant in partially edentulous jaws: a 10-year prospective multicenter study. Int J Oral Maxillofac Implants 1999;14:639–645.
18. Friberg B, Grondahl K, Lekholm U, Brånemark PI. Long-term follow-up of severely atrophic edentulous mandibles reconstructed with short Brånemark implants. Clin Implant Dent Relat Res 2000;2:184–189.
19. Deporter D, Ogiso B, Sohn DS, et al. Ultrashort sintered porous-surfaced dental implants used to replace posterior teeth. J Periodontol 2008;79:1280–1286.
20. Urdaneta RA, Daher S, Leary J, et al. The survival of ultrashort locking-taper implants. Int J Oral Maxillofac Implants 2012;27:644–654.
21. Buser D, Nydegger T, Hirt HP, et al. Removal torque values of titanium implants in the maxilla of miniature pigs. Int J Oral Maxillofac Implants 1998;13:611–619.

22. Khang W, Feldman S, Hawley CE, Gunsolley J. A multi-center study comparing dual acid-etched and machined-surfaced implants in various bone qualities. J Periodontol 2001;72:1384–1390.

23. Quinlan P, Nummikoski P, Schenk R, et al. Immediate and early loading of SLA ITI single-tooth implants: an in vivo study. Int J Oral Maxillofac Implants 2005;20:360–370.

24. Monje A, Fu JH, Chan HL, et al. Do implant length and width matter for short dental implants (6–9 mm)? A meta-analysis of prospective studies. J Periodontol 2013;84(12):1783–1791.

25. Berglundh T, Persson L, Klinge B. A systematic review of the incidence of biological and technical complications in implant dentistry reported in prospective longitudinal studies of at least 5 years. J Clin Periodontol 2002;29(Suppl 3):197–212; discussion 232–233.

26. Blanes RJ, Bernard JP, Blanes ZM, Belser UC. A 10-year prospective study of ITI dental implants placed in the posterior region. II: Influence of the crown-to-implant ratio and different prosthetic treatment modalities on crestal bone loss. Clin Oral Implants Res 2007;18:707–714.

27. Malo P, de Araujo Nobre M, Rangert B. Short implants placed one-stage in maxillae and mandibles: a retrospective clinical study with 1 to 9 years of follow-up. Clin Implant Dent Relat Res 2007;9:15–21.

28. Fugazzotto PA. Shorter implants in clinical practice: rationale and treatment results. Int J Oral Maxillofac Implants 2008;23:487–496.

29. Sivolella S, Stellini E, Testori T, et al. Splinted and unsplinted short implants in mandibles: a retrospective evaluation with 5 to 16 years of follow-up. J Periodontol 2013;84:502–512.

30. Slotte C, Grønningsaeter A, Halmoy AM, et al. Four-millimeter implants supporting fixed partial dental prostheses in the severely resorbed posterior mandible: two-year results. Clin Implant Dent Relat Res 2012;14(Suppl 1):e46–e58.

31. Annibali S, Cristalli MP, Dell'Aquila D, et al. Short dental implants: a systematic review. J Dent Res 2012;91:25–32.

32. Monje A, Chan HL, Fu JH, et al. Are short dental implants (<10 mm) effective? A meta-analysis on prospective clinical trials. J Periodontol 2013;84(7):895–904.

33. Srinivasan M, Vazquez L, Rieder P, et al. Survival rates of short (6 mm) micro-rough surface implants: a review of literature and meta-analysis. Clin Oral Implants Res 2014;25(5):539–545.

34. Pommer B, Frantal S, Willer J, et al. Impact of dental implant length on early failure rates: a meta-analysis of observational studies. J Clin Periodontol 2011;38:856–863.

35. Telleman G, Raghoebar GM, Vissink A, et al. A systematic review of the prognosis of short (<10 mm) dental implants placed in the partially edentulous patient. J Clin Periodontol 2011;38:667–676.

36. Jaffin RA, Berman CL. The excessive loss of Brånemark fixtures in type IV bone: a 5-year analysis. J Periodontol 1991;62:2–4.

37. Adell R, Eriksson B, Lekholm U, et al. Long-term follow-up study of osseointegrated implants in the treatment of totally edentulous jaws. Int J Oral Maxillofac Implants 1990;5:347–359.

38. Lindhe J, Cecchinato D, Bressan EA, et al. The alveolar process of the edentulous maxilla in periodontitis and non-periodontitis subjects. Clin Oral Implants Res 2012;23:5–11.

39. Himmlova L, Dostalova T, Kacovsky A, Konvickova S. Influence of implant length and diameter on stress distribution: a finite element analysis. J Prosthet Dent 2004;91:20–25.

40. Petrie CS, Williams JL. Comparative evaluation of implant designs: influence of diameter, length, and taper on strains in the alveolar crest. A three-dimensional finite-element analysis. Clin Oral Implants Res 2005;16:486–494.

41. Deporter D, Pilliar RM, Todescan R, et al. Managing the posterior mandible of partially edentulous patients with short, porous-surfaced dental implants: early data from a clinical trial. Int J Oral Maxillofac Implants 2001;16:653–658.

42. Renouard F, Nisand D. Short implants in the severely resorbed maxilla: a 2-year retrospective clinical study. Clin Implant Dent Relat Res 2005;7(Suppl 1):S104–S110.

43. Urdaneta RA, Leary J, Lubelski W, et al. The effect of implant size 5 × 8 mm on crestal bone levels around single-tooth implants. J Periodontol 2012;83:1235–1244.

44. Bidez MW, Misch CE. Force transfer in implant dentistry: basic concepts and principles. J Oral Implantol 1992;18:264–274.

45. McGuire MK, Nunn ME. Prognosis versus actual outcome. III. The effectiveness of clinical parameters in accurately predicting tooth survival. J Periodontol 1996;67:666–674.

46. Shillingburg HT Sumiya H, Whitsett LD, et al. Fundamentals of Fixed Prosthodontics, 3rd edn. Carol Stream, IL: Quintessence; 1997, pp 85–103, 191–192.

47. Nelson SJ. Wheeler's Dental Anatomy, Physiology, and Occlusion, 9th edn. St Louis, MO: Saunders Elsevier; 2010.

48. Grossmann Y, Sadan A. The prosthodontic concept of crown-to-root ratio: a review of the literature. J Prosthet Dent 2005;93:559–562.

49. Misch CE. Clinical Biomechanics in Implant Dentistry. Contemporary Implant Dentistry, 3rd edn. St Louis, MO: Mosby Elsevier; 2008, pp 543–555.

50. Greenstein G, Cavallaro Jr JS. Importance of crown to root and crown to implant ratios. Dent Today 2011;30:61–62, 64, 66 passim; quiz 71, 60.

51. Blanes RJ. To what extent does the crown–implant ratio affect the survival and complications of implant-supported reconstructions? A systematic review. Clin Oral Implants Res 2009;20(Suppl 4):67–72.

52. Schulte J, Flores AM, Weed M. Crown-to-implant ratios of single tooth implant-supported restorations. J Prosthet Dent 2007;98:1–5.

53. Tawil G, Younan R. Clinical evaluation of short, machined-surface implants followed for 12 to 92 months. Int J Oral Maxillofac Implants 2003;18:894–901.

54. Rokni S, Todescan R, Watson P, et al. An assessment of crown-to-root ratios with short sintered porous-surfaced implants supporting prostheses in partially edentulous patients. Int J Oral Maxillofac Implants 2005;20:69–76.

55. Urdaneta RA, Rodriguez S, McNeil DC, et al. The effect of increased crown-to-implant ratio on single-tooth locking-taper implants. Int J Oral Maxillofac Implants 2010;25:729–743.
56. Misch CE, Steignga J, Barboza E, et al. Short dental implants in posterior partial edentulism: a multicenter retrospective 6-year case series study. J Periodontol 2006;77:1340–1347.
57. Guljé F, Abrahamsson I, Chen S, et al. Implants of 6 mm vs. 11 mm lengths in the posterior maxilla and mandible: a 1-year multicenter randomized controlled trial. Clin Oral Implants Res 2013; 24(12):1325–1331.
58. Guichet DL, Yoshinobu D, Caputo AA. Effect of splinting and interproximal contact tightness on load transfer by implant restorations. J Prosthet Dent 2002;87:528–535.
59. Hauchard E, Fournier BP, Jacq R, et al. Splinting effect on posterior implants under various loading modes: a 3D finite element analysis. Eur J Prosthodont Restor Dent 2011;19:117–122.
60. Yilmaz B, Seidt JD, McGlumphy EA, Clelland NL. Comparison of strains for splinted and nonsplinted screw-retained prostheses on short implants. Int J Oral Maxillofac Implants 2011;26:1176–1182.
61. Balshi TJ, Wolfinger GJ. Two-implant-supported single molar replacement: interdental space requirements and comparison to alternative options. Int J Periodontics Restorative Dent 1997;17:426–435.
62. Vigolo P, Zaccaria M. Clinical evaluation of marginal bone level change of multiple adjacent implants restored with splinted and nonsplinted restorations: a 5-year prospective study. Int J Oral Maxillofac Implants 2010;25:1189–1194.
63. Esposito M, Cannizarro G, Soardi E, et al. A 3-year post-loading report of a randomised controlled trial on the rehabilitation of posterior atrophic mandibles: short implants or longer implants in vertically augmented bone? Eur J Oral Implantol 2011;4:301–311.
64. Esposito M, Pellegrino G, Pistilli R, Felice P. Rehabilitation of posterior atrophic edentulous jaws: prostheses supported by 5 mm short implants or by longer implants in augmented bone? One-year results from a pilot randomised clinical trial. Eur J Oral Implantol 2011;4:21–30.
65. Cannizzaro G, Felice P, Minciarelli AF, et al. Early implant loading in the atrophic posterior maxilla: 1-stage lateral versus crestal sinus lift and 8 mm hydroxyapatite-coated implants. A 5-year randomised controlled trial. Eur J Oral Implantol 2013;6:13–25.
66. Aghaloo TL, Moy PK. Which hard tissue augmentation techniques are the most successful in furnishing bony support for implant placement? Int J Oral Maxillofac Implants 2007;22(Suppl):49–70.
67. Rocchietta I, Fontana F, Simion M. Clinical outcomes of vertical bone augmentation to enable dental implant placement: a systematic review. J Clin Periodontol 2008;35:203–215.
68. Jensen SS, Terheyden H. Bone augmentation procedures in localized defects in the alveolar ridge: clinical results with different bone grafts and bone-substitute materials. Int J Oral Maxillofac Implants 2009;24(Suppl):218–236.
69. Schwarz F, Alcoforado G, Nelson K, et al. Impact of implant–abutment connection, positioning of the machined collar/microgap, and platform switching on crestal bone level changes. Camlog Foundation Consensus Report. Clin Oral Implants Res 2014;25(11):1301–1303.
70. Atieh MA, Ibrahim HM, Atieh AH. Platform switching for marginal bone preservation around dental implants: a systematic review and meta-analysis. J Periodontol 2010;81:1350–1366.
71. Urdaneta RA, Daher S, Lery J, et al. Factors associated with crestal bone gain on single-tooth locking-taper implants: the effect of nonsteroidal anti-inflammatory drugs. Int J Oral Maxillofac Implants 2011;26:1063–1078.
72. Linkevicius T, Apse P, Grybauskas S, Puisys A. The influence of soft tissue thickness on crestal bone changes around implants: a 1-year prospective controlled clinical trial. Int J Oral Maxillofac Implants 2009;24:712–719.
73. Lin GH, Chan HL, Wang HL. The significance of keratinized mucosa on implant health: a systematic review. J Periodontol 2013;84:1755–1767.
74. Urdaneta RA, Leary J, Panetta KM, Chuang SK. The effect of opposing structures, natural teeth vs. implants on crestal bone levels surrounding single-tooth implants. Clin Oral Implants Res 2014;25:e179–e188.

Answers to Self-Study Questions

A. The definition of short implants is not unequivocal, and every study has its own definition [14]. However, 10 mm is a threshold accepted by most clinicians to differentiate a "short" or "long" implant. In the early age of implant dentistry, 10- mm residual bone height was considered the minimal amount of bone required to place a "standard-length" implant. The implant, which had a length ≥10 mm, was called a standard implant or long implant. Early trials using smooth-surface implants demonstrated a higher failure rate of short implants (<10 mm) compared with long implants [15,16,17]. Years later, one study demonstrated the first long-term (mean 8 years, range 1–14 years) successful clinical outcomes (cumulative survival rate: 95.5% in 5 years; 92.3% in 10 years) of the short Brånemark system implants (247 implants in 3.75 mm × 7 mm and 13 implants in 5 mm × 6 mm) [18]. Recently, some studies defined implants ≤6 mm long as "ultrashort" implants and demonstrated successful clinical outcomes [19,20]. For these two cases, we define a short implant as an implant with a length of less than 10 mm.

Nowadays, rough-surface implants demonstrate better mechanical and biological characteristics than traditional machined-surface implants [21–23]. The length of an implant might not be a concern in most clinical situations anymore [24]. Therefore, short implants might not be considered "short" in the future. With the routine use of implants of shorter length (<10 mm), the definition of short implants seems to be changing, and it is possible that only those implants shorter than 6 mm will be considered "short" in the future.

B. As discussed in the answer to question A, the definition for short dental implant continues to evolve. The once considered standard length dental implant might now be considered too long for routine use. Many sites of implantation have insufficient bone height because of previous significant bone loss or bony defect. One could argue most edentulous sites might be applicable for a short dental implant given its comparable short- and long-term success (more details will be discussed in the answer to question C). However, the threshold of short implant placement for different clinical scenarios has yet to be defined. It is generally accepted that a short dental implant is indicated where alveolar ridge height is limited but there is sufficient width.

Both atrophic maxilla and mandible present anatomical limitations and vital structures that hamper the placement of long dental implants, including pneumatized sinus, inferior alveolar nerve, mental foramen, and lingual concavity. When facing these situations, the viable option of placing shorter dental implants should be proposed to the patients. Especially for medically compromised patients who cannot endure several surgical appointments or when a bone grafting procedure is a great challenge, such as vertical augmentation, short dental implants may serve as a better option to reduce potential complications. Short dental implants could also be the last resort if a bone grafting procedure is unsuccessful.

C. Insufficient bone height is a significant problem for implant placement. A vertical augmentation procedure to increase bone height is technically sensitive and can cause significant postoperative morbidities and complications [25]. The sinus lift procedure at the posterior maxilla is more predictable than other vertical augmentation procedures since the graft materials can be held in the sinus with sufficient blood supply from the alveolar bone and sinus membrane [6]. However, extra augmentation procedures always increase cost, morbidity, and treatment time. Short implant placement is another alternative option for these clinical situations, and there is clinical evidence supporting its predictability.

Several clinical studies have shown high success rates (ranging from 94 to 99%) and predicable clinical outcomes of placing short implants with long-term follow-up of up to 10 years [14,26–29]. One retrospective cohort study demonstrated a cumulative survival rate of 97.5% in 410 short implants (5–8 mm) during a mean 20-month follow-up period [20]. Even 4 mm short implants had predictable clinical outcomes with a 92.3% survival rate and close to 0.5 mm crestal bone change in 2 years [30]. Several systematic reviews of short implants also demonstrated high survival or success rates. One 2012 study included 6193 short implants (<10 mm) and demonstrated a cumulative survival rate of 99.1% during a mean 3.2 ± 1.7-year follow-up [31]. The success rate without any biological or biomechanical complications was 98.8% or 99.8% respectively. Another 2012 study demonstrated an estimated survival rate of 88.1% for short implants (6–9 mm) and 86.7% for standard implants (≥10 mm) in a 168-month follow-up period without statistical significant difference [32]. In the extended review of the same research group, the length or diameter of the short implants did not seem to affect the survival rate [24]. In a meta-analysis that focused on 6 mm nonsubmerged Straumann implants, the cumulative survival rate was 93.7% (follow-up range 1–8 years) [33]. The studies included in these reviews had different kinds of prostheses, including full-arch fixed prostheses, partial fixed prostheses, implant-supported overdentures, and hybrid prostheses. The results supported the use of short implant restored with various prostheses.

With regard to location of implant placement, short implants seemed to have higher failure rates in the maxilla than the mandible [31,32,34,35]. Standard implants have also shown higher failure rates in the maxilla [36,37]. The reason for the increase in failure rates for implants placed in the maxilla seems to be the low bone density [36] or haphazard trabecular orientation [38], which could reduce primary stability at placement and then increase the risk of failure. However, these studies have some limitations, such as the use of machined-surface implants or small sample sizes [31]. Therefore, more clinical trials comparing the survival of rough-surface short implants in maxilla and mandible are needed.

Finite-element studies have shown significantly higher crestal bone strains surrounding short implants when compared with long ones [39,40], and this increased strain has been theoretically correlated to crestal bone loss. However, this rationale is not supported with the available scientific evidence clinically. Changes in bone levels

surrounding short implants have been reported to be similar to bone levels on longer implants. A 2000 study demonstrated a mean crestal bone resorption of 0.9 ± 0.6 mm in 270 short implants in 10 years [18]. Another study demonstrated 0.13 ± 0.12 mm resorption of 15 short implants in 3 years [41]. Renouard et al. in 2005 demonstrated 0.44 ± 0.52 mm bone resorption of 96 short implants in 2 years [42]. One retrospective cohort demonstrated 0.36 mm and 0.04 mm average loss of crestal bone level in maxilla and mandible respectively of 97 short implants (5 mm × 8 mm) followed for an average of 5.9 years [43].

In summary, clinical studies on short implants have demonstrated high survival rates, stable bone levels, and low complication rates. These studies validate the practicability and predictability of short implants.

D. Crown height is positively related to the moment of force on the teeth or implants [44]. For natural tooth, crown-to-root ratio has been used as a clinical predictor of the prognosis of periodontally compromised teeth [45] or prognosis of the fixed restorations [46]. Crown-to-root ratio is generally about 0.6 for maxillary teeth and 0.55 for mandibular teeth [47]. A crown-to-tooth ratio of 1:1 has been suggested as the minimum threshold for successful fixed partial dentures supported on natural teeth, but there is limited scientific evidence on the subject [48]. For implant-supported restorations, it has been proposed that the larger moment of force produced by increased CIR could lead to an increase in crestal bone loss around implants [49]. Even though increased forces on short implants have been demonstrated in in vitro studies [50], the deleterious effect of increased CIR has not been replicated in clinical studies. In a systematic review, a CIR of 2 has been suggested as the maximal threshold for fixed implant-supported restorations [51]. A retrospective study of 889 implants with a mean follow-up of 2.3 years reported no significant differences between the mean CIR of failed implants (1.4:1) and the mean CIR of all implants (1.3:1) [52]. Clinical trials have demonstrated that increased CIR (in general 1–2, up to 4.95) were associated with an increase in loosening and fracture of abutments but did not lead to crestal bone resorption or implant failure [26,53–55]. In a prospective study with a mean follow-up of 46 months, short implants (5 or 7 mm, mean CIR 2.6 or 1.8) demonstrated 0.2 mm less crestal resorption than long implants (9 or 12 mm, mean CIR 1.4 or 1.0) [54]. Owing to the anatomical limitations, short implants with high CIR are usually placed in posterior areas. Also, short implants with a wide diameter (>4 mm) have been used [55]. The increase in implant diameter may compensate for the increased forces caused by increased CIR [39,40]. In summary, clinical studies have shown that increased CIR leads to an increase in prosthetic complications, but it is not correlated to an increase in implant failure or bone loss with short implants.

It has been suggested that splinting multiple short implants may help in force distribution [56,57]. In vitro model studies have demonstrated better force distribution in splinted implants than in individual implants [58–60]. It has been reported that splinting implants increases resistance to lateral loads, decreases the risk of implant component fractures [49], and reduces abutment screw loosening on screw-retained implant restorations [61]. However, splinting implants has not been shown to decrease implant failures and/or reduce bone loss in clinical studies. Clinical outcomes (survival rate, bone level changes) are similar for splinted and nonsplinted implant restorations [62]. Splinted implant restorations with high CIR have demonstrated similar crestal bone level changes to nonsplinted implants in clinical studies [54]. Therefore, splinting multiple short implants may reduce prosthetic complications, but it does not seem to improve implant survival and/or preserve crestal bone.

E. Even though the placements of short implants and long implants have shown similar complications, bone augmentation procedures, which add a new set of possible complications, are commonly needed to place longer implants.

A systematic review of short implants [31] reported biological success rates (defined as absences of persistent pain, peri-implant inflammation, peri-implant radiolucency, and implant mobility) of 98.8% (95% confidence interval (CI): 97.8–99.8%) and biomechanical success rates (defined as absence of fractured occlusal materials,

fractured or loosened prosthetic components, implant fracture, and/or prosthesis instability) of 99.9% (95% CI: 99.4–100.0%). In all selected studies reporting biological complications, the biological success ranged from 89.5% to 100%. In 1346 prosthetically restored implants of seven selected studies, only four biomechanical complications were reported in a mean follow-up period of 2.6 years.

In several randomized clinical trials, short implants (≤8 mm) did not demonstrate higher rates of biological or biomechanical complications when compared with longer implants [57,63–65].

The need for vertical augmentation procedures prior to the placement of implants increases the rate of complications associated with longer implants. From the previous reviews, the implant survival rate involving vertical augmentation procedures ranged around 90.4–83.8% (during a follow-up period of 1–5 years), which was lower than generally accepted implant survival rate [66], and vertical augmentation procedures also had high complication rates (>10%) [67,68].

In summary, in cases where short implants can be used in lieu of augmentation procedures, a significant reduction in surgical and postoperative complications can be expected. If there is sufficient bone, the complication rates of short and long implants may be similar.

F. Table 1 summarizes various factors the clinician has to pay attention to when using short implants.

At the implant/bone level, primary stability is a major concern since the surface for mechanical engagement is limited for most screw-type short dental implants. When placing short screw-type

Table 1: Concerns at Different Level for Short Dental Implant

Implant/ bone level	Primary stability
	Preserve bone around short implant
Abutment/soft tissue level	Proper abutment used to decrease bone resoprtion and prosthetic complication
	Adequate soft tissue
Prosthesis/occlusion level	Proper occlusion surface design
	Avoid parafunctional forces

dental implants into low -ensity bone such as posterior maxilla, one might consider doing undersized osteotomy for better primary stability. It is also important to make sure there is sufficient buccal and lingual bone thickness to minimize potential risk of bone resorption.

Since the implant length is short, it is also crucial to minimize crestal bone remodeling whenever possible. Animal studies have shown that subcrestal placement of the short dental implants may serve to maintain the osseointegrated surface over the rough surface [69]. Short implants (5 mm wide by 8 mm long) with an HA coating and subcrestal placement have shown very stable bone level in a retrospective cohort study during a mean follow-up of 5.9 years [43].

Short dental implant design and selection may be crucial for a successful outcome. At the abutment and soft tissue level, using a platform switching abutment may be helpful in reducing the amount of crestal bone remodeling [70]. In addition, abutment design may play a role in crestal bone stability [71]. The amount and quality of soft tissue may also play a role in maintaining the crestal bone level of dental implants. Thinner initial tissue thickness

(<2 mm) may be associated with more crestal bone remodeling [72], and a lack of keratinized tissue around dental implants is also associated with more attachment loss and significantly higher plaque and gingival index [73]. Although these factors are not specific to the placement of short dental implants, clinicians should still be aware of the potential concerns at this interface.

At the prosthesis and occlusion level, the longer crown or higher CIR would not affect the survival of the implants as discussed in the answer to question D, but may increase prosthetic complications [71]. If the implant is opposing an implant-supported fixed restoration, it is associated with more crestal bone loss compared with those occluding against natural teeth [74]. Excessive parafunctional forces are also a concern. Some possible clinical modifications can be considered: (1) Decrease lateral forces or excursive interference to the posterior implant prosthesis by adjusting occlusion. (2) Avoid cantilevers. (3) Increase the number of implants to support long spans. (4) Increase the diameters of implants to compensate unfavorable lateral force. (5) Increase the surface area of osseointegration by using rough-surfaced implants.

Acknowledgment

Clinical radiographs and photographs were supplied courtesy of Implant Dentistry Center, Boston, MA, USA.

Case 6

Platform Switching

Medical History

The patient is in good health and receives regular checkups with her physician every 4 months. No contraindications for treatment were found. There are no reported drug allergies and the patient has no medical issues.

The patient denies a history of:
- rheumatic fever, heart disease, heart surgery
- immunocompromising diseases (e.g., hepatitis, human immunodeficiency virus, acquired immune deficiency syndrome)
- prolonged bleeding or easy bruising
- endocrine abnormalities
- malignancy
- prescription medications
- prosthetic joints.

Review of Systems

- Vital signs
  - Blood pressure: 130/82 mmHg
  - Pulse rate: 62 beats/min
  - Respiration: 16 breaths/min
  - O$_2$ saturation: 99%
- Weight: 120 lbs

Social History

The patient works as a teller at a bank. She reveals that she has had a difficult time balancing a 40-hour work week, the household, and children. She also mentions not having enough time to attend to her dental checkups. She denies drinking alcohol or smoking.

Extraoral Examination

There were no significant findings. The patient has no masses or swelling, and no trismus is found. There were no masses on palpation. There was a slight deviation to the left when the patient opened her jaw. No popping or crepitus noted on opening.

Intraoral Examination

There were no masses or lesions noted on examination of the soft tissues. Gingival examination shows generalized moderate erythema.

A small amount of keratinized tissue was observed and there was limited vestibular depth in the left edentulous area. Tooth #32 had a full metal crown and was found to have class 3 mobility. Tooth #29 also had a full metal crown.

Tooth #25 was a single implant and tooth #22 had a porcelain-fused-to-metal (PFM) restoration.

The maxilla is edentulous.

Occlusion

There is a lack of vertical dimension, and the lower teeth have extruded.

Radiographic Examination

The maxillary ridge is edentulous with bilateral low sinus floors.

Tooth #32 has localized severe bone loss, with a root canal and poor adaptation of the metal crown. Due to bone loss, extraction of the tooth will be carried out.

Tooth #29 has mild bone loss, and there is recurrent decay.

Teeth #28 and #27 have direct restorations. Teeth #26, #24, #23, and #21 have root canal treatment, and tooth #22 has a PFM crown.

There is a single implant at the position of #25.

The edentulous area in the left mandible quadrant appears adequate and there is enough room to the inferior alveolar nerve to allow placement of an implant.

There has been severe bone loss in the edentulous area in the right portion of mandible and there is inadequate room to place an implant due to the proximity of the inferior alveolar canal (Figure 1).

Treatment

Although a comprehensive treatment plan was presented to the patient to address all of the issues, the patient only seeks for implant, #18–#21, #30, and #31.

Once the realistic treatment plan was consented to, the patient received oral hygiene instructions and a prophylaxis.

Preoperative Consultation

After reevaluation the surgical phase began. The medical history was reviewed, and consent forms describing benefits and risk associated with the procedure were reviewed and signed by the patient.

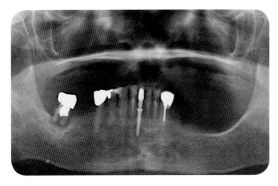

Figure 1: Preoperative panoramic radiograph of patient.

The patient was instructed to stop taking any aspirin that is more than 81 mg 7 days before the surgery.

From the day before the surgery the patient was instructed to take amoxicillin 875 mg bid for 7 days, and take ibuprofen 600 mg q6h prn for pain for 5 days.

Implant Placement

An inferior alveolar block with carbocaine 4% without epinephrine and local infiltration with septocaine 2% 1:100,000 were administered to the edentulous area. Tooth #32 due to the bone loss that caused class 3 mobility, which gave it a hopeless prognosis.

A crestal incision was made a full-thickness flap was elevated in the mandibular edentulous ridge from the extracted site to tooth #29.

Vertical incisions (about 4 mm) on the lingual and buccal ridge were made mesially and sutured with 4-0 silk to aid in retraction for better visibility.

Osteotomy was started with a lance drill at 1000 rpm with saline solution as irrigation.

The drilling sequence was carried out for both implants #30 and #31. For tooth #31 a Megagen Exfeel 5 mm × 10 mm fixture was inserted, and for #30 a Megagen Exfeel 4.5 mm × 11.5 mm implant was inserted. Both implants were placed at the level of the bone.

A postoperative radiograph was taken. The positioning of the dental implants was normal, and there was no infringement of the nerve canal.

Cover screws were placed to cover and protect the internal connection of the implant and the flap was closed to begin healing process for 2 months.

After 2 months, a second-stage surgery was performed to expose and remove the cover screws. The healing abutments were placed.

After 4 months, healing abutments were removed to continue with the restorative phase.

On the contralateral site a similar surgical protocol was used. Megagen EZ plus fixtures were placed at the level of the bone at the #18, #19, #20, and #21 sites. A postoperative radiograph revealed ideal placement with no damage to anatomical structures.

A cover screw was placed on every implant, and the flap was closed with interrupted sutures.

After 2 months the cover screws were removed and the healing abutments placed and the platform switching system used for #19, #20, and #21.

Four months later, healing abutments were removed and impressions were obtained for the final restorations.

Post-Operative Radiographic Follow-Up

See Figures 2, 3, 4, 5, 6, 7, and 8.

Discussion

Radiographic follow-up after 2 years shows the bone loss on the right side was more evident and gradual. The panoramic radiograph reveals that the bone is gradually being lost in the crestal portion that surrounds the implant neck. On other hand, in radiographs depicting the left side, the crestal bone surrounding the implant necks appears to be well maintained by the use of platform switching in the final restoration (except #21, which did not have platform switching). According to Albrektsson et al., a normal rate of bone loss around implant sites after the first year is 1 mm; after the first year the normal rate of bone loss is 0.1 mm every consecutive year [1].

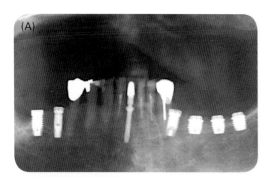

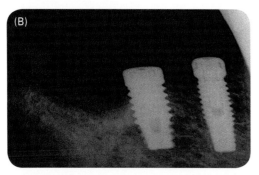

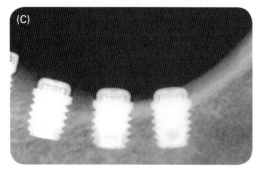

Figure 2: (A) Postoperative panoramic radiograph, showing both surgical sites with fixtures already placed. (B, C) We can appreciate how fixtures have been placed at bone level in both surgical sites; no anatomical structure has been compromised.

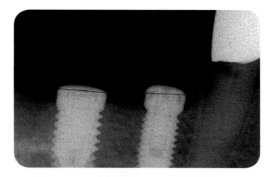

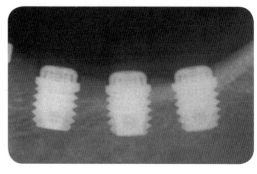

Figure 3: Two-month postoperative. Bone levels are within acceptable healing limits for this time period.

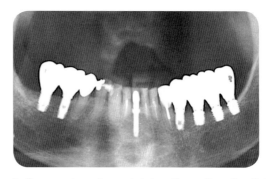

Figure 4: Panoramic radiograph taken 6 months after fixture placement compares both non-platform-switched and platform-switched sites. Note the bone loss in crestal bone surrounding implants in lower left side (0.5 mm in implant #30).

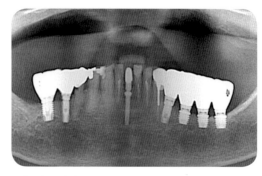

Figure 5: Patient follow-up continued 1 year after the procedure. More evident bone loss is observed in the lower left implants. Right side bone level surrounding implants looks in good condition; bone loss has not been an issue.

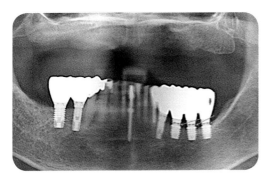

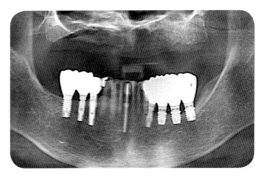

Figure 6: Follow-up on non-platform-switched implants shows greater bone loss after 2 years of final restorations placement. Green arrows indicate implant–abutment junction.

Figure 8: After 3 years of radiological follow-up. Radiological evidence shows that bone loss in non-platform-switched implants side is greater than on right side mandible where platform-switched restorations were placed.

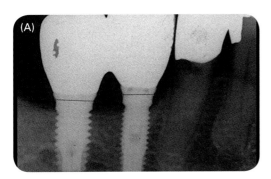

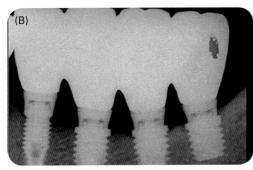

Figure 7: (A) Two years after fixture placement the bone level surrounding the implant neck in left side of mandible has been lost by up to 2 mm (red lines represent the initial bone level 2 years ago). (B) Bone level surrounding implants on right side of mandible has been kept at a good level and is associated with platform switching.

The platform switching concept was discovered by accident in 1991 when Lazzara and Porter used a smaller diameter abutment on a large diameter implant collar. Twenty-five years ago implants of 5 and 6 mm diameter did not have any matching diameter abutments. The difference in diameter between available abutments and implants was 0.9–1.9 mm. After the accidental discovery, follow-up radiographs at 1–5 years revealed little bone loss in comparison with implants fitted with matching diameter components [2].

Several investigations state that location of the implant–abutment junctions directly affects crestal bone that is in direct contact with fixture, as shown in Figure 4. The bacterial colonization of the microgap at the implant–abutment junction and the establishment of a biological width or mucosal barrier around the implant are some factors that most likely affect crestal bone level changes [3–7].

Histomorphometric studies indicate that platform switching may have other advantages besides crestal bone level preservation, such as improving esthetics by maintaining the peri-implant soft and hard tissue. This would be beneficial in esthetically demanding locations and also help achieve better primary stability [6,8].

Degidi et al. indicated that connective tissue grows in the fixture shoulder after 28 days of implantation, which provides strength and stability to the implant [9]. Because of this new tissue that grows around the fixture neck it is speculated that bacterial invasion into the implant–abutment junction is now prevented so that crestal bone around the dental implant neck can be preserved. You can see an example of this in Figure 6 on #18, #19, and #20. Li et al. conducted a radiological follow-up for 2–6 years and found less complications in platform switching [10]. This is illustrated in Figure 7 for #18, #19, and #20, which shows 0.3 mm bone loss in 2 years versus #30 and #31 showing 2 mm bone loss. Hürzeler et al. showed less bone resorption with platform switching (−0.29 ± 0.34 mm) than the control group that did not have platform switching (−2.02 ± 0.49 mm) [11,12].

Another reason for better bone maintenance around platform switching is the stress distribution. In a study published by Sahabi et al., six three-dimensional finite-element models demonstrated that, in conventional non-platform-switching models, the stress concentration was around the periphery of the uppermost surface of the implant. The neck of the implant is the area that has the deepest contact with crestal bone in conventional models. On other hand, platform-switched models showed that high stress is shifted toward the center of the implant, leaving crestal bone stress free [7]. So, how much platform difference is enough? In terms of extent of platform switching, a higher extent of platform switch has showed better stress distribution results, which means less stress in bone. However, more investigation should be done to gather information about the minimum or maximum platform extent [12].

According to Ruiz-Ramirez et al., abutment geometry influences the collagen fibers; therefore, a wider abutment will help in the formation of oblique and perpendicular orientation of collagen membrane. It also helps to create a greater connective tissue thickness [13]. This newly created connective tissue will help to achieve a natural soft tissue barrier that can also be called biological width or mucosal barrier. This natural barricade will protect the crestal bone that surrounds the implant site and give better esthetic results for the emergence profile of final restoration [2–6].

Self-Study Questions

(Answers located at the end of the case)

A. Who were the first two doctors that discovered platform switching and how did they discover it?

B. How does the microgap in the implant–abutment junction affect crestal bone level?

C. What other histomorphic advantages does platform switching have?

D. According to Degidi et al. [9], how soon can we find connective tissue and what does this provide?

E. What did Sahabi et al. [7] find in their three-dimensional finite-element study with regard to platform switching?

F. How does abutment geometry influence the collagen fibers surrounding it?

G. How does soft tissue help in bone maintenance?

References

1. Albrektsson T, Zarb G, Worthington P, Eriksson AR. The long-term efficacy of currently used dental implants: a review and proposed criteria of success. Int J Oral Maxillofac Implants 1986;1(1):11–25.
2. Lazzara RJ, Porter SS. Platform switching: a new concept in implant dentistry for controlling postrestorative crestal bone levels. Int J Periodontics Restorative Dent 2006;26:9–17.
3. Hermann FDL, Henriette DDS, Palti A. Factors influencing the preservation of the periimplant marginal bone. Implant Dent 2007;16(2):166–175.
4. Ericsson I, Persson LG, Berglundh T, et al. Different types of inflammatory reactions in peri-implant soft tissues. J Clin Periodontol 1995;22:255–261.
5. Berglundh T, Lindhe J. Dimension of the periimplant mucosa. Biological width revisited. J Clin Periodontol 1996;23(10):971–973.
6. Atieh MA, Ibrahim HM, Atieh AH. Platform switching for marginal bone preservation around dental implants: a systematic review and meta-analysis. J Periodontol 2010;81:1350–1366.
7. Sahabi M, Adibrad M, Mirhashemi FS, Habibzadeh S. Biomechanical effects of platform switching in two different implant systems: a three-dimensional finite element analysis. J Dent (Tehran) 2013;10(4):338–350.
8. Luongo R, Traini T, Guidone PC, et al. Hard and soft tissue responses to the platform-switching technique. Int J Periodontics Restorative Dent 2008;28(6):551–557.
9. Degidi M, Iezzi G., Scarano A, Piattelli A. Immediately loaded titanium implant with a tissue-stabilizing/maintaining design ('beyond platform switch') retrieved from man after 4 weeks: a histological and histomorphometrical evaluation. A case report. Clin Oral Implants Res 2008;19(3):276–282.
10. Li Q, Lin Y, Qiu LX, et al. Clinical study of application of platform switching to dental implant treatment in esthetic zone. Zhonghua Kou Qiang Yi Xue Za Zhi 2008;43(9):537–541 (in Chinese).
11. Hurzeler M, Fickl S, Zuhr O, Wachtel HC. Peri-implant bone level around implants with platform-switched abutments: preliminary data from a prospective study. J Oral Maxillofac Surg 2007;65(7 Suppl 1):33–39.
12. Singh R, Singh SV, Arora V. Platform switching: a narrative review. Implant Dent 2013;5:453–459.
13. Delgado-Ruiz RA, Calvo-Guirado JL, Abboud M, et al. Connective tissue characteristics around healing abutments of different geometries: new methodological technique under circularly polarized light. Clin Implant Dent Relat Res 2015;17(4):667–680.

Answers to Self-Study Questions

A. The platform switching concept started in 1991 when Lazzara and Porter introduced the idea that refers to the use of a smaller diameter abutment on a large-diameter implant collar.

B. Bacterial colonization of the microgap at the implant–abutment junction and the establishment of a biological width or mucosal barrier around the implant are among the factors that most likely cause crestal bone level changes.

C. Crestal bone level preservation, improving esthetics, and maintaining the peri-implant soft and hard tissue.

D. Connective tissue grows after 28 days of implantation in the implant shoulder, which provides strength and stability to the implant.

E. In conventional non-platform-switching models, the stress concentration was around the periphery of the uppermost surface of the implant. This is in the area with the deepest contact with crestal bone in conventional models. On the other hand, platform-switched models showed that high stress is shifted toward the center of the implant, leaving crestal bone stress free.

F. Abutment geometry influences the collagen fibers; therefore, a wider abutment will help in the formation of an oblique and perpendicular orientation of collagen membrane.

G. This newly created connective tissue will help in achieving a natural soft tissue barrier, which is also called the biological width or mucosal barrier. This natural barricade will protect the crestal bone that surrounds the implant site and give better esthetic results for the emergence profile of final restoration.

3

Prosthetic Design

Clinical Cases in Implant Dentistry, First Edition. Edited by Nadeem Karimbux and Hans-Peter Weber.
© 2017 John Wiley & Sons, Inc. Published 2017 by John Wiley & Sons, Inc.

Case 1

Abutment Design

CASE STORY

A 26-year-old Caucasian male presented with the chief complaint of "I am concerned with the health and esthetics of my implants." The patient displayed a uniquely high dental IQ, as he was a second-year predoctoral dental student at the time of his initial presentation. The patient had a history of congenitally missing maxillary canines and had undergone implant therapy to replace teeth #6 and #11 with implant-supported crowns at age 21 (Figure 1). Upon further

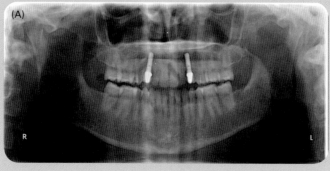

(A)

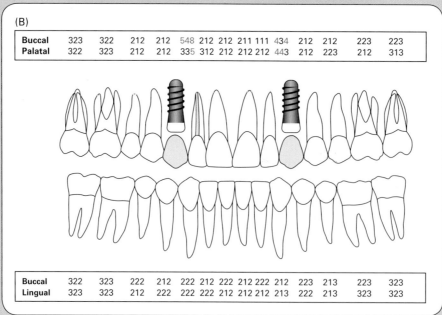

(B)

| Buccal | 323 | 322 | 212 | 212 | 548 | 212 | 212 | 211 | 111 | 434 | 212 | 212 | 223 | 223 |
| Palatal | 322 | 323 | 212 | 212 | 335 | 312 | 212 | 212 | 212 | 443 | 212 | 223 | 212 | 313 |

| Buccal | 322 | 323 | 222 | 212 | 222 | 212 | 222 | 212 | 222 | 212 | 223 | 213 | 223 | 323 |
| Lingual | 323 | 323 | 212 | 222 | 222 | 222 | 212 | 212 | 212 | 213 | 222 | 213 | 323 | 323 |

Figure 1: (A) Panoramic radiograph of patient at initial presentation. (B) Probing pocket depth measurements during the initial visit.

discussion, the patient revealed that his concern was related to the apparent chronic inflammation around his implants (Figure 2), manifested by bleeding upon routine oral hygiene procedures, such as brushing and interproximal flossing. As the patient had learned more about peri-implant health from his didactic lectures, he had recently become more concerned about the long-term prognosis of his implants and was seeking a diagnosis and treatment strategy for the source of his peri-implant inflammation.

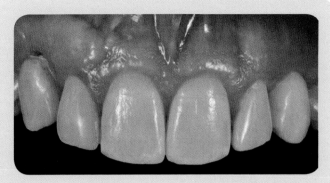

Figure 2: Preoperative clinical presentation (frontal view).

LEARNING GOALS AND OBJECTIVES

- To be able to recognize and diagnose cement-related peri-implant mucositis and peri-implantitis
- To understand the role of abutment design on the potential for excess cement around an implant-supported restoration
- To understand the effect that the surface topography of cements plays in bacterial biofilm production and proinflammatory processes
- To understand restorative approaches that can be utilized to minimize excess cement below an implant's restorative margin
- To understand the effect that the radiopacity of cements has on radiographic detection of excess peri-implant cement

Medical History

At the time of treatment the patient demonstrated no systemic health issues and was not taking any medications. The patient had a history of allergy to amoxicillin, manifested as urticaria.

Review of Systems

- Vital signs
  - Blood pressure: 126/78 mmHg
  - Pulse rate: 76 beats/min (regular)
  - Respiration: 15 breaths/min

Social History

The patient did not smoke or drink alcohol at the time of treatment.

Extraoral Examination

No significant findings were noted. The patient had no masses or swelling, and temporomandibular joint function was within normal limits. There was no facial asymmetry noted, and no signs of lymphadenopathy were found.

Intraoral Examination

- Oral cancer screening was negative.
- Soft tissue examination, including tongue and floor of the mouth, was within normal limits. Salivary status was within normal limits as well.
- Periodontal examination revealed pocket depths in the range of 1–8 mm, with bleeding on probing (BOP) limited to sites #6 and #11. Patient demonstrated excellent oral hygiene throughout dentition.
- Localized areas of gingival inflammation were noted in the peri-implant mucosa of #6 (Figure 3) and #11 (Figure 4), with visual erythema and a discontinuous marginal gingiva present on the midfacial aspect of site #6.
- Dentition demonstrated signs of enamel hypocalcification and pitting (#25 and #26) (Figure 5).

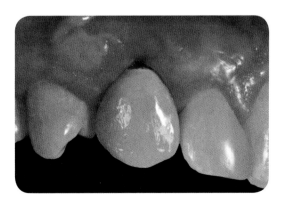

Figure 3: Preoperative presentation of implant #6 (midfacial view).

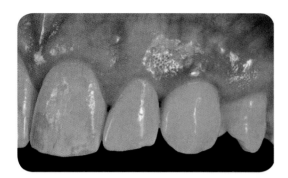

Figure 4: Preoperative presentation of implant #11 (midfacial view).

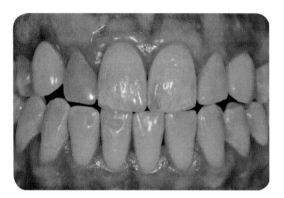

Figure 5: Preoperative presentation of centric occlusion (note anterior open bite and left unilateral crossbite; enamel hypocalcification and pitting also observed).

Occlusion

The patient's occlusion demonstrated an anterior open bite from #6 to #12, with a unilateral crossbite on the right side associated with teeth #4 and #5 (Figure 5). The patient lacked anterior disclusion protrusively and laterally, and thus demonstrated accelerated wear of the posterior occlusal surfaces.

Radiographic Examination

Posterior bitewings (Figure 6) and periapical radiographs of implants #6 (Figure 7A) and #11 (Figure 7B) were ordered. Radiographic examination of the bitewings revealed normal crestal bone levels on the natural

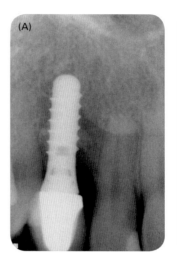
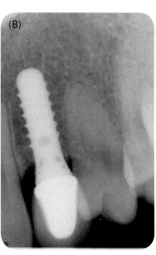

Figure 7: (A) Periapical radiograph of implant #6 demonstrating incomplete seating of the coronal restoration, excess cement on the mesial aspect of the implant body apical to the restorative platform, and vertical crestal bone loss on the mesial aspect of the implant. (B) Periapical radiograph of implant #11 demonstrating incomplete seating of the coronal restoration, excess cement on the mesial aspect of the implant body apical to the restorative platform, with stable crestal bone levels.

posterior dentition, absence of caries radiographically, and no previous restorations. Review of the implant periapical radiographs revealed soft-tissue-level implant bodies supporting incompletely seated implant crowns, visible as open radiographic margins, with excess cement noted on the mesial aspect of both implants. The mesial crestal bone level of implant #6 demonstrated ~1–2 mm of attachment loss apical to the noted excess cement. The crestal bone levels on the distal aspect of the maxillary lateral incisors demonstrated normal attachment levels.

Diagnosis

After reviewing the clinical and radiographic findings, diagnoses of cement-related peri-implantitis of implant #6 and cement-related peri-implant mucositis of implant #11 were made, consistent with recent summary reviews on this topic [1].

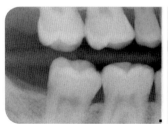
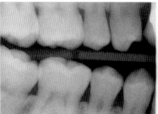
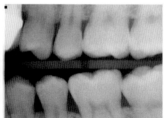
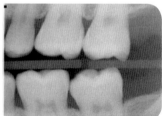

Figure 6: Bitewing radiographs of patient demonstrating stable bone levels and absence of previous restorative history.

Treatment Plan

The treatment plan for this patient consisted of amelioration of the clinical factors contributing to the observation of chronic inflammation around implants #6 and #11; namely, the removal of the incompletely seated restorations (which contributed to marginal gaps and thus inflammatory responses) and mechanical debridement and removal of the remaining excess cement along the walls of the transmucosal portion of the implant bodies. Upon achieving these two objectives, long-term provisionalization of the respective implant bodies with screw-retained interim restorations was planned. Evaluation of the peri-implant bone and mucosa would then take place over a period of 3–6 months prior to making a decision in regard to the definitive restorations.

Treatment

Diagnostic records, including mounted diagnostic casts, clinical photographs, and the aforementioned radiographs, were made prior to any surgical or prosthetic treatment began.

Upon approval of the treatment plan by the patient, implant crowns #6 and #11 were sectioned with a beaver bur and copious irrigation, with the aid of a dental operating microscope (Figure 8). Upon careful sectioning

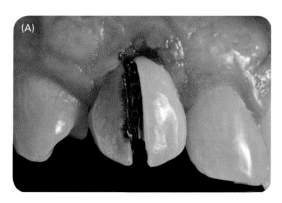

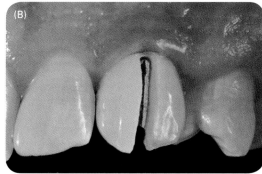

Figure 8: (A) Sectioning of implant #6 crown under dental operating microscope, paying attention to not inadvertently damaging the underlying abutment. (B) Sectioning of implant #11 crown using the same methodology.

of the crowns, with attention specifically directed to avoid damage of the underlying implant-abutments underneath, the crowns were removed with the aid of a crown-spreader and spoon excavator. The abutments were left intact (Figure 9) and subsequently removed with the aid of a Straumann solid abutment driver for regular neck (RN) solid abutments (Art No. 046.068, Straumann USA, Andover, MA, USA) (Figure 10).

A tunnel approach on the facial and mesial aspects of implant #6 was utilized to gain visual and mechanical access to the visually confirmed excess cement (Figure 11). Mechanical debridement with hand-scalers and ultrasonic scalers was utilized to physically

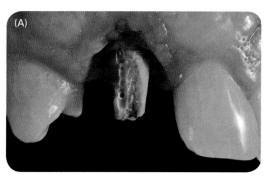

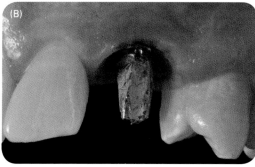

Figure 9: (A) After removal of the coronal restoration at implant #6, the underlying implant abutment is in view prior to removal. (B) View of abutment at implant #11 prior to removal

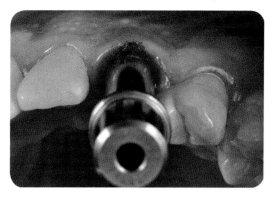

Figure 10: Use of abutment driver to remove the original restorative abutments to gain prosthetic and surgical access to the peri-implant tissues.

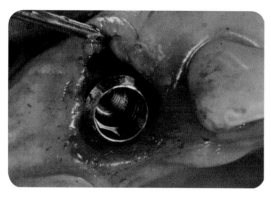

Figure 11: An envelope exposure of the midfacial aspect of implant #6 reveals visual confirmation of excess cement along the transmucosal aspect of the implant body.

remove the excess cement, which was abundant on the transmucosal collars of the implant bodies. Upon completion of mechanical removal of the excess cement (confirmed visually and tactilely), interim polyether ether ketone (PEEK) abutments (RN synOcta PEEK/ TAN temporary meso abutment, Art No. 048.668, Straumann USA, Andover, MA, USA) were modified in the transmucal and occlusal aspects to allow for proper emergence and clearance of the subsequent interim restorations. Interim, screw-retained implant-supported restorations were fabricated via a direct protocol (Figure 12), and were chosen for their retrievability and to remove excess cement as an etiology during attempted reattachment of peri-implant mucosal structures. At the conclusion of this debridement and provisionalization appointment, a bioresorbable minocycline gel (Arestin, Orapharma Inc., Bridgewater, NJ, USA) was inserted locally into the peri-implant mucosal sulcus (Figure 13) to help reduce the quantity of pathogenic bacteria in the sulcular environment and assist with healing.

Subsequent recall evaluations within 6 months of debridement and provisionalization demonstrated significant improvements in the probing depth measurements, BOP, and visual appearance of the peri-implant mucosa (Figure 14). However, due to the removal of chronic, cement-related peri-implant inflammation around implant #6, some midfacial mucosal recession was noted with exposure of the transmucosal metal collar of the soft-tissue-level implant shoulder. The patient has now been presented with the option(s) of undergoing subepithelial connective tissue grafting at site #6 and/or preparation of the implant collar, both in an effort to conceal this portion of the implant and thus to improve the esthetic integration of the restoration. The patient is currently considering both

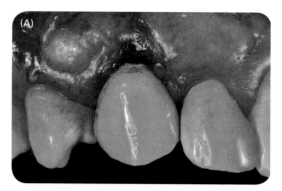

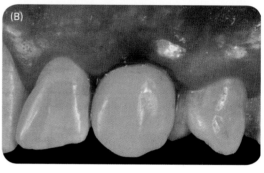

Figure 12: (A) Implant-level, screw-retained provisional restoration #6 fabricated chairside to optimize contour, remove cement-related etiology for inflammation, and allow straightforward retrieval. (B) Identical strategy employed for implant #11.

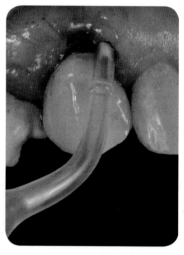

Figure 13: Application of Arestin (minocycline HCl) locally to the peri-implant sulcus to reduce pathologic bacteria and inflammation, as well as promote healing.

options and will make a definitive decision in the near future, as this case remains in progress.

Discussion

In this clinical case, the primary etiologies for peri-implantitis (implant #6) and peri-implant mucositis (implant #11) were (1) incompletely seated coronal

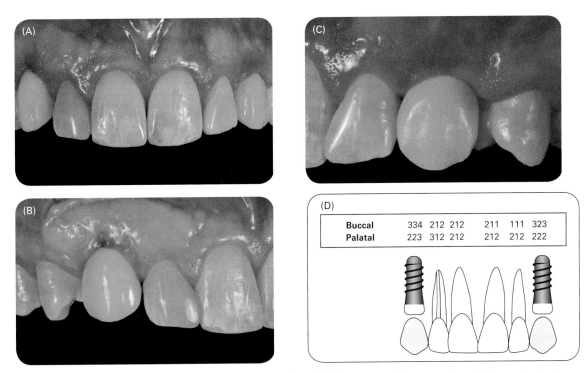

Buccal	334	212	212		211	111	323
Palatal	223	312	212		212	212	222

Figure 14: (A) Frontal view of provisional restorations 6 months after debridement and placement; note the reduction in marginal gingival inflammation at site #6, with concomitant recession of the midfacial mucosa. (B) Midfacial view of implant #6 interim restoration. (C) Midfacial view of implant #11 interim restoration. (D) Probing depths in upper front after treatment.

restorations and (2) excess luting cement apical to the prosthetic margins of the transmucosal implants.

While in North America the use of cement-retained implant crowns remains popular, it has been demonstrated that screw-retained implant-supported crowns exhibit smaller marginal gaps compared with the marginal gaps at cement-retained implant-supported crowns [2]. This is primarily attributable to the film thickness of the cement, even if the coping of the crown closely approximates the external surfaces and finish line of the transmucosal abutment [3–5]. In this specific case, the macrogaps that were created by the incomplete seating of the coronal restorations created a compartmentalized environment that was protective for the retention of bacteria, cellular debris, and other proinflammatory mediators. The presence of such a gap, especially if it is subgingival, and inaccessible for the patient to clean, can be deleterious to the long-term homeostasis of healthy peri-implant mucosa.

Additionally, and perhaps of greater significance, was the presence of excess cement apical to the prosthetic finish line and gingival margin of the implant-supported restorations. Excess cement below the suprastructure of implant-supported restorations has become increasingly correlated to peri-implantitis lesions and its associated biological complications [6–8]. These cement-related peri-implantitis sequelae are thought to occur due to a mechanism similar to what is seen with deposits (i.e., calculus and its associated biofilms) that create roughened topographies on natural teeth. Such roughened surface topographies potentially allow for bacterial colonization and biofilm formation [9,10], favoring anaerobic bacterial species (i.e., *Staphylococcus aureus* [10,11]) proliferation, and subsequent proinflammatory cytokine/chemokine-mediated soft- and hard-tissue remodeling. Evidence has demonstrated that removal of excess peri-implant cement is associated with a reduction or resolution of peri-implantitis symptoms [12].

Prosthetic strategies to minimize or eliminate excess cement include screw retention of implant-supported prostheses [13], custom abutments – that is, computer-aided design/computer-aided manufacturing (CAD/CAM) – with designs that move the prosthetic margin to an anatomically accessible location based on the peri-implant mucosal architecture, thus enabling more predictable cement removal [14], placing physical barriers such as retraction cords [15] in the peri-implant mucosal sulcus to prevent cement extrusion apically, as well as modifications of traditional clinical cementation protocols [16,17].

Self-Study Questions

(Answers located at the end of the case)

A. What is peri-implant mucositis?

B. What is peri-implantitis?

C. How does abutment design affect margin location relative to the marginal peri-implant mucosa?

D. How does an implant's abutment margin location affect the ability for predictable cement removal?

E. Is there a difference among dental cements for luting of implant-supported restorations?

References

1. American Academy of Periodontology. Peri-implant mucositis and peri-implantitis: a current understanding of their diagnoses and clinical implications. J Periodontol 2013;84:436–443.
2. Keith SE, Miller BH, Woody RD, Higginbottom FL. Marginal discrepancy of screw-retained and cemented metal-ceramic crowns on implants abutments. Int J Oral Maxillofac Implants 1999;14:369–378.
3. Wilson PR. Crown behaviour during cementation. J Dent 1992;20:156–162.
4. White SN, Yu Z, Tom JF, Sangsurasak S. In vivo marginal adaptation of cast crowns luted with different cements. J Prosthet Dent 1995;74:25–32.
5. Wu JC, Wilson PR. Optimal cement space for resin luting cements. Int J Prosthodont 1994;7:209–215.
6. Pauletto N, Lahiffe BJ, Walton JN. Complications associated with excess cement around crowns on osseointegrated implants: a clinical report. Int J Oral Maxillofac Implants 1999;14:865–868.
7. Gapski R, Neugeboren N, Pomeranz AZ, Reissner MW. Endosseous implant failure influenced by crown cementation: a clinical case report. Int J Oral Maxillofac Implants 2008;23:943–946.
8. Shapoff CA, Lahey BJ. Crestal bone loss and the consequences of retained excess cement around dental implants. Compend Contin Educ Dent 2012;33:94–96, 98–101; quiz 102, 112.
9. Salcetti JM, Moriarty JD, Cooper LF, et al. The clinical, microbial, and host response characteristics of the failing implant. Int J Oral Maxillofac Implants 1997;12:32–42.
10. Leonhardt A, Renvert S, Dahlen G. Microbial findings at failing implants. Clin Oral Implants Res 1999;10:339–345.
11. Heitz-Mayfield LJ, Lang NP. Comparative biology of chronic and aggressive periodontitis vs. peri-implantitis. Periodontol 2000 2010;53:167–181.
12. Wilson Jr TG. The positive relationship between excess cement and peri-implant disease: a prospective clinical endoscopic study. J Periodontol 2009;80:1388–1392.
13. Gervais MJ, Wilson PR. A rationale for retrievability of fixed, implant-supported prostheses: a complication-based analysis. Int J Prosthodont 2007;20:13–24.
14. Parpaiola A, Norton MR, Cecchinato D, et al. Virtual abutment design: a concept for delivery of CAD/CAM customized abutments – report of a retrospective cohort. Int J Periodontics Restorative Dent 2013;33:51–58.
15. Bennani V, Schwass D, Chandler N. Gingival retraction techniques for implants versus teeth: current status. J Am Dent Assoc 2008;139:1354–1363.
16. Dumbrigue HB, Abanomi AA, Cheng LL. Techniques to minimize excess luting agent in cement-retained implant restorations. J Prosthet Dent 2002;87:112–114.
17. Wadhwani C, Pineyro A. Technique for controlling the cement for an implant crown. J Prosthet Dent 2009;102:57–58.
18. Zitzmann NU, Berglundh T, Marinello CP, Lindhe J. Experimental peri-implant mucositis in man. J Clin Periodontol 2001;28:517–523.
19. Gualini F, Berglundh T. Immunohistochemical characteristics of inflammatory lesions at implants. J Clin Periodontol 2003;30:14–18.
20. Linkevicius T, Vindasiute E, Puisys A, et al. The influence of the cementation margin position on the amount of undetected cement. A prospective clinical study. Clin Oral Implants Res 2013;24:71–76.
21. Wadhwani C, Hess T, Faber T, et al. A descriptive study of the radiographic density of implant restorative cements. J Prosthet Dent 2010;103:295–302.
22. Pette GA, Ganeles J, Norkin FJ. Radiographic appearance of commonly used cements in implant dentistry. Int J Periodontics Restorative Dent 2013;33:61–68.

Answers to Self-Study Questions

A. Peri-implant mucositis is a condition in which the peri-implant mucosa is characterized by an inflammatory reaction. In this regard, it shares a similar etiology to peri-implantitis. However, unlike peri-implantitis, peri-implant mucositis is restricted only to the soft tissues surrounding the dental implant and does not demonstrate signs of crestal bone loss/destruction around the implant body beyond what would be considered normal bone remodeling following healing from implant surgery. Peri-implant mucositis is analogous to the process of gingivitis in natural teeth. Like gingivitis, the clinical signs and symptoms can be reversed via an improvement in oral hygiene procedures, or in the case of an acute mucositis reaction to a foreign body by the prompt removal of the offending object. Peri-implant mucositis is histologically characterized by the upregulation of T cells in the mucositis lesion and is confined to the barrier epithelium [18]. Clinical signs, such as BOP, peri-implant mucosal erythema, or suppuration, may all be signs of peri-implant mucositis.

B. Peri-implantitis, like peri-implant mucositis, is characterized by an inflammatory reaction. However, unlike peri-implant mucositis, peri-implantitis extends beyond the soft tissues and often results in destruction of the hard- and soft-tissue attachment to the implant body. In comparison with the natural dentition, peri-implantitis can be thought of as analogous to periodontitis. Unlike peri-implant mucositis, which is restricted histologically to the barrier epithelium, peri-implantitis extends further apically to the pocket epithelium. Histological analyses have demonstrated the significant presence of high numbers of plasma cells, lymphocytes, macrophages, and polymorphonuclear leukocytes [19]. Peri-implantitis, like peri-implant mucositis, can be a reversible phenomenon, as long as local and/or systemic contributing etiologies are addressed in an adequate timeframe. However, if etiological factors (such as excess cement in the clinical case presented here) are left unaddressed, crestal bone loss can occur, potentially resulting in the loss of osseointegration and failure of the endosseous implant.

C. Dental implant abutments that support a cement-retained coronal restoration (i.e., a single-tooth implant-supported crown or a multiple-unit implant-supported fixed partial denture) are typically fabricated from one of three possible designs (Figure 15). Each of these design categories has ramifications for the predictability of margin position placement relative to the adjacent peri-implant mucosa. The most rudimentary design is that of the prefabricated stock abutment. Prefabricated/stock abutments typically have a predetermined coronal collar height that provides retention and resistance form for the coronal restoration, as well as emergence width and height options, depending on the particular implant system or manufacturer. Prefabricated/stock abutments are also characterized by a flat circumferential restorative platform, which does not take into account local anatomic peri-implant mucosal variation, and are typically limited to titanium. Moving to slightly more complex designs, many implant manufacturers offer *semi-anatomic* abutments, which have prefabricated semi-anatomic design features, such as scalloped restorative platforms and various emergence height and width options as well as collar heights. Many of these semi-anatomic abutments can also be prepared (subtractive approach) within certain limits by a laboratory technician to meet the specific needs of a unique peri-implant mucosal

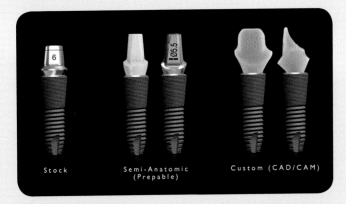

Figure 15: Schematic representation of *stock* (prefabricated) abutment (left), *semi-anatomic* (prepable) abutment (center), and *fully anatomic, patient-specific* (CAD/CAM custom) abutment (right).

architecture. Options for either titanium or zirconia abutment biomaterials are often available within this category. While offering many advanced features compared with a stock abutment, semi-anatomic abutments have inherent limitations with regard to margin placement and emergence profile customization. With the advent of CAD/CAM technology, many implant manufacturers are now offering fully customizable anatomic abutments, which allow for anatomic cutbacks from an implant restoration's planned full contour, analogous to a crown preparation. Elements such as customizable emergence width options, transmucosal topographies, abutment height, and site-specific margin location relative to the peri-implant mucosa are routinely available for modification based on the preferences of the clinician. Within CAD/CAM abutments, both gold hue and traditional titanium are often available, as well as zirconia of various hues. With regard to the aforementioned abutment design categories, abutments with greater design complexity offer the clinician much greater control over the location of the final prosthetic margin relative to the adjacent marginal gingiva.

D. A recent study by Linkevicius et al. [20] demonstrated elegantly the effect of the implant abutment margin location on the retention of excess cement in the marginal peri-implant mucosa. In their study, 53 patients were treated with single implant-supported restorations that had utilized prefabricated stock titanium abutments to support the crowns. As explained in the answer to question C, such stock abutments have a flat restorative platform circumferentially. Yet, anatomically, it is well established that alveolar ridges, and the associated mucosa, are usually scalloped, especially in the presence of an interproximal contact that supports the interdental col. The study measured the subgingival location at four sites for each of the stock abutments (mesial, distal, buccal, lingual). Cement-retained coronal restorations with an occlusal opening were subsequently cemented in place by a single experienced clinician. After clinical procedures were performed to remove excess cement, a standardized periapical radiograph was made. After tactile, visual, and radiographic means were

used to confirm cement removal, the screw-access cover was removed and the abutment–crown complex was immediately removed. The peri-implant sulcus and abutment–crown complex were subsequently photographed, and data were generated that quantified the surface area of cement covering the implant–abutment complex relative to the entire surface area. The findings of this study demonstrated that as the abutment–crown interface was located further apically from the marginal gingiva, these focal areas had a clinically and statistically significant elevation in the amount of remnants of restorative cement. Additionally, the authors demonstrated that despite the standardized radiographs demonstrating a lack of radiographic evidence of cement remnants, a majority of the abutment–crown complexes demonstrated excess cement remnants when visually evaluated after removal of the restoration from the implant fixture. The authors concluded that dental radiographs may not be considered as a reliable means by which to evaluate whether excess cement has been left in situ by the clinician during a cementation procedure. This study can inform the reader that prefabricated abutments, which typically demonstrate a uniform/flat circumferential restorative platform, may inadvertently create iatrogenic sequelae of cement-related peri-implant mucositis or peri-implantitis for the reasons mentioned. Unfortunately, prospective clinical trials have yet to evaluate if anatomically correct or site-specific CAD/CAM abutments would ameliorate this situation by placing the restorative platform in an anatomically correct, more accessible position for the clinician to access during luting procedures.

E. Recent studies [21,22] have evaluated whether there is an influence of cement formulation or type with regard to the ability of the clinician to radiographically detect excess cement apical to the abutment–crown interface. As Linkevicius et al. [20] demonstrated (see answer to question D), the majority of cases that reveal visual confirmation of excess cement in fact avert detection via traditional radiography. Wadhwani et al. [21] evaluated the relative radiographic density of commonly used dental cements for delivery of implant-supported restorations. In both their evaluations, as well as the one published by Pette et al. [22], standardized discs of various commonly used cements were prepared in thicknesses between 0.5 and 2.0 mm. The standardized cement preparations were then placed next to a standard radiographic aluminum step wedge, which was used to evaluate the relative radiopacity of the cement specimens. Standardized radiographs of both 60 and 70 kVp were then obtained and the specimens characterized using a gray-level value in comparison with the step wedge. In both studies, the authors found that the highest gray-level values were recorded consistently for the zinc-containing cements (i.e., TempBond Original, TempBond NE, and Fleck's). Cements that have been marketed as implant specific (i.e., Improv, Premier Implant Cement) could either only be detected at the thickest preparations of 2.0 mm or were undetectable at all. The findings of these early studies on this topic demonstrate that zinc-containing cements may be preferential for implant-supported restorations, given their higher relative radiopacity. Such radiographic detection (although not always sufficient) is considered critical for being able to reduce the risk of leaving cement residues behind at the time of implant restoration. Thus, it would appear to be a helpful tool to lower the incidence of cement-related biological complications.

Case 2

Screw-Retained Implant Restorations

CASE STORY

The patient is a healthy 25-year-old male dental student with a chief complaint of, "I want to have my lateral incisor before graduation." Medical history is unremarkable, and the patient is not currently taking any medications.

The patient is congenitally missing tooth #10.

LEARNING GOALS AND OBJECTIVES

- To be able to understand the guidelines for a screw-retained implant restoration
- To understand the technique and materials employed
- To understand the factors affecting the outcomes when deciding on a screw-retained over a cement-retained restoration
- To help streamline the decision-making process on the type of implant restoration to fabricate
- To help streamline the procedure, both surgical and restorative, and achieve the best possible results

Medical History

No significant data to record; unremarkable medical history.

Review of Systems

- Vital signs
  - Blood pressure: within normal limits
  - Pulse rate: within normal limits
  - Respiration: within normal limits

Social History

The patient is a nonsmoker and drinks only on social occasions.

Extraoral Examination

No significant findings were noted. The patient had no facial asymmetry, and there were no masses or swelling in any area. Lymph nodes were normal upon palpation. The temporomandibular joints were within normal limits.

Intraoral Examination

- Soft tissue exam was within normal limits.
- Periodontal examination was unremarkable.
- Oral cancer screening was negative.
- Missing tooth #10 (Figure 1).
- Minor restorative work present (amalgams and composites), as well as a porcelain-fused-to-metal (PFM) crown on #19; all in good condition.
- Evaluation of the alveolar ridge in area #10 revealed a Seibert class III defect [1].
- Presence of orthodontic brackets in both maxilla and mandible.

Occlusion

The fact that tooth #10 is missing does not create any major occlusal issue. The patient had bilateral canine guidance as well as normal anterior guidance. There were no occlusal discrepancies or interferences noted.

Radiographic Examination

A full-mouth radiographic series was ordered. The radiographic examination revealed normal bone levels.

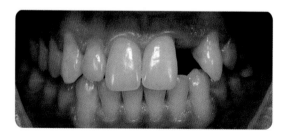

Figure 1: Pretreatment clinical view.

Radiopaque images suggested amalgam restorations on #3 and #12, a root canal treatment, a post and core and a PFM crown on #19, and composite restorations on #4, #5, #13, #20, #21, and #30. The maxillary left anterior area showed missing tooth #10 as well as an abnormal bone level at the distal interproximal area I on tooth #9 and adequate interradicular space between #9 and #11.

Diagnosis
Congenital dental agenesis of tooth #10, Seibert class III defect.

Treatment Plan
The treatment plan for this patient consisted of initial periodontal therapy that included oral prophylaxis and oral hygiene instructions to address gingival inflammation, although the patient is a dental student and is well aware and on top of his oral health, followed by a placement of an endosseous implant on the #10 site, along with a soft tissue graft of the area at the same time as the implant placement, restored by an implant-supported lithium disilicate (IPS e.max® Press) crown delivered at the implant placement.

Treatment
After the orthodontic treatment and initial periodontal therapy were finished, impressions were taken of the area as well as a face-bow and bite registration to study the case before rendering the proposed work. As with any prosthodontic procedure, the initial step is to do a diagnostic wax-up of the work needed (Figure 2); it will render all necessary information prior to any major or irreversible changes in the mouth. A full-contour wax-up of the missing tooth was done, and at that time it was noted that the space available was slightly larger than anticipated, resulting in a much larger lateral incisor compared with tooth #7. It was decided at the time that the distribution of the available space was much better utilized by slightly changing the mesial contours of tooth #11. This was accomplished by adding wax to

the mesial of #11, creating a bulkier contour without drastically changing the normal contours of a maxillary canine or creating any potential food trap that could jeopardize the final restoration, therefore obtaining a more suitable available space for a better looking lateral incisor showing better symmetry with the contralateral side (see Figure 2 for the diagnostic wax-up).

The diagnostic cast and the diagnostic wax-up were used to fabricate a radiographic template (Figure 3). After obtaining a cone beam computer tomographic study (Figure 4), implant surgical planning was completed with the use of special implant planning software (co-Diagnostix, Straumann USA, Andover, MA) (Figure 5). By combining both the digital wax-up and the cone beam computer tomography scan, a computerized rendering of the necessary work allowed the selection of the best possible final position of the implant to be placed, both from the prosthodontic and the surgical points of view. The system created a three-dimensional rendering of the proposed site of the implant as well as the proposed final position of the crown, which was originally planned as a screw-retained restoration. The accepted digital plan was then digitally transformed to aid in the fabrication of a guided surgery surgical template (Figure 6) as well as to plan the surgery.

The surgical template that was fabricated based on the three-dimensional rendering (Figure 7) demonstrated that a screw-retained restoration was possible since the access hole for the implant screw was located in the cingulum area of tooth #10. Using this surgical template on the diagnostic model before implant surgery gave us the ability to fabricate the final

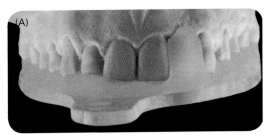
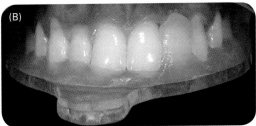

Figure 3: (A) Radiographic template on diagnostic cast. (B) Radiographic template intraorally.

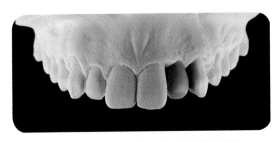

Figure 2: Diagnostic wax-up of tooth #10 (FDI #22).

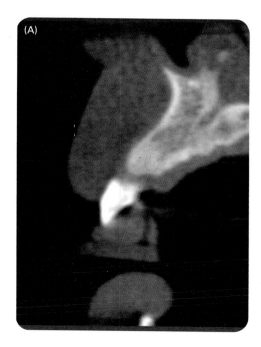

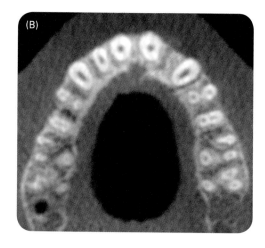

Figure 4: Cone beam computed tomography images: (A) cross-sectional of treatment site; (B) horizontal (occlusal) view.

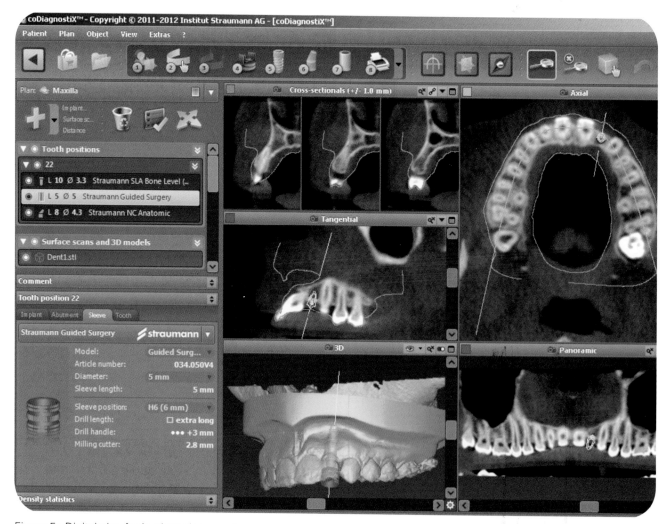

Figure 5: Digital plan for implant placement.

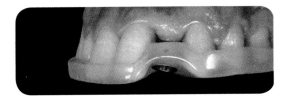

Figure 6: Guided-surgery template.

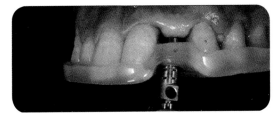

Figure 7: Implant site preparation with guided-surgery template.

crown and have it ready for delivery the day of the surgery, giving us the opportunity to manage the soft tissues with much more control.

The implant was placed without any complications using the surgical template previously fabricated and with the flapless surgery approach (Figure 8). After the implant was placed, a connective tissue graft was done to achieve the most favorable soft tissue esthetic results, and a final crown was placed the day of the surgery (Figure 9). Once healing was complete, a final impression was taken following standard clinical procedures for the fabrication of a non-preparation veneer on #11. This veneer was delivered as previously planned. The diagnostic stage had rendered a very satisfactory esthetic result from both the patient's and the dentist's view (Figures 10, 11, and 12).

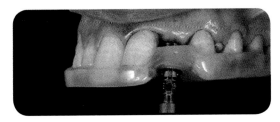

Figure 8: Implant placement with guided-surgery template.

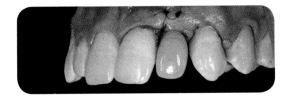

Figure 9: Final restoration placed immediately following implant surgery.

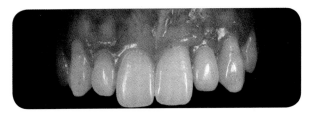

Figure 10: Final restoration and tissue healing 4 weeks after placement (frontal view).

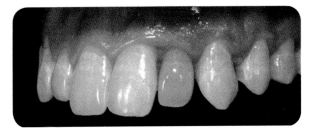

Figure 11: Final restoration and tissue healing 4 weeks after placement (lateral view).

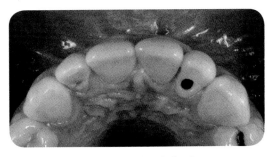

Figure 12: Final restoration (occlusal view).

Discussion

The key element in this case, or any implant case for that matter, is treatment planning. When we talk about planning we must think and visualize the final outcome before performing any major irreversible steps on our patients. A good set of initial impressions and a careful occlusal evaluation of the mounted study models give us an idea of the current condition and serve as the foundation to use for a diagnostic wax-up of the proposed work. This diagnostic wax-up serves as a visual aid of future work, so careful planning can be accomplished. In this particular situation, the wax-up not only helped in finding out the amount of available space and the contours of the final restoration, which assisted in the decision-making of fabricating the veneer for the mesial of the adjacent canine, but also helped in deciding the final position of the implant by digitally transforming the wax-up and using the software along with the CT scan. Careful planning and a thorough study of the case will render a satisfactory final restoration and help with having more control of the case through the whole process.

One of the advantages of a screw-retained implant restoration is that it is easier to control the emergence profile of the restoration and to handle the adjacent soft tissues, especially if the implant is placed in a deep subgingival position. Having a temporary restoration placed at the time of the surgery, or as in this case the final restoration, helps in contouring the soft tissues to our liking, rendering a better final result. The force of the screw as the restoration is being placed pushes the soft tissues out, and with careful control of the emergence profile of this restoration we can somehow manipulate the soft tissues for a better esthetic result.

Of course, with a cement-retained restoration we can potentially achieve the same esthetic results handling the surrounding soft tissues and emergence profile with a custom abutment provided there is a temporary restoration made at the time of the surgery. However, another advantage of a screw-retained restoration over a cement-retained one is precisely the use of cement on the latter, particularly if the implant is placed subgingivally. Most often than not on cement-retained restorations the dentist will try to place the margin of the custom abutment as subgingival as possible to prevent the abutment from showing. Then, it is very difficult to clean any excess cement after the restoration is inserted, creating a potential problem that can easily be avoided with a screw-retained restoration.

A screw-retained implant crown will have the access hole for the retentive screw visible and along the long axis of the implant underneath. In order to be able to use a screw-retained implant crown, the implant should ideally be placed in the center of the tooth if it is a posterior tooth and at the cingulum area if it is an anterior tooth. One of the disadvantages of a screw-retained restoration is that the access hole may be visible. It can be somewhat disguised with composite material after insertion, but it can be difficult to match with the surrounding porcelain. This does not necessarily post a problem on an anterior tooth because, like on this case presented, the access hole is located at the cingulum, which is not a visible area and does not pose an esthetic issue. On the other hand, it can potentially be an esthetic issue if it is a posterior tooth, especially in the mandible, which could make the access hole visible even if it is sealed with a composite restoration. This used to be more of a problem when restorations were PFM. The access hole, completely made of metal, would show through the composite plug; moreover, some technicians would leave a ring of metal around the access hole to give support for the porcelain, posing an even greater esthetic challenge. Now, with the advent of new restorative materials like zirconia or lithium disilicate, we do not seem to have that problem as much. Therefore, even if the shade of the composite plug used to seal the access to the screw does not completely match the surrounding porcelain, the fact that the framework underneath is closer to a tooth color possesses less of an esthetic challenge.

In this particular case, a novel approach was used. The final crown was delivered the same day of the surgery, avoiding the undesirable connections and disconnection of the abutment during the healing time [2]. This is a clear example of how the latest technologies in implant dentistry (computer-aided surgery) and the most esthetically advanced material (lithim disilicate) can help in the achievement of more predictable results in the esthetic area.

Even though this case had a big esthetic component being an anterior tooth, both the surgical and restorative components were greatly handled by the same dentist. The end result was outstanding because of the skill level of the dentist and careful planning, including at a diagnostic stage, securing a good final outcome. This is why the diagnostic stage is so important; it is the only way to ensure a good final result before doing any irreversible change in the patient's mouth. This proves that, with careful planning, the restoration of a missing tooth with an implant and crown can become manageable for any clinician with adequate experience and lead to a good esthetic and functional results.

Self-Study Questions

(Answers located at the end of the case)

A. What are the guidelines for a screw-retained implant restoration?

B. What are the advantages of a screw-retained over a cement-retained restoration?

C. What are the disadvantages of a screw-retained restoration?

D. How does one decide between a screw-retained and cement-retained restoration?

E. What steps should be taken for a screw-retained restoration?

F. Can the same dentist perform both the surgical and restorative portions of the treatment?

G. How can I show the patient the end result before starting the treatment?

H. What is the best way to control the soft tissues surrounding the implant?

I. How important is retrievability?

References

1. Seibert JS. Reconstruction of deformed partially edentulous ridges using full thickness onlay grafts: part I – technique and wound healing. Compend Contin Educ Dent 1983;4:437–453.

2. Degidi M, Nardi D, Piattelli A. One abutment at one time: non-removal of an immediate abutment and its effect on bone healing around subcrestal tapered implants. Clin Oral Implants Res 2011;22(11):1303–1307.

Answers to Self-Study Questions

A. One of the main guidelines is the implant's position; considerations need to be taken if the tooth that is being restored is an anterior or posterior tooth since the screw-retained restoration will have the hole to access the screw. Ideally, for an anterior tooth the access hole is on the lingual area close to the cingulum level, and for a posterior tooth the ideal position of the access hole is in the center of the occlusal table. In both situations the location of the access hole is where it would make more sense esthetically, particularly for an anterior tooth. The same applies when considering function. Since the implant is centrally positioned, the forces would be directed along the long axis of the implant, improving on the force distribution being applied.

Another consideration is implant depth and the condition and thickness of the surrounding soft tissues. Creating a proper emergence profile could be difficult if the implant is positioned close to the gingival margin and could create an esthetic complication. As a general rule, the deeper the implant is positioned the more control one has of the emergence profile and the soft tissues.

Another guideline is retrievability. A common problem with implant restorations is screw loosening. Tightening the screw to the recommended torque will secure the restoration in place, but it is common for the screw to become loose at some point. Having direct access to the screw solves the problem easily.

B. When an implant is in a deep subgingival position more often than not the surrounding soft tissues will offer resistance to the seating of the crown, particularly if no temporary restoration has been in place controlling the emergence profile, and sometimes, even having a temporary restoration, the emergence profile of said temporary might not be exactly the same as the permanent, presenting us with the challenge of the soft tissues offering resistance to the seating of the crown. One of the advantages of a screw-retained restoration is that the force used to seat the restoration is applied by tightening the screw and not by finger pressure. By slowly tightening the screw we can slowly make the tissues get used to the new emergence profile and control the seating of the crown.

Another advantage of a screw-retained restoration is the fact that no cement is needed. Using the same example as earlier, if the implant is placed deep subgingivally and the plan is for a cement-retained restoration, efforts will be made so that the finish line of the abutment used will be as subgingival as possible to avoid any esthetic complications. Once the crown is cemented, it is very difficult to confirm that all excess cement is removed, especially when the margins are subgingival. More often than not some cement may remain unseen, creating constant irritation of the surrounding soft tissues that would not be the case if the restoration is screw-retained.

C. One of the disadvantages is the access hole for the restoration and how visible it would be. Another disadvantage is that the implant has to be placed for easy access to the access hole and conspicuously enough that it can be slightly disguised with the composite seal. If the plan is for a screw-retained restoration and the implant is positioned in such a way that the access hole would be in the middle of the buccal surface of an esthetically visible tooth, then a screw-retained restoration is certainly not the best option.

D. Making this decision can sometimes be difficult because there are many variables to consider, but with careful planning the decision-making process can be made simpler. During the diagnostic stage while evaluating the available space, the information obtained by the CT scan can give us the final position of the planned implant based on the available bone. Knowing this final position beforehand can give us an idea of the type of restoration that can be made. In this particular case this gave us the liberty to fabricate the final restoration even before the implant was placed. Based on the advantages and benefits of a screw-retained restoration, it is probably the best option to consider whenever possible.

E. The steps traditionally taken for any implant restoration are careful evaluation of properly mounted study casts, diagnostic wax-up to evaluate the available space, fabrication of a radiographic stent, CT scan study, fabrication of the surgical template based on the information obtained from the CT scan, surgical placement of the implant following the surgical protocol, delivery of the provisional restoration, final impressions, and delivery of the final restorations.

F. As seen in this particular case, the same dentist can perform both the surgical and the restorative aspects of the treatment provided that the dentist has the necessary training required for placing implants and has an understanding of the restorative portions of the treatment. Currently, the implant manufacturing companies offer surgical training for dentists interested in placing their own implants. As long as careful planning is involved and the dentist has a clear understanding of their limitations, performing both aspects of treatment is perfectly viable.

G. The best possible way to show the patient and to visualize the end result is with a diagnostic wax-up done on properly mounted study casts. Although it is not absolutely necessary, it helps in visualizing the case better, especially for the patient, if the wax used is tooth colored.

H. The best way to control the surrounding soft tissues is to provide the patient with a temporary restoration that has the best possible emergence profile and anatomical features, either at the time of the surgical placement of the implant or at the implant uncovering second stage. Even though for this case no temporary was made and instead the final restoration was delivered at the time of the surgery, the purpose of the final restoration was the same: to control the soft tissues. The decision as to when to provide a temporary restoration is usually based on the dentist's preference, the evaluation of the tooth being restored, the esthetics of the case, and the occlusion. Furthermore, careful evaluation of the quality and quantity of bone at the time of the surgery may influence this decision. By providing a temporary restoration not only are the soft tissues being handled but also an occlusion is being established. Even if the tooth is left out of occlusion, to a certain degree some amount of function is being achieved. If the amount and quality of bone available are sufficient and primary stability is achieved, this small amount of function may not be an issue. On the other hand, if primary stability is achieved but the amount or the quality of available bone is not the best, then it is probably better to deliver the temporary at the implant uncovering second phase of the treatment.

I. This subject has received substantial attention with respect to advantages and disadvantages of implant restorations. Some believe that implant restorations should be treated like restorations cemented onto teeth, meaning cutting a crown off if there is an underlying problem, such as screw loosening or other maintenance. Others believe that with the improvements in implant design the screw-loosening problem has been eliminated because implants do not behave like teeth and with careful planning restorations can be made to be retrievable. As clinicians, we should try to plan for this possibility. For continued maintenance of the patients or for patients that move geographically, it is much simpler when there is no doubt about the method of retention and no guesswork is involved as to which type of cement was used or the condition of the underlying abutment. Certainly, the advances in implant design have helped to reduce the incidence of screw loosening;, but as with any mechanical interface, it still occurs.

If screw loosening occurs under a cement-retained restoration and the type of cement used is unknown, the best way to correct the problem is to destroy the crown to gain access to the abutment and screw, rendering the restoration unserviceable and requiring it to be remade. If the same problem occurs for a screw-retained restoration, the solution is as simple as removing the composite plug, gaining access to the screw, and retightening or better yet replacing the screw with a new one applying the recommended torque.

Case 3

Choice of Restorative Materials

CASE STORY

An 80-year-old Caucasian male presented with a chief complaint of, "My anterior tooth fractured recently." The examination showed that the approximately 20-year-old crown on tooth #9 had fractured subgingivally (Figures 1 and 2). To keep all treatment options open, emergency root canal treatment had been performed. A temporary removable denture was provided to replace the fractured tooth.

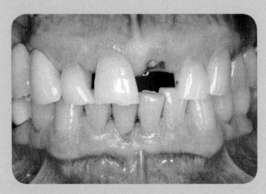

Figure 1: Preoperative presentation – facial view.

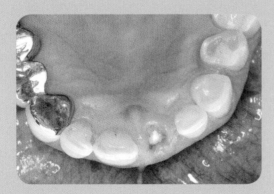

Figure 2: Preoperative presentation – occlusal view.

LEARNING GOALS AND OBJECTIVES
- To identify the indications for different dental materials in anterior and posterior restorations
- To understand the limitations of every material
- To understand when a provisional phase is needed

Medical History

The patient reported a history of hypertension, which is controlled with medication (ramipril). The patient reported no allergies.

Review of Systems
- Vital signs
  - Blood pressure: 125/72 mmHg
  - Pulse rate: 82 beats/min (regular)
  - Respiration: 17 breaths/min

Social History

The patient is a nonsmoker and drinks occasionally (a glass of wine once a month).

Extraoral Examination

During the extraoral examination, there were no significant findings. The patient had no masses, swelling, or asymmetries. Palpation of the temporomandibular joint did not reveal any clicking or crepitation. Movement and opening range of the mandible were within normal limits, and the patient reported no discomfort. The patient had a low smile line.

Intraoral Examination
- The soft tissues, including tongue and floor of the mouth, were within normal limits.
- Periodontal examination revealed pocket depths in the range of 2–3 mm (Figure 3).

(A)

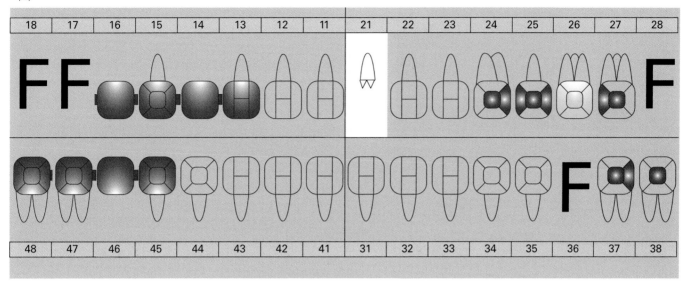

(B)

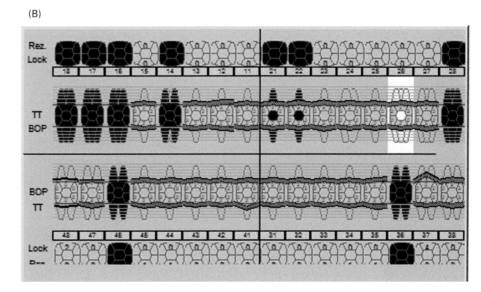

Figure 3: (A) Dental charting.
(B) Periodontal charting.

- The gingiva was of thick biotype.
- All teeth showed positive vitality except the remaining root of #9.
- Evaluation of the alveolar ridge in the area of #9 revealed no deformities. The remaining root was partially covered by the surrounding gingiva.
- Teeth #8 and #10 were free from caries and restorations.
- Multiple restorations in the form of single crowns and fixed partial dentures were present.

Occlusion

There were no occlusal disharmonies or interferences. Anterior overbite and overjet were both measured as 2 mm.

Radiographic Examination

A panoramic radiograph (Figure 4) and a full mouth radiographic series were ordered (see Figure 5 for the patient's periapical radiograph of the area of interest). In general, marginal bone levels were within normal limits. The root of tooth #9 showed no periapical pathology.

Diagnosis

Based on the classification of the American College of Prosthodontists [1], the diagnosis for this case is a moderately compromised partial edentulous patient with edentulous areas in two sextants in both arches (class II) and a remaining root #9.

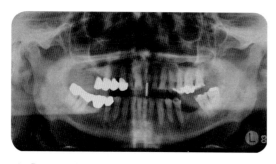

Figure 4: Panoramic radiograph with a reference pin in area of tooth #9.

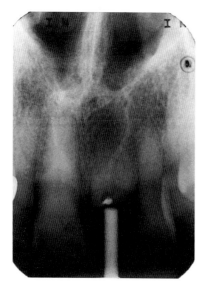

Figure 5: Periapical radiograph depicting the remaining root #9 and a reference pin.

Treatment Plan

The treatment plan for this patient consisted of the extraction of tooth #9 followed by an immediate implant placement. The tooth was to be restored with a provisional restoration after osseointegration of the implant. The provisional restoration would also serve to create the emergence profile for the final restoration in the surrounding peri-implant mucosa. Subsequently, a full-ceramic restoration on a custom abutment was to be delivered.

Treatment

The remaining root of tooth #9 was extracted atraumatically using local anesthesia with the help of a periotome. After extraction the alveolar walls were examined thoroughly using a periodontal probe. The buccal plate was well preserved with no deficiencies and an estimated thickness of 1 mm. An implant (4.1 mm diameter × 10 mm length) was placed with the

help of a surgical template. The implant showed high primary stability. The gap between the implant and the buccal plate was filled with xenograft bone particles. A soft tissue graft from the palate assured primary wound closure. The temporary removable partial denture was adjusted to allow unharmed healing. Antibiotics (amoxicillin, 1000 mg) were prescribed three times a day for 1 week. The sutures were removed after 10 days.

After 3 months, the second stage surgery was performed and a healing abutment was inserted. As the diameter and cross-section of the implant were different from the estimated crown and there was an excess of peri-implant mucosa (Figures 6 and 7), the soft tissue had to be conditioned. Additionally, in the esthetic area, the provisional was used to test the shape of the final crown. To condition the soft tissue the provisional was realigned chairside in several steps using a flowable composite (Figures 8, 9, and 10). The crown was extended apically, mesially, and distally until the desired emergence profile and crown shape were achieved (Figures 11 and 12). After 3 months (Figures 13 and 14) the final impression was taken with a customized impression coping. Owing to the esthetic area, a zirconia-based full-ceramic restoration was delivered (Figures 15, 16, and 17). The clinical (Figures 18 and 19) and radiographic (Figure 20) follow-up after 6 months showed sound and stable peri-implant tissues without any signs of inflammation.

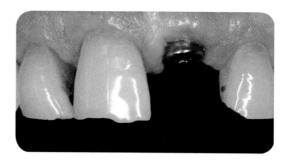

Figure 6: Healing abutment – facial view.

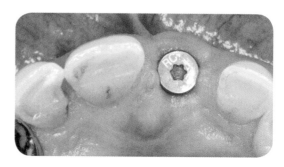

Figure 7: Healing abutment – occlusal view.

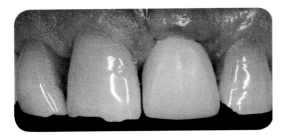

Figure 8: Soft tissue conditioning by using a provisional crown – first step.

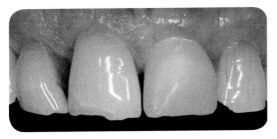

Figure 9: Soft tissue conditioning by relining the provisional crown – second step.

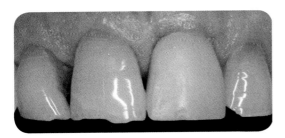

Figure 10: Soft tissue conditioning and adjusting the shape of the provisional crown – third step.

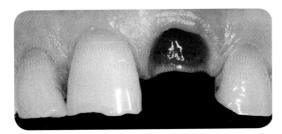

Figure 11: Emergence profile – facial view.

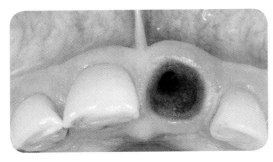

Figure 12: Emergence profile – occlusal view.

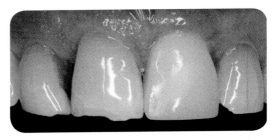

Figure 13: Stable peri-implant soft tissue after 3 months – facial view.

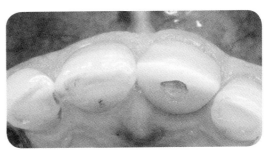

Figure 14: Stable peri-implant soft tissue after 3 months – occlusal view.

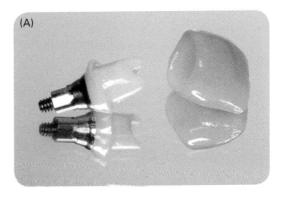

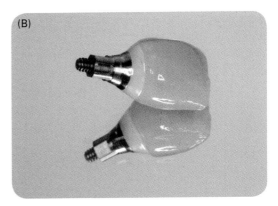

Figure 15: (A) Zirconia-based abutment and (B) full-ceramic crown.

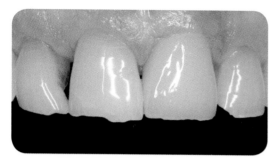

Figure 16: Final crown – facial view.

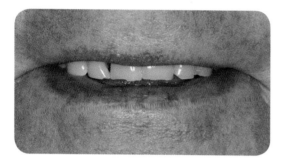

Figure 17: Final crown – smile profile.

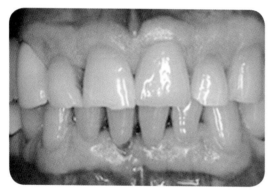

Figure 18: Follow-up at 6 months – facial view.

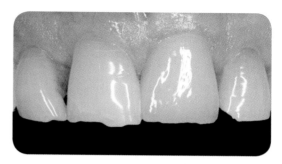

Figure 19: Follow-up at 6 months – detail.

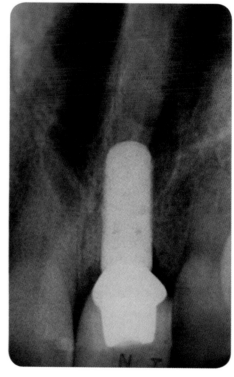

Figure 20: Periapical radiograph after crown delivery.

Discussion

As there was a lot of excess peri-implant mucosa after the second stage, a provisional crown had to condition the soft tissue before taking the final impression. If the restoration puts too much pressure on the peri-implant tissue, a retraction could result, which could have an effect on the esthetic outcome. Clinically, an overload of pressure could be detected by persistent anemia of the soft tissue. Any anemic areas around the relined provisional should be supported by blood again within 10 min, which means the mucosa should be pink again. Therefore, the provisional was relined three times by

extending its form to give the soft tissue the time to adjust. Finally, the desired emergence profile similar to the adjacent tooth was achieved.

As the restoration is located in the esthetic area, a metal-free restoration was chosen. Porcelain-fused-to-metal was the material of choice for many decades and achieves very good esthetic results. However, all-ceramic materials are more esthetically pleasing. Additionally, the peri-implant mucosa reacts very favorably to this biocompatible material. There is no risk of grayish discoloration of the peri-implant mucosa due to metallic materials.

Self-Study Questions

(Answers located at the end of the case)

A. When is provisionalization absolutely necessary?

B. Which types of restorative materials are available for final implant-supported single crowns?

C. In which region are esthetic aspects important, and which material takes these aspects into account?

D. Is it possible to combine different materials in the same patient?

E. Can computer-assisted design (CAD)/computer-assisted manufacturing (CAM) technologies be utilized for implant-supported restorations?

References

1. McGarry TJ, Nimmo A, Skiba JF, et al. Classification system for partial edentulism. J Prosthodont 2002;11(3):181–193.
2. Higginbottom F, Belser U, Jones JD, Keith SE. Prosthetic management of implants in the esthetic zone. Int J Oral Maxillofac Implants 2004;19(Suppl):62–72.
3. Jung RE, Zembic A, Pjetursson BE, et al. Systematic review of the survival rate and the incidence of biological, technical and esthetic complications of single crowns on implants reported in longitudinal studies with a mean follow-up of 5 years. Clin Oral Implants Res 2012;23(Suppl 6):2–21.
4. Zarone F, Russo S, Sorrentino R. From porcelain-fused-to-metal to zirconia: clinical and experimental considerations. Dent Mater 2011;27(1):83–96.
5. Buser D, Belser U, Lang NP. The original one-stage dental implant system and its clinical application. Periodontol 2000 1998;17(1):106–118.
6. Gallucci GO, Grütter L, Nedir R, et al. Esthetic outcomes with porcelain-fused-to-ceramic and all-ceramic single-implant crowns: a randomized clinical trial. Clin Oral Implants Res 2011;22(1):62–69

7. Wittneben JG, Weber HP. Prosthodontic considerations and treatment procedures. In: WittnebenJG, WeberHP (eds), ITI-Treatment Guide, Vol. 6: Extended Edentulous Spaces in the Esthetic Zone. Berlin: Quintessence; 2012, pp 65–90.
8. Glauser R, Sailer I, Wohlwend A, et al. Experimental zirconia abutments for implant-supported single-tooth restorations in esthetically demanding regions: 4-year results of a prospective clinical study. Int J Prosthodont 2004;17(3):285–290.
9. Kohal RJ, Att W, Bächle M, Butz F. Ceramic abutments and ceramic oral implants. An update. Periodontol 2000 2008;47(1):224–243.
10. Raptis NV, Michalakis KX, Hirayama H. Optical behavior of current ceramic systems. Int J Periodontics Restorative Dent 2006;26(1):31–41.
11. Hämmerle CHF, Stone P, Jung RE, et al. Consensus statements and recommended clinical procedures regarding computer-assisted implant dentistry. Int J Oral Maxillofac Implants 2009;24(Suppl):126–131.
12. Kapos T, Ashy LM, Gallucci G, et al. Computer-aided design and computer-assisted manufacturing in prosthetic implant dentistry. Int J Oral Maxillofac Implants 2009;24(Suppl):110–117.

Answers to Self-Study Questions

A. Provisional restorations help to establish function and esthetics to allow for a predictable result of the final crown. In addition, a provisional implant-supported crown plays an important role in conditioning the peri-implant soft tissue [2]. The cross-section of the crown is usually different than the supporting implant. Accordingly, the peri-implant soft tissue has to be adapted without any harm to allow for a predictable esthetic outcome. Taking into account these factors, a provisional crown is essential in the esthetic area. The provisional crown provides the clinician and patient the possibility to evaluate the shape and color as well as the cleansability and function of the future restoration.

B. Implant-supported single crowns demonstrate high survival rates of 96.3% after 5 years and 89.4% after 10 years [3]. Porcelain-fused-to-metal crowns have been utilized for many years with very good clinical results. The underlying metallic framework allows for good stability, and sufficient esthetics is achieved with veneering ceramics [4]. In the posterior region with high bite forces, porcelain-fused-to-metal is currently the material of choice.

Especially in anterior sites, the reestablishment of esthetics is the focus of the restoration [5]. Nowadays, different all-ceramic materials offer a valuable treatment alternative. All-ceramic restorations seem to have a similar success rate to ceramo-metal restorations [6]. Zirconia-based restorations may replace metal-based restorations due to their promising high mechanical stability.

However, the decision for one material or the other is always influenced by functional and mechanical aspects, such as bruxism or limited interocclusal space [7].

C. Esthetic aspects have to be considered, especially in visible areas. These are most likely located in the anterior region. However, an esthetic assessment has to be determined individually for every patient. According to the smile line, some patients display not only the incisors and the canines, but also the premolars and even the first molar. If the patient even displays most parts of the gingiva, the esthetic demands become greater for the clinician. Any subgingivally located metallic component may cause a grayish discoloration of the peri-implant tissue [8,9]. Furthermore, all-ceramic materials react physically similar to the natural tooth to the incident light. The light is transmitted and partially diffused through because of its translucency [10]. This fact makes the restoration look more natural. Thus, all-ceramic materials are recommended in anterior areas.

D. Yes, it is possible to combine different crown materials in the same patient. The choice for the adequate material should be based on functional, technical, and esthetic demands.

E. Modern digital technologies show great promise in tooth-supported prosthetics. CAD and CAM technologies may replace the conventional workflow, such as casting of the restoration by means of manual work. The restoration is designed digitally and afterwards milled automatically out of prefabricated blanks. These technologies have been used in implant dentistry for customized abutments as well as for frameworks of crowns and fixed partial dentures. But utilizing the hardware and software requires experience and continuing education. In the hand of clinically experienced practitioners and laboratory technicians, CAD/CAM-fabricated restorations could be implemented in individual case assessment [11]. Currently, there are no long-term studies that could recommend the routine use in implant dentistry [12].

4

Soft Tissue Management

Clinical Cases in Implant Dentistry, First Edition. Edited by Nadeem Karimbux and Hans-Peter Weber.
© 2017 John Wiley & Sons, Inc. Published 2017 by John Wiley & Sons, Inc.

Case 1

Free Gingival Grafts

CASE STORY

A 45-year-old woman of Asian descent presented with a minimal band of keratinized gingiva on the buccal aspects of implants #28 and #30 (Figures 1 and 2). Past dental therapy rendered to this patient at sites #28, #29, and #30 included a ridge augmentation procedure along with implant placement. Because this patient had a small band of keratinized gingiva at these sites to begin with (Figures 3 and 4), a treatment plan that included a surgical procedure to augment the keratinized gingiva around implants #28 and #30 was presented.

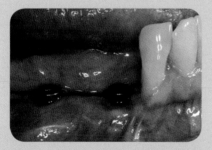

Figure 1: Buccal view of implants #28 and #30

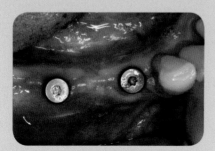

Figure 2: Occlusal view of implants #28 and #30

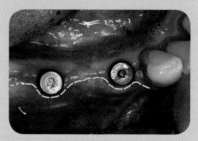

Figure 3: Buccal view of implants #28 and #30 with dotted yellow line delineating the mucogingival junction (MGJ) and revealing the lack of adequate keratinized gingiva around implants #28 and #30

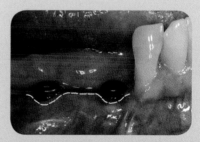

Figure 4: Occlusal view of implants #28 and #30 with dotted yellow line delineating the MGJ and revealing the lack of adequate keratinized gingiva around implants #28 and #30

LEARNING GOALS AND OBJECTIVES

- To be able to identify the lack of keratinized gingiva around dental implants
- To understand the importance of keratinized gingiva around dental implants
- To understand the potential problems associated with the lack of keratinized gingiva around dental implants
- To understand the role of free gingival grafts in augmenting keratinized gingiva around dental implants

Medical History

The patient had hypercholesterolemia that was controlled by simvastatin and diet. The patient reported no other medical conditions and had no known allergies to medications.

Review of Systems

- Vital signs
  - Blood pressure: 128/84 mmHg
  - Pulse rate: 72 beats/min
  - Respiration: 15 breaths/min

Social History

The patient never used tobacco and very rarely drank alcohol. Patient denied using recreational drugs.

Extraoral Examination

There were no abnormal masses and swellings upon palpation. Masticatory muscles and temporomandibular joints were normal.

Intraoral Examination

- Oral cancer screening was negative.
- Soft tissues, including hard and soft palate, buccal mucosa, gingiva, floor of the mouth and tongue, were normal.
- Plaque accumulation was minimal in general.
- Gingiva was healthy in general but deficient on the buccal aspects of implants #28 and #30 (Figures 1–4).
- Periodontal charting (Figure 5) showed probing pocket depths of ≤3 mm throughout the entire dentition. There was generalized gingival recession due to previous destruction of periodontal attachment. Bleeding on probing was minimal. Probing pocket depths around implants were not measured.

Occlusion

No occlusal disharmonies or interferences were detected.

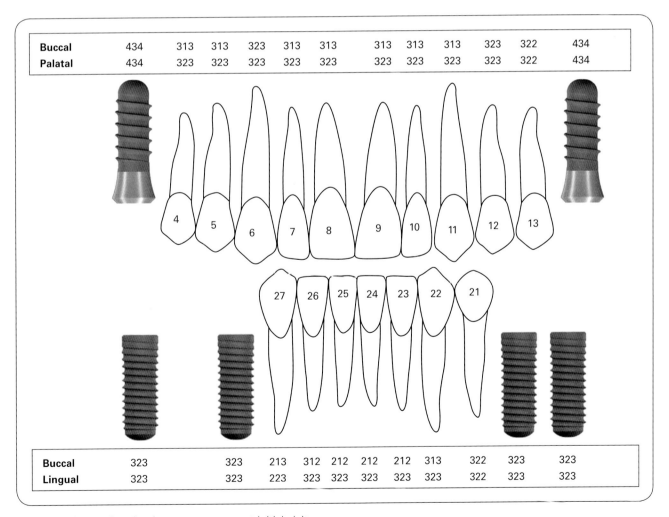

Buccal	434	313	313	323	313	313	313	313	313	323	322	434
Palatal	434	323	323	323	323	323	323	323	323	323	322	434

Buccal	323	323	213	312	212	212	212	313	322	323	323
Lingual	323	323	223	323	323	323	323	323	322	323	323

Figure 5: Probing pocket depth measurements at initial visit

Radiographic Examination

Radiographic finding at sites #28, #29, and #30 appeared to be normal. There was no crestal bone loss around implants #28 and #30.

Diagnosis and Prognosis

The patient was diagnosed with partial edentulism and plaque-induced gingivitis on reduced periodontium prior to the start of dental implant therapy. This diagnosis was based on (1) the history of previous periodontal therapy that had rendered the patient's periodontal disease at a maintainable state, (2) the presence of clinical attachment loss due to previous periodontal destruction, and (3) probing pocket depths of 3 mm or less with some bleeding on probing. Pertaining to the mucogingival conditions around dental implants, a diagnosis of inadequate attached keratinized gingiva on the buccal aspects of implants #28 and #30 was given (Figures 1–4).

The prognosis of the patient's periodontal condition was considered to be favorable based on Kwok and Caton's [1] periodontal prognostic classification system because (1) both local and systemic factors that could lead to periodontal destruction were either absent or controllable, (2) the patient's oral hygiene was quite good, and (3) the patient attended regular periodontal maintenance visits every 3 months. Even though Kwok and Caton's periodontal prognostic classification system was intended for assigning prognosis to natural dentition [1], this system could also be helpful in evaluating the prognosis of dental implants. Owing to the lack of attached keratinized gingiva on implants #28 and #30, it would be difficult for the patient to control plaque because each time when the patient brushed around the implants the alveolar mucosa (mobile tissues) on the buccal aspects of the implants would move with the bristles of the toothbrush, resulting in ineffective plaque removal. As such, a questionable prognosis was given to implants #28 and #30 because inadequate keratinized gingiva on the buccal aspects of implants was a local factor that prevented effective plaque removal by the patient [1].

Treatment Plan

The following treatment plan and treatment sequence were discussed with the patient.
- Diagnostic phase – comprehensive periodontal examination, radiographic examination.
- Disease control phase – oral hygiene instruction, oral prophylaxis.

- Surgical phase – free gingival graft (FGG) at the buccal aspects of implants #28 and #30 to augmented keratinized gingiva.
- Reevaluation phase – follow up of FGG healing and assessment of the patient's ability to remove plaque around implants.
- Maintenance phase – periodic implant maintenance visit once every 3–6 months depending on the patient's ability to control plaque.

Treatment Rendered

After the disease control phase was completed, a soft tissue grafting involving placement of an FGG on the buccal aspects of implants #28 and #30 and the edentulous ridge at site #29 was performed (see Figures 6, 7, and 8 for a description of the procedure). One capsule of 2% lidocaine 1 : 100,000 was given for buccal and lingual infiltration at sites #28, #29, and #30. An incision was made at the MGJ from sites #28 to #30 and a partial-thickness flap was raised, leaving the underlying periosteum intact. After measuring the soft tissue grafting area required at the recipient site, a

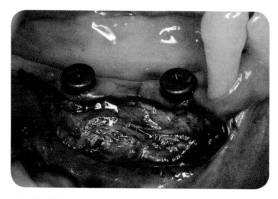

Figure 6: Recipient site preparation: incision was made at MGJ around implants #28 and #30, and split thickness flap was raised leaving the underlying periosteum.

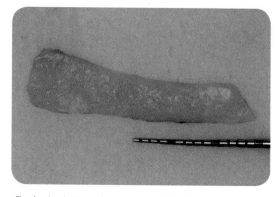

Figure 7: A gingival graft measured 30x7x1.25mm was harvested.

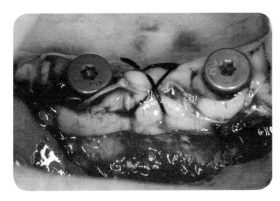

Figure 8: Gingival graft was stabilized on the buccal aspects of implants #28 and #30 using sutures.

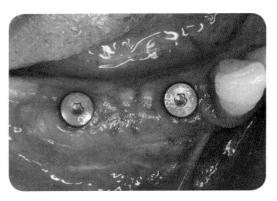

Figure 10: Two week post-operative visit showed good healing of gingival graft at the recipient site (occlusal view).

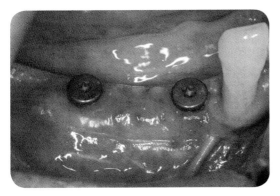

Figure 9: Two week post-operative visit showed good healing of gingival graft at the recipient site (buccal view).

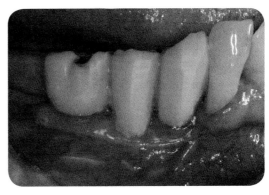

Figure 11: Four month post-operative visit demonstrated maturation of the gingival graft with well defined MGJ that is continuous with MGJ on adjacent tooth #27. Adequate attached keratinized gingiva around implants #28 and #30 was obtained. Provisional implant restoration 28 × 30 was in place.

$30 \times 7 \times 1.25$ mm^3 FGG was harvested from the right palate and transferred to the recipient site where it was secured with chromic gut and silk sutures. Every attempt was made to ensure the stability and the immobility of the FGG at the recipient site to maximize contact between the periosteum and the connective tissue layer of the FGG for blood supply. The immobility of the FGG was tested by pulling the buccal mucosa and detecting any FGG movements. By 2 weeks postoperatively the FGG had become vascularized and blended well with the surrounding soft tissues (Figures 9 and 10). The patient returned at 4 months with provisional restorations and had an adequate band of attached keratinized gingiva on the buccal aspects of implants #28 and #30 (Figure 11).

Discussion

The main purpose of performing an FGG procedure in this case was to augment the attached keratinized gingiva on the buccal aspects of implants #28 and #30. With an adequate zone of keratinized gingiva, the patient's ability to remove plaque from around the implants would be greatly enhanced (see self-study question C). Because the patient already presented with sufficient vestibular depth, no vestibuloplasty was required (see Chapter 4 Case 3 – Vestibuloplasty and Frenectomy). Therefore, a narrow band of gingival graft measuring 7 mm corono-apically was harvested (Figure 7). If an increase in the vestibular depth was desired in this situation, a wider graft (e.g., 15 mm corono-apically) would have been obtained to deepen the vestibule. A $30 \times 7 \times 1.25$ mm^3 gingival graft was harvested here, so after suturing it to the recipient bed the most apical extent of the graft will be at the MGJ of the adjacent tooth #27. This allowed a continuity of the MGJ from the natural teeth to the implants so that no abrupt change of MGJ position is noted, thereby making gingiva more natural looking (Figures 9 and 11).

An FGG procedure can be done at different stages of the dental implant therapy. If a patient presents with a severely resorbed alveolar ridge in mandible, the amount of keratinized gingiva is oftentimes very limited and confined to the crestal area. In this scenario, the clinician has several options in regard to the timing of augmenting the keratinized gingiva. First, an FGG procedure can be performed prior to ridge augmentation. With a wider zone of keratinized gingiva, the clinician will have an easier time suturing the flaps at the time of ridge augmentation (suturing alveolar mucosa can be challenging). Also, with thicker gingival tissues the chances of the underlying barrier membrane or titanium mesh perforating through the soft tissue are reduced.

Second, an FGG procedure can also be carried out after ridge augmentation and implant placement and before implant restoration (as demonstrated in the case presented here). The advantage of this approach is that the clinician will know how much keratinized gingiva is required to be augmented around implants and can hence harvest a gingival graft with appropriate size, taking into account the graft shrinkage [2,3]. In addition, if a vestibuloplasty is needed, the clinician will be able to deepen the vestibule simultaneously with the same FGG procedure. Moreover, because it is not uncommon to encounter frenal attachments that may have formed over the incisions made during ridge augmentation procedures, by augmenting the keratinized gingiva at this time these aberrant frenal attachments can also be removed simultaneously with the same FGG procedure.

Third, an FGG procedure can also be performed after implant restorations are completed. One of the disadvantages of this approach is the access to the surgical site. For example, if a patient presents with no keratinized gingiva between the cresto-interproximal areas of two adjacent implants, with implant restorations already in place the clinician will have

difficulty in accessing this interproximal area to prepare the recipient bed and to stabilize the graft. Sometimes, the clinician may need to remove the restoration in order to access the cresto-interproximal sites. Perhaps the most common reason for augmenting keratinized gingiva after the completion of implant restorations is where plaque accumulation around implant restorations has led to gingival inflammation and possibly gingival recession with implant thread exposure, resulting in a minimal amount of residual keratinized gingiva (see Figures 14, 15, 16, and 17). In these situations an FGG procedure can be utilized to augment the keratinized gingiva (see Figure 16). It is important to note that, in addition to gingival grafts, there are other surgical procedures (e.g., subepithelial connective tissue grafting, tissue allografting) that can be used in augmenting the keratinized gingiva and covering exposed implant threads (see Chapter 4 Case 1 and 2).

There are a few items that clinicians should keep in mind when performing gingival grafting procedures. First, one should make an effort to remove all loose tissue fibers and muscle attachments in the submucosa of the recipient sites so the gingival grafts that are to be sutured to the recipient beds will not be mobile. Second, clinicians should understand the expected shrinkage of the gingival grafts, with thinner grafts having higher shrinkage than the thicker grafts [2,3]. Third, when placing gingival grafts on the recipient beds, clinicians should ensure that the connective tissue side, rather than the keratinized epithelial side, of the grafts is in contact with the vascular periosteum bed.

Self-Study Questions

(Answers located at the end of the case)

A. What is keratinized gingiva?

B. What is the importance of keratinized gingiva around natural teeth and dental implants? What are the differences of the soft tissue attachment apparatus between natural teeth and dental implants?

C. What are some clinical issues that may arise with insufficient keratinized gingiva around dental implants?

D. What is an FGG?

E. What are the indications of FGGs in dental implant therapy?

F. What will patients experience after FGG procedures?

G. What are the potential complications associated with FGG procedures?

References

1. Kwok V, Caton JG. Commentary: prognosis revisited: a system for assigning periodontal prognosis. J Periodontol 2007;78(11):2063–2071.
2. Sullivan HC, Atkins JH. Free autogenous gingival grafts. I. Principles of successful grafting. Periodontics 1968;6:121–129.
3. Mörmann W, Schaer F, Firestone AR. The relationship between success of free gingival grafts and transplant thickness. Revascularization and shrinkage – a one year clinical study. J Periodontol 1981;52:74–80.
4. Fiorellini JP, Kim DM, Ishikawa SO. The gingiva. In: Newman MG, Takei HH, Klokkevold PR, Carranza FA (eds), Carranza's Clinical Periodontology, 10th edn. St Louis, MO: Saunders Elsevier; 2006, pp 46–67.
5. Romanos GE, Bernimoulin JP. Collagen as a basic element of the periodontium: immunohistochemical aspects in the human and animal. 1. Gingiva and alveolar bone. Parodontologie 1990;4:363–375.
6. Berglundh T, Lindhe J, Ericsson I, et al. The soft tissue barrier at implants and teeth. Clin Oral Implants Res 1991;2:81–90.
7. Sculean A, Gruber R, Bosshardt DD. Soft tissue wound healing around teeth and dental implants. J Clin Periodontol. 2014;41(Suppl 15):S6–S22.
8. Berglundh T, Lindhe J, Marinello C, et al. Soft tissue reaction to de novo plaque formation on implants and teeth. An experimental study in the dog. Clin Oral Implants Res 1992;3:1–8.
9. Lindhe J, Berglundh T, Ericsson I, et al. Experimental breakdown of peri-implant and periodontal tissues. A study in the beagle dog. Clin Oral Implants Res 1992;3:9–16.
10. Toijanic JA, Ward CB, Gewerth ME, Banakis ML. A longitudinal clinical comparison of plaque-induced inflammation between gingival and peri-implant soft tissues in the maxilla. J Periodontol 2001;72:1139–1145.
11. Greenstein G, Cavallaro J. The clinical significance of keratinized gingiva around dental implants. Compend Contin Educ Dent 2011;32:24–31.
12. Wennström JL, Derks J. Is there a need for keratinized mucosa around implants to maintain health and tissue stability? Clin Oral Implants Res 2012;23(Suppl 6):136–146.
13. Gobbato L, Avila-Ortiz G, Sohrabi K, et al. The effect of keratinized mucosa width on peri-implant health: a systematic review. Int J Oral Maxillofac Implants 2013;28:1536–1545.
14. Lin GH, Chan HL, Wang HL. The significance of keratinized mucosa on implant health: a systematic review. J Periodontol 2013;84:1755–1767.
15. Lang NP, Berglundh T; Working Group 4 of Seventh European Workshop on Periodontology. Periimplant diseases: where are we now? – Consensus of the Seventh European Workshop on Periodontology. J Clin Periodontol 2011;38(Suppl 11):178–181.
16. Nevins M, Cappetta EG. Mucogingival surgery: the rationale and long-term results. In: Nevins M, Mellonig JT (eds), Periodontal Therapy: Clinical Approaches and Evidence of Success, volume 1. Chicago, IL: Quintessence; 1988, pp 279–290.
17. Evian CI, al-Maseeh J, Symeonides E. Soft tissue augmentation for implant dentistry. Compend Contin Educ Dent 2003;24:195–198.
18. Nabers JM. Free gingival grafts. Periodontics 1966; 4:243–245.
19. Mlinek A, Smukler H, Buchner A. The use of free gingival grafts for the coverage of denuded roots. J Periodontol 1973;44:248–254.
20. Matter J. Free gingival grafts for the treatment of gingival recession. A review of some techniques. J Clin Periodontol 1982;9:103–114.
21. Griffin TJ, Cheung WS, Zavras AI, Damoulis PD. Postoperative complications following gingival augmentation procedures. J Periodontol 2006;77:2070–2079.
22. Brasher WJ, Rees TD, Boyce WA. Complications of free grafts of masticatory mucosa. J Periodontol 1975; 46:133–138.
23. Larato DC. Palatal exostoses of the posterior maxillary alveolar process. J Periodontol 1972;43:486–489.
24. Soehren SE, Allen AL, Cutright DE, Seibert JS. Clinical and histologic studies of donor tissues utilized for free grafts of masticatory mucosa. J Periodontol 1973;44:727–741.
25. Ruben MP, Kon S, Goldman HM, et al. Complications of the healing process after periodontal surgery. J Periodontol 1972;43:339–346.

Answers to Self-Study Questions

A. Keratinized gingiva is a part of the oral mucosa that surrounds the necks of the teeth and covers parts of the alveolar bone that houses teeth [4]. It extends from the gingival margin to the MGJ. Keratinized gingiva is lined by keratinized epithelium, and the parts of keratinized gingiva that are tightly bound to the underlying alveolar bone or the cementum of teeth are known as the *attached* keratinized gingiva. The width of attached keratinized gingiva is defined as the distance from the MGJ to the bottom of the gingival sulcus/periodontal pocket. The *unattached* keratinized gingiva does not attach to alveolar bone and cementum. The width of unattached keratinized gingiva is defined as the distance from the bottom of the gingival sulcus/periodontal pocket to the gingival margin.

B. The attached keratinized gingiva around natural dentition harbors gingival fibers made of type I collagen [5]. These collagen fibers provide a mechanical seal to the gingiva and together function as a barrier against oral microbiota. The attached keratinized gingiva also has the ability to resist friction that arises during mastication when food particles are being passed apically from the occlusal table over the keratinized gingiva to the oral vestibule. In addition, because of its firm attachment to the underlying structures, the attached keratinized gingiva is not mobile and hence allows effective plaque removal with cleaning devices such as toothbrushes and flosses.

The attachment apparatus of the attached keratinized gingiva surrounding a dental implant is different from those surrounding a natural tooth. The gingival fibers of a natural tooth are inserted perpendicularly to the cementum [4]. In contrast, the connective tissue fibers surrounding a dental implant for the most part run parallel to the implant and do not attach to the implant titanium surface [6]. Moreover, a significant part of the attachment apparatus around a dental implant consists of long junctional epithelium rather than connective tissue attachment [7]. Because of these structural differences, the attachment apparatus around dental implants is more susceptible to tissue breakdown than that found around natural dentition in the presence of plaque accumulation [8–10].

The importance of keratinized gingiva on implant health has been a subject of debate over the past years. Some review articles concluded that there is insufficient evidence supporting the need of keratinized gingiva for peri-implant tissue stability [11,12]. However, other systematic reviews reported that more plaque accumulation and tissue inflammation are associated with inadequate peri-implant keratinized gingiva [13,14]. Because the organization of the attachment apparatus around implants renders peri-implant soft tissues more susceptible to breakdown in the presence of plaques [8–10], presumably it is important to have adequate width of attached keratinized gingiva around dental implants.

C. When there is an insufficient amount of keratinized gingiva around dental implants, the majority of the peri-implant soft tissues will be made of alveolar mucosa [4]. Because alveolar mucosa is a mobile tissue, it is difficult for the patient to keep a plaque-free environment around implants. The peri-implant alveolar mucosa will move with the toothbrush bristles when the patient brushes their implants. Therefore, inadequate peri-implant keratinized gingiva may lead to increased plaque retention and gingival inflammation. Since the soft tissue attachment apparatus around implants appears to be less resistant to gingival inflammation [8–10] (see answer to self-study question B), the patient is more likely to develop peri-implant mucositis and peri-implantitis [15].

Furthermore, in situations where implants are placed in severely atrophic alveolar ridges with inadequate peri-implant keratinized gingiva, the peri-implant vestibular spaces are often limited, not allowing dental hygiene devices (e.g., toothbrush) enough room to remove plaque and food debris. Figure 12 demonstrates a lack of adequate keratinized gingiva on the buccal aspects of implants #29 and #30, and a lack of vestibule as revealed by the mucosal folds (arrows) that formed around the embrasures between tooth #28, implant #29, and implant #30. There is food debris and plaque accumulation around the implants (Figure 12). Removal of implant restorations #29 and #30 demonstrates a complete lack of buccal keratinized gingiva (Figure 13). Figure 14 shows inadequate keratinized gingiva on the buccal aspects of implant #25 and a frenal attachment (arrow) that interferes with effective plaque control. The implant threads are exposed and covered by plaques and calculus,

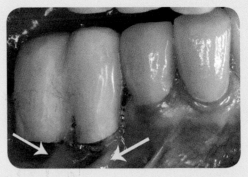

Figure 12: The mucosal folds (yellow arrows) on the buccal alveolar mucosa are imprints of the embrasures between tooth #28, implant #29 and implant #30. The mucosal folds indicate that there is a very close contact between the alveolar mucosa and the buccal surface of implant restorations #29 and #30, suggesting a lack of adequate peri-implant vestibular space.

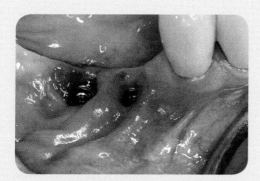

Figure 13: A lack of buccal peri-implant keratinized gingiva is more clearly demonstrated when implant restorations are removed.

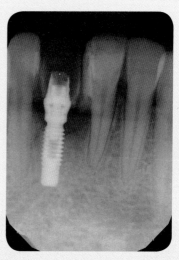

Figure 15: Peri-implant crestal bone loss on the mesial aspect of implant #25 is evident. Note the amount of calculus that can be seen on the radiograph.

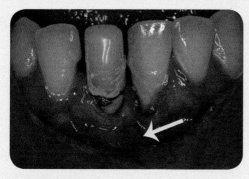

Figure 14: Implant #25 has a minimal width of keratinized gingiva and is surrounded by plaque and calculus. An aberrant frenal attachment on the mesial aspects of implant #25 (yellow arrow) may also have prevented effective plaque control.

which are visible also on the radiograph (Figure 15). Factors such as insufficient peri-implant keratinized gingiva, inadequate peri-implant vestibular space, and unfavorable peri-implant frenal attachments prevent effective plaque removal and may lead to peri-implant mucositis and/or peri-implantitis (see Chapter 4 Case 3 – Vestibuloplasty and Frenectomy).

D. An FGG procedure is a type of mucogingival surgery used to correct soft tissue deformities around natural dentition [16] and dental implants [17]. An FGG itself refers to the gingival graft that is harvested from donor tissue consisting of keratinized epithelium and a dense lamina propria [2]. The graft is harvested from the same patient and hence is considered to be an autograft. Any intraoral sites that contain sufficient tissue volume with these tissue characteristics can serve as donor sites for gingival grafts. Examples of donor sites are hard palates, maxillary tuberosities, and keratinized gingiva on edentulous alveolar ridges.

E. There are several indications for performing an FGG procedure around natural dentition. First, an FGG helps to increase the zone of keratinized gingiva around teeth [2,18]. Second, an FGG can be utilized to treat gingival recession defects and cover exposed roots for esthetic concerns and dentinal hypersensitivity [19,20]. Third, an FGG helps to increase vestibular depth (see Chapter 4 Case 3 – Vestibuloplasty and Frenectomy). These indications can also be applied to dental implants. As shown in Figures 14, 15, 16, and 17, an FGG can be used to cover exposed implant threads (similar to covering gingival recession around teeth), to increase the zone of attached keratinized gingiva, and to deepen the vestibule with simultaneous removal of frenal attachment. Figure 17 demonstrates that treatment with an FGG on the buccal aspect of implant #25 helps

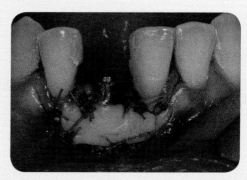

Figure 16: A FGG is stabilized on the buccal aspect of implant #25 with sutures.

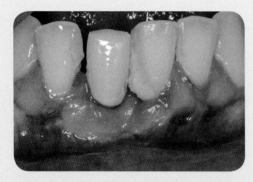

Figure 17: Post-operative healing at 4 weeks shows complete coverage of the exposed implant threads (see Figure 14 for pre-operative photograph). Implant #25 now has an adequate amount of buccal keratinized gingiva. Aberrant frenal attachment on the mesial aspects of implant #25 has also been removed. Note that FGG also achieves root coverage on the buccal aspects of tooth #24. Patient was given further instructions on plaque control and was placed on 3-month hygiene visits.

to create healthier peri-implant soft tissues that are important in the overall health of a dental implant.

F. Following FGG procedures, patients will typically experience some swelling and discomfort in the form of pain and soreness peaking around 48–72 h postoperatively. There may also be some minor bleeding. These events are parts of the normal healing process and can be minimized by applying a cold compress, such as an ice pack, for the first 48 h after surgery (off and on every 10–15 min), taking pain medications (starting nonsteroidal anti-inflammatory drugs such as ibuprofen prior to surgery may help reduce inflammation), and applying gauze with firm pressure at the bleeding site for 20–30 min. Patients should refrain from disturbing the surgical sites by touching or eating/chewing in these areas. Disturbances to the donor sites may lead to unwanted bleeding. Disturbances to the recipient sites where gingival grafts are stabilized by sutures may result in failure of the grafts because initially the grafts depend solely on diffusion from the recipient beds for survival (this phenomenon is known as plasmatic circulation) [2].

G. Although they are relatively uncommon, complications during or following FGG procedures can occur [21]. Most of the reported complications are as follows. First, excessive or prolonged intra-/postoperative bleeding at the donor sites can occur if the incisions are made too deep into the palatal

tissues where a palatal vessel may be severed [22]. It is also important to conduct thorough medical histories to identify patients with clotting deficiencies or bleeding disorders. To control bleeding, pressure should be applied to the bleeding sites for 20–30 min. If greater palatine artery/vein and/or its branches are severed, compress sutures tightened over this vasculature may help slow down the bleeding. Administration of 1:50,000 epinephrine available in some local anesthetic solutions could also reduce bleeding. Moreover, hemostatic agents such as Gelfoam® (absorbable collagen sponge) and Surgicel® (cellulose polymer) can be applied to the bleeding sites to encourage hemostasis.

Second, bony exposure can happen at the donor site postoperatively [22]. Clinicians need to determine the thickness of the gingival grafts to be harvested and measure the thickness of the donor tissues (e.g., palatal tissue thickness) to avoid leaving denuded bone or a very thin layer of periosteum that may result in tissue necrosis [22]. Clinicians should also be aware of the prevalence of palatal exostoses in the posterior maxillary alveolar processes when harvesting palatal donor tissues [23]. Bone sounding with a periodontal probe after local anesthesia of the donor site is a useful technique to measure the thickness of donor tissue.

Third, the discrepancy of color matching between the grafts and the adjacent gingiva of the recipient sites may occur with grafts thicker than 1.25 mm or in individuals whose keratinized gingiva contain physiologic pigmentation [22]. The color matching problem could potentially be minimized by harvesting thinner grafts (0.75–1.25 mm) and making beveled incisions at the attached gingiva [24]. Fourth, if the muscle fibers and the loose tissues in the submucosa were not adequately removed at the recipient sites, the overlying gingival grafts will be "movable" and thus not offering the physical seal that attached gingiva offers [2] (refer to answer to self-study question B). Fifth, delayed healing of both donor and recipient sites may happen with excess granulation tissues occurring at the margin of the graft or the flap [22,25]. Lastly, failure of the graft union could potentially occur if grafts are placed over a large area of denuded bone at the recipient sites [22,24]. Without periosteum, the blood supply to the grafts will be limited, leading to necrosis of the overlying grafts.

Case 2

Subepithelial Connective Tissue Graft

CASE STORY
A 24-year-old Caucasian male presented with a chief complaint of "I don't like the appearance of the gum around my front implant, or the restoration itself" (Figure 1). Owing to trauma sustained in a car accident 5 years ago, tooth #8 was assigned a hopeless prognosis. The patient received immediate implant placement with immediate provisionalization from his previous dentist. The patient visited his dentist regularly and shared his concern regarding the esthetics of the implant site. He was told that there was nothing to do in order to improve the appearance of the tissue discoloration associated with a grayish hue on the facial peri-implant mucosa (Figure 2).

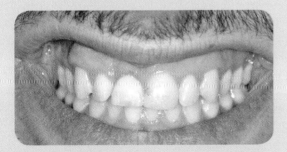

Figure 1: Preoperative presentation (facial view).

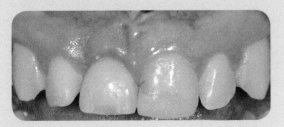

Figure 2: Preoperative presentation (intraoral view).

Medical History
The medical history was noncontributory and there were no contraindications to surgical treatment. The patient was not taking any medication and had no known allergies.

Review of Systems
- Vital signs
  - Blood pressure: 120/80 mmHg
  - Pulse rate: 72 beats/min (regular)
  - Respiration: 12 breaths/min

Social History
The patient did not smoke or drink alcohol at the time of treatment.

Extraoral Examination
A comprehensive extraoral examination consisting of assessment of temporomandibular joint function, facial asymmetries, and other alterations of normality by observation and palpation was conducted. No significant findings were noticed.

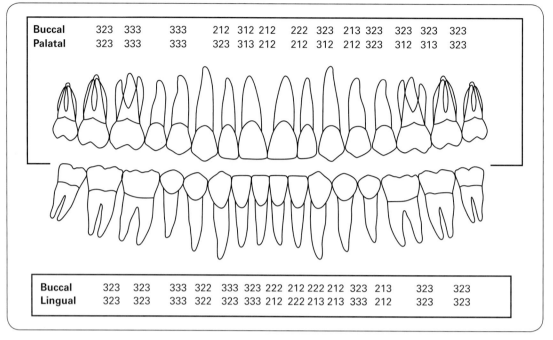

Buccal	323	333	333	212	312	212	222	323	213	323	323	323	323
Palatal	323	333	333	323	313	212	212	312	212	323	312	313	323

Buccal	323	323	333	322	333	323	222	212	222	212	323	213	323	323
Lingual	323	323	333	322	323	333	212	222	213	213	333	212	323	323

Figure 3: Probing depth measurements at the initial visit.

Intraoral Examination

- Intra- and extraoral exam was within normal limits; oral cancer screening was negative.
- Probing depths were in the range of 2–3 mm (Figure 3).
- Signs of gingival inflammation (bleeding on probing 15%) and grayish facial hue was observed on the facial of #8 implant (Figure 2).
- Shorter clinical crown on #8 implant-supported restoration was also observed (Figure 4).
- Oral hygiene: full mouth plaque score was <20%. He reported brushing and flossing regularly, at least once a day.

Occlusal analysis

Occlusion was stable. Interocclusal relationship was an Angle class I. There were no occlusal discrepancies or interferences.

Radiographic Examination

A full mouth radiographic series was obtained. Figure 4 is the periapical radiograph of the area of interest. Radiographic examination of this site revealed normal marginal bone levels. A localized cone bean computer tomography (CBCT) scan (Scanora 3D Nahkelantie 160, 04300 Tuusula, Finland) with a reduced field of view (6 cm × 6 cm) was obtained in order to identify the residual amount of bone at the facial aspect of the

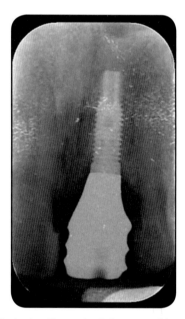

Figure 4: Periapical radiograph of the area of interest.

implant. The CBCT scan showed the presence of adequate bone circumferentially around #8 implant (Figure 5).

Diagnoses

- Peri-implant mucositis around #8 implant.
- Abnormal color of the peri-implant mucosa on #8.

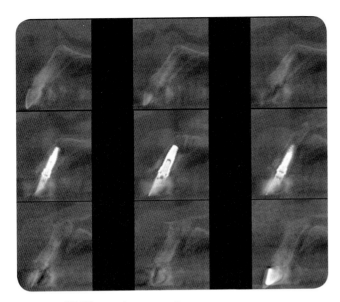

Figure 5: CBCT scan image captures.

- Ridge deficiency confined to the mucosal tissue on the facial aspect of #8 implant (Figure 6).
- Peri-implant mucosa excess, leading to a short clinical crown, on #8 implant.

Treatment Plan

The treatment plan for this patient consisted of initial-phase therapy that included oral prophylaxis and oral hygiene instructions to address the peri-implant mucositis. Upon completion of the disease control phase, the corrective phase was initiated by the performance of a subepithelial connective tissue graft (SeCTG) procedure. The indication of this surgical intervention was indicated to correct the facial tissue volume deficiency on #8 implant. After maturation of the grafted site (between 12 and 16 weeks postsurgically), the emergence profile of the provisional crown was modified in order to achieve an ideal soft tissue profile around the implant and to match the gingival contour of the adjacent/contralateral central incisor. After adequate time for mucosal stabilization (approximately 3 months) the definitive crown was delivered.

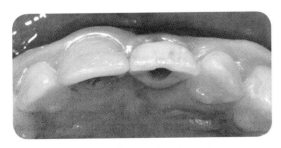

Figure 6: Pre-op presentation (occlusal view).

Treatment

Following initial-phase therapy aimed at controlling the peri-implant mucosal inflammation, the patient presented for the SeCTG. The implant-supported crown on #8 was replaced with a healing abutment in order to gain better access to the surgical area. After obtaining local anesthesia at the surgical site, a full-thickness buccal pouch was created. The connective tissue graft was harvested from the palate (Figure 7). Briefly, an access incision was made buccal to the implant and extended mesially and distally to the adjacent teeth (#7 and #9). The incision was made through the periosteum to allow for the creation of a subperiosteal tunnel, exposing the facial osseous plate. The tunnel was extended one tooth apart from the implant site, both in the mesial and distal directions, in order to mobilize the mucosal margins and to facilitate coronal repositioning of the flap. A microsurgical periosteal evator (De mini flat tip, Karl Schumacher 108 Lakeside Drive, Southampton, PA, USA) was used to create the subperiosteal tunnel. The elevator was introduced through the facial access incision and inserted between the periosteum and bone to elevate the periosteum, creating the subperiosteal tunnel. It is important to extend the tunnel sufficiently beyond the mucogingival margin as well as through the gingival sulci of the teeth of interest to allow for low-tension coronal repositioning of the gingiva. Additionally, the subperiosteal tunnel was extended interproximally under each papilla, without making any surface incisions through the papillae. The graft was then secured under the tunnel with an external horizontal mattress suture (Vicryl, Ethicon, New Jersey, USA) (Figure 8). A provisional crown was then delivered and the patient was instructed not to brush or bite directly on the surgical area. The only postoperative medication prescribed was 800 mg ibuprofen tablets to be taken TID for the first 3 days after surgery. Sutures were removed at 1 week. Healing was normal at 2 weeks (Figure 9).

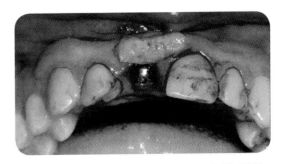

Figure 7: Subepithelial connective tissue graft (SeCTG).

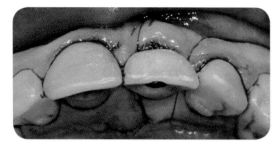

Figure 8: Graft and suture in place.

After 3 months of healing (Figure 10), the emergence profile of the provisional crown was modified in order to achieve an ideal soft tissue profile around the implant and to match the gingival contour of #9 (Figure 10). After adequate time for soft tissue stabilization (additional 3 months) the definitive crown was delivered (Figure 11).

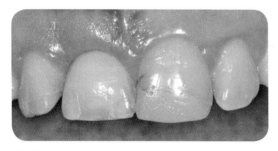

Figure 9: Postoperative aspect at 2 weeks.

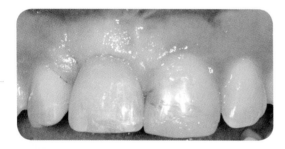

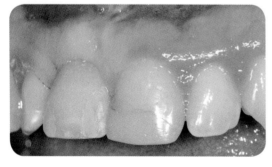

Figure 10: The emergence profile of the provisional crown was modified in order to achieve an ideal soft tissue profile around the implant.

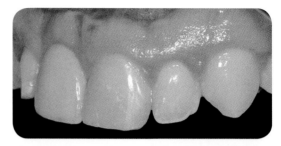

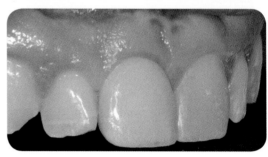

Figure 11: Final crown delivery.

Discussion

The natural appearance of an implant-supported restoration and the stability of the surrounding mucosal architecture are the foundation for a successful treatment outcome, particularly in the esthetic zone [1]. In this case the primary etiology of the mucosal discoloration over the facial of #8 implant was primarily due to inadequate soft tissue thickness. If an implant is placed in its correct three-dimensional position and is completely surrounded by bone up to the implant–abutment junction, the soft tissue discoloration and the color-change effect on the marginal peri-implant soft tissue is the result of inadequate mucosa thickness [2]. Jung et al. demonstrated that the restorative materials have a significant influence on soft tissue color appearance. Potentially unpleasant color appearance can be corrected with increasing mucosa thickness. In another study, Bressan et al. [3] reported that the presence of a different abutment closer to the soft tissue might affect the esthetic appearance of the peri-implant soft tissue and alter its color and appearance. For this reason the peri-implant mucosal color is different from the gingival color around natural teeth, regardless of the type of restorative material selected. The thickness of the peri-implant soft tissue appears to be a crucial factor in the impact of color alterations on the peri-implant mucosa.

Therefore, critical thresholds of mucosal thickness in the esthetic zone should be carefully considered. Interestingly, it has been shown that the color change induced by titanium may still cause a visible difference even with a mucosal thickness up to 2 mm [4]. On the other hand, with a minimum thickness of 3 mm no visible differences were identified independently of the abutment material tested. Therefore, a thick peri-implant biotype is always recommended in order to achieve an ideal esthetic result, particularly in anterior segments. In the case presented here, the 1-year follow-up photograph (Figure 12) shows stable tissue contour and adequate soft tissue scalloping with no presence of inflammation or discoloration of the peri-implant mucosa.

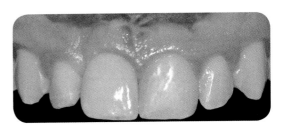

Figure 12: At 1 year post-op.

Self-Study Questions

(Answers located at the end of the case)

A. What is an SeCTG?

B. Is an SeCTG different from a free gingival graft (FGG)?

C. What is the gingival/mucosa biotype?

D. May the soft tissue thickness influence crestal bone changes around implants?

E. Is the SeCTG able to induce keratinization?

F. Is there a minimum keratinized mucosa thickness needed to maintain peri-implant health?

G. What are the main factors that influence the esthetic outcomes of an implant-supported restoration?

References

1. Kan JY, Rungcharassaeng K, Lozada JL, Zimmerman G. Facial gingival tissue stability following immediate placement and provisionalization of maxillary anterior single implants: a 2- to 8-year follow-up. Int J Oral Maxillofac Implants 2011;26(1):179–187.
2. Jung RE, Sailer I, Hämmerle CH, et al. In vitro color changes of soft tissues caused by restorative materials. Int J Periodontics Restorative Dent 2007;27(3).251–257.
3. Bressan E, Paniz G, Lops D, et al. Influence of abutment material on the gingival color of implant-supported all-ceramic restorations: a prospective multicenter study. Clin Oral Implants Res 2011;22(6):631–637.
4. Park SE, Da Silva JD, Weber HP, Ishikawa-Nagai N. Optical phenomenon of periimplant soft tissue. Part I. Spectrophotometric assessment of natural tooth gingival and peri-implant mucosa. Clin Oral Implant Res 2007;18:569–574.
5. Langer B, Calagna L. The subepithelial connective tissue graft. J Prosthet Dent 1980;44(4):363–367.
6. Allen EP, Gainza CS, Farthing GG, Newbold DA. Improved technique for localized ridge augmentation. A report of 21 cases. J Periodontol 1985;56(4):195–199.
7. Sullivan HC, Atkins JH. Free autogenous gingival grafts. I. Principles of successful grafting. Periodontics 1968;6(3):121–129.
8. Olsson M, Lindhe J. Periodontal characteristics in individuals with varying form of the upper central incisors. J Clin Periodontol 1991;18(1):78–82.
9. Gobbato L, Tsukiyama T, Levi Jr PA, et al. Analysis of the shapes of maxillary central incisors in a Caucasian population. Int J Periodontics Restorative Dent 2012;32(1):69–78.
10. Stellini E, Comuzzi L, Mazzocco F, et al. Relationships between different tooth shapes and patient's periodontal phenotype. J Periodontal Res 2013;48(5):657–662.
11. Hermann JS, Buser D, Schenk RK, et al. Biologic width around one- and two-piece titanium implants. Clin Oral Implants Res 2001;12(6):559–571.
12. Cochran DL, Hermann JS, Schenk RK, et al. Biologic width around titanium implants. A histometric analysis of the implanto-gingival junction around unloaded and loaded nonsubmerged implants in the canine mandible. J Periodontol 1997;68(2):186–198.
13. Iacono VJ. Dental implants in periodontal therapy. J Periodontol 2000;71:1934–1942.
14. Lindhe J, Berglundh T. The interface between the mucosa and the implant. Periodontol 2000 1998;17:47–54.
15. Linkevicius T, Apse P, Grybauskas S, Puisys A. The influence of soft tissue thickness on crestal bone changes around implants: a 1-year prospective controlled clinical trial. Int J Oral Maxillofac Implants 2009;24(4):712–719.

16. Karring T, Lang NP, Loe H. The role of gingival connective tissue in determining epithelial differentiation. J Periodontal Res 1975;10:1–11.
17. Lin GH, Chan HL, Wang HL. The significance of keratinized mucosa on implant health: a systematic review. J Periodontol 2013;84(12): 1755–1767.
18. Wennström JL, Derks J. Is there a need for keratinized mucosa around implants to maintain health and tissue stability? Clin Oral Implants Res 2012;23(Suppl 6):136–146.
19. Gobbato L, Avila-Ortiz G, Sohrabi K, et al. The effect of keratinized mucosa width on peri-implant health: a systematic review. Int J Oral Maxillofac Implants 2013;28(6):1536–1545.

Answers to Self-Study Questions

A. An SeCTG is one of the options that may be indicated to correct a mucogingival deformity [5], such as an alveolar ridge deficiency or to perform a root coverage procedure. The graft is typically harvested from the masticatory mucosa of the hard palate and/or the tuberosity. SeCTGs are composed of glandular tissue, fatty tissue and connective tissue, in different proportions depending on the location and individual patient features. The full-thickness inlay graft technique [6], which is presented in this case, was indicated to correct the soft tissue defect by adding an average of 2–4 mm thickness.

B. FGGs of the palatal mucosa are harvested to augment the width of keratinized tissue in dentate patients or around dental implants [7]. An FGG may also be utilized in conjunction with vestibuloplasty to increase the supportive area of a removable denture base. A typical FGG consists of fatty tissue, connective tissue, and epithelium. This graft is stabilized with sutures to cover the recipient site, which has been previously de-epithelized to expose the underlying connective tissue. As mentioned earlier, the SeCTG is harvested from the hard palate or tuberosity. The SeCTG typically does not contain any epithelium, but on occasion there can be a thin collar along one edge. The recipient site is prepared by elevating a partial-thickness flap underneath which the connective tissue graft is placed; finally, the partial-thickness flap is sutured back into its original position or coronally advanced, depending on the therapeutic goal. Nonsubmerged grafts (FGGs) are no longer justified in the coverage of recession defects for esthetic purposes. The procedure is uncomfortable for the patient because of the denuded palatal donor site, and the match with the surrounding tissues is unpredictable.

C. Seibert and Lindhe in 1989 proposed the term "periodontal biotype" to designate distinct features (i.e., flat–thick and scalloped–thin) of the periodontium, including the underlying alveolar bone. The term "periodontal biotype" has been discussed and described in the literature by many authors [8]. Recent research has revealed that the morphologic characteristics of the gingiva and periodontium are related to the dimensions of the alveolar process, the shape of the teeth [9], and the eventual inclination and position of the fully erupted teeth. Thus, a tooth with a tapered crown form and minute proximal contact areas it seems is generally associated with a thin periodontal biotype, including a thin bony housing. Teeth with a short but wide crown and with large contact areas, however, are usually associated with a thick periodontal biotype and a thick bony housing [10].

D. The influence biologic width formation on crestal bone loss around implants has been intensely discussed in recent years [11]. It was observed that the healthy peri-implant mucosa formed a barrier around the implant–abutment interface that is comprised of two zones: one including a junctional epithelium and one zone comprised of a collagen-rich but cell-poor connective tissue [12]. This soft tissue extension is usually referred to as the biologic width around implants, and it serves as a protective mechanism for the underlying bone. Some have suggested that if a minimal mucosal dimension is not available, bone loss may occur to ensure the proper development of the biologic width [13]. These findings are consistent with prior tooth-related studies, which showed that the establishment of biologic width after tooth crown lengthening involved crestal bone loss. However, data regarding the relationship between mucosal thickness (buccolingual dimension) and marginal bone loss around implants are scarce. In an animal experiment, Lindhe and Berglundh [14] reported that the preexisting presence of surrounding thin tissues may induce marginal bone loss during formation of the peri-implant mucosal seal. Observations in another histologic study showed that implants surrounded by consistently thin mucosa tended to have angular bone defects, while a wide mucosa biotype prevailed at implant sites with an even alveolar pattern [15]. However, the evidence provided by well-designed animal studies is limited, which in turn reduces the generalizability of the aforementioned results to clinical practice [15]. In addition, clinical research regarding the effects of tissue thickness on bone stability around implants in humans is lacking.

In a recent controlled clinical trial, Linkevicius et al. [15] tested the influence of gingival tissue thickness on marginal bone loss around placed implants; they recommended to avoid a supracrestal implant placement if a thin mucosal biotype is present. Based on this evidence, it is recommended to consider the thickening of thin mucosa prior to implant placement in order to minimize the occurrence of complications.

E. In 1975 Karring et al. [16] published an experimental study in monkeys where they tested the ability of gingival connective tissue in determining epithelial differentiation. The results suggested that gingival connective tissue is capable of inducing formation of a keratinized gingival epithelium per se. Based on the findings in this study it can be inferred that the epithelium of the graft develops through the migration of nonkeratinized epithelial cells of the surrounding alveolar mucosa and that, upon passing the junction between the two types of connective tissue, the gingival connective tissue induces their differentiation into cells with the same characteristics as those of keratinized gingival epithelium.

F. The absence of periodontal ligament, and connective tissue attachment around dental implants, may make peri-implant tissues more susceptible to the development of a robust inflammatory response when exposed to dental plaque accumulation and microbial invasion. For these reasons, it may be logical to think that the presence of a cuff-like mucosal barrier, provided by a band of peri-implant keratinized

mucosa, is an essential requisite to ensure successful long-term maintenance of peri-implant tissues from both biological and esthetic standpoints. However, there is a lack of strong evidence with regard to risk/benefits of absence/presence of keratinized mucosa at dental implants. As of today there are three systematic reviews [17–19] observing that limited keratinized mucosa around implants (<2 mm) is associated with clinical parameters of inflammation. In clinical situations where proper plaque control is performed, data suggest that the presence of keratinized mucosa around implants may not be of importance. However, on the basis of the selected evidence, the predictive value of keratinized mucosa is limited. There is a need for adequately powered, prospective longitudinal clinical trials to elucidate the importance of keratinized mucosa in the maintenance of peri-implant health.

G. Esthetics encompasses not only implant-supported restorations that mimic nature, but also healthy peri-implant tissues with an adequate architecture. Papilla loss and facial gingival recession represent esthetically challenging situations. Studies have been conducted to identify the etiologies of tissue loss, and techniques have been developed to prevent or minimize its occurrence. The preservation or reproduction of a natural mucogingival architecture surrounding dental implants placed in the anterior maxilla is challenging for the restorative dentist, particularly when patients present with a high lip line upon smiling. The challenge arises from the loss of mucogingival tissue as a result of bone remodeling after tooth extraction/loss. The selection of a dental implant system that allows a proper biological response of the hard and soft tissues in a particular clinical scenario represents the first step for the achievement of an adequate esthetic result. Additionally, a proper surgical technique, ideal three-dimensional implant positioning, and soft tissue management are necessary for a natural outcome. Finally, the selection of the proper prosthetic solution, both in terms of material and contour, which is often overlooked, contributes significantly to the achievement of a proper shade and shape of the peri-implant mucosa. The utilization of custom abutments that allow for an ideal emergence profile is critical for the achievement of proper esthetic results, particularly in those sites with thin biotype.

Case 3

Vestibuloplasty and Frenectomy

CASE STORY

A 48-year-old Asian woman presented with a lack of adequate vestibular depth around implant #14. The patient underwent horizontal ridge augmentation, maxillary sinus bone augmentation, and implant placement at site #14. Owing to the severe loss of vertical bone height at site #14, implant #14 was placed about 4–6 mm apical to the cementoenamel junction (CEJ) of #13 (Figure 1). Therefore, the level of the implant–abutment junction was close to the depth of the surrounding vestibule. Although there was a band of 2–3 mm keratinized gingiva on the buccal aspect of implant #14, the vestibule was very shallow (Figure 2). Consequently, when the patient was at rest the alveolar mucosa surrounding the keratinized gingiva impinged closely against the healing abutment of implant #14, leaving no vestibule (Figure 2). In addition, there was a frenum-like structure attaching to #13 that might have made the patient's oral hygiene home care more difficult (Figure 3).

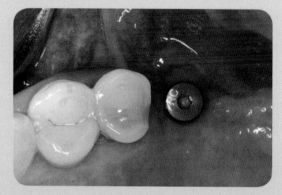

Figure 2: A band of 2–3 mm keratinized gingiva was present on buccal of implant #14. However, owing to the lack of vestibule, the buccal alveolar mucosa surrounding implant #14 constantly impinged upon implant healing abutment, resulting in an "excessive" tissue fold in the mucosa.

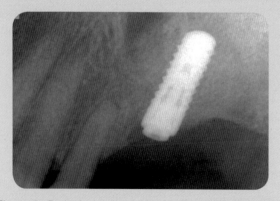

Figure 1: Periapical radiograph of implant #14 showed the implant platform 4–6 mm apical to CEJ of tooth #13.

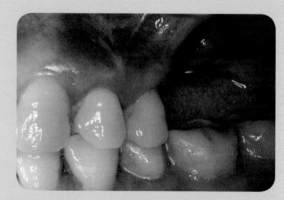

Figure 3: A frenum-like structure attached to tooth #13 might prevent effective plaque control. The "excessive" tissue fold in the buccal mucosa of implant #14 was also evident.

LEARNING GOALS AND OBJECTIVES

- To be able to identify the lack of vestibule and abnormal frenal attachments around dental implants
- To understand the potential complications associated with insufficient vestibules or abnormal frenal attachments around dental implants
- To understand the treatment options available for creating adequate vestibular depth and removing abnormal frenal attachments around dental implants

Medical History

The patient was well nourished with no acute distress at the time of examination. The patient reported no significant medical history and no allergies to medications.

Review of Systems

- Vital signs
  - Blood pressure: 126/76 mmHg
  - Pulse rate: 65 beats/min
  - Respiration: 14 breaths/min

Social History

The patient never smoked and drank alcoholic beverages only on social occasions. The patient denied using recreational drugs.

Extraoral Examination

No abnormal swellings and masses were detected. Lymph nodes were normal upon palpation. Temporomandibular joints and muscles of mastication appeared normal.

Intraoral Examination

- Oral cancer screening was negative.
- Soft tissues, including buccal mucosa, tongue, floor of the mouth, and hard/soft palate, were all normal.
- Plaque accumulation was visible at posterior teeth and mandibular anterior teeth.
- Gingiva in general was healthy except at implant site #14, where there was insufficient keratinized gingiva with a lack of vestibule. There was a frenum-like attachment buccal of tooth #13.
- Periodontal charting (Figure 4) showed no probing pocket depths greater than 3 mm except around implant #14, which had some pocket depths of 4 mm with bleeding on probing. No tooth mobility, furcal involvement, gingival recession, and mucogingival defect were detected.

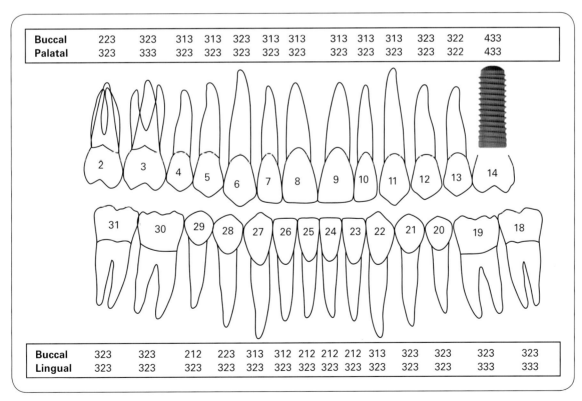

Buccal	223	323	313	313	323	313	313	313	313	313	323	322	433	
Palatal	323	333	323	323	323	323	323	323	323	323	323	322	433	

Buccal	323	323	212	223	313	312	212	212	212	313	323	323	323	323	
Lingual	323	323	323	323	323	323	323	323	323	323	323	323	333	333	

Figure 4: Probing pocket depth measurements at initial visit.

Occlusion

There were no occlusal discrepancies.

Radiographic Examination

The periapical radiograph showed loss of vertical alveolar ridge height and evidence of sinus bone augmentation at site #14 (Figure 1). The implant platform of #14 was placed about 4–6 mm apical to th CEJ of tooth #13 due to loss of ridge height.

Diagnosis and Prognosis

The patient was diagnosed with plaque-induced gingivitis according to the American Academy of Periodontology [1] and peri-implant mucositis at implant #14 due to the presence of bleeding on probing and the absence of detectable peri-implant bone loss [2]. In addition, the patient was diagnosed with a lack of adequate vestibule around implant #14 and an aberrant frenum-like attachment buccal of tooth #13.

Although Kwok and Caton's periodontal prognostic classification system was intended for assigning prognosis to natural dentition [3], this system could also be useful in assigning prognosis to dental implants. By using this prognosis system, implant #14 was assigned with a questionable prognosis because of the difficulty in controlling plaque around implant #14 due to a lack of vestibular depth and a proximal aberrant frenal-like attachment.

Treatment Plan

The following treatment plan and treatment sequence were discussed with the patient.
- Diagnostic phase – comprehensive periodontal examination, radiographic examination.
- Disease control phase – oral hygiene instruction, oral prophylaxis.
- Surgical phase – vestibuloplasty at implant #14 and labial frenectomy at tooth #13.
- Reevaluation phase – follow up on healing of vestibuloplasty and frenectomy up to 1 year.
- Maintenance phase – periodic implant maintenance visit once every 3–6 months depending on patient's plaque control.

Treatment Rendered

Following the disease control phase when patient's oral hygiene had been optimized, vestibuloplasty on buccal of implant #14 and frenectomy on tooth #13 were performed in conjunction with a gingival graft (Figure 5A–D). A horizontal incision was made slightly

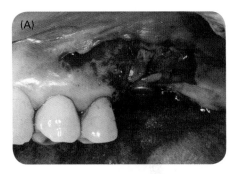
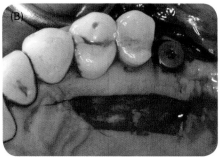
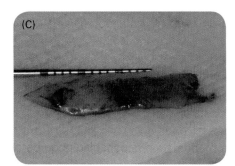
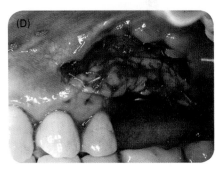
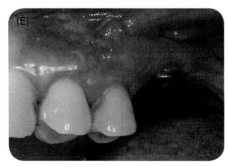
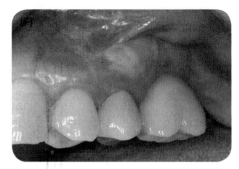

Figure 5: Vestibuloplasty and frenectomy with gingival graft at tooth #13 and implant #14. (A) A split-thickness flap was raised at mucogingival junction. (B) A gingival graft was harvested from the left palate. (C) Gingival graft was measured about 25 mm × 7 mm. (D) Gingival graft was sutured at recipient site with multiple single interrupted sutures going through the graft and the periosteum. (E) Three-week postoperative visit showed uneventful healing. (F) Vestibule had been deepened with the absence of frenum-like attachment at 4-month follow-up visit. An adequate band of keratinized gingiva was present at the buccal aspect of implant #14.

coronal to the mucogingival junction buccal to tooth #13 and implant #14, and a split-thickness flap was raised, leaving periosteum as the recipient bed for the gingival graft. Mobile tissues over the periosteum, especially at tooth #13 where a frenum-like structure was attached, were removed. A 1.5 mm thick 25 mm × 7 mm gingival graft was then harvested from the left palate and placed over the prepared periosteum bed at sites #13 and #14. The gingival graft was sutured with multiple single interrupted sutures that engaged both the periosteum and the graft. After stabilizing the gingival graft, the buccal vestibule was pulled manually to check for any mobility of the graft to ensure graft stability. At the 3-week postoperative visit, healing at the surgical site appeared normal with evidence of an adequate band of keratinized gingiva over tooth #13 and implant #14 (Figure 5E). Four months postoperatively, buccal gingiva at sites #13 and #14 exhibited signs of complete keratinization with a band of 7–10 mm keratinized tissue, an adequate vestibular depth, and the absence of labial frenum (Figure 5F).

Discussion

A combination of a frenum-like structure and a lack of adequate vestibule at the buccal aspect of sites #13 and #14 made it difficult for the patient to effectively remove plaque due to the limited space available for hygiene instrumentation (e.g., toothbrush and floss). As such, vestibuloplasty and frenectomy were indicated in this situation. Vestibuloplasty and frenectomy were performed in conjunction with a gingival graft because, in addition to vestibule deepening and frenum removal, a wide band of keratinized gingiva on the buccal aspect

of implant #14 was desired. Clinicians could also perform vestibuloplasty and frenectomy without gingival grafts by making incisions within the keratinized gingiva and apically position the gingival flap (see answer to self-study question D). Both vestibuloplasty and frenectomy could be done prior to or after implant restoration. In this case, surgical procedures were carried out prior to implant #14 restoration to permit better visualization and access during the surgery.

Factors that might have led to an aberrant frenum-like attachment and a shallow vestibule at sites #13 and #14 were as follows (see answer to self-study question C). First, this patient initially presented with a severely pneumatized left maxillary sinus and Seibert class III alveolar ridge defect [4] that required sinus bone augmentation and horizontal ridge augmentation. It is not uncommon for patients who had severely resorbed alveolar ridges to present with limited keratinized gingiva. Second, the need to coronally advance the soft tissue flap for primary closure during the bone augmentation procedures might have led to the formation of a shallow vestibule. Third, the frenum-like structure at site #13 might have been a scar tissue that had formed during the bone augmentation procedure. To regain the lost vestibule and keratinized gingiva, clinicians could apically position the keratinized gingiva at the time of implant surgery or perform a gingival graft before, at, or after the implant fixture placement. Regardless of the types of surgical approach taken, clinicians should inform the patient about the possible need for vestibuloplasty and frenectomy whenever extensive ridge augmentation procedures are indicated as part of the implant therapy.

Self-Study Questions

(Answers located at the end of the case)

A. What is a vestibule? What is a frenum?

B. What are some clinical issues that may arise with insufficient vestibular depths and aberrant frenal attachments around dental implants?

C. What may lead to shallow vestibules and aberrant frenal attachments around dental implants?

D. How are vestibuloplasty and frenectomy performed?

E. What are some potential contraindications to vestibuloplasty and frenectomy?

References

1. Armitage GC; Research, Science and Therapy Committee of the American Academy of Periodontology. Diagnosis of periodontal diseases. J Periodontol 2003; 74(8):1237–1247.
2. Lang NP, Berglundh T; Working Group 4 of Seventh European Workshop on Periodontology. Periimplant diseases: where are we now? – Consensus of the Seventh European Workshop on Periodontology. J Clin Periodontol 2011;38(Suppl 11):178–181.
3. Kwok V, Caton JG. Commentary: prognosis revisited: a system for assigning periodontal prognosis. J Periodontol 2007;78(11):2063–2071.
4. Seibert JS. Reconstruction of deformed, partially edentulous ridges, using full thickness onlay grafts. Part II. Prosthetic/periodontal interrelationships. Compend Contin Educ Dent 1983;4:549–562.
5. Heitz-Mayfield LJ. Peri-implant diseases: diagnosis and risk indicators. J Clin Periodontol 2008;35(8 Suppl):292–304.
6. Kuboki Y, Hashimoto F, Ishibashi K. Time-dependent changes of collagen crosslinks in the socket after tooth extraction in rabbits. J Dental Res 1988;67:944–948.
7. Devlin H, Hoyland J, Newall JF, Ayad S. Trabecular bone formation in the healing of the rodent molar tooth extraction socket. J Bone Mineral Res 1997;12:2061–2067.
8. Amler MH, Johnson PL, Salman I. Histological and histochemical investigation of human alveolar socket healing in undisturbed extraction wounds. J Am Dent Assoc 1960;61:32–44.
9. Devlin H, Sloan P. Early bone healing events in the human extraction socket. Int J Oral Maxillofac Surg 2002;31:641–645.
10. Machtei EE. The effect of membrane exposure on the outcome of regenerative procedures in humans: a meta-analysis. J Periodontol 2001;72:512–516.
11. Ochsenbein C. Newer concept of mucogingival surgery. J Periodontol 1960;31:175–185.
12. Wilderman MN, Wentz FM, Orban BJ. Histogenesis of repair after mucogingival surgery. J Periodontol 1961;31:283–299.
13. Staffileno H, Wentz FM, Orban BJ. Histologic study of healing of split thickness flap surgery in dogs. J Periodontol 1962;33:56–69.
14. Wilderman MN. Repair after a periosteal retention procedure. J Periodontol 1963;34:484–503.
15. Medeiros Júnior R, Gueiros LA, Silva IH, et al. Labial frenectomy with Nd:YAG laser and conventional surgery: a comparative study. Lasers Med Sci 2015;30(2):851–856.
16. Kovacevska G, Tomov G, Baychev P, et al. Er:YAG laser assisted vestibuloplasty: a case report. J Surg 2013; 1:59–62.
17. Ho DK, Elangovan S, Shih S. Chapter 5: Mucogingival therapy – case 5: frenectomy and vestibuloplasty. In: Karimbux N (ed.), Clinical Cases in Periodontics, 1st edn. Ames, IA: John Wiley & Sons, Inc.; 2012, pp 197–203.

Answers to Self-Study Questions

A. A vestibule in the oral cavity is the space between the teeth and the inside of the cheeks and lips. An oral vestibule provides room for temporary storage of food particles during mastication. Vestibules with adequate depth facilitate oral hygiene home care by providing space for hygiene instrumentation (e.g., toothbrush, floss). A frenum in the oral cavity is a tissue fold that attaches the inside of the lips, cheeks, or floor of the mouth to alveolar mucosa, gingiva, and/or the underlying periosteum. A frenum restricts the mobility of the tissues that it attaches to. For example, a lingual frenum restricts the mobility of the tongue.

B. Insufficient vestibular depths around dental implants hinder the ability of patients to practice good plaque control because of the lack of space for hygiene instrumentation. High frenal attachments around dental implants may act as barriers that prevent thorough cleansing of implant restorations and peri-implant tissues. In addition, if the peri-implant gingiva where the frenum attaches to is thin, the pulling force exerted through the frenum to the thin gingiva may result in gingival recession around dental implants (Figure 6). All these situations lead to greater plaque retention. Therefore, the risk of developing peri-implant mucositis and peri-implantitis is increased because poor oral hygiene due to inadequate plaque removal is a risk indicator for peri-implant diseases [5]. Gingival inflammation resulting from plaque accumulation around implants has the potential to negatively affect peri-implant hard and soft tissues, thereby jeopardizing the functionality and the esthetics of the implant restorations.

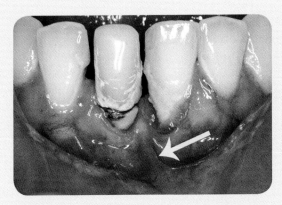

Figure 6: A combination of aberrant frenal attachment (yellow arrow), frenal pull, ill-fitting restoration, and plaque/calculus accumulation due to poor oral hygiene leads to peri-implantitis around implant #25.

C. The alveolar processes in the jaws are tooth-dependent structures that will undergo significant structural changes following tooth loss. The dynamics and the magnitude of these changes have been investigated in both dog [6,7] and human studies [8,9]. These investigations have identified the key processes of tissue modeling and remodeling after tooth extraction that eventually lead to a reduction on the overall ridge dimensions with significant changes in both the buccal and lingual bone crests. Reduction in both ridge height and width then results in the reduction of vestibular depth.

Guided bone regeneration procedures are performed to increase the alveolar ridge width and height. Mucoperiosteal releasing incisions are often required in these procedures to coronally advance the soft tissue flaps for primary closure that is critical to new bone formation [10]. However, in advancing the flaps coronally, the vestibule depths are shortened. The shortening of the vestibular depth is even more evident when coronally advancing flaps over alveolar ridges that already have severe loss of height and shallow vestibule to begin with.

Aberrant frenal attachments may appear in the form of scar tissues resulting from previous surgical procedures that involved vertical releasing incisions (Figure 3). Alternatively, aberrant frenal attachments sometimes can just be what the individual is born with (e.g., frenum attachments very close to the free gingival margin). It is important for clinicians to communicate to patients the potential needs for frenum removal or repositioning around dental implants to facilitate plaque control.

D. Vestibuloplasty is a surgical procedure utilized to "restore" the alveolar ridge height by apically positioning the soft tissues attaching to the buccal or lingual aspects of the ridge. Vestibuloplasty can be performed in a few different ways. In the denudation technique, all of the soft tissues from the gingival margin to the mucogingival junction are removed, leaving the underlying alveolar bone exposed to the oral cavity [11]. The goal of this procedure is to remove and replace the existing gingiva with a new and wider zone of attached gingiva. In so doing, the vestibule is deepened. However, some adverse effects, such as extensive bone resorption and severe patient discomfort during healing, are observed [12].

In split-flap vestibuloplasty, only the superficial part of the oral mucosa is removed, leaving bone covered by the periosteum [13,14]. Here, a horizontal incision is made slightly coronal to the mucogingival junction with respect of the amount of the residual keratinized tissue. In the instance of a complete absence of keratinized gingiva, the horizontal incision is made just below the free gingiva margin down to the periosteum. Two vertical incisions are often needed to better expose the underlying periosteum, thereby facilitating the reflection and the apical positioning of the flap. A deep split-thickness flap is raised, leaving only the periosteum as the protection of the underlying ridge and the recipient bed for the gingival graft if vestibuloplasty is to be performed in combination with gingival graft (see Chapter 4 Case 1 – Free Gingival Grafts). Any mobile tissues and frena should be removed (frenectomy) over the periosteum in order to avoid the recurrence of the soft tissue deformity during healing. If gingival grafting is expected, the graft is to be harvested from the palate or the maxillary tuberosity and to be stabilized by means of multiple single interrupted or internal mattress sutures that engage both the periosteum and the graft. The flap is positioned apically to the planned depth of the vestibule. A surgical pack may be used to protect the surgical site and the newly exposed zone of periosteum if a gingival graft is not performed.

Frenectomy is performed by the complete removal of the frenal attachments that house fibrous tissues. Similar to vestibuloplasty, clinicians have the choice of leaving or not leaving a layer of periosteum over the bone. A gingival graft can also be placed over the area where the frenum was.

Both vestibuloplasty and frenectomy can be done using scalpel blades or soft tissue lasers [15,16]. In summary, vestibuloplasty and frenectomy can be performed either with a split-thickness or a full-thickness flap in conjunction with or without gingival grafts.

Please consult the case on Frenectomy and Vestibuloplasty in *Clinical Cases in Periodontics* for more information on how to perform vestibuloplasty and frenectomy [17].

E. Because vestibuloplasty and frenectomy can induce secondary intention healing when the underlying periosteums are left exposed, it is not uncommon for the surgical sites to develop scar (keloid) tissues whose color may be different from the surrounding tissue color. In addition, the new mucogingival junction formed at the surgical site may not align with adjacent mucogingival junction. For these reasons, vestibuloplasty and frenectomy may be relatively contraindicated in areas with high esthetic demands. Furthermore, if the area of vestibuloplasty and frenectomy is in close proximity to delicate anatomical structures such as the mental foramen, it may be contraindicated to perform such procedures with sharp instruments to prevent structural damage such as nerve damage.

5

Ridge Site Preparation

Case 1

Xenograft Membrane: Porcine Derived

CASE STORY

A 48-year-old African American female presented with a chief complaint of "I don't feel comfortable with my anterior bridge, it always bleeds. I want to change it." The patient lost teeth #8 and #9 due to trauma 10 years ago. She had a four-unit fixed partial denture (FPD) fabricated and placed from tooth #7 to tooth #10 to restore the edentulous area. However, this restoration had open margins and it was overcontoured (Figures 1 and 2). The patient visited her dentist regularly for uninterrupted dental care and reported that she brushed and floss at least once a day. She had multiple composite restorations.

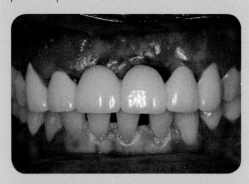

Figure 1: Initial presentation.

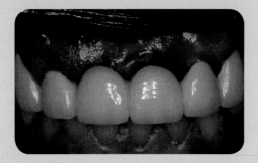

Figure 2: Initial presentation maxillary anteriors.

LEARNING GOALS AND OBJECTIVES

■ To be able to understand the concept of using a resorbable barrier membrane for guided bone regeneration (GBR)
■ To learn the different uses of resorbable barrier membranes (DynaMatrix®) in periodontal surgeries
■ To understand the factors affecting the outcomes of periodontal surgeries using a resorbable barrier membrane (DynaMatrix)

Medical History

At the time of treatment the patient presented with hypertension, controlled with medications (lisnopril 5 mg/day).

Review of Systems

• Vital signs
  ○ Blood pressure: 132/86 mmHg
  ○ Pulse rate: 86 beats/min
  ○ Respiration: 15 breaths/min

Social History

The patient is a former smoker (10 years ago); she was not smoking or drinking alcohol at the time of starting the treatment.

Extraoral Examination

No significant findings were noted. The patient had no masses or swelling and the temporomandibular joint was within normal limits. Facial asymmetry was noted and her lymph nodes were normal on palpation.

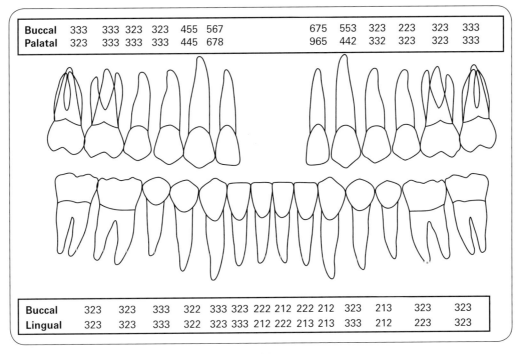

Buccal	333	333	323	323	455	567		675	553	323	223	323	333
Palatal	323	333	333	333	445	678		965	442	332	323	323	333

Buccal	323	323	333	322	333	323	222	212	222	212	323	213	323	323
Lingual	323	323	333	322	323	333	212	222	213	213	333	212	223	323

Figure 3: Probing pocket depth measurements during the initial visit.

Intraoral Examination

- Oral cancer screening was negative.
- Soft tissue exam, including her tongue and floor of the mouth, were within normal limits.
- Periodontal examination revealed pocket depths in the range of 2–3 mm except in the upper anterior area, where she recorded between 6 and 9 mm (Figure 3).
- Localized areas of gingival inflammation noted in areas #7 and 10 (see Figures 1 and 2).
- Periapical abscess between teeth #6 and 7 with labial exudate (see Figure 2).
- Evaluation of the alveolar ridge in areas #8 and #9 revealed both horizontal and vertical ridge resorption (Figure 4).
- Extensive restorations in the form of single crowns and FPDs.

Occlusion

There were no occlusal discrepancies or interferences noted (Figures 1 and 2).

Radiographic Examination

A full mouth radiographic series was ordered (see Figure 5 for patient's periapical radiograph of the area of interest). Radiographic examination revealed normal bone levels except for the maxillary anterior area. Widening of the periodontal ligament were noted around #7 and #10. Open margins and recurrent decay were noted in teeth #7 and #10.

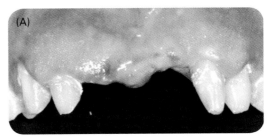
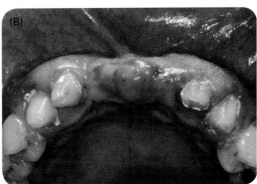

Figure 4: (A) Maxillary anteriors after #6-X-X-X-11 FPD removal. (B) Occlusal view of anterior maxilla.

Diagnosis

The diagnosis made according to American Academy of Periodontology was plaque-induced gingivitis with localized severe periodontitis in areas #6 and #11, irreversible pulpitis teeth #7 and #10, and #8–#9 edentulous area (Seibert class III) (Figure 4).

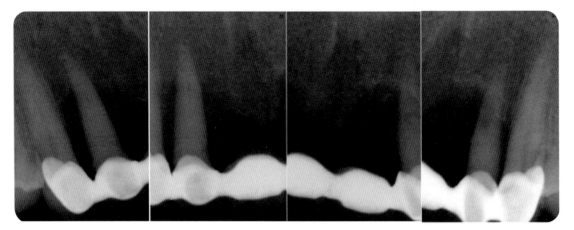

Figure 5: Periapical radiographs #6–#11.

Treatment Plan

The initial phase therapy included an oral prophylaxis with systemic antibiotic (amoxicillin 500 mg) and oral hygiene instructions to address gingival inflammation. This was followed by extraction of teeth #7 and #10. A GBR procedure was used to augment the buccopalatal deficiency of the alveolar ridge in area #7–#10. After adequate healing of the grafted site (4 months), the implants were placed in sites #7 and #10. The implants were restored with a four-unit implant-supported FPD after an adequate time for osseointegration (3 months). Teeth #6 and #11 were restored with single-unit crowns. An alternative treatment plan of a fixed bridge 6-X-X-X-X-11 was presented to the patient but she opted for the implant-supported bridge.

Treatment

After the initial-phase therapy, the patient presented for the extraction of teeth #7 and #10. Atraumatic extraction was performed using a periotome and universal forceps after obtaining profound anesthesia at the surgical site using local anesthetic; no flaps were reflected during the procedure. Sutures were placed to approximate the edges of the soft tissue. The sutures were removed after 2 weeks, and another 6 weeks of healing was allowed. In 8 weeks the patient presented for the #7–#10 GBR procedure. After using local anesthetic, full-thickness buccal and palatal flaps were reflected. The incision was midcrestal at sites #7 to #10, which extended to the adjacent teeth as sulcular incisions. Decortication was performed on the underlying bone using a small round bur to facilitate entry of blood cells from bone into the healing graft (Figure 6). Periosteal

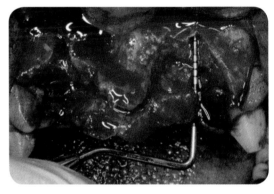

Figure 6: Area #7–#10 bone defect after flap reflection.

fenestration of the buccal flap was obtained to improve the coronal mobility of the flap to achieve tension-free primary closure. The size of the membrane was determined based on the defect size and trimmed accordingly. The membrane extended beyond the defect by at least 3 mm.

Bone allograft particles were saturated in distilled deionized water and then packed into the defect. The membrane was tucked underneath the buccal and palatal flaps to completely cover the bone graft particles. The flaps were positioned and sutured in place using nonresorbable sutures. Horizontal mattress sutures were used initially to approximate the flaps, followed by several interrupted sutures to achieve primary closure (Figure 7). A temporary restoration (Essix retainer) was provided to the patient on the day of the surgery, making sure that there was at least 2 mm relief from the surgical site. After 2 weeks, all the sutures were removed except the horizontal mattress sutures, which were kept for another 2 weeks. The area was gently swabbed with chlorhexidine before

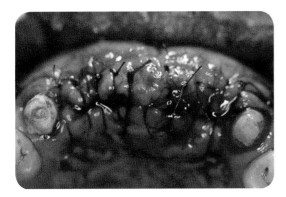

Figure 7: Flap closure (primary).

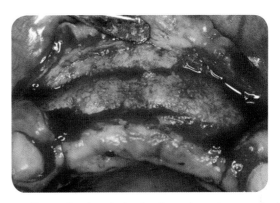

Figure 9: Flap reflection during implant placement surgical procedure.

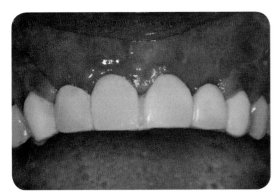

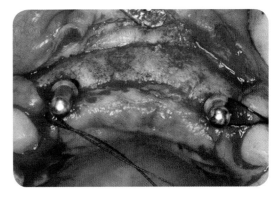

Figure 10: Implant placement surgical procedure.

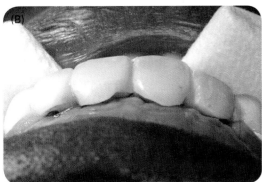

Figure 8: (A, B) Temporary restoration at 4 weeks post-GPR procedure.

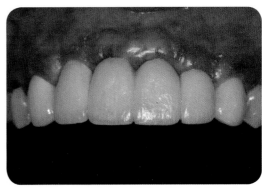

Figure 11: Final restoration (implant-supported FPD #7–#10).

and after the suture removal procedure. The adjacent teeth were debrided gently using hand instruments, and a temporary FPD #7–#11 was provided at the same appointment (Figure 8).

After 4 months of healing, significant buccal bone gain was noted, and two tapered implants (3.5 mm diameter × 13 mm height) were placed (according to manufacturer's instruction) without the need for any additional grafting (Figures 9 and 10). At 3 months following placement the implants were restored with a four-unit implant-supported FPD (Figures 11–13).

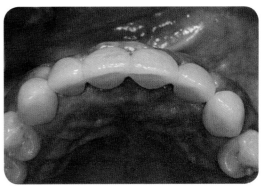

Figure 12: Final restoration (implant-supported FPD #7–#10).

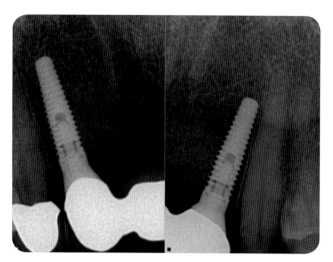

Figure 13: Periapical radiographs of #7and #10 final restoration.

Discussion

In this case, the primary etiology of the localized gingival inflammation is the poor margins and overcontoured restoration (FPD) and the violation of the biological width. These factors paired with the lack of optimal home dental care can increase the severity of the inflammation, which will cause the breakdown of tooth-supporting tissues. Ridge resorption in area #8 and #9 was due to previous tooth extraction and trauma. The rate of resorption is more on the buccal side, which leads to a thin ridge. Other possible factors that could lead to the ridge deformity is past history of periodontal disease in the extracted teeth (#8, #9).

Seibert classified ridges based on their topography into three classes. Class I denotes horizontal (buccolingual/-palatal) deficiency, while classes II and III denote vertical and a combination of horizontal and vertical deficiencies respectively. In this case a majority of resorption occurred horizontally, but slight crestal resorption was noted, making it into a Seibert class III situation [1].

Ridge augmentation procedures are a group of techniques employed to increase the buccopalatal or apico-coronal dimension of the alveolar ridge. Several techniques are available, with GBR being one of them. Each technique has its advantages and disadvantages, and predictability varies based on the case type. The clinical situation dictates the technique of choice. Historically, GBR was performed using a barrier membrane alone, but using bone grafts along with a membrane for GBR has currently become a standard of care. GBR has been shown to be a very reliable technique to gain horizontal (buccopalatal/-lingual) dimension to facilitate implant insertion, which we were able to accomplish in this patient.

Like any periodontal surgical procedures, the patient's systemic factors, such as uncontrolled diabetes or hypertension, will strongly negatively influence the outcome of this technique. Therefore, proper patient and site selection are important to increase the likelihood of success. The patient in this case is a nonsmoker with a controlled hypertension. The patient's oral hygiene was optimal throughout the treatment and she was seeing her dentist regularly for periodontal recall, which is another factor that needs to be weighed in.

Severe ridge deformities often impair both esthetics and function. Soft tissue, hard tissue, or combination augmentation may be attempted to reduce these defects; soft tissue reconstruction is useful in treating some mild cases. Severe defects may require a staged approach of hard and soft tissue augmentation [2]. The selection of the surgical treatment also depends on the type of prosthetic treatment. For example, when an FPD is planned, soft tissue augmentation is preferred [3], whereas hard tissue augmentation is preferred when dental implant therapy is selected.

Self-Study Questions

(Answers located at the end of the case)

A. What does implant site preparation mean?

B. What are the surgical procedures used in implant site preparation?

C. What are the different barrier membranes used in GBR for implant site preparation?

D. What is the waiting time after GBR implant site preparation?

E. Is there a difference in survival rate of implant placed in augmented site or in nonaugmented native bone?

F. What are the planning steps before implant site preparation?

G. What is the composition of DynaMatrix membranes?

H. What are indications for the use of DynaMatrix?

I. What are the possible postoperative complications of using a resorbable barrier membrane (DynaMatrix)?

J. What is the management of exposed resorbable barrier membrane (DynaMatrix)?

References

1. Lindhe JKT. Clinical Periodontology and Implant Dentistry, 4th edn. Hoboken, NJ: Wiley-Blackwell; 2003.
2. Seibert JS, Salama H. Alveolar ridge preservation and reconstruction. Periodontol 2000 1996;11:69–84.
3. Miller Jr PD. Periodontal plastic surgery. Curr Opin Periodontol 1993:136–143.
4. American Academy of Periodontology. Guidelines for management of patients with periodontal disease. J Mich Dent Assoc 2006;88(10):24.
5. Miller N, Penaud J, Foliguet B, et al. Resorption rates of 2 commercially available bioresorbable membranes. A histomorphometric study in a rabbit model. J Clin Periodontol 1996;23(12):1051–1059.
6. Juodzbalys G, Raustia AM, Kubilius R. A 5-year follow-up study on one-stage implants inserted concomitantly with localized alveolar ridge augmentation. J Oral Rehabil 2007;34(10):781–789.
7. Duskova M, Leamerova E, Sosna B, Gojis O. Guided tissue regeneration, barrier membranes and reconstruction of the cleft maxillary alveolus. J Craniofac Surg 2006;17(6):1153–1160.
8. Wang HL, Boyapati L. "PASS" principles for predictable bone regeneration. Implant Dent 2006;15(1):8–17.
9. Chen ST, Wilson Jr TG, Hämmerle CH. Immediate or early placement of implants following tooth extraction: review of biologic basis, clinical procedures, and outcomes. Int J Oral Maxillofac Implants 2004;19(Suppl):12–25.
10. Bell RB, Blakey GH, White RP, et al. Staged reconstruction of the severely atrophic mandible with autogenous bone graft and endosteal implants. J Oral Maxillofac Surg 2002;60(10):1135–1141.
11. Adell R, Lekholm U, Brånemark P-I. Surgical procedures. In: Brånemark P-I, Zarb GA, Albrektsson T (eds), Tissue-Integrated Prostheses: Osseointegration in Clinical Dentistry. Chicago, IL: Quintessence; 1985, pp 211–232.
12. Kahnberg KE, Nystrom E, Bartholdsson L. Combined use of bone grafts and Brånemark fixtures in the treatment of severely resorbed maxillae. Int J Oral Maxillofac Implants 1989;4(4):297–304.
13. Keller EE, Van Roekel NB, Desjardins RP, Tolman DE. Prosthetic-surgical reconstruction of the severely resorbed maxilla with iliac bone grafting and tissue-integrated prostheses. Int J Oral Maxillofac Implants 1987;2(3):155–165.
14. Nystrom E, Kahnberg KE, Gunne J. Bone grafts and Brånemark implants in the treatment of the severely resorbed maxilla: a 2-year longitudinal study. Int J Oral Maxillofac Implants 1993;8(1):45–53.
15. Jensen SS, Terheyden H. Bone augmentation procedures in localized defects in the alveolar ridge: clinical results with different bone grafts and bone-substitute materials. Int J Oral Maxillofac Implants 2009;24(Suppl):218–236.
16. Shah KC, Lum MG. Treatment planning for the single-tooth implant restoration – general considerations and the pretreatment evaluation. J Calif Dent Assoc 2008;36(11):827–834.
17. Nevins M, Nevins ML, Camelo M, et al. The clinical efficacy of DynaMatrix extracellular membrane in augmenting keratinized tissue. Int J Periodontics Restorative Dent 2010;30(2):151–161.
18. Kim DM, Nevins M, Camelo M, et al. The feasibility of demineralized bone matrix and cancellous bone chips in conjunction with an extracellular matrix membrane for alveolar ridge preservation: a case series. Int J Periodontics Restorative Dent 2011;31(1):39–47.
19. Saroff SA. The use of DynaMatrix extracellular membrane for gingival augmentation and root coverage: a case series. J Implant Adv Clin Dent 2011;3(3):19–30.

Answers to Self-Study Questions

A. Hard and soft tissues often need to be "prepared" (regenerated/restored) to allow implants to be placed in an ideal position functionally and esthetically with an adequate amount of osseous support [4]. There are a variety of hard tissue defects, ranging in complexity from bone dehiscence to horizontal or vertical defects or a combination of both [1]. Augmentation procedures for implant site preparation will vary depending on the complexity of the defect. There are many different types of augmentation materials with different biological properties. These properties and other local environmental and systemic factors can affect the outcome of the augmentation procedure [4]. Major soft tissue defects are easily managed prior to implant placement where minor defects could be addressed at the time of implant placement [4].

B. A healthy and adequate osseous ridge is necessary to place an implant for full function and esthetics. If this situation is not present, osseous augmentation prior to implant placement is indicated [4]. This augmentation procedure will depend on the complexity of the defect. GBR is a common augmentation technique where a barrier membrane is used to separate the grafted site from the overlying soft tissue. Distraction osteogenesis and sinus floor elevation procedures are also used in improving the width and the height respectively in defected alveolar ridges [4].

C. Historically, GBR and grafting techniques began with impractical Millipore (paper) filter barriers [5]. Expanded polytetrafluoroethylene membranes were first used by in 1984 and were considered the standard for GBR [6] with excellent outcomes. This kind of nonresorbable membrane must be removed during a second surgery 4–6 weeks after the initial procedure. Oftentimes nonresorbable membranes can get exposed during this healing time and contaminated, resulting in early removal affecting the outcome of the regeneration procedure. Resorbable membranes were developed to avoid these limitations [5]. These membranes are either animal derived or synthetic polymers. They are

gradually hydrolyzed or enzymatically degraded [7] and, therefore, do not require a second surgical stage of membrane removal. Their sources are varied, beginning in early years with cow collagen, polylactic acid, polyglycolide, Vicryl, artificial skin, and freeze-dried dura mater. Recently developed synthetic membranes often combine different materials [8].

Collagen membranes are commonly used in GBR procedures and are of either type I or II collagen from cows or pigs. They are often cross-linked and take between 4 and 40 weeks to resorb, depending on the type. Collagen absorbable barrier membranes do not require surgical removal. These membranes inhibit migration of epithelial cells, stabilize particulate graft materials, and prevent blood loss by promoting platelet aggregation leading to early clot formation and wound stabilization [5,6]. These mebranes may also facilitate primary wound closure via fibroblast chemotactic properties [6].

D. An important consideration during implant site preparation is how much healing time is needed before proceeding with the implant placement. Incorporation of the graft material into the recipient site and formation of vital bone in the developed site will vary in duration. Several studies have suggested waiting 4–6 months before implant placement. However, the healing time after implant site preparation will vary depending on many factors, such as patient factors (habits, systemic conditions), the graft material used, and the size of the developed site [9,10]. However, some other studies showed that implants can be placed simultaneously with the graft (one-stage surgery) if an adequate bone is available to provide primary implant stability [11–14].

E. Implants placed in partially edentulous patients who had either vertical or horizontal augmentation have a comparable survival rate with implant places in nonaugmented native bone. In 12–60 months' follow-up data after implant loading, an implant placed in a vertically augmented ridge had 95–100% survival rate, whereas an implant placed in a horizontally augmented site had 96.9–100% survival rate [15].

F. Before proceeding to the augmentation procedure, multiple planning steps need to be considered; assessment of the available bone and bone volume needed to accommodate the prospective implant and restoration is a major step in the planning for an augmentation procedure [16]. A diagnostic wax-up of the final prosthesis will also be helpful in presenting the final outcome to the patient; this diagnostic wax-up can be transformed later to a surgical guide. Cone-beam computed tomography is also used in planning the augmentation procedure for implants site preparation, where the surgical guide can be used to indicate the implant position and determine the amount of augmentation needed to reach the desired position [16].

G. DynaMatrix extracellular membrane is a xenograft derived from porcine small intestinal submucosa that facilitates soft tissue healing and remodeling into natural tissue (http://www. keystonedental.com/dynamatrix). DynaMatrix retains its natural composition of collagen types I, III, VI, glycosaminoglycan (hyaluronic acid, chondroitin sulfate A and B, heparin, and heparin sulfate), proteoglycans, growth factors (fibroblast growth factor-2, transforming growth factor-β), and fibronectin. The active proteins and molecules found within DynaMatrix communicate with the body by signaling surrounding tissue to grow across the scaffold. These active proteins also support the natural healing process by attracting cells and nutrients to the wounded area.

H. Alveolar ridge augmentation is one of the major indications for DynaMatrix membrane, it will prevent downgrowth of soft tissue, promoting selective osteogenic cells to proliferate to form the bone without soft tissue interference. DynaMatrix membrane has many other indications, such as soft tissue augmentation, lateral window closer during sinus lift procedure, and ruptured sinus membrane repair during sinus lift procedure [17].

I. Early membrane exposure can occur in the first days after ridge augmentation procedures. Membrane exposure can impair the regenerative outcomes, resulting in compromised bone quality and quantity [17]. Soft tissue dehiscence resulting in spontaneous membrane exposures have been reported to range from 28% to 40% [15]. Furthermore, most bioabsorbable barrier membranes are not intended to be left exposed during the healing period [18].

J. DynaMatrix is enzyme and infection resistant and can be left exposed in the surgical site. Spontaneous exposure of the membranes has been commonly reported after using it in alveolar bone augmentation procedures; however, it appears that despite exposure this membrane can still serve as a barrier. In a recent study, ridge preservation sockets did not receive primary coverage over the membrane (membrane left exposed). This site still obtained similar clinical and radiographic findings when compared with the primary flap closure technique [19].

Case 2

Guided Bone Regeneration

CASE STORY

A 53-year-old Caucasian female presented with a chief complaint of "I don't like the spaces in the right side of my mouth and I need something fixed to fill in those spaces." The patient lost tooth #5 recently due to recurrent caries and she lost tooth #4 several years ago. The patient had a three-unit fixed partial denture fabricated and placed from #3 to #5. At the time of extraction of #5 the bridge was sectioned between pontic #4 and abutment #5. Therefore, when she presented to the clinic, she had a mesially cantilevered pontic #4 attached to abutment tooth #3 (Figures 1 and 2). The patient visited her dentist regularly for uninterrupted dental care and reported that she brushed and flossed at least once a day. She had extensive restorations placed throughout her mouth in the forms of single crowns or fixed partial dentures.

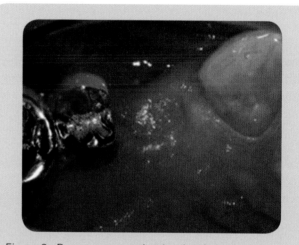

Figure 2: Pre-op presentation (occlusal view).

LEARNING GOALS AND OBJECTIVES

- To be able to understand the concept of guided bone regeneration (GBR)
- To understand the technique and the materials employed in GBR
- To understand the factors affecting the outcomes following GBR treatment and also the potential early complications associated with this technique

Medical History

At the time of treatment the patient presented with type II diabetes, controlled with medications (glyburide and metformin). Her last HbA1c level was 6.5, measured a few weeks before her initial exam. The patient was also hypertensive, controlled with medications (lisinopril). In addition, she was prophylactically taking low-dose aspirin (81 mg/day).

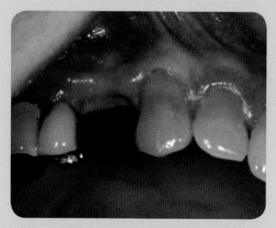

Figure 1: Pre-op presentation (facial view).

Review of Systems

- Vital signs
  - Blood pressure: 128/68 mmHg
  - Pulse rate: 86 beats/min (regular)
  - Respiration: 15 breaths/min

Social History

The patient did not smoke or drink alcohol at the time of treatment.

Extraoral Examination

No significant findings were noted. The patient had no masses or swelling, and the temporomandibular joint was within normal limits. There was no facial asymmetry noted and her lymph nodes were normal on palpation.

Intraoral Examination

- Oral cancer screening was negative.
- Soft tissue exam, including her tongue and floor of the mouth, were within normal limits.
- Periodontal examination revealed pocket depths in the range of 2–3 mm (Figure 3).
- Localized areas of gingival inflammation noted.
- Evaluation of the alveolar ridge in the areas #4 and #5 revealed both horizontal and vertical resorption of bone (Figure 4).
- Extensive restorations in the form of single crowns and fixed partial dentures.

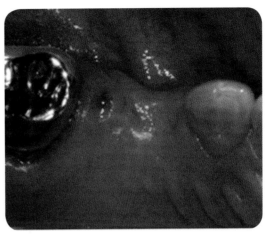

Figure 4: Pre-op presentation after pontic removal (occlusal view)

Occlusion

There were no occlusal discrepancies or interferences noted.

Radiographic Examination

A full mouth radiographic series was ordered (see Figure 5 for patient's periapical radiograph of the area of interest). Radiographic examination revealed normal bone levels. There was a slight loss of bone noted in the crestal bone height at #5 site. The height of bone between the crestal

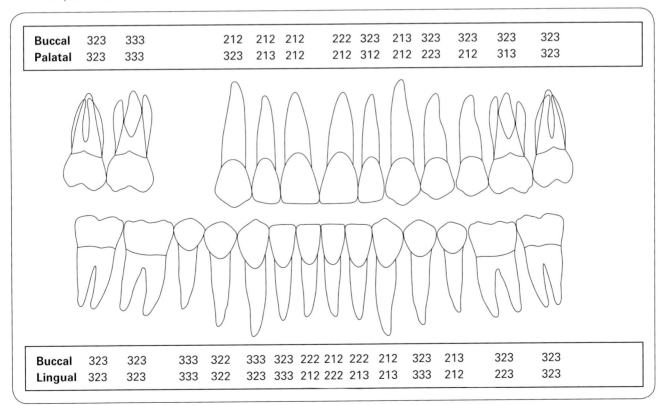

Buccal	323	333		212	212	212	222	323	213	323	323	323	323
Palatal	323	333		323	213	212	212	312	212	223	212	313	323

Buccal	323	323	333	322	333	323	222	212	222	212	323	213	323	323
Lingual	323	323	333	322	323	333	212	222	213	213	333	212	223	323

Figure 3: Probing pocket depth measurements during the initial visit.

bone and maxillary sinus and the mesio-distal space between #3 and #6 seemed adequate for placement of dental implants of standard diameter and height.

Diagnosis

American Academy of Periodontology diagnosis of plaque-induced gingivitis with mucogingival conditions and deformities on edentulous ridge was made.

Treatment Plan

The treatment plan for this patient consisted of initial-phase therapy that included oral prophylaxis and oral hygiene instructions to address gingival inflammation. This was followed by a GBR procedure to augment the bucco-palatal deficiency of the alveolar ridge. After adequate healing of the grafted site, the implants were installed. After adequate time for osseointegration, the implants were restored.

Treatment

After the initial-phase therapy, the patient presented for GBR. The pontic was separated and removed prior to surgery (Figure 4). After achieving adequate anesthesia at the surgical site using local anesthetic, full-thickness buccal and palatal flaps were reflected. The incision was mid-crestal at sites #4 and #5, which extended to the adjacent teeth as sulcular incisions. Decortication was performed on the underlying bone using a small round bur to facilitate entry of cells from bone into the healing graft (Figure 6B). The periosteum of the buccal flap was scored to improve the coronal mobility of the flap to achieve tension-free primary (complete) closure. The size of the membrane was determined based on the defect size and trimmed accordingly. The membrane extended beyond the defect by at least 3 mm.

Bone allograft particles were saturated in distilled deionized water and then packed onto the defect

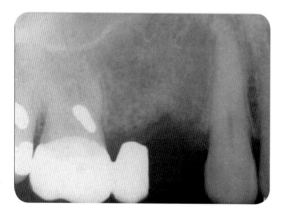

Figure 5: Periapical radiograph depicting the crestal bone levels at sites, #4 and #5.

(Figure 6D). The membrane was tucked underneath the buccal and palatal flaps to completely cover the bone graft particles (Figure 6E). The flaps were positioned and sutured in place using nonresorbable sutures. Horizontal mattress sutures were used initially to approximate the flaps, followed by several interrupted sutures to achieve primary closure. After 2 weeks, the sutures were removed and the area was dabbed with chlorhexidine. The adjacent teeth were debrided gently using hand instruments. After 4 months of healing, significant buccal bone gain was noted and two implants (3.5 mm diameter × 11 mm height) were placed (according to manufacturer's instruction) without the need for any additional grafting. Two months following placement, the implants were restored (Figure 7).

Discussion

In this case, the primary etiology of ridge resorption was tooth extraction. Tooth extraction can lead to resorption of the ridge (more so on the buccal aspect), and the majority of resorption occurs during the first 6 months. Other possible factors that lead to ridge deformity include trauma, developmental, cyst or tumor resection, and current or past history of periodontal disease. Ridge augmentation procedures are a group of techniques employed to increase the buccopalatal or apico-coronal dimension of the alveolar ridge. Several techniques are available and GBR being one of them (refer to answers to self-study questions A, B, C, and D). Each technique has its advantages and disadvantages, and predictability varies based on the case type. The clinical situation dictates the technique of choice. Historically, GBR was performed using a barrier membrane alone, but currently using bone grafts along with membrane for GBR has become a standard of care (refer to answer to self-study question E). GBR has been shown to be a very reliable technique to gain horizontal (buccopalatal/-lingual) dimension to facilitate implant insertion, which we were able to accomplish in this patient (refer to answer to self-study question F). Like any periodontal surgical procedures, the patient's systemic factors, such as smoking or uncontrolled diabetes, will strongly negatively influence the outcome of this technique (refer to self-study question G). Therefore, proper patient and site selection are important to increase the likelihood of success. The patient in this case is a nonsmoker and a diabetic with good glycemic control. The patient's oral hygiene was optimal throughout the treatment, and she was seeing her dentist regularly for periodontal recall, which is another factor that needs to be weighed in.

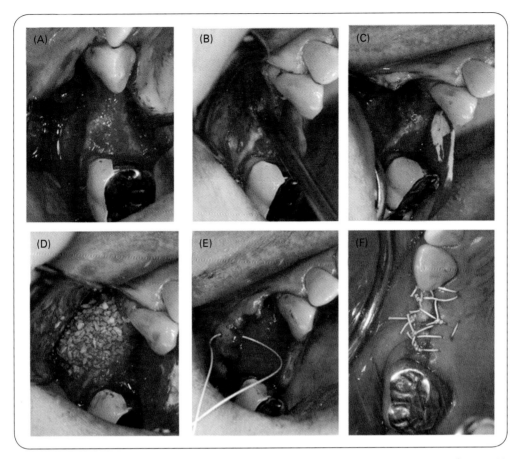

Figure 6: GBR performed after reflecting a full-thickness flap (A), decorticating the underlying bone (B), followed by placement of membrane (C) and bone allograft particles (D). Flaps were approximated and sutured to achieve primary closure of the surgical site (E, F).

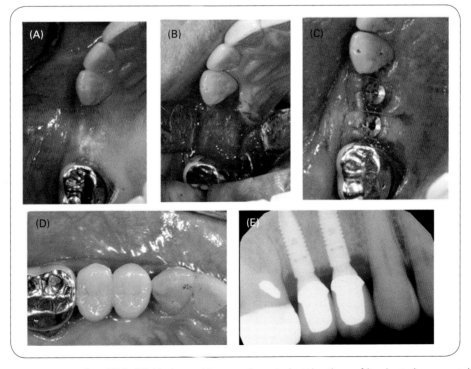

Figure 7: (A) Four months post-op after GBR. (B) Horizontal bone gain noted at the time of implant placement. Implants (C) placed and (D) restored. (E) Periapical radiograph showing the restored implant.

Self-Study Questions

(Answers located at the end of the case)

A. What is GBR?

B. Is GBR different from guided tissue regeneration (GTR)?

C. Is GBR the same technique as ridge/socket preservation?

D. How does GBR work?

E. What are the materials required to perform GBR procedures?

F. How predictable is GBR?

G. What are the factors that influence the GBR outcome?

H. What are the potential early complications that lead to failure or diminished outcome of GBR?

I. What are the recent advances in bone tissue engineering that have the potential to improve GBR outcomes?

References

1. Buser D, Dula K, Belser U, et al. Localized ridge augmentation using guided bone regeneration. 1. Surgical procedure in the maxilla. Int J Periodontics Restorative Dent 1993;13(1):29–45.
2. Buser D, Dula K, Hess D, et al. Localized ridge augmentation with autografts and barrier membranes. Periodontol 2000 1999;19:151–163.
3. Darby I. Periodontal materials. Aust Dent J 2011;56(Suppl 1):107–118.
4. Clementini M, Morlupi A, Canullo L, et al. Success rate of dental implants inserted in horizontal and vertical guided bone regenerated areas: a systematic review. Int J Oral Maxillofac Surg 2012;41(7):847–852.
5. Hämmerle CH, Jung RE, Feloutzis A. A systematic review of the survival of implants in bone sites augmented with barrier membranes (guided bone regeneration) in partially edentulous patients. J Clin Periodontol 2002;29(Suppl 3):226–231; discussion 232–233.
6. Park SH, Wang HL. Clinical significance of incision location on guided bone regeneration: human study. J Periodontol 2007;78(1):47–51.
7. Li J, Wang HL. Common implant-related advanced bone grafting complications: classification, etiology, and management. Implant Dent 2008;17(4):389–401.
8. Rios HF, Lin Z, Oh B, et al. Cell- and gene-based therapeutic strategies for periodontal regenerative medicine. J Periodontol 2011;82(9):1223–1237.
9. Elangovan S, Srinivasan S, Ayilavarapu S. Novel regenerative strategies to enhance periodontal therapy outcome. Expert Opin Biol Ther 2009; 9(4):399–410.

Answers to Self-Study Questions

A. GBR is one of the surgical techniques that are employed to augment alveolar bone [1]. Collectively, these techniques are called ridge augmentation procedures. Unlike other techniques to augment the ridge, such as autogenous block bone graft, GBR is relatively non-invasive, and the fact that GBR predominantly employs bone graft substitutes rather than patient's own bone eliminates the need for a second surgical site to harvest bone. Historically, GBR was employed to augment ridge for improving the ridge topography prior to complete denture fabrication or as pontic site development for improved esthetics. Currently, GBR is primarily employed in cases where bone volume gain is a requisite to facilitate dental implant placement [2].

B. Though both procedures work on similar principles of selective cellular exclusion and space maintenance, they differ from each other by their target tissue of regeneration. GTR is employed around the roots of periodontitis-affected teeth to achieve regeneration of the lost periodontium – namely, new periodontal ligament, new bone, and new cementum – over a previously diseased root surface. Therefore, the primary goal of GTR is to achieve both soft and hard tissue regeneration, whereas GBR is primarily performed to generate new bone (hard tissue) over the patient's existing bone. It is important to remember that procedures performed to augment bone around dental implants either at the time of placement or thereafter are also termed GBR.

C. Although bone is the target tissue to be regenerated when considering GBR or ridge/socket preservation techniques, both the techniques differ in their timing of implementation in the overall treatment sequence as well as in their primary objective. GBR is usually performed as a separate procedure (to augment the alveolar ridge) after extraction and before or at the same time when placing dental implants. Ridge/socket preservation, on the other hand, is performed at the time of tooth extraction to limit the physiological resorption of the ridge that normally occurs following extraction.

D. As mentioned before, GBR works by the principles of selective cellular exclusion and space maintenance. To accomplish these objectives, membranes and bone graft particles are employed. The role of membrane is to act as a barrier and prevent the epithelial and connective tissue cells from the overlying flap proliferating and occupying the space that is created for bone regeneration. If not excluded, epithelial cells (which have higher cellular kinetics than bone cells) will populate the space, leading to soft tissue fill and poor outcomes. In addition, the membrane also helps maintain space. The role of bone grafts is to specifically maintain space and to act as a scaffold for the native bone precursor cells to attach, proliferate, and differentiate into bone-forming cells (osteoblasts) that produce bone matrix (osteoid), which eventually mineralizes to form mature bone.

E. Bone grafts and membrane are the two main components of GBR. As listed in Table 1, based on the source, bone graft particles can be autografts,

Table 1: GBR armamentarium

Bone graft substitutes
- Autografts (procured from the same individual)
- Allografts (procured from the same species)
- Xenografts (procured from a different species)
- Alloplasts (synthetic)

Membranes
- Resorbable (made from collagen of different species)
- Nonresorbable (synthetic)

Tacking screws
- Resorbable (synthetic polymer based)
- Nonresorbable (metal based)

Tenting screws

allografts, xenografts, or alloplasts. Currently, allografts and xenografts are the most commonly employed bone graft materials for GBR. Based on the biodegradability of the membranes, they can be either resorbable or nonresorbable. Though clinicians use nonresorbable membranes in select clinical situations, a large majority of GBR procedures currently utilize resorbable membranes (to avoid the morbidity associated with surgical removal of nonresorbable membranes). In select clinical situations that require effective long-term cellular exclusion and space maintenance, tacking screws that approximates the edges of the membrane effectively to the underlying bone and tenting screws that provide additional support to the membrane from underneath are utilized. More information about periodontal biomaterials for regenerative applications can be obtained from a recent descriptive review [3].

F. GBR is shown to be a predictable technique to gain bone in atrophic areas to allow for implant placement. Current scientific evidence in the form of systematic reviews clearly indicates that implants placed in augmented bone are no different from implants in native bone, with regard to their survival rates [4,5]. However, clinical trials with well-defined success criteria and a long-term follow-up are required to accurately determine the success rate of implants placed in GBR augmented bone [4,5].

G. The following factors influence the treatment outcome following GBR [1,6].

Patient-specific factors. Factors such as compliance, presence of habits (such as smoking), or other underlying systemic disorders that negatively affect the outcome should be carefully considered during the treatment planning and modified as needed.

Clinician-specific factors. Surgical factors such as proper flap design, considerations for maximal blood supply to the site, attaining passive primary flap closure, and achieving immobilization of the graft during healing are critical in determining the success of GBR. Proper patient and site selection are vital, requiring a thorough patient evaluation. For example, ridge augmentation techniques other than GBR (such as distraction osteogenesis or block grafts) should be considered in cases where significant combined vertical and horizontal augmentation is required. Selecting the biomaterials based on the extent and topography of the defect and the prevailing scientific evidence is equally important.

H.

1. *Premature exposure of membrane or screws.* Factors such as flap tension, muscle pull, or poor compliance might lead to early exposure of the membrane or screws (if used). Nonresorbable membranes when exposed can become a nidus of infection, which is not so much the case with resorbable membranes. Newer nonresorbable membranes made with a specific pore size were shown to be biocompatible, even when they are exposed to the oral cavity. The effect of membrane exposure on GBR outcome is controversial, with a handful of studies demonstrating its deleterious effect [7].

2. *Loss of the graft.* Early exposure of resorbable membrane may lead to premature disintegration or collapse, leading to loss of bone graft particles [7].

3. *Infection of the graft.* Factors such as nonsterile practices during surgery or a systemic condition such as diabetes or any immunocompromised states can predispose an individual to infection at the surgical site. Systemic antibiotics and topical antibiotic mouth rinse are usually prescribed after GBR to reduce the incidence of graft infection.

4. *Hemorrhage from the surgical site.* Excessing bleeding from the surgical site can be attributed to improper incisional design or systemic conditions like hypertension or the usage of anticoagulants.

I. The following are the advances that have been shown to be effective in regenerating bone in either preclinical or clinical studies, both in the fields of dentistry and orthopedics:

1. Protein therapy (e.g., bone morphogenetic protein-2, platelet-derived growth factor-BB)
2. Cell therapy (e.g., somatic or stem cell delivery).
3. Gene therapy (viral and nonviral delivery of genes that encode for bone inducing proteins).
4. Biomimetic scaffold (scaffold that incorporate active bone anabolic peptides or molecules).
5. Combinations of the above four.

Some of the products are already in clinical use, while some are still in development [8,9].

Case 3

Growth Factors

CASE STORY

A 45-year-old Caucasian male presented with some purulence around #24, #25, and #26 (Figure 1). Teeth #24 and #25 had class III mobility while #26 had class II mobility. Tooth #24 had undergone apicoectomy in the past due to failed endodontic therapy. A periapical radiograph revealed a considerable area of radiolucency surrounding the apices of #24, #25, and #26 with significant loss of alveolar bone (Figure 2). Clinical exam revealed probing depths up to 8–9 mm around #24, #25, and #26 with calculus build-up, and some purulence could be seen on the buccal gingiva near the apex of #24 (Figure 1).

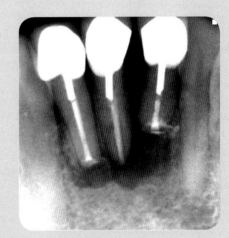

Figure 2: Periapical radiograph revealing radiolucent areas surrounding the apices of #24, #25, and #26.

LEARNING GOALS AND OBJECTIVES

■ To understand the role of tissue engineering in implant site development.
■ To understand the role growth factors in guided bone regeneration (GBR) procedures.
■ To understand the benefits and the risks of utilizing growth factors in GBR procedures

Medical History

The patient reported excellent health with no known medical conditions. He denied taking any medications and has no known allergies to any drugs.

Review of Systems

• Vital signs
  ○ Blood pressure: 126/78 mmHg
  ○ Pulse rate: 67 beats/min
  ○ Respiration: 14 breaths/min

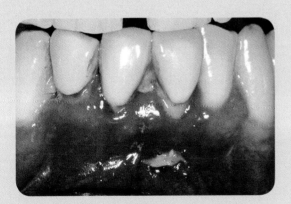

Figure 1: Clinical photograph demonstrating erythematous gingiva around #24, #25, and #26 with purulence present on the buccal gingiva near the apex of #24.

Social History

The patient never smoked, but drank alcoholic beverages once or twice a month. He denied using any recreational drugs.

Extraoral Examination

No detectable abnormal masses or swellings around the head and neck areas were noted. Examination of masticatory muscles and temporomandibular joints was within normal limits.

Intraoral Examination

- Soft tissues, including hard/soft palate, buccal mucosa, floor of the mouth, and tongue, were normal.
- Oral cancer screening was negative.
- Generalized plaque accumulation was evident with localized calculus build-up at mandibular anterior area.
- Gingiva was in general coral pink with localized areas of erythema in the mandibular anterior area where suppuration upon probing was observed.
- Periodontal probing depths of mostly 2–3 mm except for the mandibular anterior area where #24 and #25 had 8–9 mm of probing depth and #26 had 5–6 mm of probing depth (Figure 3).
- Teeth #24 and #25 presented with class III mobility, while class II mobility was detected for #26. Bleeding on probing was observed around mandibular incisors.

Occlusion

No occlusal interference was noted.

Radiographic Examination

A periapical radiograph of the mandibular anterior showed a significant region of radiolucency surrounding #24, #25, and #26 (Figure 2).

Diagnosis and Prognosis

Based on the clinical and radiographic examinations, the patient was diagnosed with localized severe chronic periodontitis with possible combined endoperiodontal lesion at #24, #25, and #26 [1].

The individual tooth prognoses prior to treatments were questionable for #24 and hopeless for #25 and #26 basing on McGuire's prognostic classification system [2].

Treatment Plan

The following treatment plan and treatment sequence were discussed with the patient based on the patient's desire to receive dental implant therapy.

- Diagnostic phase – comprehensive periodontal and restorative examinations, including radiographic examination.
- Disease control phase – oral hygiene instruction, extraction of #24, #25, and #26 due to questionable-to-hopeless prognoses, scaling and root planing of #23 and #26, and adult prophylaxis on the rest of dentition.

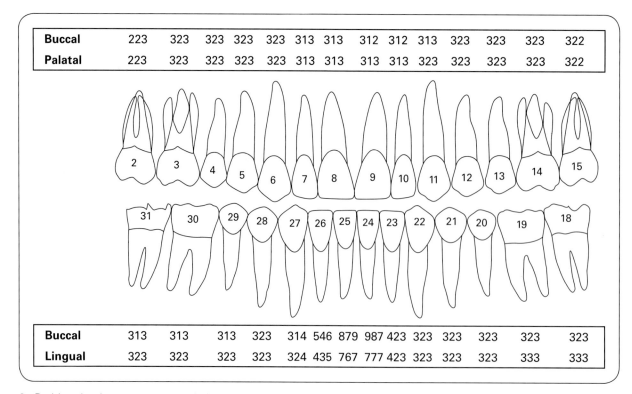

Buccal	223	323	323	323	323	313	313	312	312	313	323	323	323	322
Palatal	223	323	323	323	323	313	313	313	313	323	323	323	323	322

Buccal	313	313	313	323	314	546	879	987	423	323	323	323	323	323
Lingual	323	323	323	323	324	435	767	777	423	323	323	323	333	333

Figure 3: Probing depth measurements during initial visit.

- Surgical phase – alveolar ridge augmentation at sites #24, #25 and #26, and implant placement #24 and #26 to support a #24-X-#26 implant prosthesis.
- Maintenance phase – delivery of occlusal guard, and periodic implant prosthesis maintenance every 4–6 months depending on patient's plaque control.

Treatment Rendered

Teeth #24, #25, and #26 had questionable-to-hopeless prognoses and were extracted during disease control phase to eliminate infection. Amoxicillin was prescribed prior to removal of these teeth. The sockets were thoroughly curetted. There was a complete loss of buccal bone and partial loss of lingual bone around the incisors. Because of the extensive nature of the infection and the severity of gingival inflammation, it was decided not to perform simultaneous GBR procedure at the time of extraction. Inflamed gingiva typically appeared to be fragile, so it was not ideal to perform GBR because the risk of barrier membrane exposure would be higher. Given the nature of the radiolucency around the apices of #24, #25, and #26, the granulation tissues surrounding the mandibular incisors were collected and sent for pathological analysis. A diagnosis of apical radicular (periapical) cyst was given. No further action was recommended by the oral pathology service pertaining to this site.

A healing period of 4 months was allowed before initiating a GBR procedure. This period allowed osteoids to form and soft tissue to mature [3], and both elements were essential in GBR flap management. As expected, this patient presented at 4 months with a Seibert class III deficiency in the mandibular anterior area with loss of both ridge width and height [4] (Figures 4, 5, 6, and 7).

GBR to augment mainly the width of alveolar ridge in the mandibular anterior area was attempted using a combination therapy that included allograft particulates

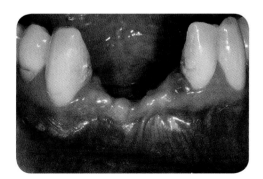

Figure 4: Buccal clinical photograph showing loss of some ridge height at mandibular anterior area.

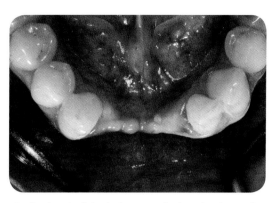

Figure 5: Occlusal clinical photograph showing loss of some ridge width at mandibular anterior area.

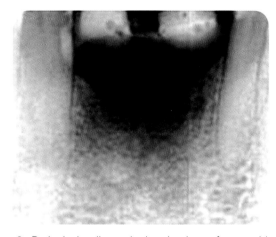

Figure 6: Periapical radiograph showing loss of some ridge height at mandibular anterior area.

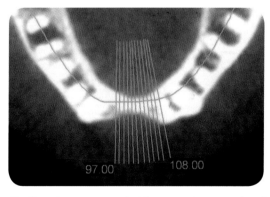

Figure 7: Cone beam computed tomography scan showing loss of some ridge width at mandibular anterior area.

(freeze-dried bone allograft (FDBA), Biomet 3i), a titanium-reinforced expanded polytetrafluoroethylene (ePTFE) membrane (Gore-Tex®, GORE), and recombinant human platelet-derived growth factor-BB (rhPDGF-BB) (Gem 21S®, Osteohealth) [5–7] (Figures 8, 9, 10, 11, 12, 13, 14, and 15). The patient was placed on methylprednisolone (Medrol Dosepak) 1 day prior

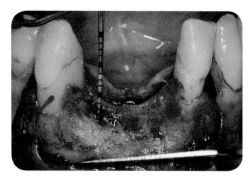

Figure 8: Buccal clinical photograph of mandibular anterior area following full-thickness flap elevation.

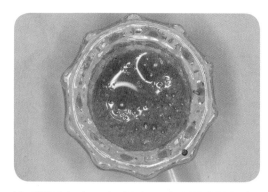

Figure 12: FDBA hydrated with 0.5 mL rhPDGF-BB.

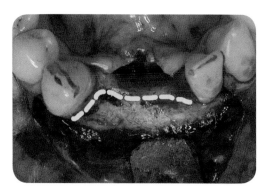

Figure 9: Occlusal clinical photograph showing narrow ridge width at the crest.

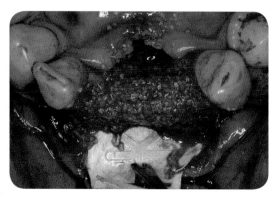

Figure 13: Placement of rhPDGF-BB-hydrated FDBA at grafted site with ePTFE membrane stabilized on the buccal aspect of the ridge with fixation screws (not visible here).

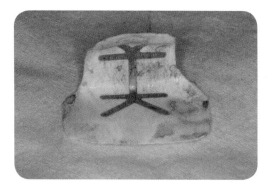

Figure 10: Trimmed titanium-reinforced ePTFE membrane.

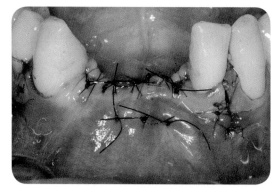

Figure 14: Buccal clinical photograph showing flap closure.

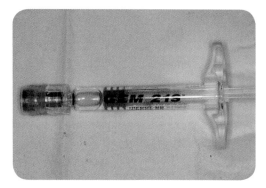

Figure 11: Gem 21S (Osteohealth) syringe containing rhPDGF-BB.

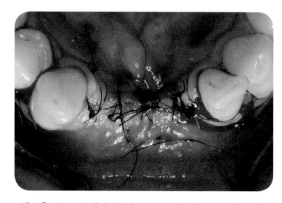

Figure 15: Occlusal clinical photograph showing flap closure.

to the surgery to control postoperative swelling. After raising a full-thickness flap, the residual ridge was decorticated with a small carbide bur to allow progenitor cells and nutrients from the bone marrow space to gain access to the grafted area. The titanium-reinforced ePTFE membrane was trimmed to fit the bone-grafted area leaving about 2 mm distance from the membrane to the flap margins and the adjacent teeth. This membrane was then fixated at the buccal apical aspect because the stability of the grafts was critical in the bone formation. Meanwhile, FDBA (Biomet 3i) was soaked with 0.5 mL rhPDGF-BB for about 15 min, as FDBA had been shown to act as a biocompatible matrix for rhPDGF-BB [8]. FDBA particulates hydrated with rhPDGF-BB were then transferred to the grafted area where they were packed until an ideal ridge contour was achieved. The ePTFE membrane was then positioned over the bone grafts. Periosteal release of buccal and lingual flaps was performed to coronally advance the flap to achieve tension-free primary closure of the surgical site. Amoxicillin and hydrocodone 7.5 mg/acetaminophen 300 mg (Vicodin ES) were prescribed to the patient to prevent infection and to control pain respectively. Care was taken to adjust the temporary prosthesis to ensure no unwanted pressure impinging at the bone-grafted area.

The patient presented at the 2-week postoperative visit with normal healing of the surgical site (Figure 16). Complete soft tissue closure of the flap was evident. At 6 months postaugmentation, the periapical radiograph showed signs of radiographic bone fill at the grafted area (Figure 17). Upon full reflection of the flap at the time of implant placement, clinically there was a significant amount of ridge width gain at the previously deficient mandibular anterior alveolar ridge (Figures 18

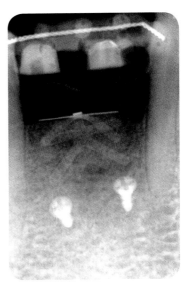

Figure 17: Six-month postoperative radiograph showing signs of radiographic bone fill at the grafted area and the presence of ePTFE membrane with two fixation screws in place.

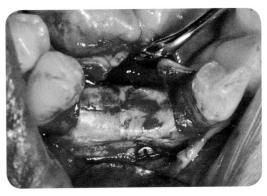

Figure 18: Clinical photograph at 6 months showing the presence of ePTFE membrane clinically upon full-thickness flap reflection.

and 19). There was an adequate ridge width to place prosthetically driven implant placement (#24 and #26) without additional bone grafting (Figures 20 and 21).

Discussion

In this scenario, a staged approach was taken to first remove infected incisors and subsequently wait for 4 months prior to performing the GBR procedure. A period of 4 months of healing postextraction was allowed because it was known from a human histological study examining the osteogenic activity of the extraction sockets that at 4 months after extraction the bony trabeculae in the sockets would have already become mineralized [3]. Alternatively, clinicians could

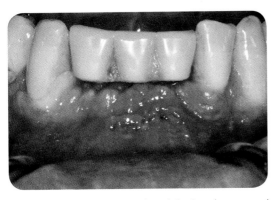

Figure 16: Two-week postoperative visit showing normal soft tissue healing at the grafted area without exposure of the ePTFE membrane.

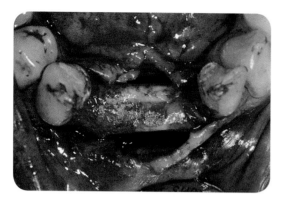

Figure 19: Occlusal clinical photograph showing adequate bone width gain at the previously bone-grafted area.

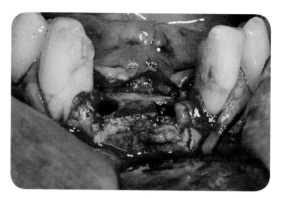

Figure 20: Clinical photograph showing the osteotomy sites for implants #24 and #26.

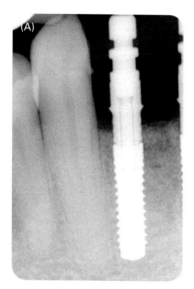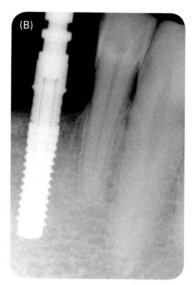

Figure 21: Periapical radiographs showing the placement of implants (A) #24 and (B) #26.

also enter as early as 8 weeks postextraction to perform the GBR procedure. By 8 weeks, osteoids (immature, nonmineralized bone) would have already formed in the sockets [3], and soft tissues overlying the sockets would have obtained adequate tensile strength required for the GBR procedures. Flap reflection at 8 weeks, however, may sometimes be more challenging because of the intertwining of connective tissues and osteoids in the sockets, and oftentimes osteoids are inevitably removed during flap reflection.

Apart from the staged approach, it is also feasible to perform GBR procedures simultaneously at the time of extraction. One advantage of this approach is to preserve buccal ridge contour at the extraction sites [9] because the majority of ridge resorption happens during the first 3 months following extraction [10], with horizontal hard and soft tissue dimensional changes occurring to a greater extent than that of

vertical dimensions [11]. Nevertheless, disadvantages of this approach include (1) the need to perform more coronal flap advancement to achieve primary closure, leading to shallower vestibule, (2) more likelihood for barrier membrane exposure, and (3) the possibility of bone graft infection leading to poorer bone quality if granulation tissues are not adequately removed. In this case, an attempt was not made to perform extraction and simultaneous GBR because of the severity of the infection and the fragility of the inflamed gingiva that made it difficult to maintain flap closure, especially given our intended use of nonresorbable ePTFE membrane. In addition, our decision to first obtain pathological diagnosis of the apical granulation tissues also prevented us from doing simultaneous GBR.

Given the abundance and the quality of the alveolar bone in the anterior mandible, it was also feasible to place dental implants without an additional GBR procedure. One could potentially place the implants at a more apical position so that the implant platform would be mostly surrounded by alveolar bone, and if not then a simultaneous buccal bone augmentation at the time of implant placement could be performed. However, placing implants at a more apical position next to natural teeth presented with some problems. First, the discrepancy between the implant platform and cementoenamel junction of the adjacent tooth might lead to the formation of a periodontal pocket that could prevent effective plaque control. Second, if implants were placed more apically and also very close to the natural teeth (less than 1.5 mm), the interproximal bone, and hence the papilla between the tooth and the implant, might be lost because of bone remodeling [12]. Third, the implant prosthesis might appear longer in the vertical dimension than that of the adjacent tooth, causing a potentially nonesthetic outcome. In the case presented here, by performing a separate GBR procedure we were able to allow the implants to be placed at a more coronal position and still be surrounded by bone.

The concept of tissue engineering has revolutionized the way medical treatments are rendered to the patients. The components of tissue engineering, when applied to implant dentistry, include the following: the cells, the scaffolds on which the cells migrate, and the growth factors that recruited cells (see answer to self-study question A). The combination therapy used in this GBR procedure reflected this concept of tissue engineering. The nonresorbable ePTFE barrier membrane provided a seal to discourage connective tissue and epithelial cells from entering into the bone grafted area, thereby favoring bone cells to populate the site [13]. The titanium-reinforced membrane also offered structural rigidity for maintaining space at the bone grafted site [14]. FDBA was osteoconductive and acted as a scaffold to allow migration of bone cells and other progenitor cells required for bone formation. rhPDGF-BB is a growth factor that recruited progenitor cells, stimulated cell division, and facilitated the formation of new blood vessels critical in new bone formation [15,16]. In summary, the intention of the combination therapy was to maximize the likelihood of new bone formation required for dental implant therapy.

rhPDGF-BB has been approved by the US Food and Drug Administration (FDA) for the treatment of intrabony periodontal defects, furcation periodontal defects, and gingival recession associated with periodontal defects. However, clinicians have also utilized rhPDGF-BB for various intraoral bone grafting procedures, including ridge preservation following extraction [7,17] and ridge augmentation [5,6]. Nevertheless, the use of rhPDGF-BB for bone grafting at edentulous sites, such as the clinical case demonstrated here, is considered to be off-label use.

Self-Study Questions

(Answers located at the end of the case)

A. What is tissue engineering?

B. What are growth factors and which growth factors are available for use in implant dentistry for site development?

C. What are rhPDGF-BB and recombinant human bone morphogenetic protein (rhBMP)-2?

D. What are the available delivery systems (carriers) for growth factors?

E. How are growth factors used in GBR procedures?

F. Does using growth factors in GBR procedures enhance the quality and quantity of bone formation?

G. What are some of the concerns of using growth factors in GBR procedures?

H. What is platelet-rich plasma (PRP)?

References

1. Armitage GC; Research, Science and Therapy Committee of the American Academy of Periodontology. Diagnosis of periodontal diseases. J Periodontol 2003;74:1237–1247.

2. McGuire MK, Nunn ME. Prognosis versus actual outcome. II. The effectiveness of clinical parameters in developing an accurate prognosis. J Periodontol 1996;67:658–665.

3. Evian CI, Rosenberg ES, Coslet JG, Corn H. The osteogenic activity of bone removed from healing extraction sockets in humans. J Periodontol 1982:53:81–85.

4. Seibert JS. Reconstruction of deformed, partially edentulous ridges, using full thickness onlay grafts. Part II. Prosthetic/periodontal interrelationships. Compend Contin Educ Dent 1983;4:549–562.

5. Nevins M, Camelo M, Nevins ML, et al. Growth factor-mediated combination therapy to treat large local human alveolar ridge defects. Int J Periodontics Restorative Dent 2012;32:263–271.

6. Ho DK, Fu MM, Kim DM. Vertical ridge augmentation of atrophic posterior mandible using platelet-derived growth factor: two case reports. J Oral Implantol 2015;41(5):605–609.

7. Nevins ML, Reynolds MA, Camelo M, et al. Recombinant human platelet-derived growth factor BB for reconstruction of human large extraction site defects. Int J Periodontics Restorative Dent 2014;34:157–163.

8. Nevins M, Hanratty J, Lynch SE. Clinical results using recombinant human platelet-derived growth factor and mineralized freeze-dried bone allograft in periodontal defects. Int J Periodontics Restorative Dent 2007;27:421–427.

9. Pietrokovski J, Massler M. Alveolar ridge resorption following tooth extraction. J Prosthet Dent 1967;17:21–27.

10. Schropp L, Wenzel A, Kostopoulos L, Karring T. Bone healing and soft tissue contour changes following single-tooth extraction: a clinical and radiographic 12-month prospective study. Int J Periodontics Restorative Dent 2003;23:313–323.

11. Tan WL, Wong TL, Wong MC, Lang NP. A systematic review of post-extractional alveolar hard and soft tissue dimensional changes in humans. Clin Oral Implants Res 2012;23(Suppl 5):1–21.

12. Choquet V, Hermans M, Adriaenssens P, et al. Clinical and radiographic evaluation of the papilla level adjacent to single-tooth dental implants. A retrospective study in the maxillary anterior region. J Periodontol 2001;72:1364–1371.

13. Linde A, Alberius P, Dahlin C, et al. Osteopromotion: a soft-tissue exclusion principle using a membrane for bone healing and bone neogenesis. J Periodontol 1993;64(11 Suppl):1116–1128.

14. Jovanovic SA, Nevins M. Bone formation utilizing titanium-reinforced barrier membranes. Int J Periodontics Restorative Dent 1995;15:56–69.

15. Hughes FJ, Turner W, Belibasakis G, Martuscelli G. Effects of growth factors and cytokines on osteoblast differentiation. Periodontol 2000 2006;41:48–72.

16. Hollinger JO, Hart CE, Hirsch SN, et al. Recombinant human platelet-derived growth factor: biology and clinical applications. J Bone Joint Surg Am 2008;90(Suppl 1):48–54.

17. Nevins ML, Camelo M, Schupbach P, et al. Human histologic evaluation of mineralized collagen bone substitute and recombinant platelet-derived growth factor-BB to create bone for implant placement in extraction socket defects at 4 and 6 months: a case series. Int J Periodontics Restorative Dent 2009;29:129–139.

18. Spector M. Basic principles of scaffolds in tissue engineering. In: Lynch SE, Marx RE, Nevins M, Wisner-Lynch LA (eds). Tissue Engineering: Application in Oral and Maxillofacial Surgery and Periodontics, 2nd edn. Hanover Park, IL: Quintessence; 2008, pp 26–36.

19. McGuire MK, Nunn ME. Evaluation of the safety and efficacy of periodontal applications of a living tissue-engineered human fibroblast-derived dermal substitute. I. Comparison to the gingival autograft: a randomized controlled pilot study. J Periodontol 2005;76:867–880.

20. McGuire MK, Scheyer ET, Nunn ME, Lavin PT. A pilot study to evaluate a tissue-engineered bilayered cell therapy as an alternative to tissue from the palate. J Periodontol 2008;79:1847–1856.

21. Hovey LR, Jones AA, McGuire M, et al. Application of periodontal tissue engineering using enamel matrix derivative and a human fibroblast-derived dermal substitute to stimulate periodontal wound healing in class III furcation defects. J Periodontol 2006;77:790–799.

22. Nasr HF, Aichelmann-Reidy ME, Yukna RA. Bone and bone substitutes. Periodontol 2000 1999;19:74–86.

23. Jung RE, Thoma DS, Hammerle CH. Assessment of the potential of growth factors for localized alveolar ridge augmentation: a systematic review. J Clin Periodontol 2008;35(8 Suppl):255–281.

24. Stavropoulos A, Wikesjö UM. Growth and differentiation factors for periodontal regeneration: a review on factors with clinical testing. J Periodontal Res 2012;47:545–553.

25. Urist MR. Bone: formation by autoinduction. Science 1965;150:893–899.

26. Urist MR, Strates BS. Bone morphogenetic protein. J Dent Res 1971;50:1392–1406.

27. Chen TL, Bates RL, Dudley A, et al. Bone morphogenetic protein-2b stimulation of growth and osteogenic phenotypes in rat osteoblast-like cells: comparison with TGF-β1. J Bone Miner Res 1991;6:1387–1393.

28. Wang EA, Israel DI, Kelly S, Luxenberg DP. Bone morphogenetic protein-2 causes commitment and differentiation in C3H10T1/2 and 3T3 cells. Growth Factors 1993;9:57–71.

29. Urist MR, Huo YK, Brownell AG, et al. Purification of bovine bone morphogenetic protein by hydroxyapatite chromatography. Proc Natl Acad Sci U S A 1984;81:371–375.

30. Howell TH, Fiorellini J, Jones A, et al. A feasibility study evaluating rhBMP-2/absorbable collagen sponge device for local alveolar ridge preservation or augmentation. Int J Periodontics Restorative Dent 1997;17:124–139.

31. Fiorellini JP, Howell TH, Cochran D, et al. Randomized study evaluating recombinant human bone morphogenetic protein-2 for extraction socket augmentation. J Periodontol 2005;76:605–613.

32. Boyne PJ, Marx RE, Nevins M, et al. A feasibility study evaluating rhBMP-2/absorbable collagen sponge for

maxillary sinus floor augmentation. Int J Periodontics Restorative Dent 1997;17:11–25.

33. Triplett RG, Nevins M, Marx RE, et al. Pivotal, randomized, parallel evaluation of recombinant human bone morphogenetic protein-2/absorbable collagen sponge and autogenous bone graft for maxillary sinus floor augmentation. J Oral Maxillofac Surg 2009;67:1947–1960.

34. Jung RE, Glauser R, Schärer P, et al. Effect of rhBMP-2 on guided bone regeneration in humans. Clin Oral Implants Res 2003;14:556–568.

35. De Freitas RM, Susin C, Spin-Neto R, et al. Horizontal ridge augmentation of the atrophic anterior maxilla using rhBMP-2/ACS or autogenous bone grafts: a proof-of-concept randomized clinical trial. J Clin Periodontol 2013;40:968–975.

36. Simion M, Fontana F, Rasperini G, Maiorana C. Vertical ridge augmentation by expanded-polytetrafluoroethylene membrane and a combination of intraoral autogenous bone graft and deproteinized anorganic bovine bone (Bio Oss). Clin Oral Implants Res 2007;18:620–629.

37. Nevins M, Camelo M, De Angelis N, et al. The clinical and histologic efficacy of xenograft granules for maxillary sinus floor augmentation. Int J Periodontics Restorative Dent 2011;31:227–235.

38. Nevins M, Kirker-Head C, Nevins M, et al. Bone formation in the goat maxillary sinus induced by absorbable collagen sponge implants impregnated with recombinant human bone morphogenetic protein-2. Int J Periodontics Restorative Dent 1996;16:8–19.

39. Uludag H, D'Augusta D, Palmer R, et al. Characterization of rhBMP-2 pharmacokinetics implanted with biomaterial carriers in the rat ectopic model. J Biomed Mater Res 1999;46:193–202.

40. Jensen OT, Kuhlke KL, Leopardi A, et al. BMP-2/ACS/allograft for combined maxillary alveolar split/sinus floor grafting with and without simultaneous dental implant placement: report of 21 implants placed into 7 alveolar split sites followed for up to 3 years. Int J Oral Maxillofac Implants 2014;29:e81–e94.

41. Jung RE, Windisch SI, Eggenschwiler AM, et al. A randomized-controlled clinical trial evaluating clinical and radiological outcomes after 3 and 5 years of dental implants placed in bone regenerated by means of GBR techniques with or without the addition of BMP-2. Clin Oral Implants Res 2009;20:660–666.

42. Marx RE, Carlson ER, Eichstaedt RM, et al. Platelet-rich plasma: growth factor enhancement for bone grafts. Oral Surg Oral Med Oral Pathol Oral Radiol Endod 1998;85:638–646.

43. Kassolis JD, Rosen PS, Reynolds MA. Alveolar ridge and sinus augmentation utilizing platelet rich plasma in combination with freeze-dried bone allograft. Case series. J Periodont 2000;71:1654–1661.

44. Eskan MA, Greenwell H, Hill M, et al. Platelet-rich plasma assisted guided bone regeneration for ridge augmentation: a randomized, controlled clinical trial. J Periodontol 2014;85(5):661–668.

45. Khairy NM, Shendy EE, Askar NA, El-Rouby DH. Effect of platelet rich plasma on bone regeneration in maxillary sinus augmentation (randomized clinical trial). Int J Oral Maxillofac Surg 2013;42:249–255.

46. Shanaman R, Filstein MR, Danesh-Meyer MJ. Localized ridge augmentation using GBR and platelet rich plasma: three case reports. Int J Periodont Restor Dent 2001;21:343–345.

47. Cabbar F, Güler N, Kürkcü M, et al. The effect of bovine bone graft with or without platelet-rich plasma on maxillary sinus floor augmentation. J Oral Maxillofac Surg 2011;69:2537–2547.

48. Marx RE. Platelet-rich plasma: evidence to support its use. J Oral Maxillofac Surg 2004;62:489–496.

Answers to Self-Study Questions

A. Tissue engineering is a therapeutic field in regenerative medicine that uses biology and engineering to restore and/or enhance tissue functions. When applied to implant dentistry and clinical periodontology, tissue engineering helps to facilitate healing and promote true regeneration of tissues in more predictable and less invasive manners [18].

Tissue engineering consists of three elements: scaffolds, cells, and growth factors [18]. Scaffolds are matrices that provide a framework, permitting cells to migrate from surrounding tissues to the defect areas such as bone-grafted sites. Scaffolds may also function as carriers that deliver growth factors or exogenous cells to the defect sites. Moreover, sometimes scaffolds also provide structural integrity needed for space maintenance at the grafted areas. Cells are required for any biologic activities including tissue regeneration and can be autogenic (from the host) or allogenic (from another individual of the same species). Examples of the use of allogenic cells in clinical periodontology include live cell therapies utilized in soft tissue grafting [19,20] and periodontal regenerative procedures [21]. Both differentiated (e.g., osteoblasts, fibroblasts) and undifferentiated cells (e.g., progenitor cells to osteoblasts) are required for tissue regeneration. Growth factors are regulators essential for cellular functions. When all three elements are present, with appropriate environment and time given for healing the regeneration of tissues is made possible.

B. Growth factors are naturally occurring molecules produced by the body to induce and direct cellular activities. Specifically, growth factors can function as chemotactic agents by recruiting cells, mitogens by inducing cell proliferation, and morphogens by stimulating cell differentiation. As such, growth factors are *osteoinductive* (osteoinduction is a process by which molecules such as growth factors contained in the bone grafting materials convert the neighboring cells in the host to bone-forming osteoblasts, which produce new bone [22]).

Regenerative medicine has utilized the technology of recombinant protein therapeutics in laboratories to synthesize growth factors that can carry out the biological functions of naturally occurring growth factors. To date, the two recombinant human growth factors available for dental applications are rhPDGF-BB and rhBMP-2. Only rhBMP-2 is approved for implant site development at this time. There are currently other growth factors being developed for use in dentistry, such as bone morphogenetic protein-7, basic fibroblast growth factor, vascular endothelial growth factor (VEGF), growth/differentiation factors-5, and insulin-like growth factors [23,24].

C. rhPDGF-BB is a synthetic protein molecule mimicking naturally occurring platelet-derived growth factor (PDGF)-BB. PDGF is mainly produced, stored, and released by platelets at the sites of injury and has been shown to participate in the healing of soft tissues and the regeneration of osseous structures [15,16]. PDGF chemotactically recruits gingival fibroblasts and mitogenically induce their proliferation essential in wound healing of connective tissues [15,16]. PDGF also induces angiogenesis, a process by which new blood vessels are formed supplying nutrients to the grafted area [16]. In 2005, FDA approved rhPDGF-BB, marketed as Gem 21S growth factor enhanced matrix (Osteohealth), for use in intrabony periodontal defects, furcation periodontal defects, and gingival recession associated with periodontal defects.

rhPDGF-BB has also been widely used in off-labeled manners by many clinicians for various intraoral bone grafting procedures, such as socket grafting [7,17] and ridge augmentation procedures [5,6].

rhBMP-2 is a synthetic protein molecule that exerts biological functions of naturally occurring bone morphogenetic protein (BMP)-2. BMP-2 is a morphogen known for its capability to induce new bone formation [25,26] by inducing the differentiation of mesenchymal cells to osteoblasts [15,27,28]. BMPs are present in very small amounts estimated to be 1–2 µg/kg of cortical bone in human body [29]. The US FDA has approved rhBMP-2, marketed as INFUSE® bone graft (BioHorizon), for dental application in localized alveolar ridge augmentation at extraction sockets [30,31] and maxillary sinus bone augmentation procedures [32,33]. Like rhPDGF-BB, off-label use of rhBMP-2 has also been popular among clinicians for ridge augmentation procedures [34,35].

D. In general, growth factors require appropriate delivery systems, also known as carriers, to be delivered to the target sites and to maximize their effects on surrounding tissues. An ideal delivery system should exhibit the following characteristics: (1) safety without toxicity to host, (2) lack of immunogenicity, (3) host biocompatibility, (4) appropriate bioresorbable rate not interfering with tissue regeneration, (5) optimal release kinetics that allow gradual growth factor release over a period of time, (6) structural integrity to maintain space at grafted site, (7) scaffolds for cell migration, proliferation, and differentiation, and (8) easy handling properties [18].

To date, β-tricalcium phosphate (β-TCP) is the only US FDA-approved delivery system for rhPDGF-BB. β-TCP is an alloplast made of calcium salt and phosphoric acid. Other materials that have been shown to be carriers for rhPDGF include FDBA particulates, demineralized FDBA particulates, and xenograft particulates [5,36,37].

The only US FDA-approved delivery system for rhBMP-2 is an absorbable collagen sponge (ACS) derived from type I collagen in bovine tendon. Studies have demonstrated the safety, feasibility, and efficacy of utilizing ACS as the carrier for rhBMP-2 in bone augmentation procedures [38,39].

Although ACS exhibits many positive features of an ideal carrier, it lacks structural integrity and is resorbed by the host in a relatively short period of time. Because of these disadvantages, other materials, such as bone xenografts [34] and bone allografts [40], have been used in combination with rhBMP-2 and ACS.

E. rhPDGF-BB (Gem 21S growth factor enhanced matrix, Osteohealth) is supplied in the form of liquid (0.5 mL) in a syringe at the concentration of 0.3 mg/mL. Carriers such as FDBA particulates are hydrated with rhPGDF-BB for about 15 min with proper aseptic technique to allow rhPDGF to adhere to the carriers. Subsequently, rhPDGF-hydrated FDBA particulates are placed on the bony defect sites and packed with moderate pressure. Excessive bleeding should be controlled prior to application of rhPDGF-BB to reduce the washing out of rhPDGF by blood. rhPDGF-hydrated carriers are then covered by a barrier membrane, and the overlying mucoperiosteal flap is sutured to achieve primary closure without tension (see Figures 8, 9, 10, 11, 12, 13, 14,14, and 15).

rhBMP-2 (INFUSE bone graft, BioHorizon) comes in a concentration of 1.5 mg/mL with different loading doses ranging from 1.05 to 12.0 mg. rhBMP-2 is supplied as lyophilized powder that needs to be reconstituted in sterile water for 15 min. Reconstituted rhBMP-2 solution is then uniformly applied onto the ACS in sterile field. A period of 15 min is allowed for the rhBMP-2 protein to bind to the collagen sponge. The rhBMP-2-soaked ACS is then applied to the defect area with gentle pressure. Mucoperiosteal flap overlying rhBMP-2/ACS is then sutured to achieve primary closure (see Figures 22, 23, 24, and 25).

F. Jung and colleagues in their systematic review examined the clinical, histological, and radiographic outcomes of utilizing PDGF-BB or BMP-2 in GBR procedures [23,41]. Owing to the limited number and differing levels of available studies, it was not possible to conclude on this subject. Nevertheless, the authors noted that in general the use of these growth factors in GBR procedures may be considered beneficial. Further well-controlled randomized clinical trials are required to answer this question.

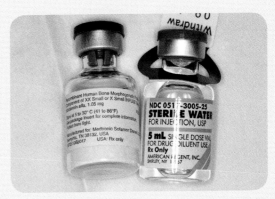

Figure 22: rhBMP-2 (INFUSE bone graft) in the form of lyophilized powder (left) is to be reconstituted in sterile water (right) for 15 min.

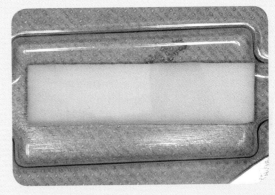

Figure 23: ACS placed on sterilized tray.

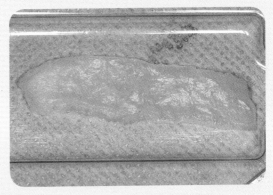

Figure 24: ACS soaked with reconstituted rhBMP-2.

G. Growth factors such as PDGF and BMP-2 are present in the body at physiologic concentrations adequate to exert their biological effects. Because of the needs to utilize rhPDGF-BB and rh-BMP2 in high concentrations to produce desirable outcomes, one concern of using these recombinant human growth

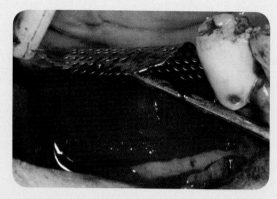

Figure 25: rhBMP-2/ACS placed on edentulous ridge.

factors is the possibility of causing carcinogenic and immunological events in the hosts. The formation of excess bone at unintended sites has also posed another concern. The US FDA mandates that both rhPDGF-BB and rhBMP-2 not be used in pregnant women because the potential impacts of these protein molecules on the developing fetus have not been adequately investigated.

Although there are few reports of adverse events in dentistry pertaining to the use of rhPDGF-BB and rhBMP-2, it is important to understand their potential in causing side effects. For example, rhBMP-2 may cause sinusitis when used for maxillary sinus bone augmentation, as well as edema due to inflammation elicited by rhBMP-2 that could result in facial swelling and paresthesia if swelling is exerting pressure against a nerve [30,32].

H. PRP is blood plasma containing concentrates of platelets obtained by autologous blood draw. PRP contains all three PDGF isomers (PDGF-AA, PDGF-AB, and PDGF-BB), VEGF, transforming growth factors β-1 and β-2, EGF, and cell adhesion molecules such as vitronectin, fibrin, and fibronectin critical for wound healing [42].

PRP has been shown to be effective in promoting osseous regeneration in dental applications [42–45]. However, other reports also exist to question the overall benefits of PRP in bone formation [46,47]. The apparent controversy seems to arise from how PRP is collected and prepared. For example, centrifugation of blood must be precise to separate platelets from red blood cells in high platelet concentration and without damaging or lysing the platelets otherwise these platelets will be unable to secrete bioactive growth factors [48]. In addition, it is very critical to apply PRP in the clotted state to the surgical site because clotting triggers the granules in platelets to fuse with cell membrane, thereby allowing them to release their growth factors [48].

Acknowledgments

We would like to thank Dr. Caleb Kim for providing us the preoperative clinical photograph (Figure 1) and Dr. Chie Hayashi for the follow-up clinical photographs after ridge augmentation (Figures 18, 19, 20, and 21).

Case 4

Alveolar Ridge Preservation: Allograft

CASE STORY

A 54-year-old Caucasian female presented at a periodontics clinic referred from her general dentist. Her chief complaint was "I would like to replace my broken front tooth." She is seen as a regular patient. She has a history of generalized slight chronic periodontitis and is currently enrolled in a periodontal maintenance program consisting of periodic recalls every 6 months with a hygienist and comprehensive annual exams with a periodontist. Upon initial functional and limited intraoral examination, it was noticed that the maxillary right lateral incisor was decoronated (Figures 1 and 2). The patient declared that the porcelain-fused-to-metal (PFM) crown fractured while she was eating. She did not report any symptoms; her main concern was essentially esthetic, but she was not interested in modifying the maxillary diastema present at the midline.

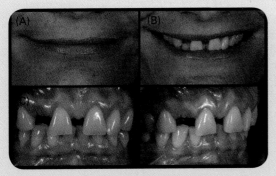

Figure 1: (A) Frontal extraoral view of relaxed smile. (B) Frontal extraoral view of forced smile, demonstrating a low smile line. (C) Frontal intraoral view of anterior zone in occlusion. (D) Lateral intraoral view from the right of anterior zone in occlusion.

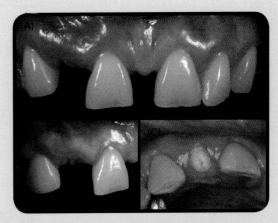

Figure 2: (A) Frontal intraoral view of the anterior maxillary esthetic zone. (B) Lateral intraoral view of the site of interest (maxillary right lateral incisor). (C) Occlusal view of the site of interest.

LEARNING GOALS AND OBJECTIVES

- To discuss different therapeutic modalities for the management of an extraction site in the anterior esthetic zone in order to maximize the chance of achieving a successful outcome when an implant-supported restoration is planned
- To understand the indications and clinical effectiveness of alveolar ridge preservation (ARP)
- To review some of the critical factors that may affect the outcomes of ARP

Medical History

This patient had a history of depression and bipolar disorder. She was hospitalized when she was 27 for a C-section. Upon initial examination, she was taken bupropion (100 mg twice per day), citalopram hydrobromide (20 mg once per day), and a multivitamin complex in a daily basis. On the basis of this information, surgical treatment was not contraindicated.

Review of Systems
- Vital signs
  - Blood pressure: 117/74 mmHg
  - Pulse rate: 67 beats/min
  - Respiration: 14 breaths/min

Social History

The patient has never smoked. She declares being an occasional drinker, for a maximum of approximately 20–30 g of alcohol per day.

Extraoral Examination

A comprehensive extraoral examination consisting of an assessment of temporomandibular joint function, facial asymmetries, and other alterations of normality by observation and palpation was conducted. No significant findings were noticed.

Intraoral Examination

- Exam of the intraoral mucosa, tongue, hard/soft palate, and tonsils revealed no remarkable findings.
- Oral hygiene – full mouth plaque score was 8%. She claimed brushing three times per day and flossing at least once per day on a regular basis.
- Comprehensive periodontal exam reveals the presence of generalized slight attachment loss (Figure 3). The patient declared that she was diagnosed with generalized slight chronic periodontitis about 20 years ago, which was treated and arrested with nonsurgical therapy.
- Maxillary right lateral incisor was fractured (chief complaint).

Occlusal analysis

Interocclusal relationship was an Angle class I. Overbite was 3 mm and overjet was 2 mm. There were no occlusal discrepancies or interferences. However, the patient has a history of parafunctional habits, evidenced by obvious tooth wear (Figures 1 and 2), which may have been implicated as a precipitating factor in the fracture of the crown on the maxillary right lateral incisor.

Radiographic Examination

A complete mouth radiographic series was obtained 9 months prior to the initial consultation in the periodontics clinic (Figure 4). The periapical radiograph of the tooth of interest (prior to the coronal fracture) revealed the presence of a periapical lesion and approximately

10% of interproximal bone loss following a horizontal pattern (Figure 5). The root morphology was tapered, with a slight apex dilaceration toward the distal. A cone beam computer tomography (CBCT) scan (i-CAT Next Generation, Hatfield, PA, USA) of the upper arch was obtained following clinical examination, in order to plan the management of the extraction site, with particular interest in a precise measurement of the facial bone morphology and thickness. The CBCT scan showed the extension and distribution of the periapical lesion in three dimensions. The facial bone thickness was approximately 1 mm, which is typically associated with a thin biotype (Figure 6).

Diagnoses

These diagnoses were established following the American Academy of Periodontology Classification for Periodontal Diseases and Conditions [1]:
- gingivitis associated with dental plaque only;
- history of generalized slight chronic periodontitis;
- gingival recession;
- mucogingival deformity on the facial of the mandibular left second premolar (keratinized gingiva width is 1 mm plus no attached gingiva);
- horizontal alveolar ridge deficiency on mandibular left first molar site;
- maxillary right lateral incisor fracture (chief complaint).

Treatment Plan

The treatment plan for this patient consisted of initial disease control therapy that included oral prophylaxis and reinforcement of oral hygiene instructions to address the isolated sites of gingival inflammation. Upon completion of the disease control phase, at approximately 2 months from the initial consultation, the corrective phase was initiated.

To address the chief complaint, a multidisciplinary consultation involving an endodontist, a periodontist, and her general dentist took place, where different treatment options for the chief complaint were presented to the patient, including:

1. Tooth reconstruction, involving endodontic therapy, crown lengthening, cast post/core, and PFM crown.
2. Tooth extraction and replacement with a fixed partial denture.
3. Tooth extraction, ARP, and replacement with implant-supported restoration.
4. Orthodontic tooth extrusion, subsequent tooth extraction, and replacement with implant-supported restoration.
5. Tooth extraction and immediate implant placement for an implant-supported restoration.

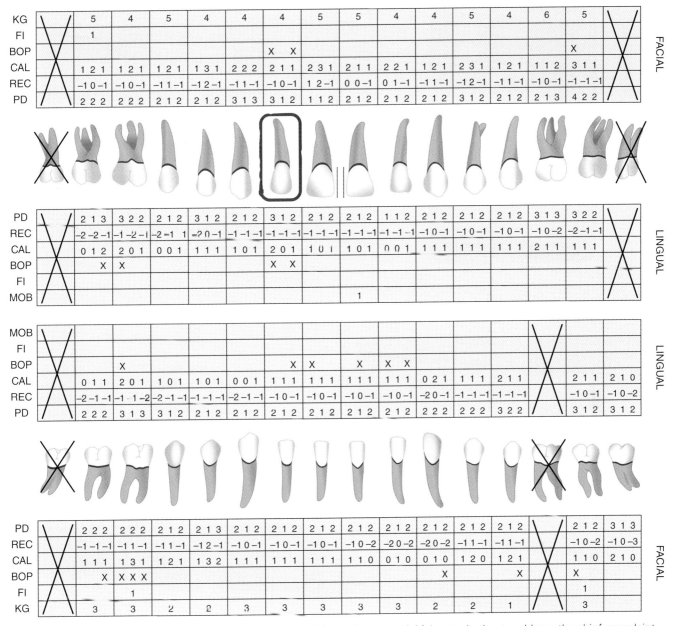

FACIAL

KG	✕	5	4	5	4	4	4	5	5	4	4	5	4	6	5	✕
FI		1														
BOP						X X								X		
CAL		1 2 1	1 2 1	1 2 1	1 3 1	2 2 2	2 1 1	2 3 1	2 1 1	2 2 1	1 2 1	2 3 1	1 2 1	1 1 2	3 1 1	
REC		−1 0 −1	−1 0 −1	−1 1 −1	−1 2 −1	−1 1 −1	−1 0 −1	1 2 −1	0 0 −1	0 1 −1	−1 1 −1	−1 2 −1	−1 1 −1	−1 0 −1	−1 −1 −1	
PD		2 2 2	2 2 2	2 1 2	2 1 2	3 1 3	3 1 2	1 1 2	2 1 2	2 1 2	2 1 2	3 1 2	2 1 2	2 1 3	4 2 2	

LINGUAL

PD	✕	2 1 3	3 2 2	2 1 2	3 1 2	2 1 2	3 1 2	2 1 2	2 1 2	1 1 2	2 1 2	2 1 2	2 1 2	3 1 3	3 2 2	✕
REC		−2 −2 −1	−1 −2 −1	−2 −1 1	−2 0 −1	−1 −1 −1	−1 −1 −1	−1 −1 −1	−1 −1 −1	−1 −1 −1	−1 0 −1	−1 0 −1	−1 0 −1	−1 0 −2	−2 −1 −1	
CAL		0 1 2	2 0 1	0 0 1	1 1 1	1 0 1	2 0 1	1 0 1	1 0 1	0 0 1	1 1 1	1 1 1	1 1 1	2 1 1	1 1 1	
BOP		X X				X X										
FI																
MOB									1							

LINGUAL

MOB	✕													✕		
FI																
BOP		X				X X	X	X X								
CAL		0 1 1	2 0 1	1 0 1	1 0 1	0 0 1	1 1 1	1 1 1	1 1 1	1 1 1	0 2 1	1 1 1	2 1 1		2 1 1	2 1 0
REC		−2 −1 −1	−1 1 −2	−2 −1 −1	−1 −1 −1	−2 −1 −1	−1 0 −1	−1 0 −1	−1 0 −1	−1 0 −1	−2 0 −1	−1 −1 −1	−1 −1 −1		−1 0 −1	−1 0 −2
PD		2 2 2	3 1 3	3 1 2	2 1 2	2 1 2	2 1 2	2 1 2	2 1 2	2 1 2	2 2 2	2 2 2	3 2 2		3 1 2	3 1 2

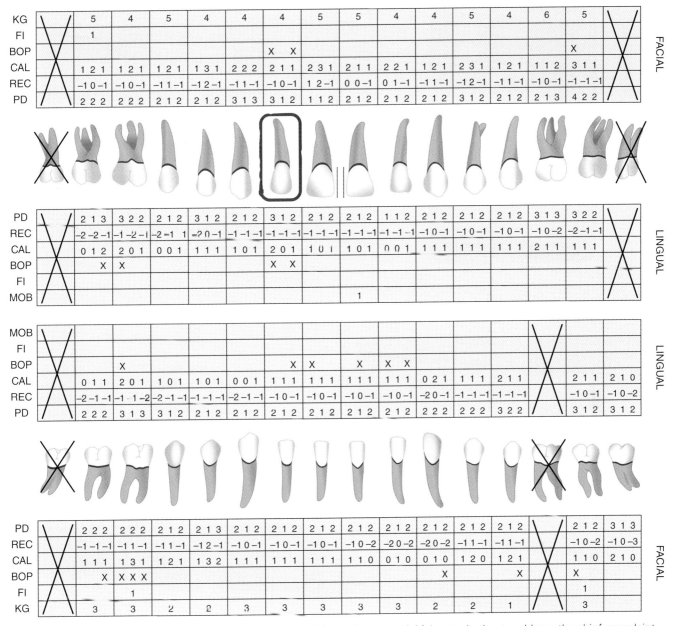

FACIAL

PD	✕	2 2 2	2 2 2	2 1 2	2 1 3	2 1 2	2 1 2	2 1 2	2 1 2	2 1 2	2 1 2	2 1 2	2 1 2	✕	2 1 2	3 1 3
REC		−1 −1 −1	−1 1 −1	−1 1 −1	−1 2 −1	−1 0 −1	−1 0 −1	−1 0 −1	−1 0 −2	−2 0 −2	−2 0 −2	−1 1 −1	−1 1 −1		−1 0 −2	−1 0 −3
CAL		1 1 1	1 3 1	1 2 1	1 3 2	1 1 1	1 1 1	1 1 1	1 1 0	0 1 0	0 1 0	1 2 0	1 2 1		1 1 0	2 1 0
BOP		X	X X X								X		X		X	
FI			1												1	
KG		3	3	2	2	3	3	3	3	2	2	1			3	

Figure 3: Periodontogram depicting the periodontal status of the patient upon initial consultation to address the chief complaint.

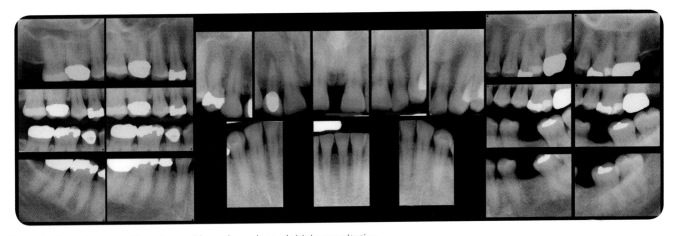

Figure 4: Complete mouth radiographic series prior to initial consultation.

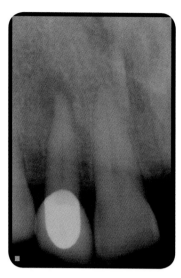

Figure 5: Periapical radiograph of the site of interest prior to initial consultation. Note the periapical radiolucency, compatible with chronic periapical pathosis.

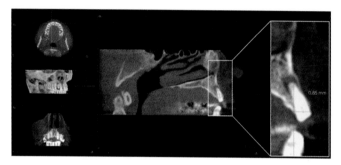

Figure 6: Images of the CBCT scan upon initial consultation.

Patient decided against options 1, 2, and 4. Option 1 involved expenses higher or comparable to other options that would be more conservative with the surrounding periodontal tissues in a predictable way. Option 2 was the least conservative one since the adjacent teeth would have to be prepared to a certain extent, irrespective of the restorative option chosen. In spite of being the most conservative and also possibly the most predictable alternative, option 4 entailed higher expenses, longer treatment time, and wearing orthodontic appliances, which was refused by the patient. Between options 3 and 5, the patient was advised by the dental team to select option 3. This recommendation was made mainly because of the thin bone (<1 mm) present on the facial aspect of the lateral incisor, as illustrated in Figure 6, which could potentially affect the esthetic outcomes should the remodeling of the alveolar ridge result in a significant reduction in height and width. The patient accepted this proposal.

Treatment

Tooth Extraction and Alveolar Ridge Preservation

After isolation of the surgical field, the patient was asked to rinse with an antimicrobial solution (e.g., chlorhexidine 0.12% for 15–20 s). Following the application of a topical anesthetic gel containing benzocaine 20%, a local anesthetic was administered on the facial and palatal mucosa applying an infiltrative technique for a total of half a carpule of 4% articaine and one carpule of 2% lidocaine, both containing a 1 : 100,000 concentration of epinephrine. After achieving local anesthesia, the surgical act was initiated with a minimally traumatic tooth extraction technique using a periotome, a straight elevator, and a mini-forceps (Figure 7). Tooth extraction was uneventful (Figure 8). The alveolar socket was carefully curetted to eliminate any remnants of the periapical lesion and then profusely irrigated with sterile saline. At this point, the socket was carefully inspected to verify the integrity of the alveolar bone. The alveolus was indeed constituted by four bony walls, with a minimal facial fenestration (possible 2 mm × 2 mm) at the apex. Careful elevation of the facial and lingual mucosa was done with a blunt instrument, in order to create a pouch that would permit the insertion and stabilization of an occlusive nonabsorbable membrane (Figure 9). In this case a combination allograft consisting of a mixture of freeze

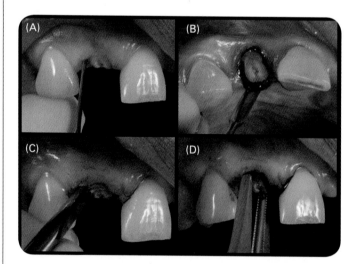

Figure 7: Intraoral photographs illustrating the process of minimally traumatic extraction. (A) Lateral view demonstrating the use of a periotome to sever the supracrestal connective tissue attachment. (B) Occlusal view demonstrating the use of the periotome on the palatal aspect of the periodontal mucosa. (C) Lateral view showing the use of a straight elevator to luxate the remaining tooth structure. (D) Lateral view depicting the use of a mini-forceps.

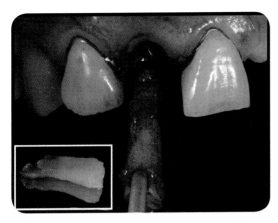

Figure 8: Lateral view of the site at the moment of extraction. Inset: detail of the extracted tooth; note the periapical lesion attached to the root apex.

dried bone allograft (FDBA) and demineralized FDBA (DFDBA) was used to fill the socket up to the crestal bone (Figure 10). Then, the membrane was tucked into the facial pouch to completely cover the grafted site. A cross mattress suture using a nonabsorbable material was done over the socket in order to stabilize the soft tissue and prevent the dislodgement of the membrane in the early stages of healing (Figure 11).

Postoperative Care, Evaluation of Outcomes, and Implant Placement Planning

General verbal and written postoperative instructions were provided to the patient. Additionally, the

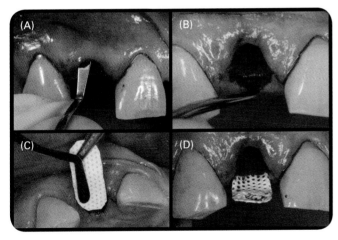

Figure 9: (A, B) Images demonstrating the use of a blunt instrument to reflect the mucosa approximately 3 mm apically on the facial and palatal aspect respectively. (C) Custom-shaped nonabsorbable (dense polytetrafluoroethylene (d-PTFE)) membrane being tucked in the palatal pouch created between the alveolar bone and the mucosa. (D) Membrane stabilized in the palatal pouch. Note the smooth side is placed against the soft tissue.

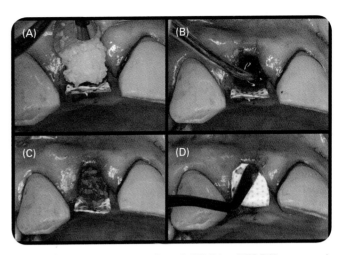

Figure 10: (A) Combination allograft (FDBA + DFDBA) was used to fill the socket. (B) A bone condenser was utilized to pack the bone grafting material into the dental alveolus. (C) The bone graft filled the socket up to the alveolar crest. (D) The membrane was then tucked under the mucoperiosteal mini-flap.

patient was instructed in the gentle application of a cotton swab soaked in a disinfecting solution (e.g., chlorhexidine 0.12%) over the membrane, which was recommended to be done twice a day during the first 2 weeks, in order to prevent plaque accumulation. To minimize the chance of a postsurgical infection,

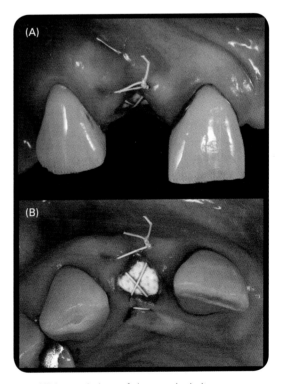

Figure 11: (A) Lateral view of the surgical site upon completion of the procedure. (B) Occlusal view of the site. A cross mattress suture using 5-0 d-PTFE suturing material was used to stabilize the soft tissues over the membrane.

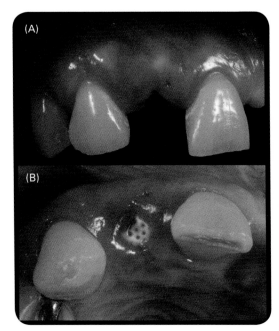

Figure 12: (A) Lateral and (B) occlusal views of the site at 2 weeks after the surgical procedure. The suture was removed at this visit.

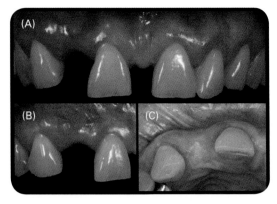

Figure 13: (A) Frontal view of the anterior maxillary esthetic zone at 14 weeks postoperatively. (B) Lateral view. (C) Occlusal view.

an antibiotic was prescribed (i.e., amoxicillin 500 mg three times per day for 7 days; in case of allergies to penicillins, an alternative is clindamycin 300 mg three times per day for 10 days). Nonsteroidal anti-inflammatory medication (i.e., ibuprofen 400 mg three or four times per day until symptoms disappear) was also prescribed.

The patient returned at 2 weeks after the intervention for a postoperative visit. The patient reported no symptoms, and no signs of infection were observed. The site was inspected and the suture was removed (Figure 12). The non-absorbable membrane was gently removed using cotton forceps, no anesthesia was required for this procedure. Oral hygiene instructions were reviewed and the patient was dismissed. At 14 weeks the patient returned to the clinic for evaluation of clinical outcomes and planning the implant placement. The mucosa presented a mature aspect; no signs of infection in the extraction site or gingival inflammation on the adjacent teeth were observed, and the papillary height appeared to be well preserved. However, some degree of horizontal ridge remodeling was evident (Figure 13). A second CBCT scan (i-CAT Next Generation, Hatfield, PA, USA) of the upper arch was obtained to assess the bone volume available for implant placement. The radiographic exam revealed that the bone density of the grafted area

appeared to resemble that of the native surrounding bone. Although bone remodeling had occurred, the placement of an implant of approximately 3.5 mm in diameter and 11 mm in height, which was considered as standard for this anatomical location, was feasible (Figure 14). A comparative volumetric analysis reveals the net contour loss over the healing period of 14 weeks, which was approximately 6% (Figure 15). Implant placement was planned virtually and a computer-generated guide was subsequently ordered, in order to minimize the risk of inadequate implant placement and maximize the preservation of the facial bone (Figure 16).

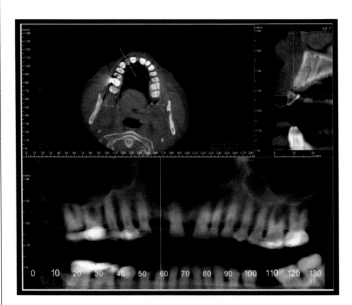

Figure 14: CBCT scan image depicting a panoramic and a sagittal view of the site of interest at approximately 14 weeks from the time of tooth extraction. The patient was wearing a radiographic guide to visualize the ideal contour of the prosthetic crown.

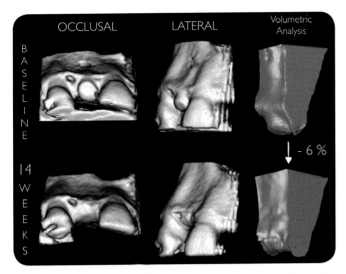

Figure 15: Comparison of the volumetric reconstruction of the alveolar ridge prior to tooth extraction and 14 weeks after tooth extraction and ARP, including two constant regions of interest that were used for volumetric reduction calculations (right). The estimated net bone contour reduction was 6%.

Implant Placement

The same protocol, in terms of surgical preparation and local anesthesia, described earlier was followed in this intervention. The computer-generated guide was tried-in to verify its stability and adaptation (Figures 17 and 18). Briefly, a straight midcrestal incision over keratinized mucosa extending intrasulcularly into the midline of both adjacent teeth was done after the demarcation of the implant position using a soft-tissue punch through the surgical guide. A full-thickness flap was elevated and the drilling sequence recommended by both the

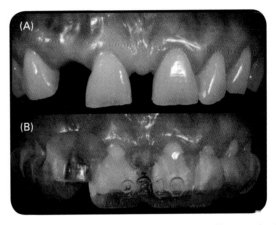

Figure 17: (A) Frontal view of the anterior maxillary esthetic zone at the time of implant placement (17 weeks after tooth extraction). (B) Frontal view of the same area while the patient is wearing a computer-generated surgical guide.

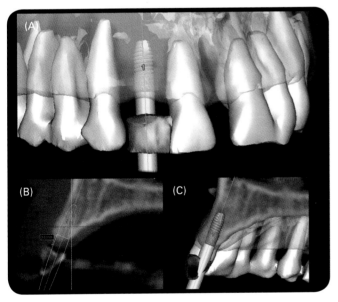

Figure 16: (A) Virtual implant placement in a volumetric reconstruction of the hard tissues of the premaxilla after cleaning up the data from the second CBCT scan. (B) Sagittal section at the implant midline. Note the subcrestal position of the implant platform to keep a distance of approximately 3 mm from the planned cementoenamel junction in order to have an adequate emergence profile. (C) Sagittal view integrating the volumetric reconstruction, the radiographic image, and the ideal implant position with respect to the planned prosthetic crown.

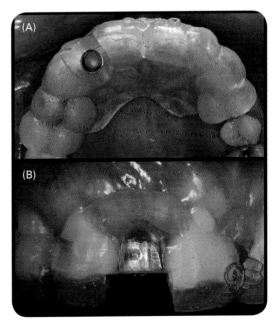

Figure 18: (A) Occlusal view of the anterior segment of the maxillary arch with the tooth-supported, computer-generated surgical guide in place. (B) Lateral view with surgical guide in place.

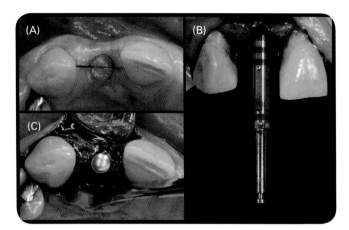

Figure 19: (A) Occlusal view of the site of interest after initial incisions were made. Note that, aside from a supracrestal incision, a soft-tissue punch was used through the surgical guide to mark the exact implant placement and facilitate the adaptation of the mucosa around the healing abutment. (B) Occlusal view of the final drill into the osteotomy. (C) Lateral view of the handpiece implant driver immediately after implant placement.

implant and surgical guide manufacturers was followed (Figure 19). The implant was placed with primary stability (i.e., approximately 35 N cm^2) and a 3 mm tall, straight healing abutment was inserted at 25 N cm^2. A double-sling suture around the healing abutment and a single interrupted suture to stabilize the papilla between the canine and the first premolar were given using 4-0 PTFE suturing material (Figure 20). A periapical radiograph of

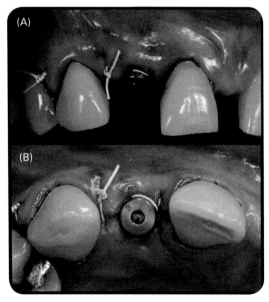

Figure 20: (A) Lateral view of the surgical site upon completion of the implant placement surgical procedure. (B) Occlusal view of the site. A double-sling suture around the healing abutment and a single interrupted suture to stabilize the papilla between the canine and the first premolar were given using 4-0 PTFE suturing material.

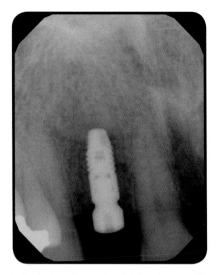

Figure 21: Periapical radiograph obtained immediately after implant placement.

the site was obtained prior to dismissing the patient (Figure 21). This radiograph confirmed the slightly subcrestal position of the implant and the parallelism to the adjacent teeth, as planned. The patient was provided with general postoperative instructions and was scheduled for a postoperative visit at 2 weeks.

Discussion

Alveolar bone resorption is a direct and naturally occurring consequence of tooth loss [2,3]. Current evidence indicates that tooth extraction triggers an irreversible process of remodeling that affects the periodontal structures, resulting in horizontal and vertical reduction of the alveolar ridge volume, mainly affecting the hard tissue [4,5]. Interestingly, tooth extraction ranks in the top five of the most frequently performed dental services in the USA [6]. Therefore, understanding how to manage the extraction site to minimize the extent of alveolar bone remodeling should be a fundamental component in the skill set of general dentists and specialists alike. This is of particular importance when the extraction site is located in the esthetic zone and an implant-supported restoration is planned, as in the case presented.

When tooth extraction is considered or indicated in the context of a multidisciplinary treatment plan, multiple therapeutic options for the management of the extraction site are available nowadays, including common alternatives such as tooth extraction alone, tooth extraction and ridge preservation through socket grafting, immediate implant placement or orthodontic extrusion with delayed implant placement, among others [7,8]. Obviously, identifying the ideal treatment option for a certain clinical scenario is not always an easy task. Therefore, careful case selection is warranted via a meticulous analysis of the key local, systemic, and behavioral factors, as well as patient preferences, that may determine the treatment plan and the short- and long-term outcomes [9,10].

In the case described here, the patient did not present any systemic contraindication for surgery (e.g., smoking, uncontrolled diabetes, bone metabolic disorders). The analysis of critical local factors should include the periodontal, endodontic, and occlusal status of the tooth indicated for extraction, the facial width of keratinized mucosa, and the periodontal biotype. The latter plays a preponderant role in the decision-making process of whether to perform immediate implant placement or perform ridge preservation for delayed implant placement, since a thin biotype (<1–1.5 mm of facial bone) has been consistently associated with increased ridge resorption in recent studies [11–13]. This factor is of special importance to obtain predictable results in the esthetic zone, since the average thickness of the facial bone is <1 mm, according to several investigations in this topic [14–16]. In the case presented here, the facial bone thickness was approximately 1 mm (Figure 6). Therefore, the patient was advised to discard immediate implant placement, in spite of the presence of a low smile line (Figure 1).

Preservation of the alveolar ridge should start with a careful, minimally traumatic tooth extraction technique (Figure 7). This step is fundamental to minimize the damage to the periodontal structures, hence retaining the possibility of attempting the preservation of the alveolar ridge, instead of ridge reconstruction according to guided bone regeneration principles. In general, ridge reconstruction is indicated when, upon tooth extraction, the integrity of the alveolar bone is highly compromised, such as in cases where a dehiscence is present, either as a result of previous unadverted periodontal destruction or as the result of a traumatic extraction.

Finally, it is worth noting that a subepithelial connective tissue graft or a dermal allograft could be indicated concomitant to ARP or at the time of implant placement in order to augment deficient facial soft tissue or prevent horizontal soft tissue volume loss, in order to maximize the chances of obtaining an esthetic result [17]. This additional therapy was not performed in this case since the esthetic soft tissue component of the suite was not compromised at the time of implant placement. However, its indication should not be ruled out in similar clinical scenarios until the peri-implant tissues mature around the implant-supported restoration (either provisional or definitive), in case additional horizontal reduction should occur.

Self-Study Questions

(Answers located at the end of the case)

A. What is ARP?

B. What are the indications/contraindications of ARP?

C. What is the clinical efficacy of ARP?

D. Does ARP via socket grafting completely prevent ridge resorption postextraction in a predictable manner?

E. Is there any biomaterial or technique that has been associated with superior outcomes?

F. What are the success and survival rates of implants placed in sites that underwent ARP at the time of tooth extraction?

References

1. Armitage GC. Development of a classification system for periodontal diseases and conditions. Ann Periodontol 1999;4:1–6.
2. Jahangiri L, Devlin H, Ting K, Nishimura I. Current perspectives in residual ridge remodeling and its clinical implications: a review. J Prosthet Dent 1998;80:224–237.
3. Van der Weijden F, Dell'Acqua F, Slot DE. Alveolar bone dimensional changes of post-extraction sockets in humans: a systematic review. J Clin Periodontol 2009;36:1048–1058.
4. Araujo MG, Lindhe J. Ridge alterations following tooth extraction with and without flap elevation: an experimental study in the dog. Clin Oral Implants Res 2009;20:545–549.

5. Schropp L, Wenzel A, Kostopoulos L, Karring T. Bone healing and soft tissue contour changes following single-tooth extraction: a clinical and radiographic 12-month prospective study. Int J Periodontics Restorative Dent 2003;23:313–323.
6. American Dental Association. Survey of dental services rendered. http://catalog.ada.org/login/login.aspx?URL=/members/sections/professionalResources/05_sdsr.pdf (accessed February 23, 2014).
7. Darby I, Chen ST, Buser D. Ridge preservation techniques for implant therapy. Int J Oral Maxillofac Implants 2009;24(Suppl):260–271.
8. Ishikawa T, Salama M, Funato A, et al. Three-dimensional bone and soft tissue requirements for optimizing esthetic results in compromised cases with multiple implants. Int J Periodontics Restorative Dent 2010;30:503–511.
9. Avila G, Galindo-Moreno P, Soehren S, et al. A novel decision-making process for tooth retention or extraction. J Periodontol 2009;80:476–491.
10. Greenstein G, Cavallaro J, Tarnow D. When to save or extract a tooth in the esthetic zone: a commentary. Compend Contin Educ Dent 2008;29:136–145; quiz 146, 158.
11. Barone A, Ricci M, Tonelli P, et al. Tissue changes of extraction sockets in humans: a comparison of spontaneous healing vs. ridge preservation with secondary soft tissue healing. Clin Oral Implants Res 2013;24(11):1231–1237.
12. Leblebicioglu B, Salas M, Ort Y, et al. Determinants of alveolar ridge preservation differ by anatomic location. J Clin Periodontol 2013;40:387–395.
13. Spinato S, Galindo-Moreno P, Zaffe D, et al. Is socket healing conditioned by buccal plate thickness? A clinical and histologic study 4 months after mineralized human bone allografting. Clin Oral Implants Res 2014;25:e120–e126.
14. Braut V, Bornstein MM, Belser U, Buser D. Thickness of the anterior maxillary facial bone wall-a retrospective radiographic study using cone beam computed tomography. Int J Periodontics Restorative Dent 2011;31:125–131.
15. Huynh-Ba G, Pjetursson BE, Sanz M, et al. Analysis of the socket bone wall dimensions in the upper maxilla in relation to immediate implant placement. Clin Oral Implants Res 2010;21:37–42.
16. Januario AL, Duarte WR, Barriviera M, et al. Dimension of the facial bone wall in the anterior maxilla: a cone-beam computed tomography study. Clin Oral Implants Res 2011;22:1168–1171.
17. Migliorati M, Amorfini L, Signori A, et al. Clinical and aesthetic outcome with post-extractive implants with or without soft tissue augmentation: a 2-year randomized clinical trial. Clin Implant Dent Relat Res 2015;17(5):983–995.
18. Lin S, Schwarz-Arad D, Ashkenazi M. Alveolar bone width preservation after decoronation of ankylosed anterior incisors. J Endod 2013;39:1542–1544.
19. Salama M, Ishikawa T, Salama H, et al. Advantages of the root submergence technique for pontic site development in esthetic implant therapy. Int J Periodontics Restorative Dent 2007;27:521–527.
20. Baumer D, Zuhr O, Rebele S, et al. The socket-shield technique: first histological, clinical, and volumetrical observations after separation of the buccal tooth segment – a pilot study. Clin Implant Dent Relat Res 2015;17(1):71–82.
21. Hurzeler MB, Zuhr O, Schupbach P, et al. The socket-shield technique: a proof-of-principle report. J Clin Periodontol 2010;37:855–862.
22. Kan JY, Rungcharassaeng K. Proximal socket shield for interimplant papilla preservation in the esthetic zone. Int J Periodontics Restorative Dent 2013;33:e24–e31.
23. Brugnami F, Caiazzo A. Efficacy evaluation of a new buccal bone plate preservation technique: a pilot study. Int J Periodontics Restorative Dent 2011;31:67–73.
24. Poulias E, Greenwell H, Hill M, et al. Ridge preservation comparing socket allograft alone to socket allograft plus facial overlay xenograft: a clinical and histologic study in humans. J Periodontol 2013;84:1567–1575.
25. Horváth A, Mardas N, Mezzomo LA, et al. Alveolar ridge preservation. A systematic review. Clin Oral Investig 2013;17(2):341–363.
26. Morjaria KR, Wilson R, Palmer RM. Bone healing after tooth extraction with or without an intervention: a systematic review of randomized controlled trials. Clin Implant Dent Relat Res 2014;16:1–20.
27. Ten Heggeler JM, Slot DE, Van der Weijden GA. Effect of socket preservation therapies following tooth extraction in non-molar regions in humans: a systematic review. Clin Oral Implants Res 2011;22:779–788.
28. Vignoletti F, Matesanz P, Rodrigo D, et al. Surgical protocols for ridge preservation after tooth extraction. A systematic review. Clin Oral Implants Res 2012;23(Suppl 5):22–38.
29. Vittorini Orgeas G, Clementini M, De Risi V, de Sanctis M. Surgical techniques for alveolar socket preservation: a systematic review. Int J Oral Maxillofac Implants 2013;28:1049–1061.
30. Weng D, Stock V, Schliephake H. Are socket and ridge preservation techniques at the day of tooth extraction efficient in maintaining the tissues of the alveolar ridge? Eur J Oral Implantol 2011;4:59–66.
31. Chan HL, Lin GH, Fu JH, Wang HL. Alterations in bone quality after socket preservation with grafting materials: a systematic review. Int J Oral Maxillofac Implants 2013;28:710–720.
32. Barone A, Orlando B, Cingano L, et al. A randomized clinical trial to evaluate and compare implants placed in augmented versus non-augmented extraction sockets: 3-year results. J Periodontol 2012;83:836–846.

Answers to Self-Study Questions

A. ARP involves the clinical management of the alveolar ridge to minimize the dimensional changes that typically occur after tooth extraction. There are a plethora of ARP techniques described in the literature. The majority of them involve the application of a socket filler after tooth extraction, generally a bone substitute (i.e., allografts, xenografts, or alloplastic materials) and covering the access to the socket with some type of biocompatible material (e.g., collagen sponge, absorbable collage membrane, nonabsorbable barrier, calcium sulfate). This ridge preservation approach is known as socket grafting. ARP therapy by socket 'filling' or 'grafting' emerged in the mid-1980s as a therapeutic alternative rationalized upon the notion that filling the space left by the extracted tooth would emulate a 'root retention effect' for alveolar bone volume preservation. Socket filling gained popularity over the years owing to its conceptual attractiveness and technical simplicity. But not all ridge preservation techniques involve tooth extraction, since root submersion is a predictable approach to preserve the alveolar bone dimensions in clinical scenarios when a tooth is nonrestorable [18,19]. Other modalities of ridge preservation described in the literature are the 'socket-shield technique' [20–22] and the overbuilding of the facial bone [23,24].

ARP and ridge preservation are generally acknowledged as exchangeable terms. However, ARP should not be referred as 'socket preservation,' since an attempt to preserve the socket (or alveolus) is not made; on the contrary, it is expected to fill with mature bone.

B. ARP is generally indicated in clinical scenarios where a tooth is nonrestorable and/or is planned for extraction and the maintenance of the alveolar ridge volume is critical for the overall treatment plan. The most common indication is in extraction sites where immediate implant placement is contraindicated (e.g., highly esthetic area, severe chronic infections), but a future implant-supported restoration is planned. In these scenarios, ARP may be crucial to avoid the need of advanced implant site development approaches that would increase the total treatment morbidity, cost, and time.

C. Recent systematic reviews have explored the clinical efficacy of ARP on techniques in terms of bone width and height changes compared with tooth extraction alone [25–30]. Only two of these systematic reviews performed a quantitative analysis [28,29]. Vignoletti et al. [28] found that, after a variable healing period of 6–24 months, average alveolar bone loss in terms of width and height were reduced 1.8 mm and 1.5 mm respectively, compared with sites that did not receive any intervention after tooth extraction. On the other hand, Vittorini Orgeas et al. [29] found that, after a variable healing period of 3–12 months, average alveolar bone loss in terms of width and height were reduced 1.3 mm and 0.7 mm respectively, compared with sites where tooth extraction alone was performed. These dimensional differences between both studies can be explained by the differences in the selected literature based on the specific eligibility criteria of each systematic review. Nevertheless, the findings were coincidental in the apparent beneficial effect of ARP therapy in preventing alveolar bone loss after tooth extraction.

D. Although ARP therapy may aid in preventing alveolar bone loss after tooth extraction, it is not always a predictable strategy to fully prevent alveolar bone resorption [26,27]. Hence, some degree of alveolar bone volumetric reduction should be expected after tooth extraction, even if ARP is performed simultaneously. The extent of bone resorption is variable, depending on individual patient factors, such as the periodontal biotype. In the case here, where ARP was done, the estimated net volume loss was approximately 6% after a healing period of 14 weeks.

E. A variety of outcomes (e.g., clinical, radiographic, histologic, quality of life) can be designated to determine whether ARP therapy has been effective or not. Current evidence indicates there is no particular biomaterial or technique that has been consistently associated with superior and predictable outcomes in terms of dimensional stability of the alveolar ridge, either clinically or radiographically [28]. Interestingly, a recent systematic review has been conducted focused on the assessment of histomorphometric outcomes after ARP using different biomaterials. A certain degree of variability in vital bone formation was observed in response to the use of various socket filling materials, such as allografts, xenografts, and alloplastic materials; however, no biomaterial showed significantly superior results compared with the rest [31].

F. According to recent studies aimed at answering this clinically significant question, implants placed in sites that underwent ridge preservation exhibit similar survival and success rates as implants placed in sites that did not receive this type of therapy. Barone et al. conducted a randomized controlled trial aimed at determining implant survival rates, among other parameters of interest, for implants placed in sites that received ARP via socket grafting with a xenograft compared with implants placed in extraction sites that healed naturally. Each group was comprised of 20 subjects who received one implant each. Cumulative implant survival rate in both groups was approximately 95% after 3 years, with no significant differences in any of the other parameters analyzed [32].

Acknowledgments

We would like to thank Barry Bartee and Shane Shuttlesworth (Osteogenics Biomedical Inc., Lubbock, TX, USA), Rachel Miller (Materialise Dental), and Adam Van Pelt (http://www.omfsolutions.com) for their valuable assistance and support in the development of the case presented. G.A. would like to specially thank the American Academy of Periodontology Foundation (AAPF) for the support provided to pursue an academic career in periodontics as a full-time faculty.

Case 5

Alveolar Ridge Preservation: Alloplast

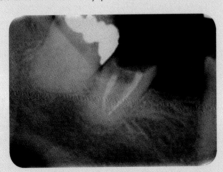
Medical History
The patient had a history of nonmetastasized breast cancer. Radiation and chemotherapy in combination with surgery were performed to treat the cancer. Both radiation and chemotherapy were terminated in March 2013. Citalopram was prescribed for depression.

The patient also reported that she had a fear of the dentist and dental procedures. Ativan was requested by the patient prior any dental treatment.

Review of Systems
• Vital signs
  ○ Blood pressure: 95/65 mmHg
  ○ Pulse rate: 74/min
  ○ Respiration: 16 breaths/min

Social History
The patient is a current smoker with a half pack per day for almost 30 years. She tried smoking cessation on several occasions but it was not successful. The patient denied any substance abuse.

Extraoral Examination
On facial inspection, her face looked normal with no asymmetry, no scars, and no swelling. On palpation, there were no lymphadenopathy, masses, or temporomandibular joint tenderness.

Intraoral Examination
• Floor of the mouth: within normal limits.
• Tongue: within normal limits.
• Buccal and lingual mucosa: within normal limits.
• Hard and soft palate: within normal limits.

Periodontal Examination
• Gingival tissue was within normal limits. The tissue was pink, there was minimal erythema, stippling was

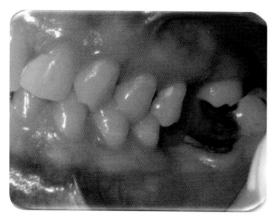

Figure 2: Mandibular left posterior region (lateral view).

present, and there was minimal bleeding on probing (Figure 2).
- Pocket depths between 1 and 3 mm (Figure 3).
- Localized recession of 1 mm.

Occlusion

There were no occlusal discrepancies or interferences noted.

Radiographic Examination

A periapical radiograph was ordered and reviewed for tooth #31 (Figure 1). The crown of the tooth had fractured due to dental caries, which extended below the level of the alveolar crest of bone. The root canal filling material appeared about 3 mm short of the radiographic apex of the tooth. There was a widening of the periodontal ligament space at the periapical region of tooth #31. A computed tomography scan was also ordered (Figure 4).

Diagnosis

American Academy of Periodontology diagnosis of plaque-induced gingivitis was made.

Treatment Plan

Initial consultation with the patient's primary care physician was made. The physician confirmed that the patient could undergo the tooth extraction. The patient's oncologist confirmed that her radiotherapy was localized to the chest area and did not involve the head and neck region. The patient had minimal probing depths. However, phase 1 therapy was performed, oral hygiene instructions were given, and her compliance and maintenance were reassessed. The patient was advised to limit the amount of cigarette smoking to a minimum during the treatment period to avoid healing complications.

Prior to seeing the patient, restorative and endodontic consultations were obtained. Tooth #31 was deemed nonrestorable due to the extent of the fracture and caries (Figures 1 and 2). Extraction and implant placement were proposed to the patient. However, owing to her limited finances, the patient agreed to have the tooth extracted and graft the socket to prepare the site for future dental implant in #31. In the

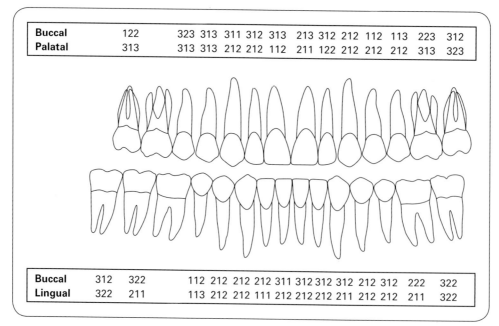

Buccal	122		323	313	311	312	313	213	312	212	112	113	223	312
Palatal	313		313	313	212	212	112	211	122	212	212	212	313	323

Buccal	312	322	112	212	212	212	311	312	312	312	212	312	222	322
Lingual	322	211	113	212	212	111	212	212	212	211	212	212	211	322

Figure 3: Probing pocket depth measurements during the initial visit.

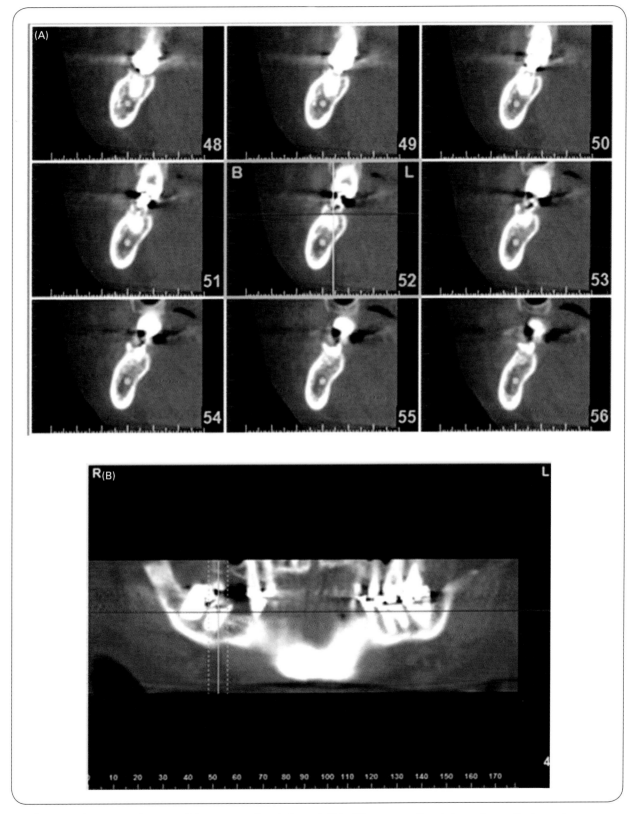

Figure 4: Computed tomography scan: (A) cross-sectional view of #31; (B) cross-sectional view of mandibular arch.

meantime, the patient will receive a free short dental implant on edentulous area #30 as part of a clinical trial.

Treatment

The patient presented on time for her surgery. An inferior alveolar nerve block with local anesthesia was given (Figure 5). The roots of tooth #31 were separated with a high-speed crisscross surgical bur. A combination of elevators and forceps was used to remove the roots (Figure 6). The socket was thoroughly debrided with curettes and irrigated with saline. A midcrestal incision was made for the edentulous area #30. A full-thickness flap was elevated using a Buser elevator. A 6.5 mm × 5 mm short implant was placed (Figure 7). Calcium phosphate particulate bone graft was packed into the socket with a condenser (Figures 8 and 9). Mini vertical incisions were placed on the buccal and lingual aspects of the flaps at the mesial and distal aspects of #31 to coronally advance the flap. Using a 5.00 Nylon suture, primary flap closure was accomplished using simple interrupted loops (Figure 10). Postoperative instructions and medications were printed and given to the patient. A baseline periapical radiograph was

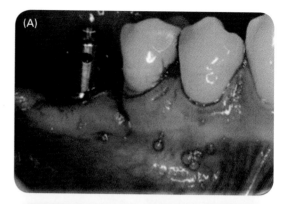

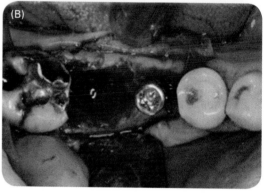

Figure 7: Implant placement on #30 after tooth extraction on #31. MIS implant system with diameter of 4.2 mm and length of 6 mm with internal hex connection: (A) lateral view; (B) occlusal view.

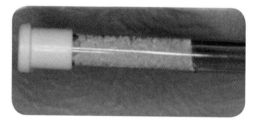

Figure 8: β-TCP preparation.

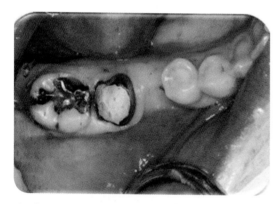

Figure 5: Preoperative occlusal view.

ordered (Figure 11). The patient returned in 3 weeks for the removal of the sutures (Figure 12). The sutures were removed and the patient was advised to start brushing the teeth in the lower right quadrant with a soft tooth brush. A 2-week postoperative visit revealed normal healing (Figure 13). The 4-week follow-up showed normal healing (Figure 14). Postoperative radiographs were also exposed (Figure 15). She will return for the final restoration of the crown on implant #30 in 4 months.

Discussion

The prognosis of tooth #31 in this case was based on the restorability. Tooth #31 was deemed nonrestorable

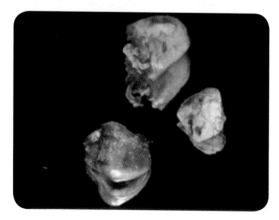

Figure 6: Atraumatic extraction of #31.

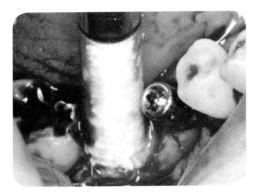

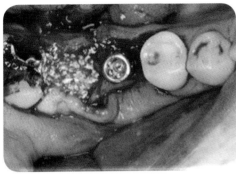

Figure 9: β-TCP application.

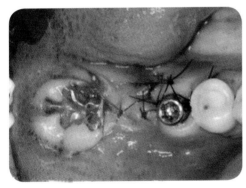

Figure 10: Primary closure after grafting the socket with β-TCP. Sutured with Nylon suture 5-0 with P3 needle.

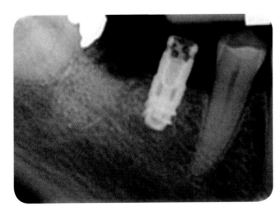

Figure 11: Baseline postoperative radiographs.

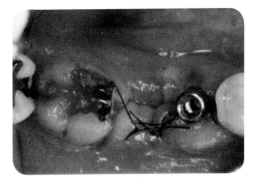

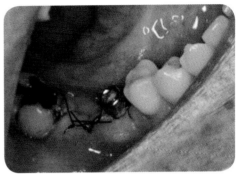

Figure 12: One-week follow-up.

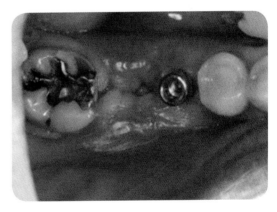

Figure 13: Two-week follow-up.

due to the extent of the fracture, caries, and inadequate endodontics treatment.

A number of studies have shown the benefit of socket preservation. Without socket or alveolar ridge preservation, a sinus lift or other ridge augmentation procedure may then be required to recreate adequate bone support for the implant.

Similar to other regenerative procedure, cigarette smoking has a negative effect on the treatment outcome. Therefore, smoking cessation should be considered. For this patient, the guideline using 5As (*Ask* about current smoking status every visit, *Advise* to quit and provide information on how beneficial quitting is, *Assess* willingness to quit, *Assist* with

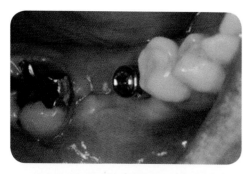

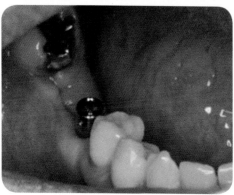

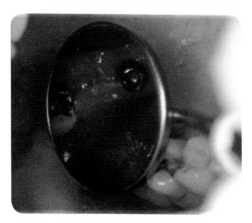

Figure 14: Four-week follow-up.

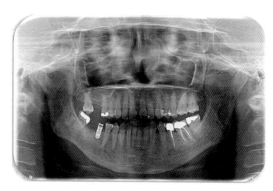

Figure 15: Postoperative panoramic radiograph.

finding resources and making a plan to quit, *Arrange* for follow-ups) from the American Academy of Family Physicians was followed. This is not only a benefit for patient in this specific surgical outcome, but also for overall health.

Various materials for socket preservation/ridge preservation/ridge augmentation have been studied. Autogenous bone graft is considered the gold standard owing to it osteogenic, osteoinductive, and osteoconductive properties. However, the alternative materials were chosen due to the limited amount of bone and morbidity of the donor site. β-Tricalcium phosphate (TCP) is resorbable, synthetic bone substitute. When compared with allogenic bone graft, β-TCP resorbs more slowly. It can act as a scaffold or space maintainer over a longer period of time. In this case, the patient did not want to have any human or animal products placed and has a desire to have the implant placed in the future; therefore, β-TCP was selected.

Self-Study Questions

(Answers located at the end of the case)

A. What is guided bone regeneration (GBR) and socket preservation?

B. What is the rationale of socket preservation and GBR?

C. What are the indications?

D. What are the complications associated with GBR and socket preservation?

E. What are the recent advances in GBR and socket preservation techniques?

F. What are the predictabilities of GBR and socket preservation?

G. What are the different materials required for GBR and socket preservation?

References

1. Hammerle CH, Araujo MG, Simion M. Evidence-based knowledge on the biology and treatment of extraction sockets. Clin Oral Implants Res 2012;23(Suppl 5): 80–82.
2. McAllister BS, Haghighat K. Bone augmentation techniques. J Periodontol 2007;78(3):377–396.
3. Schropp L, Wenzel A, Kostopoulos L, Karring T. Bone healing and soft tissue contour changes following single-tooth extraction: a clinical and radiographic 12-month prospective study. Int J Periodontics Restorative Dent 2003;23:313–323.
4. Lang NP, Pun L, Lau KY, et al. A systematic review on survival and success rates of implants placed immediately into fresh extraction sockets after at least 1 year. Clin Oral Implants Res 2012;23(Suppl 5): 39–66.
5. Becker W, Becker BE, Caffesse R. A comparison of demineralized freeze-dried bone and autologous bone to induce bone formation in human extraction sockets. J Periodontol 1994;65:1128–1133.
6. Froum S, Cho SC, Rosenberg E, et al. Histological comparison of healing extraction sockets implanted with bioactive glass or demineralized freeze-dried bone allograft: a pilot study. J Periodontol 2002;73:94–102.
7. Machtei EE. The effect of membrane exposure on the outcome of regenerative procedures in humans: a meta-analysis. J Periodontol 2001;72:512–516.
8. Rios HF, Lin Z, Oh B, et al. Cell- and gene-based therapeutic strategies for periodontal regenerative medicine. J Periodontol 2011;82:1223–1237.
9. Nevins M, Camelo M, Nevins ML, et al. Periodontal regeneration in humans using recombinant human platelet-derived growth factor-BB (rhPDGF-BB) and allogenic bone. J Periodontol 2003;74:1282–1292.
10. Sarment DP, Cooke JW, Miller SE, et al. Effect of rhPDGF-BB on bone turnover during periodontal repair. J Clin Periodontol 2006;33:135–140.
11. Intini G, Andreana S, Intini FE, et al. Calcium sulfate and platelet-rich plasma make a novel osteoinductive biomaterial for bone regeneration. J Transl Med 2007;5:13.
12. Bateman J, Intini G, Margarone J, et al. Platelet-derived growth factor enhancement of two alloplastic bone matrices. J Periodontol 2005;76:1833–1841.
13. Kim YJ, Lee JY, Kim JE, et al. Ridge preservation using demineralized bone matrix gel with recombinant human bone morphogenetic protein-2 after tooth extraction: a randomized controlled clinical trial. J Oral Maxillofac Surg 2014;72:1281–1290.
14. Esposito M, Grusovin MG, Papanikolaou N, et al. Enamel matrix derivative (Emdogain) for periodontal tissue regeneration in intrabony defects. A Cochrane systematic review. Eur J Oral Implantol 2009;2:247–266.
15. Vignoletti F, Matesanz P, Rodrigo D, et al. Surgical protocols for ridge preservation after tooth extraction. A systematic review. Clin Oral Implants Res 2012;23 (Suppl 5): 22–38.
16. Avila-Ortiz G, Elangovan S, Kramer KW, et al. Effect of alveolar ridge preservation after tooth extraction: a systematic review and meta-analysis. J Dent Res 2014;93(10):950–958.
17. Perelman-Karmon M, Kozlovsky A, Liloy R, Artzi Z. Socket site preservation using bovine bone mineral with and without a bioresorbable collagen membrane. Int J Periodontics Restorative dent . 2012;32:459–465.
18. Barone A, Aldini NN, Fini M, et al. Xenograft versus extraction alone for ridge preservation after tooth removal: a clinical and histomorphometric study. J Periodontol 2008;79:1370–1377.
19. Kim YK, Yun PY, Lee HJ, et al. Ridge preservation of the molar extraction socket using collagen sponge and xenogeneic bone grafts. Implant Dent 2011;20:267–272.
20. Vittorini Orgeas G, Clementini M, De Risi V, de Sanctis M. Surgical techniques for alveolar socket preservation: a systematic review. Int J Oral Maxillofac Implants 2013;28:1049–1061.
21. Toloue SM, Chesnoiu-Matei I, Blanchard SB. A clinical and histomorphometric study of calcium sulfate compared with freeze-dried bone allograft for alveolar ridge preservation. J Periodontol 2012;83:847–855
22. Mardas N, Chadha V, Donos N. Alveolar ridge preservation with guided bone regeneration and a synthetic bone substitute or a bovine-derived xenograft: a randomized, controlled clinical trial. Clin Oral Implants Res 2010;21:688–698.

Answers to Self-Study Questions

A. In 2012, the Osteology Consensus Report [1] defined the terms ridge preservation and ridge augmentation as follows:

"Ridge preservation = preserving the ridge volume within the envelope existing at the time of extraction

Ridge augmentation = increasing the ridge volume beyond the skeletal envelope existing at the time of extraction."

According to The American Academy of Periodontology, "*Guided tissue (bone) regeneration* is procedures attempting to regenerate lost periodontal structures through differential tissue responses. *Guided bone regeneration* typically refers to ridge augmentation or bone regenerative procedures; guided tissue regeneration typically refers to regeneration of periodontal attachment. Barrier techniques, using materials such as expanded polytetrafluoroethylene, polyglactin, polylactic acid, calcium sulfate and collagen, are employed in the hope of excluding epithelium and the gingival corium from the root or existing bone surface in the belief that they interfere with regeneration" [2].

While socket preservation or alveolar ridge preservation is a procedure to reduce alveolar bone resorption after tooth extraction, GBR after tooth extraction is aiming to direct the growth of new bone at sites having insufficient volumes or dimensions of bone rather than preserve the bone. Therefore, this term is usually used when buccal dehiscence is detected. However, a bone grafting material or scaffold with or without membrane is placed in the socket of an extracted tooth at the time of the extraction.

B. The significant loss of alveolar ridge dimension is an inevitable situation in many cases after tooth extraction as a result of normal alveolar bone remodeling. The postextraction bone loss is more pronounced on the buccal aspect of the ridge. The major changes of an extraction site occurred during 1 year, although mainly within the first 3 months [3]. In the Osteology Consensus Report in 2012, based on the systematic review by Lang et al. [4], a mean horizontal reduction in width of 3.8 mm and a mean vertical reduction in height of 1.24 mm of alveolar ridge within 6 months after tooth extraction may be expected [1].

Studies have shown that with a bone augmentation procedure, either socket preservation or GBR, the loss in bone volume is minimized. This facilitates subsequent placement of dental implants in the future [3,5,6].

C. According to Osteology Consensus Report [6] the indications for ridge preservation were identified as follows.
- Implant placement is planned at a time point later than tooth extraction; that is:
  i. when immediate or early implantation is not recommendable;
  ii. when patients are not available for the immediate or early implant placement (such as pregnancy, holidays);
  iii. when primary stability of an implant cannot be obtained;

  iv. in adolescent people.
- Contouring of the ridge for conventional prosthetic treatment.
- Provided the cost/benefit ratio is positive.
- Reducing the need for elevation of the sinus floor.

D. Like other surgical procedures, common postoperative complications that can occur include bleeding, swelling, bruising, and infection. Other less common complications can involve nerve or blood vessel injuries.

The use of collagen membrane has been shown to reduce the rate of membrane exposure in regenerative procedures. However, exposure can happen in some cases. According to the meta-analysis by Machtei [7], membrane exposure in the regenerative procedure around the tooth has only a minimal negative effect compared with the nonexposed site.

E. Recently, a wide variety of therapeutic strategies have evolved in the field of tissue regeneration. Cell- and gene-based therapies, for example, are being utilized and continuously tested [8].
- *Platelet-derived growth factor* (PDGF) is a growth factor that is secreted by platelets. It has chemotactic and mitogenic properties on osteoblasts and also can stimulate osteoblast type I collagen synthesis. In animal studies, PDGF promotes wound healing, stimulates periodontal ligament and bone cells, and, as a result, regenerates periodontium. Recently, PDGF has been demonstrated to induce periodontal tissue regeneration in humans [9,10].
- *Platelet-rich plasma* (PRP) and calcium sulfate have been shown by Intini et al. [11] to be able to induce bone regeneration. PRP is derived from autologous blood and is defined as a certain volume of plasma that has a platelet concentration several fold above the physiologic levels. Calcium sulfate, as a carrier, is able to activate the platelets, which results in various biologically active factors released from activated platelets that promote tissue regeneration [12]. Therefore, this calcium sulfate–platelet has been suggested for clinical use in bone regenerative therapy.

- Bone morphogenetic protein (BMP)-2, differentiation factor, has also been tested. In a recent clinical trial, the use of recombinant human BMP-2 with demineralized bone material did not show a significant difference from demineralized bone material alone in terms of the alveolar bone width and height. No adverse events were observed both locally and systemically [13].
- *Emdogain* and other growth factors. Enamel matrix derivative (EMD) is an extract of enamel matrix and contains amelogenins of various molecular weights. Amelogenins are involved in the formation of enamel and periodontal attachment formation during tooth development by promoting the migration of mesenchymal cells onto a root surface previously exposed, which is an essential step preceding formation of cementum. The clinical benefit of EMDs over conventional regenerative procedure is somewhat controversial [14].

F. Numerous studies have showed the benefit of socket and ridge preservation. Meta-analysis results showed that a ridge preservation procedure significantly reduces the loss of alveolar bone in both height and width when compared with the healing of the untreated control socket [15].
- Horizontal bone loss: ranging from +3.25 to −2.50 mm in treated group versus −0.16 to −4.50 mm in control group.
- Vertical bone loss: ranging from −2.48 to +1.3 mm in treated group versus −0.3 to −3.75 mm in control group.

This result suggests that ridge preservation therapies limit the dimensional changes (vertical and horizontal) of the alveolar ridge after tooth extraction. However, some degrees of alveolar bone loss both horizontally and vertically should still be expected. The variability in bone augmentation outcome is observed throughout the studies. The reason, however, is unknown [15,16].

In some cases, therefore, additional augmentation procedure may be needed. Therefore, patient should be informed and aware.

G. Various bone grafts and substitutes, including autogenous bone graft, allograft, alloplast, xenograft, and membrane barrier, have been suggested for grafting the postextraction site. All of these have a wide range of technique sensitivity and cost [16]. The following is known about xenografts and alloplasts.
- *Xenografts.* Extraction sites augmented with bovine bone mineral with resorbable membranes showed better outcomes in terms of the amount of bone volume compared with sites augmented with bovine bone mineral solely or without graft [17,18]. Besides resorbable membranes, collagen sponge with xenograft significantly reduced alveolar bone loss compared with xenograft alone. This suggested that while xenografts prevent the resorption of the alveolar ridge, the collagen sponge blocks the penetration of soft tissues to the socket, and thus it has the advantage of the enhancement of bone fill [19]. Theoretically, the use of membrane barriers could enhance the bone healing process, and minimize bone resorption. However, one meta-analysis showed that the use of membrane alone results in a better clinical outcome compared with membrane plus bone graft or graft alone [20]. Therefore, the use of membrane may be considered case by case.
- *Alloplasts.* One of the first alloplasts used in dentistry was calcium sulfate, which has shown osteoconductive properties. Despite the fact that it has a non-osteoinductive property, study has shown that calcium sulfate is as effective as freeze-dried bone allograft in preservation of an extraction socket/ridge [21]. Recent human controlled trials compared the potential of a biphasic ceramic bone substitute (which is composed of a combination of hydroxyapatite and β-TCP) and a bovine xenograft, both in combination with a collagen membrane. Similar amounts of newly formed bone were found to be produced [22].

The scientific evidence, however, does not provide clear guidelines in regard to the type of biomaterial [15].

Case 6

Alveolar Ridge Preservation: Xenograft

CASE STORY

Initial Presentation
A 33-year-old female patient was referred for an extraction and implant placement of tooth #9.

History
Tooth #9 was endodontically treated by a general dentist due to extensive dental caries that involved the pulp of her tooth. About a year later the tooth was retreated by an endodontist in attempt to retrieve a broken instrument in the middle part of the root. During the fabrication of a custom made post and core, the provider realized that there was not enough remaining coronal tooth structure to provide fracture resistance form for the final restoration (Figure 1). The patient was then referred for the extraction and implant placement of tooth #9.

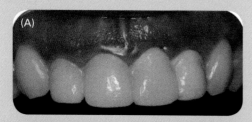

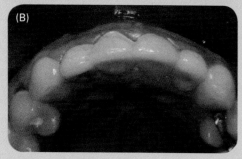

Figure 1: Preoperative photograph of the maxillary anterior dentition: (A) facial view; (B) occlusal view.

LEARNING GOALS AND OBJECTIVES
■ To be able to understand the concept of alveolar ridge augmentation at the time of tooth extraction
■ To be able to understand the technique and the materials used during alveolar ridge augmentation at the time of tooth extraction
■ To be able to understand the factors affecting the outcomes following alveolar ridge augmentation treatment and also the potential early complications associated with this technique

Medical History
- Last physical exam: January 2012
- Current major illnesses: none reported
- Current medications: none reported
- Hospitalizations: none reported
- Past illnesses: none reported
- Know allergies: none reported

Review of Systems
- Vital signs
  ○ Blood pressure: 128/68 mmHg
  ○ Pulse rate: 77 beats/min
  ○ Respiration: 16 breaths/min

Social History
She denies smoking or substance abuse. The patient drinks three glasses of red wine per week.

Extraoral Examination
The patient's face looks normocephalic. There are no scras, no masses, and no asymmetries on gross visual inspection. No lymphadenopathy, no clicking or crepitation of the temporomandibular joint upon opening.

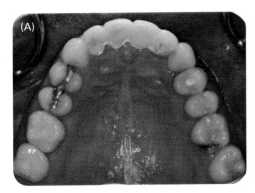

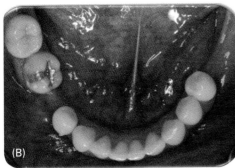

Figure 2: Intraoral examination: (A) maxillary teeth; (B) mandibular teeth.

Intraoral Examination

See Figure 2.
- Oral cancer screening: negative.
- Floor of the mouth: within normal limits.
- Buccal and lingual mucosa: within normal limits.
- Hard and soft palate: within normal limits.

Periodontal Examination

A comprehensive periodontal evaluation was completed. The patient has flat gingival biotype. All her periodontal parameters were within normal limits. Figure 3 shows the patient's periodontal charting at the time of initial periodontal evaluation.

Occlusion

There were no occlusal discrepancies or interferences noted at the time of examination.

Radiographic Examination

There was a very thin amount of tooth structure in the coronal third of the root of tooth #9. The bone level on the mesial and distal aspects of tooth #9 looked normal with no signs of bone loss (Figure 4A). A cone beam computed tomography (CBCT) scan was ordered, which showed a radiolucent lesion in the middle of the buccal plate of bone of tooth #9 (Figure 4B).

Diagnosis

An American Academy of Periodontology diagnosis of plaque-induced gingivitis was made.

Treatment Plan

After thorough evaluation of the patient's clinical and radiographic parameters, tooth #9 was extracted and ridge augmentation was performed at the time of tooth extraction. Implant placement was performed 7 months after the augmentation. The implant will be restored after 3 months.

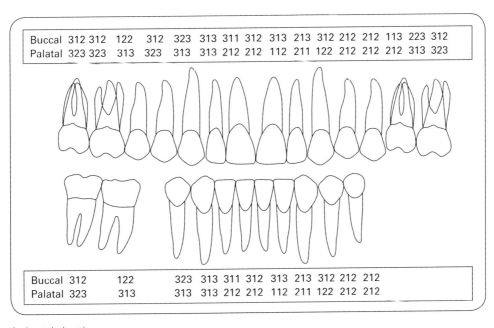

Figure 3: Initial periodontal charting.

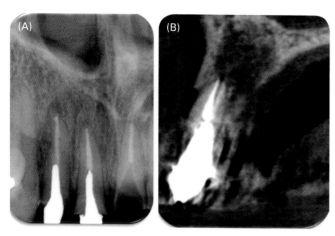

Figure 4: Pretreatment radiographs. (A) Periapical radiograph showing tooth #9 with severe loss of tooth structure due to extensive post-space preparation. Notice the severely thin coronal third of the root. (B) CBCT image of tooth #9 showing remarkable radiolucency and remarkable loss of the continuity of the buccal bone.

Treatment

Accompanied by her husband, the patient presented on time for her surgery. She took 0.5 mg of tirazolam orally for sedation 1 h before the surgery. Her blood pressure was 122/82 mmHg and her pulse was 82 beats per minute (measured from the right arm seated). The patient was advised to start rinsing with 0.12% chlorhexidine mouth rinse the day before and morning of the surgery for 2 min both after breakfast and before bedtime. Local infiltration anesthesia for the labial and palatal mucosa of teeth #8, #9, and #10 administered (lidocaine 2% with 1:100,000 of epinephrine).

The treatment started with the removal of the provisional bridge. A curved hemostat was used to remove the cemented post and core (Figure 5). A flapless tooth extraction was performed using the Benex root extraction system (Figure 6). Upon evaluation of the socket walls with a UNC periodontal probe, a fenestration defect was detected on the facial aspect of the socket (Figures 7 and 8). At this point, a full-thickness flap was raised (Figure 9) to prepare the site for guided bone regeneration. This was accomplished using a series of intrasulcular incisions around teeth #7, #8, #10, and #11 (two teeth on either side of the socket). The rational for extending the flap horizontally was to avoid using vertical incisions in the esthetic zone as well as to have better visibility and access to the bony defect. After flap elevation with a Buser elevator, a 3 mm × 3 mm fenestration defect was explored in the mid part of

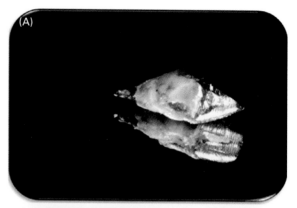

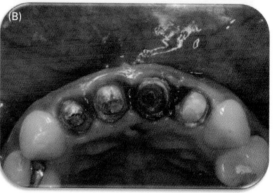

Figure 5: (A) The cemented customized post and core removed prior to the extraction of tooth #9. Notice the width of the post. (B) After the removal of the post and core. Notice the thinness of the coronal part of the root.

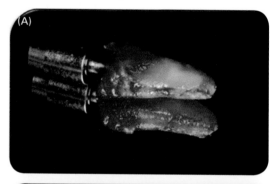

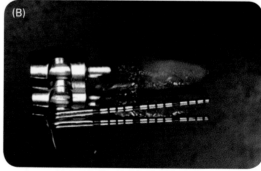

Figure 6: Tooth #9 removed with the Benex root extractor. (A) The Benex root extractor attached to the root of the tooth. (B) Measuring root length with a UNC periodontal probe for future reference.

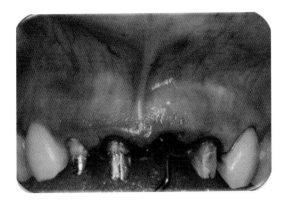

Figure 7: Evaluation of the socket walls with a UNC periodontal probe.

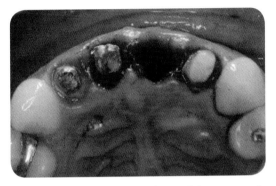

Figure 8: Occlusal view of the socket and the surrounding tissue prior to flap elevation.

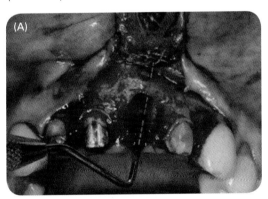

Figure 9: Socket exploration after flap elevations. (A) Notice the facial fenestration on the facial aspect of the socket. (B) Occlusal view.

the labial plate of bone. Thorough debridement and irrigation of the socket walls was performed with a Luca curette and saline respectively.

The width (mesiodistal distance) and thickness (buccolingual distance) of the edentulous ridge were measured using the UNC periodontal probe A 20 mm × 30 mm cross-linked collagen membrane was trimmed and tried on the facial aspect of the socket (Figure 10). The membrane was then tucked under the most apical part of the buccal flap (Figure 11). A deproteinized particulate bone matrix graft was used to fill the socket. An additional layer of bone graft particles was also placed on the facial aspect between the membrane and the outer surface of the labial plate of bone (Figure 12).

Since there was no intention to achieve primary closure, neither periosteal nor vertical releasing incisions were needed. The flaps were approximated and sutured in two layers using a CV 5.00 Gore Tex suture (Figure 13). At first, a horizontal mattress suture was used to allow for tension-free approximation of the

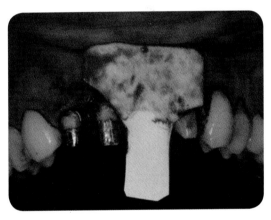

Figure 10: Trying in the cross-linked collagen membrane.

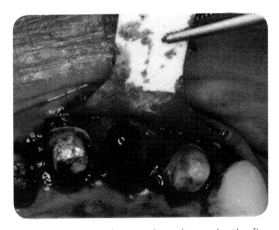

Figure 11: Collagen membrane adaptation under the flap prior to grafting.

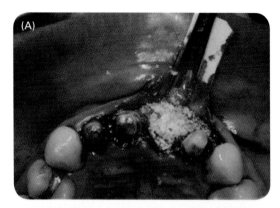

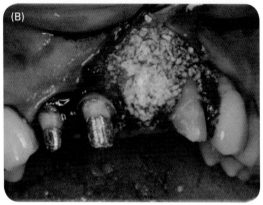

Figure 12: (A) Bio-Oss bone particles packed into the socket. (B) Bio-Oss packed on the facial aspect between the outer aspect of the buccal plate of bone and collagen membrane.

flaps. This will also help stabilize the membrane against the grafted site. A second layer of simple interrupted loops was placed to stabilize the flaps and gain further approximation. A small part of the collagen membrane over the center of the socket was left exposed to heal with secondary intention. This area will be protected by the pontic of the new provisional restoration.

A prefabricated provisional bridge was cemented into the abutment teeth with a temporary luting agent. Standard postoperative instructions were given to the patient both verbally and in writing.

The patient returned for sutures removal after 3 weeks (Figures 14 and 15). The provisional bridge was removed and the sutures were removed.

The patient returned 9 months later for the implant placement of site #9. There was more keratinized tissue over the area that was left to heal with secondary intention (Figure 16). A CBCT scan was taken and revealed enough bone for the vertical and horizontal placement of the implant (Figure 17). Local infiltration anesthesia (lidocaine 2% with 1:100,000 of epinephrine) was accomplished. Using a #15 surgical blade, a midcrestal incision was made followed by an intrasulcular incision around tooth #8 and a mini vertical releasing incision on #10. Full-thickness flaps were elevated (Figure 18).

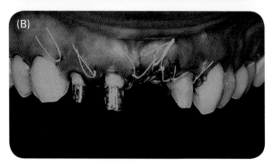

Figure 13: Flaps approximated with nonresorbable sutures: (A) occlusal view; (B) facial view.

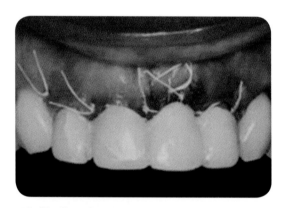

Figure 14: Healing after 3 weeks.

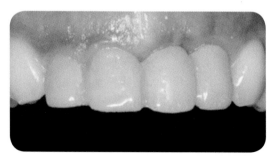

Figure 15: Healing after 6 weeks.

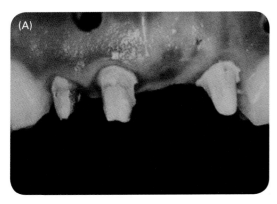
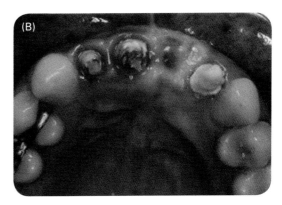

Figure 16: Tissue healing and maturation after 9 months: (A) facial view; (B) occlusal view.

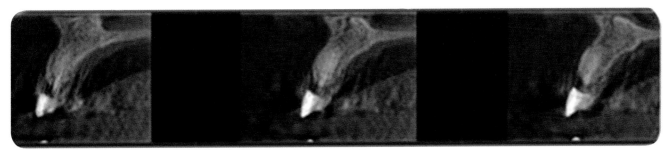

Figure 17: CBCT views 9 months after ridge augmentation.

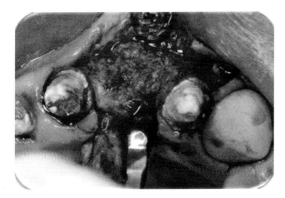

Figure 18: Flap elevation for implant bed preparation. Notice how xenografts maintain the volume of the tissue.

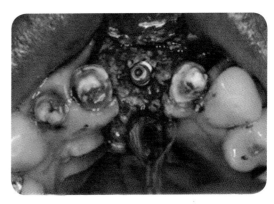

Figure 19: Occlusal view after implant placement. Notice the amount of bone on the facial aspect of the implant.

The implant osteotomy was prepared with the 3i surgical implant system. A 3.25 mm × 11.5 mm 3i implant was placed (Figure 19). A 3.4 mm × 4 mm healing abutment was also placed (Figure 20). The flaps were approximated and sutured together using a 6.00 polypropylene suture (Figure 21). The provisional restoration adjusted and cemented back with temporary cement and a periapical radiograph was taken (Figure 22). Postoperative instructions and pain medication prescriptions were given to the patient. The patient will return for follow-up and suture removal. A porcelain-fused-to-metal crown will be fabricated after the osseointegration of the implant in 3–6 months.

Discussion

Dental implant placement in the esthetic zone presents a major challenge to the surgeon and the restorative dentist. There are several implant placement protocols that have been thoroughly documented in the literature;

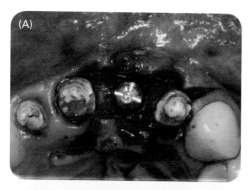

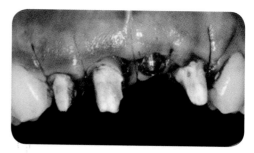

Figure 21: Flaps approximated with 6.00 polypropylene sutures.

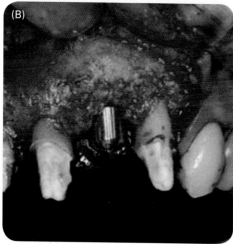

Figure 20: The placement of the healing abutment: (A) occlusal view; (B) facial view.

namely, immediate, early, and delayed implant placement. However, the choice to pursue one approach over another is dependent on a variety of patient- and clinician-related factors. The overall health, age, habits, and socio-economic status of the patient are amongst the patient-related factors that could influence the treatment decision process. On the other hand, some of the clinician-related factors include the surgical and restorative skills and comfort level of the surgeon and the restorative dentist. In this case, owing to the presence of bony fenestration in the middle of the labial plate of bone together with the patient's limited finances at the time of tooth extraction, the decision was to have the extraction and guided bone regeneration done at the same time. The rationale for selecting a slow resorbing bone graft is because of the fact that the patient was planning on visiting her family overseas and was not sure about her return date. Indeed, the patient returned after 9 months, and we can see from the CBCT images and the clinical photographs how the xenograft maintained the space and the volume for the implant placement. The rationale for selecting one biomaterial over another is still a matter of debate, and clearly there is no scientific evidence in the literature to prove that one biomaterial is suitable for all clinical situations. More details about this are available in the self-study and critical review of the literature section of this book.

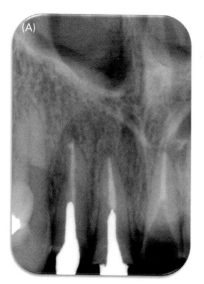
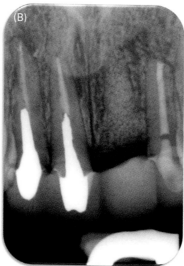
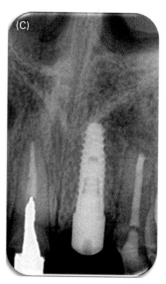

Figure 22: Periapical radiographs (A) before, (B) after guided bone regeneration, and (C) after implant placement.

Self-Study Questions

(Answers located at the end of the case)

A. What is guided bone regeneration?

B. What is the difference between guided bone regeneration and alveolar ridge preservation?

C. What are the indications of alveolar ridge preservation?

D. What are the complications associated with guided bone regeneration and socket preservation?

E. What are the different types of membranes used for guided bone regeneration?

F. What are the advantages and disadvantages of the different membranes?

G. What are the different types of bone grafting materials that can be used for grafting?

H. What are the benefits of alveolar ridge preservation at the time of tooth extraction?

I. Flapless versus flapped bone grafting at the time of tooth extraction: which approach to choose?

J. What kind of biomaterials should be used in simultaneous extraction with alveolar ridge preservation?

K. Is primary wound closure required for alveolar ridge preservation at the time of tooth extraction?

L. What are the recent advances in guided bone regeneration and socket preservation techniques?

References

1. Hurley LA, Stinchfield FE, Bassett AL, Lyon WH. The role of soft tissues in osteogenesis. An experimental study of canine spine fusions. J Bone Joint Surg Am 1959;41-A:1243–1254.
2. Hämmerle, CH, Araújo MG, Simion M; Osteology Consensus Group 2011. Evidence-based knowledge on the biology and treatment of extraction sockets. Clin Oral Implants Res 2012;23(Suppl 5):80–82.
3. Chiapasco M, Abati S, Romeo E, Vogel G. Clinical outcome of autogenous bone blocks or guided bone regeneration with e-PTFE membranes for the reconstruction of narrow edentulous ridges. Clin Oral Implants Res 1999;10(4):278–288.
4. Hutmacher DW, Kirsch A, Ackermann KL, Hürzeler MB. A tissue engineered cell-occlusive device for hard tissue regeneration – a preliminary report. Int J Periodontics Restorative Dent 2001;21:49–59.
5. Cafesse RG, Nasjleti CE, Morrison EC, Sanchez R. Guided tissue regeneration: Comparison of bioabsorbable and non-bioabsorbable membranes. Histologic and histometric study in dogs. J Periodontol 1994;65:583–591.
6. Burchardt H. The biology of bone graft repair. Clin Orthop 1983;174:28–42.
7. Schwartz Z, Mellonig JT, Carnes Jr DL, et al. Ability of commercial demineralized freeze-dried bone allograft to induce new bone formation. J Periodontol 1996;67:918–926.
8. Thaller SR, Hoyt J, Borjeson K, et al. Reconstruction of calvarial defects with anorganic bovine bone mineral (Bio-Oss) in a rabbit model. J Craniofac Surg 1993;4:79–84.
9. Furusawa T, Mizunuma K. Osteoconductive properties and efficacy of resorbable bioactive glass as a bone grafting material. Implant Dent 1997;6:93–101.
10. Araujo M, Lindhe J. Dimensional ridge alterations following tooth extraction. An experimental study in the dog. J Clin Periodontol 2005;32:212–218.
11. Vignoletti F, Matesanz P, Rodrigo D, et al. Surgical protocols for ridge preservation after tooth extraction. A systematic review. Clin Oral Implants Res 2012;23(Suppl 5):22–38.
12. Kim DM, De Angelis N, Camelo M, et al. Ridge preservation with and without primary wound closure: a case series. Int J Periodontics Restorative Dent 2013;33(1):71–78.
13. Rios HF, Lin Z, Oh B, et al. Cell- and gene-based therapeutic strategies for periodontal regenerative medicine. J Periodontol 2011;82(9):1223–1237.

Answers to Self-Study Questions

A. The concept of bone regeneration was first described in the orthopedic literature by Hurley et al. in 1959 [1]. This procedure is intended to regenerate bone solely in edentulous areas and extraction sites as part of future dental implant site development.

B. In 2012, the Osteology Consensus Report [2] defined the terms ridge preservation and ridge augmentation as follows:
- Ridge preservation = preserving the ridge volume within the envelope existing at the time of extraction.
- Ridge augmentation = increasing the ridge volume beyond the skeletal envelope existing at the time of extraction.

C. According to the report by Hämmerle et al. [2], alveolar ridge augmentation is indicated during the following situations:
1. where immediate implant placement is not possible;
2. where early implant placement is not possible;
3. where implant primary stability cannot be achieved;
4. where ridge contour is not feasible to achieve a restoratively driven implant placement;
5. where the patient cannot afford implant placement at the time of tooth extraction.

D. Like other surgical procedures, common postoperative complications include bleeding; swelling, bruising, and infection may be expected. Loss of keratinized tissue and early membrane exposure are frequently encountered when using nonresorbable membranes. Other less common complications are nerve injuries. In a study by Chiapasco et al. [3] comparing the clinical outcomes of guided bone regeneration (polytetrafluoroethylene plus particulate bone) with that of autogenous block grafting, the incidence of postoperative infection was higher in the guided bone regeneration treatment patients than with the autogenous block graft patients. This was attributed to the larger number of patients who presented with postoperative early membrane exposure as a result of wound dehiscence.

E. Barrier membranes are categorized into resorbable and nonresorbable membranes [4]. Resorbable barriers, such as collagen membranes, can be hydrolyzed by the body over a period of few weeks [5]. On the other hand, nonresorbable barrier membranes do not resorb and are not affected by the body's hydrolytic enzymes and they need to be removed with a surgical procedure.

F.

Membrane type	Resorbable	Nonresorbable
Resorption time	Few weeks	None
Need for removal	Not required	Surgery required to remove it
Mechanical properties	Reasonable	Excellent
Membrane exposure	More forgiving	Least forgiving

G.

Bone graft	Autograft	Allograft	Xenograft	Alloplast
Source	Oneself	Human tissue banks	Bovine, porcine, equine	$CaSO_4/CaPO_4$
Osteoinductive	Yes [6]	No [7]	No [8]	No [9]
Osteoconductive	Yes	Yes	Yes	Yes
Osteogenic	Yes	No	No	No

H. In 2005 an experimental study by Araujo et al. [10] showed significant alteration in the vertical and horizontal dimensions of the alveolar bone a few weeks after tooth extraction. Alveolar ridge deficiency may compromise dental implant placement into the edentulous ridges. Thus, the need for a bone augmentation procedure at the time of tooth extraction has been studied in the literature. A systematic review by Vignoletti et al. [11] showed that bone augmentation at the time of tooth extraction has resulted in significantly less horizontal and vertical alveolar bone loss than nonaugmented sites.

I. A surgeon can perform flapless versus a flapped procedure at the time of extraction. A flapless procedure might be a viable option in situations where all the socket walls are intact. On the contrary, a flapped bone grafting is essential if there is a bony defect, as in the case of apical fenestrations and dehiscences. It is also indicated when one or more of the extraction socket walls are missing at the time of extraction.

J. Until today, the scientific evidence that we have is not conclusive on this issue, but it seems that all the most commonly used materials (autografts, allografts, xenografts, and synthetic materials) that we have in our armamentarium are capable of producing enough bone augmentation for implant placement. Materials should be chosen based on individual patients and the risk factors evaluated before the plan for guided bone regeneration.

K. Kim et al. in 2013 [12] studied the effect of primary wound closure on the percentage of bone formation and the amount of the residual bone grafts after teeth extraction and ridge preservation procedures. They concluded that the amounts of new bone formation and the residual bone graft are not affected by the absence of primary wound closure at the time of ridge preservation.

L. Recently, a wide variety of therapeutic strategies have evolved in the field of tissue regeneration. Cell- and gene-based therapies [13], for example, are being utilized and continuously tested as potential means to engineer lost tissue due to disease. Amongst the currently available proteins for this purpose are platelets-derived growth factor, bone morphogenetic protein-2, and fibroblast growth factor. Other growth and differentiation factors are still being tested for approval by the regulatory agencies to be available for use in the future.

Case 7

Guided Bone Regeneration: Non-Resorbable Membrane

CASE STORY

A 58-year-old Caucasian male presented to the clinic with a chief complaint of wanting to restore his fractured tooth #20 and missing teeth #18 and #19. According to patient, #18 and #19 were extracted a few years ago due to caries and #20 had a dental history of root canal treatment, post and core placement, and restored by a single crown. He had several other dental restorations, including composite and amalgam restorations and fixed partial dentures.

LEARNING GOALS AND OBJECTIVES

- To understand the role of a barrier membrane for guided bone regeneration (GBR)
- To know the principles of using a barrier membrane in GBR
- To understand the different types of barrier membranes and proper membrane selection
- To learn basic surgical techniques using barrier membranes
- To learn the common complications associated with barrier membranes and how to manage them

Medical History

The patient presented with gout, arthritis, hypertension, hypercholesterol, and type 2 diabetes. His HbA1c measurement was 6.8.

He was taking naproxen 500 mg twice a day for pain control, allopurinol 300 mg once per day for gout, lisinopril 40 mg once per day for hypertension, simvastatin 40 mg once per day for hypercholesterolemia, metformin 1000 mg twice per day for type 2 diabetes, and prophylactic low-dose aspirin (81 mg) once per day. The patient did not report any known drug allergies.

Review of Systems

- Vital signs
  - Blood pressure: 131/77 mmHg
  - Pulse rate: 76 beats/min
  - Respiration: 14 breaths/min

Social History

According to the patient, he had no history of smoking and alcohol use.

Extraoral Examination

No significant findings. There was no facial asymmetry. The extraoral soft tissue and the temporomandibular joint were within normal limits. No lymph node enlargement was noted upon palpation.

Intraoral Examination

- Intraoral soft tissue examination was within normal limits.
- Periodontal examination revealed full mouth probing depths equal to or less than 3 mm (Figure 1).
- Slight gingival inflammation with subgingival calculus was noted.
- Generalized attrition on the anterior teeth.
- Evaluation of the residual ridge over #18 and #19 indicated horizontal and vertical ridge deformity (Seibert classification III).
- Tooth #20 was a residual root with an exposed metal post (Figure 2).
- Tooth #21 had Miller class I mobility.

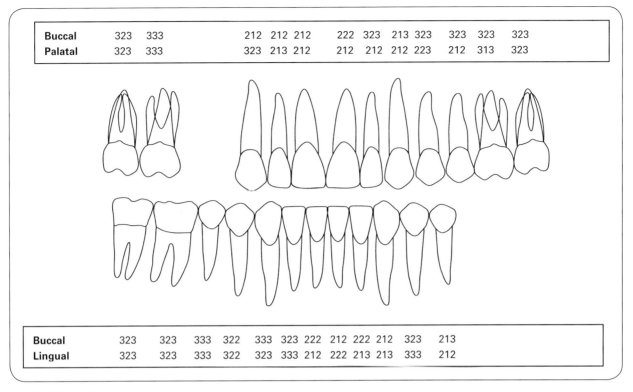

Buccal	323	333		212	212	212		222	323	213	323	323	323	323
Palatal	323	333		323	213	212		212	212	212	223	212	313	323

Buccal	323	323	333	322	333	323	222	212	222	212	323	213
Lingual	323	323	333	322	323	333	212	222	213	213	333	212

Figure 1: Probing pocket depth measurements during the initial visit.

Occlusion

There were no occlusal discrepancies, but fremitus was noted on #8 and #10.

Radiographic Examination

A peripheral radiographs showed an apical radiolucency around #20 residual root with the periodontal ligament (PDL) space widening (Figure 3). A widened PDL was also noted around #21. There was a radiolucency beneath the class II composite restoration of #21.

Diagnosis

American Academy of Periodontology diagnosis of gingivitis associated with dental plaque only without other local contributing factors with mucogingival deformities and conditions on the edentulous ridge (vertical and horizontal ridge deficiency). Secondary caries was found on #21.

Treatment Plan

The treatment plan for the patient included periodontal phase I therapy: oral hygiene instructions, supra- and

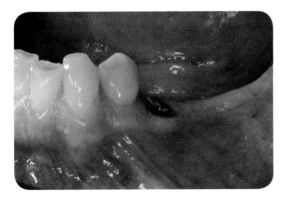

Figure 2: Preoperative presentation (facial view).

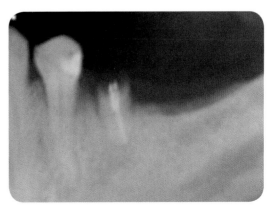

Figure 3: Periapical radiograph of the surgical area.

subgingival scaling, and occlusal adjustment. Afterwards, extraction of unrestorable #20 along with a GBR procedure were planned to augment the alveolar ridge deficiency for future implant placement #18, #19, #20. Tooth #21 was restored with a composite filling.

Treatment

After periodontal phase I therapy, the patient presented to the clinic for #20 extraction and the GBR procedure. After achieving profound local anesthesia, #20 was extracted atraumatically with a periotome and forceps (Figure 4). A crestal incision was made on the edentulous area, extended to the sulcular incision of the extraction site. Two vertical incisions were made at #21 mesiobuccal and mesiolingual line angles. A buccal flap was reflected by using the double-flap technique [1] (Figure 5). The full-thickness lingual flap was reflected afterwards. Decortication was performed on residual underlying bone by using a surgical round carbide bur (Figure 6). A nonresorbable titanium-reinforced expanded polytetrafluoroethylene (ePTFE) barrier membrane was trimmed according to the defect size. At least 2 mm distance from the membrane

margin to #21 was left to avoid bacterial contamination. Particulate freeze-dried bone allograft (FDBA) was saturated in sterilized saline. The graft material was placed onto the bone defect afterwards. The membrane was trimmed and adapted on the defect and secured by bone tacks (Figure 7). Two horizontal mattress sutures were used to approximate the periosteal layer of the double flap to secure the membrane and graft material (Figure 8). Subsequently, the outer buccal musosal flap

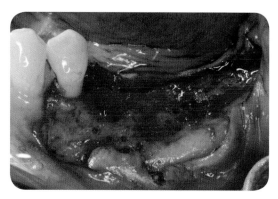

Figure 6: Post-alveolar bone decortication.

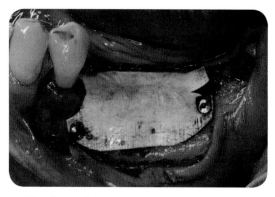

Figure 7: Titanium-reinforced ePTFE membrane placement with bone tacks.

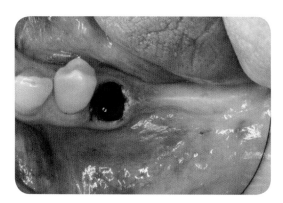

Figure 4: Post-#20 extraction site at the time of GBR (occlusal view).

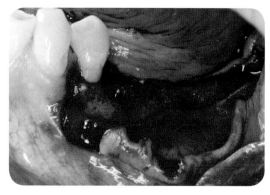

Figure 5: After flap elevation.

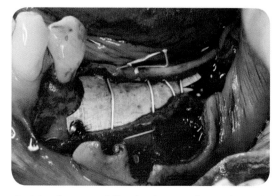

Figure 8: Membrane stabilization by suturing periosteal layer of the double flap using horizontal mattress sutures.

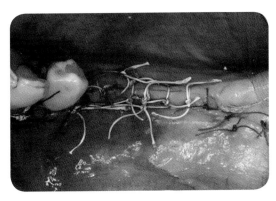

Figure 9: Tension-free primary flap closure was achieved.

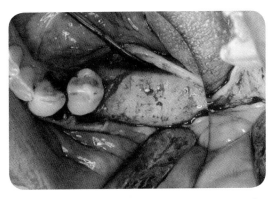

Figure 10: Post-membrane removal at reentry surgery for implant placement #18, #19, #20. Successful bone regeneration was achieved beneath the space created by barrier membrane.

was coronally advanced and sutured to the lingual flap with tension-free primary closure (Figure 9).

Sutures were removed 2 weeks postoperatively. There was no membrane exposure or other complications over the 6 months postoperative healing period. Upon reentry at 6 months post-GBR, bone tacks and nonresorbable barrier membrane were removed. The ridge was successfully augmented within the space created by the barrier membrane, thus provide a sufficient bone width and height for implant placement #18, #19, #20 (Figure 10).

Discussion

For GBR, barrier membranes serve as a barrier to prevent soft tissue ingrowth into the intended space for bone augmentation. Barrier membranes can be divided into two main categories (resorbable/ nonresorbable) according to the resorbability of the membrane. Nonresorbable membranes are more rigid than resorbable membranes and possess superior space maintenance ability over time. In other words, a nonresorbable membrane does not collapse as easily as a resorbable membrane when a large bone

augmentation is intended. In this case, a titanium-reinforced ePTFE membrane was selected because vertical augmentation was attempted in addition to horizontal augmentation. The titanium framework allows surgeons to bend the membrane into an adequate shape based on the required amount of augmentation. Precautions should be taken when configuring the membrane to ensure membrane coverage is 3 mm beyond the defect margin, and at least 2 mm away from adjacent teeth. Primary closure during the healing optimizes the outcome of GBR [2]. The trimmed membrane was adapted and stabilized on the ridge with bone tacks. A periosteal releasing incision is commonly used for flap advancement. However, it is a major challenge when used for vertical ridge augmentation. For the case shown, flap advancement and primary tension-free flap closure was achieved with the double-flap technique by utilizing a partial-thickness flap to separate the mucosal flap from the underlying periosteum on the alveolar bone [3]. No membrane exposure was detected during the postoperative healing phase. The successful outcome was achieved at the 6 months' reentry.

Self-Study Questions

(Answers located at the end of the case)

A. What is the effect of diabetes on bone formation following GBR?

B. What is the role of the barrier membrane in GBR?

C. What are the characteristics that barrier membranes should possess for GBR?

D. What are the types of barrier membranes available for GBR?

E. What are the materials used for GBR in conjunction with a barrier membrane?

F. Are there differences in treatment outcome between resorbable and nonresorbable membranes?

G. What are the clinical principles of using a barrier membrane for GBR?

H. Are the membranes always needed to be primarily covered by a soft tissue flap?

I. What are the most common postoperative complications related with membrane use for GBR and how should one manage them?

J. What is the survival or success rate of implants placed in sites treated by GBR?

References

1. Hur Y, Tsukiyama T, Yoon TH, Griffin T. Double flap incision design for guided bone regeneration: a novel technique and clinical considerations. J Periodontol 2010;81(6):945–952.
2. Machtei EE. The effect of membrane exposure on the outcome of regenerative procedures in humans: a meta-analysis. J Periodontol 2001;72(4):512–516.
3. Ogata Y, Griffin TJ, Ko AC, Hur Y. Comparison of double-flap incision to periosteal releasing incision for flap advancement: a prospective clinical trial. Int J Oral Maxillofac Implants 2013;28(2):597–604.
4. Santana RB, Xu L, Chase HB, et al. A role for advanced glycation end products in diminished bone healing in type 1 diabetes. Diabetes 2003;52(6):1502–1510.
5. Follak N, Klöting I, Merk H. Influence of diabetic metabolic state on fracture healing in spontaneously diabetic rats. Diabetes Metab Res Rev 2005;21(3):288–296.
6. Retzepi M, Lewis MP, Donos N. Effect of diabetes and metabolic control on de novo bone formation following guided bone regeneration. Clin Oral Implants Res 2010;21(1):71–79.
7. Lee SB, Retzepi M, Petrie A, et al. The effect of diabetes on bone formation following application of the GBR principle with the use of titanium domes. Clin Oral Implants Res 2013;24(1):28–35.
8. Hardwick R, Scantlebury TV, Sanchez R, et al. Membrane design criteria for guided bone regeneration of the alveolar ridge In: BuserD, DahlinC, SchenkRK (eds), Guided Bone Regeneration in Implant Dentistry. Chicago, IL: Quintessence; 1994, pp 101–136.
9. Gottlow J. Guided tissue regeneration using bioresorbable and non-resorbable devices: initial healing and long-term results. J Periodontol 1993;64(11 Suppl):1157–1165.
10. Buser D, Bragger U, Lang NP, Nyman S. Regeneration and enlargement of jaw bone using guided tissue regeneration. Clin Oral Implants Res 1990;1(1): 22–32.
11. Bartee BK, Carr JA. Evaluation of a high-density polytetrafluoroethylene (d-PTFE) membrane as a barrier material to facilitate guided bone regeneration in the rat mandible. J Oral Implantol 1995;21(2):88–95.
12. Walters SP, Greenwell H, Hill M, et al. Comparison of porous and non-porous Teflon membranes plus a xenograft in the treatment of vertical osseous defects: a clinical reentry study. J Periodontol 2003;74(8):1161–1168.
13. Simion M, Jovanovic SA, Trisi P, et al. Vertical ridge augmentation around dental implants using a membrane technique and autogenous bone or allografts in humans. Int J Periodontics Restorative Dent 1998;18(1):8–23.
14. Chiapasco M, Zaniboni M, Boisco M. Augmentation procedures for the rehabilitation of deficient edentulous ridges with oral implants. Clin Oral Implants Res 2006;17(Suppl 2):136–159.
15. Jung RE, Glauser R, Schärer P, et al. Effect of rhBMP-2 on guided bone regeneration in humans. Clin Oral Implants Res 2003;14(5):556–568.
16. Jung RE, Windisch SI, Eggenschwiler AM, et al. A randomized-controlled clinical trial evaluating clinical and radiological outcomes after 3 and 5 years of dental implants placed in bone regenerated by means of GBR techniques with or without the addition of BMP-2. Clin Oral Implants Res 2009;20 (7):660–666.
17. Simion M, Scarano A, Gionso L, Piattelli A. Guided bone regeneration using resorbable and nonresorbable membranes: a comparative histologic study in humans. Int J Oral Maxillofac Implants 1996;11(6):735–742.

18. Zitzmann NU, Naef R, Schärer P. Resorbable versus nonresorbable membranes in combination with Bio-Oss for guided bone regeneration. Int J Oral Maxillofac Implants 1997;12(6):844–852.

19. Fugazzotto PA. GBR using bovine bone matrix and resorbable and nonresorbable membranes. Part 1: histologic results. Int J Periodontics Restorative Dent 2003;23(4):361–369.

20. Melcher A, Dreyer C. Protection of the blood clot in healing circumscribed bone defects. J Bone Joint Surg 1962;44-B(2):424–430.

21. Waasdorp J, Feldman S. Bone regeneration around immediate implants utilizing a dense polytetrafluoroethylene membrane without primary closure: a report of 3 cases. J Oral Implantol 2013;39(3):355–361.

22. Yun JH, Jun CM, Oh NS. Secondary closure of an extraction socket using the double-membrane guided bone regeneration technique with immediate implant placement. J Periodontal Implant Sci 2011;41(5):253–258.

23. Simion M, Trisi P, Maglione M, Piattelli A. A preliminary report on a method for studying the permeability of expanded polytetrafluoroethylene membrane to bacteria in vitro: a scanning electron microscopic and histological study. J Periodontol 1994;65(8):755–761.

24. Fiorellini JP, Nevins ML. Localized ridge augmentation/preservation. A systematic review. Ann Periodontol 2003;8(1):321–327.

25. Donos N, Mardas N, Chadha V. Clinical outcomes of implants following lateral bone augmentation: systematic assessment of available options (barrier membranes, bone grafts, split osteotomy). J Clin Periodontol 2008;35(8 Suppl):173–202.

Answers to Self-Study Questions

A. Diabetes mellitus is defined as a metabolic disorder manifested by an abnormally high level of blood glucose. This hyperglycemia results from either insulin deficiency due to the body's failure to produce insulin (type 1) or insulin resistance (type 2), a condition in which cells fail to use insulin in the liver or muscle tissue, or a combination of types 1 and 2. It is well documented that diabetes mellitus is associated with impaired bone healing [4,5]. It has been shown that diabetes has negative effects on bone formation and osseointegration following GBR as well. Studies suggest that insulin-mediated glycemic control can improve the predictability of GBR [6,7].

B. GBR techniques have been used for vertical and horizontal ridge augmentations to enable dental implant placement in atrophic maxilla and mandible. The role of the barrier membrane in GBR is to create and maintain a space for osteogenic cells from adjacent bone marrow migrating into the site to regenerate bone tissue. It serves as a barrier to exclude rapid-growing epithelial and connective tissue cells into the intended site, and to facilitate bone ingrowth.

C. An ideal barrier membrane should possess the following characteristics [8]:
1. *Biocompatibility and integration with the host tissue.* The barrier membrane should be biocompatible, causing no or limited inflammation, immune response, and foreign-body reaction. When the barrier membrane is composed of resorbable material, the host tissue reactions resulting from the resorption should be minimal, reversible, and should not negatively influence regeneration of the desired tissues [9].
2. *Cell occlusiveness.* The barrier membrane should demonstrate the ability to exclude soft tissue and nonosteogenic cells from migrating into the space intended specifically for new bone formation.
3. *Space creation and maintenance ability.* The barrier membrane should be capable of creating and maintaining a space for bone regeneration. It is essential for the barrier membrane to maintain its shape and integral features during the healing period of GBR.
4. *Clinical manageability.* For clinical application, the barrier membrane should be easy to trim and adapt in different configurations of alveolar ridge deficiency.

D. According to the degradation characteristics, barrier membranes can be categorized into two types: nonresorbable and resorbable (Figures 11, 12, and 13).
1. *Nonresorbable membrane.* These barrier membranes can sustain their barrier and space maintenance ability for a longer period of time than a resorbable membrane can. However, a reentry surgery is indicated to remove the membrane since it cannot be degraded by the human body.

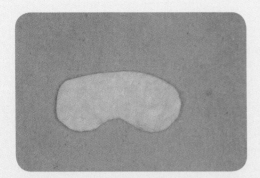

Figure 11: Resorbable collagen membrane.

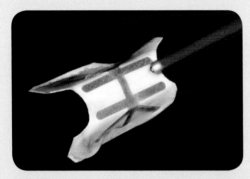

Figure 12: Nonresorbable titanium reinforced ePTFE membrane.

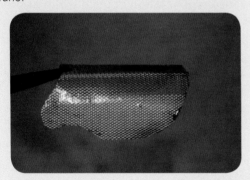

Figure 13: Titanium mesh.

Expanded polytetrafluoroethylene (ePTFE) was first introduced as a nonresorbable membrane and it has been used widely by clinicians, demonstrating favorable result of new bone formation. However, ePTFE membranes have been recently discontinued and are no longer available in the market. Currently, the available nonresorbable membranes are a high-density polytetrafluoroethylene (dPTFE) and PTFE. Both types of nonresorbable membrane have shown a similar clinical outcome of bone regeneration in a few animal and human studies

[10–12]. Some of these membranes have a titanium framework to reinforce the space maintenance ability of the membrane.
2. *Resorbable membrane.* These membranes have the benefit of being biodegradable; hence, a second surgery for membrane removal is not needed. In comparison with nonresorbable membranes, resorbable membranes have a higher compliance ability that allows better adaptation around the bone defect area (Table 1). For resorbable membranes, the majority are made of collagen (bovine or porcine derived), polylactic acid, polyglycolic acid (synthetic), or acellular dermal matrix (human).

E. GBR can be performed using a membrane alone, but the addition of bone grafting materials with membrane results in an improved amount of bone regeneration [13]. When bone graft materials are used, they are placed under the membrane, which helps in space creation and maintenance. Different types of bone grafting material can be used for GBR. Autograft is considered to be the gold standard because of its capability for osteogenesis, osteoinduction, and osteoconduction; those characteristics are the biologic mechanisms that provide a rationale for GBR.

Osteogenesis refers to the formation and development of bony tissue, and it occurs when vital osteoblasts originating from autografts contribute to new bone growth. Osteogenesis only occurs with autografts. Osteoinduction implies the recruitment of osteoprogenitor cells and stimulation of these cells to differentiate into osteoblasts, which are responsible for new bone formation. Bone morphogenetic proteins (BMPs) are a group of growth factors that are known to be osteoinductive and have been well studied in animals and humans. Osteoconduction refers to the ability of bone graft materials to serve as a scaffold for osteoblasts to form new bone. All bone graft materials need to be osteoconductive at the minimum.

In addition to autografts, other materials that have been used successfully with predictable outcomes are allografts (FDBA, demineralized FDBA), xenografts (bovine, porcine), and alloplasts (hydroxyapatite, calcium phosphate) [14].

The use of growth factors for GBR has been investigated recently. The recombinant human BMPs (rhBMPs) are human proteins that stimulate bone

Table 1: Comparison between Resorbable and Nonresorbable Membrane Usage for GBR

	Nonresorbable membrane	Resorbable membrane
Biocompatibility	• Biocompatible • Need for membrane removal surgery	• Highly biocompatible • No need for membrane removal surgery • Resorption process of membrane may cause inflammation and negatively affect bone regeneration
Membrane function	• Controlled time of barrier function	• Uncontrolled time of barrier function
Space-making ability	• Fair: when used alone • Good: with bone graft materials • Excellent: with titanium reinforcement and supporting material (bone graft materials, bone tacks, tenting screw)	• Poor: easy to collapse • Fair: with supporting material (bone graft materials, bone tacks, tenting screw)
Clinical manageability	• Moderate to difficult	• Easy to moderate
Surgical complications	• Frequent • With membrane exposure, increased risk of infection	• Less frequent • More forgiving to membrane exposure compared with nonresorbable
Indications for use	• Vertical augmentation • Large defect, critical-size defect	• Horizontal augmentation • Small defect

formation. Clinical trials supported the potential use of rhBMP-2 [15,16]. However, the use of rhBMP-2 is limited and only approved by the US Food and Drug Administration for sinus augmentations and localized alveolar ridge augmentations for defects associated with extraction sockets. Further research is necessary to determine the effectiveness of rhBMP-2 and its ideal carrier material.

F. A histologic study showed that more bone volume gain was achieved by using nonresorbable ePTFE membrane compared with resorbable poly(lactic acid)/poly(glycolic acid) membrane [17]. The unfavorable outcome of resorbable membrane may be due to the fact that there was no bone graft used in the study. Without the support of bone graft, resorbable membrane tends to collapse, resulting in compromised outcome of bone regeneration.

In contrast, a split mouth study in humans in which bone graft was utilized along with membranes for GBR showed similar clinical results between nonresorbable and resorbable membrane [18].

In the situation that sufficient membrane support can be achieved, resorbable membranes are generally preferred by clinicians because there is better soft tissue healing and lower complication rates when compared with nonresorbable membranes. Additionally, the use of a resorbable membrane does not require a second surgical stage for membrane removal. A resorbable membrane is commonly used for horizontal augmentation.

For large- or critical-size defects, a titanium-reinforced nonresorbable membrane is considered to be the most reliable way to increase the predictability of regenerated hard tissues [19] (Figure 12). Therefore, titanium-reinforced nonresorbable membranes are preferred when performing GBR for vertical augmentation as well. Titanium mesh has also been used when treating these large defects (Figure 13).

G.
1. *Stability of the wound.* The membrane should be stable without any micro-movement [20]. The stability can be achieved by using bone tacks/screws to fix the membrane onto the bone surface. Periosteal sutures are also utilized to stabilize the membrane and graft material over the alveolar bone (Figure 8).

2. *Membrane configuration.* The membrane margin should be at least 3 mm away from the bone defect margin to create a closed space to prevent soft tissue invasion. The margin of the membrane should be at least 2 mm away from the adjacent teeth to avoid bacterial contamination from the tooth.

3. *Membrane adaptation.* The membrane should be well adapted around the defect area. A sharp corner or margin of membrane should be trimmed to prevent flap perforation (Figure 14).

H. A meta-analysis indicated that both resorbable and nonresorbable membrane exposure during healing had a significant negative effect on GBR around dental implants [2]. Recently, several studies support that dPTFE membrane is impervious to bacteria and can withstand exposure in GBR [21,22]. Further studies are recommended to investigate the effect of dPTFE membrane exposure in the outcome of bone augmentation.

I. Premature membrane exposure is the most commonly reported complication related to membrane use for GBR (Figures 15 and 16).

   Exposure of resorbable membrane to the oral cavity resulted in faster resorption of the membrane, but less clinical complications were observed compared with nonresorbable membrane exposure. Conversely, when nonresorbable membranes were exposed, food debris and bacteria could easily attach to the exposed membrane surface, leading to the contamination of the healing tissues and consequently compromising the clinical result. Bacteria would penetrate the ePTFE membrane to infect the regenerated site by approximately

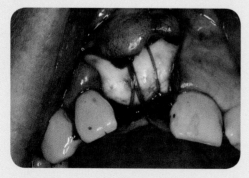

Figure 14: GBR with a resorbable membrane.

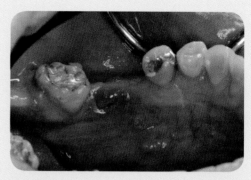

Figure 15: ePTFE membrane exposure with pus drainage.

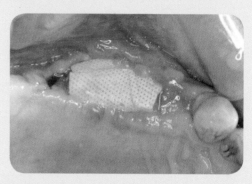

Figure 16: ePTFE membrane exposure without pus drainage.

3–4 weeks, according to an in vivo study [23]. When premature membrane exposure happened, an intense oral hygiene regimen with 0.12% chlorhexidine gluconate rinse twice a day to reduce plaque formation around exposed membrane should be performed and the patient should be followed up on a weekly basis. If purulent exudate or infection signs present at the membrane exposure site, the membrane should be removed as early as possible. Administration of systemic antibiotics (e.g., amoxicillin or amoxicillin with clavulanic acid) is also suggested.

J. Membrane use for GBR enables an increase in bone volume to facilitate optimal installation of dental implants. A systematic review indicated that the survival rate of implants placed in sites treated by GBR is similar to implants placed in native bone [24]. Another systematic review concluded that horizontal bone augmentation resulted in similar implant survival rates between augmented sites (91.7–100%) and pristine sites (93.2–100%) [25]. Although available data are limited, vertical augmentation using the GBR technique has been successfully performed, and clinical and histological data support its use.

Case 8

Ridge Split and Expansion

CASE STORY

A 65-year-old woman was referred for implant placement in the maxillary left side with a chief complaint of "I would like to fix my missing teeth." Teeth #11 through #14 had been extracted 3 years before and the patient was not wearing any denture (Figures 1 and 2). Mandibular posterior sextants were restored with implant-supported crowns. The patient claims to brush her teeth two or three times daily; she flosses once a day, but she does not use any mouth rinse.

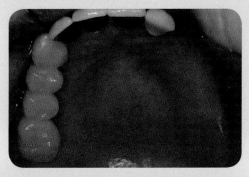

Figure 1: Occlusal view of the maxillary arch.

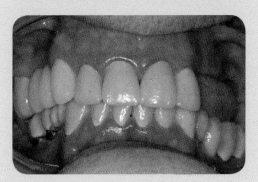

Figure 2: Preoperative occlusal view.

LEARNING GOALS AND OBJECTIVES

- To understand the indications and contraindications of the ridge split technique
- To understand the sequence of the ridge split technique
- To understand the limitations and potential complications of this technique

Medical History

The patient is prehypertensive and allergic to penicillin. She also has rheumatoid arthritis and her medications include methotrexate, Celebrex, and adalimumab.

Review of Systems

- Vital signs
  - Blood pressure: 124/78 mmHg
  - Pulse rate: 81 beats/min (regular)

Social History

The patient drinks four or five glasses of wine per week and she denies a history of smoking.

Extraoral Examination

There are no significant findings. There are no masses or swelling, and the temporomandibular joint is within normal limits.

Intraoral Examination

- There is no lymphadenopathy and an oral cancer screening is negative.
- The band of attached gingiva is adequate and stippling is present around teeth.
- Probing depths around implant sites were >4 mm (Figure 3).

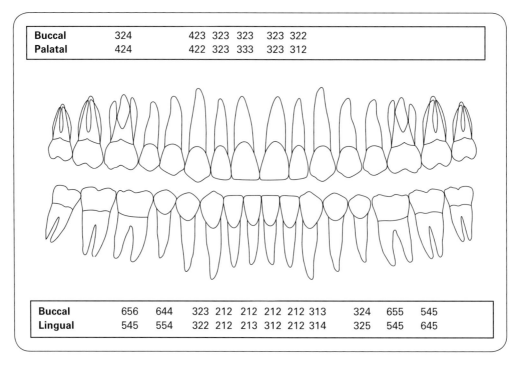

| Buccal | 324 | | 423 | 323 | 323 | | 323 | 322 |
| Palatal | 424 | | 422 | 323 | 333 | | 323 | 312 |

| Buccal | 656 | 644 | 323 | 212 | 212 | 212 | 212 | 313 | | 324 | 655 | 545 |
| Lingual | 545 | 554 | 322 | 212 | 213 | 312 | 212 | 314 | | 325 | 545 | 645 |

Figure 3: Probing pocket depth measurements.

- Tooth-implant splinted restorations were present in the mandibular posterior sextant.
- A hard tissue and soft tissue examination was completed.

Occlusion

The patient presents with a normal molar relationship on the right side and there are no interferences in excursive movements.

Radiographic Examination

An examination of a panoramic radiograph revealed bone loss of edentulous area in maxillary left side (Figure 4). Bone loss around mandibular dental implants was also observed. A computed tomographic (CT)

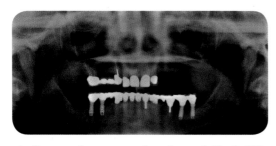

Figure 4: Preoperative panoramic radiograph. Teeth #11 through #14 were extracted 3 years ago. Mandibular posterior sextants are restored with implant-supported crowns.

image (Figure 5) revealed adequate bone height for implant placement, but a narrow ridge of 3–4 mm at the crest. The CT scan also revealed a posterior pneumatized maxillary sinus.

Diagnosis

The patient has partial edentulism and is diagnosed as ADA type II due to slight periodontitis.

Treatment Plan

The treatment plan for this patient includes an initial phase of scaling with polishing with oral hygiene instructions and ridge split with implant placement in the maxillary left side.

Treatment

After the initial consult and the diagnostic phase, the patient received initial therapy of scaling and polishing. The patient was able to maintain good oral hygiene in follow-up visits. Study models of maxillary and mandibular arch were fabricated. Since the patient wanted to avoid a sinus elevation procedure, it was decided not to place an implant in the area of tooth #14. Therefore, three implants were planned for the edentulous area of #11 through #13.

At the time of the surgery, local infiltrative anesthesia was administered (lidocaine 2%,

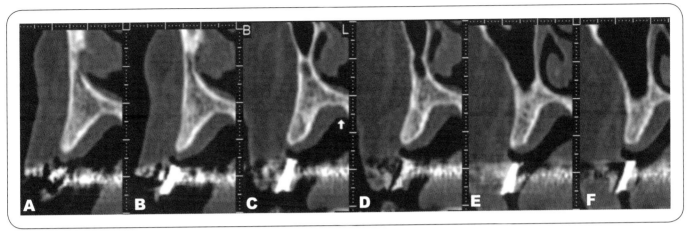

Figure 5: Preoperative CT examination of sites for implant placement. Cross-sectional images of (A, B) #11 area, (C, D) #12 area, and (E, F) #13 area.

epinephrine 1 : 100,000). A full-thickness mucoperiosteal flap was raised, confirming the presence of a narrow crest ridge previously observed in the CT scan. The initial osteotomy was performed on midcrestal bone using a #15 scalpel. Chisels of increasing width and a mallet were used to further enlarge the osteotomy 3 mm shorter than the final length of the implants to be placed (Figures 6 and 7).

Approximately 2–3 mm of expansion was achieved without performing vertical incisions in the bone (Figure 8). To prepare the osteotomy site for implant placement, sequential surgical burs according to standard implant placement protocol were used up to the final length of implants (10 mm) (Figure 9). Implants presented initial primary stability, the cover screws were placed, and the implants submerged for a healing

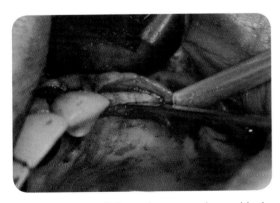

Figure 6: Initial ridge splitting using narrow bone chisel.

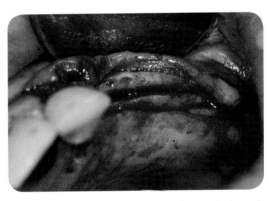

Figure 8: Ridge expansion of 2–3 mm of buccal plate after splitting the ridge with chisel.

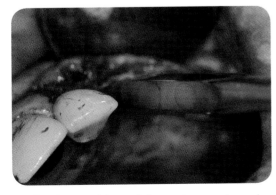

Figure 7: Continuous ridge splitting and expansion using wider bone chisel.

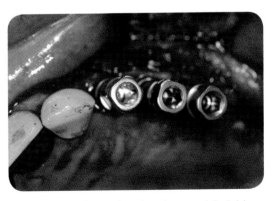

Figure 9: Dental implants placed at the expanded ridge.

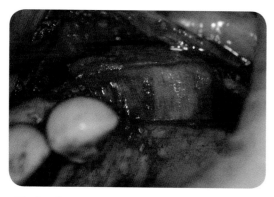

Figure 10: Gap between expanded cortical plates was grafted with particulate bone and covered with resorbable membrane.

period of 6 months. The widened space between cortical plates was filled with a mix of bovine anorganic bone filler, Bio-Oss, and demineralized freeze-dried bone allograft and covered with a bioresorbable collagen membrane (Bio-Guide) (Figure 10). The tissue was approximated and the patient was instructed not to wear any denture or place pressure on the healing site.

Second-stage surgery was performed 6 months later, healing abutments were placed, and the soft tissue allowed to heal for an additional 5 weeks (Figure 11). Splinted porcelain-fused-to-metal crowns supported by custom gold abutments then were delivered (Figure 12).

Discussion

The split ridge technique results in immediate expansion of the ridge, allowing simultaneous placement of implants in a narrow crestal ridge [1,2]. Chiapasco et al. evaluated the success of different surgical techniques

for ridge reconstruction and success rates of implants placed in the augmented areas [3]. The surgical success of split ridge and the implant survival rates were as high as guided bone regeneration and onlay graft procedure with the advantage of a shorter treatment time.

Several authors have suggested the use of a partial-thickness flap to help immobilize the displaced buccal cortical plate [4–6]. In the present case, the use of a full-thickness flap helped to avoid excessive bleeding, resulting in better visualization of the operating site and better handling of the surgical steps. In case of thin connective tissue, the partial-thickness flap procedure becomes extremely difficult and the remaining tissue over the alveolar bone is too thin to protect the bone adequately. In case of buccal plate fracture, the mobile plate may be retained with bone fixation screws [7]. Finally, when the primary stability of the implants is compromised, implants are placed only after the healing period of the augmented site.

In the maxilla, the osteotomy of the crest may be achieved with chisels and without the assistance of surgical burs. A mallet may be used to expand the plates without vertical osteotomy. The split ridge technique to expand a mandibular ridge may involve additional steps compared with the expansion of a maxillary ridge. In the mandible, the initial osteotomy is achieved using a surgical carbide bur on the alveolar crest and two vertical osteotomies. Additionally, an apical osteotomy connecting both verticals with a round bur allows the expansion and minimizes any chance of bone fracture. Instead of a mallet, hand motion is used with the chisels, resulting in slow bone expansion. To separate the ridge gently, Chiapasco et al. reported 45 cases using a wedge-type device with two surgical steel arms hinged apically and a

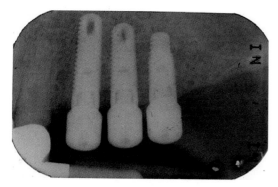

Figure 11: Periapical radiographic examination at uncovering phase 6 months after the implant placement.

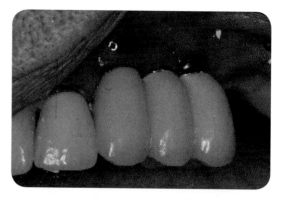

Figure 12: Final restoration with porcelain-fused-to-metal crowns.

transversal screw, which allows a progressive activation of the device [3]. Alternatively, the ridge may be split by using modulated-frequency piezoelectric energy scalpels [8].

Each case needs to be carefully assessed before considering the split ridge technique with simultaneous implant placement. Anatomical limitations such as

maxillary labial concavities may jeopardize ideal implant placement, and dense cortical plate may result in buccal wall fracture [9].

The correct indication associated with careful clinical maneuver of the ridge splitting technique allows predictable placement of implants even in narrow alveolar ridges.

Self-Study Questions

(Answers located at the end of the case)

A. What are the advantages of the split ridge technique?

B. What are the limitations of the split ridge technique?

C. What are the potential complications of the split ridge technique?

References

1. Simion M, Baldoni M, Zaffe D. Jawbone enlargement using immediate implant placement associated with a split-crest technique and guided tissue regeneration. Int J Periodontics Restorative Dent 1992;12:463–473.
2. Summers RB. The osteotome technique: part 2 – the ridge expansion osteotomy (REO) procedure. Compend Contin Educ Dent 1994;15:422–426.
3. Chiapasco M, Zaniboni M, Boisco M. Augmentation procedures for the rehabilitation of deficient edentulous ridges with oral implants. Clin Oral Implant Res 2006;17:136–159.
4. Scipioni A, Bruschi GB, Calesini G. The edentulous ridge expansion technique: a five-year study. Int J Periodontics Restorative Dent 1994;14:451–459.
5. Guirado JL, Yuguero MR, Carrión del Valle MJ, Zamora GP. A maxillary ridge-splitting technique followed by immediate placement of implants: a case report. Implant Dent 2005;14:14–20.
6. Ferrigno N, Laureti M. Surgical advantages with ITI TE implants placement in conjunction with split crest

technique. 18-month results of an ongoing prospective study. Clin Oral Implant Res 2005;16:147–155.
7. Basa S, Varol A, Turker N. Alternative bone expansion technique for immediate placement of implants in the edentulous posterior mandibular ridge: a clinical report. Int J Oral Maxillofac Implants 2004;19:554–558.
8. Vercellotii T. Piezoelectric surgery in implantology: a case report – a new piezoelectric ridge expansion technique. Int J Periodontics Restorative Dent 2000;20:358–365.
9. Bravi F, Bruschi GB, Ferrini A. A 10-year multicenter retrospective clinical study of 1,715 implants placed with edentulous ridge expansion technique. Int J Periodontics Restorative Dent 2007;27:557–565.
10. Koo S, Dibart S, Weber HP. Ridge-splitting technique with simultaneous implant placement. Compend Contin Educ Dent 2008;29:106–110.
11. Li J, Wang HL. Common implant-related advanced bone grafting complications: classification, etiology and management. Implant Dent 2008;17:389–401.

Answers to Self-Study Questions

A. This approach allows simultaneous placement of an implant even in atrophic ridges by creating self-space-making defects, and implant stabilization is achieved by placing implants at the most apical nonfractured portion of the jaw [1,10]. Therefore, overall treatment time may be shortened. Since this technique does not require a donor site, morbidity related to a second donor site is eliminated.

B. Adequate bone height should be available because the splitting of the crest does not increase bone volume vertically. A ridge with less than of 3 mm of width may not be indicated for this procedure since a minimum of 3 mm of bone width is desired to insert instruments between cortical plates for splitting and expansion. This technique is not indicated when the alveolar ridge is overangulated, especially in the maxillary anterior areas, which may compromise the esthetic outcome. Also, when a single site is planned, this technique is difficult to perform due to limited space, especially in mandible.

C. The major potential complication is fracture of the buccal plate [7]. This is more prone to occur in mandibular cases due to the thickness of cortical bone. Modifications of the conventional split technique should be considered, such as vertical and apical osteotomies. In case of fracture, bone fixation screws can be used to stabilize the buccal plate. Since this technique requires augmentation with particulate bone and biological membranes, complications related to guided bone regeneration may also occur [11]:
• hemorrhage;
• infection (fistula and abscess);
• prolonged pain;
• incision line opening an early exposure of membrane;
• flap sloughing.

6

Sinus Site Preparation

Clinical Cases in Implant Dentistry, First Edition. Edited by Nadeem Karimbux and Hans-Peter Weber.
© 2017 John Wiley & Sons, Inc. Published 2017 by John Wiley & Sons, Inc.

Case 1

Lateral Window Technique

LEARNING GOALS AND OBJECTIVES

■ To understand the principles of the lateral window technique for sinus augmentation
■ To learn important anatomic landmarks associated with the lateral window technique
■ To learn the basic surgical steps for the lateral window technique
■ To identify the proper case selection for the lateral window approach
■ To become familiar with common intra- and postoperative complications associated with the lateral window technique and how to manage them

Medical History

The patient had a history of hypertension, hypercholesterolemia and type II diabetes, all of which were well controlled with medications: lisinopril (20 mg QD), simvastatin (80 mg QD), and metformin (500 mg BID) respectively. His latest HbA1c reading was 6.7. He had no history of sinusitis. The patient reported no allergies to any medications and foods.

Review of Systems

- Vital signs
  - Blood pressure: 126/67 mmHg
  - Pulse rate: 64 beats/min
  - Respiration: 14 breaths/min

Social History

According to the patient, he had no history of smoking. He was a social drinker who drank alcohol occasionally. The patient is married with a son and two daughters. The patient was punctual and very motivated for the treatment.

Extraoral Examination

No significant findings were present. The extraoral soft tissue, temporomandibular joint, lymph node, and muscles were within normal limits.

Intraoral Examination

- Oral cancer screening was negative.
- Intraoral soft tissue examinations, including tongue and floor of the mouth, were within normal limits.
- Existing teeth were #5–#12, #21–#28.
- Periodontal examination revealed full mouth probing depths in the range of 1–3 mm (Figure 1). Bleeding on probing was not noted.
- There was no caries, but staining was present on all teeth.

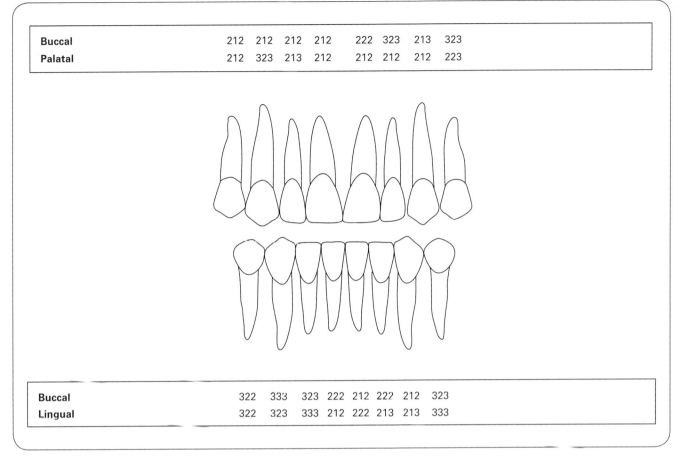

Buccal	212	212	212	212		222	323	213	323	
Palatal	212	323	213	212		212	212	212	223	

Buccal	322	333	323	222	212	222	212	323	
Lingual	322	323	333	212	222	213	213	333	

Figure 1: Probing pocket depth measurements during the initial visit.

- Evaluation of the residual ridge over #18 and #19 and #29 and #30 indicated successful augmentation after GBR without complications.
- The patient had a single implant restoration on #11.
- Cervical composite restorations on #5, #6, #12, and #21 were evident.
- Generalized occlusal attrition was present.
- Generalized 1–2 mm facial gingival recession.
- The patient's oral hygiene was good (Figure 2).

Occlusion
- There were no occlusal discrepancies or interferences.
- Overjet: 8 mm
- Overbite: 6 mm

Radiographic Examination
A full mouth radiographic series and a panoramic radiograph were obtained (Figure 3). There was generalized moderate horizontal bone loss.

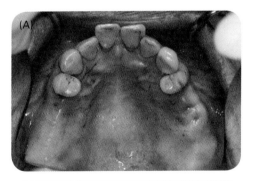
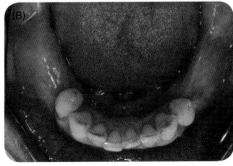

Figure 2: Preoperative occlusal view: (A) maxilla; (B) mandible.

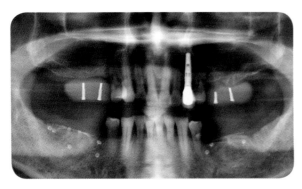

Figure 3: Preoperative presentation panoramic radiograph.

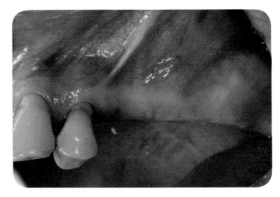

Figure 4: Preoperative presentation (facial view).

Pneumatization of the maxillary sinus was noted on both right and left sinuses. The alveolar bone height from the crest to the floor of the sinus in the implant locations (#3, #4, #13, #14) ranged from 3 to 5 mm. A single implant restoration on #11 and cervical composite restorations on #5, #6, #12, and #21 were evident. The sites treated with GBR using nonresobable membrane and tacks were evident bilaterally on the posterior mandible.

Diagnosis

American Academy of Periodontology diagnosis of generalized moderate chronic periodontitis with mucogingival deformities and conditions around teeth (facial gingival recession) was made. Also, the diagnosis of pneumatization of the maxillary sinus (right and left) was given.

Treatment Plan

The treatment plan for the patient included initial periodontal therapy: oral hygiene instructions, oral prophylaxis, and stain removal. After reevaluation of initial therapy, maxillary sinus augmentation procedures with the lateral window technique in the right and left posterior regions were planned. After 6 months of adequate healing time, implants were placed at #3, #4, #13, and #14. For the augmented sites in the posterior mandible, implants were placed at #19, #20, #29, and #30 following removal of the nonresorbable membrane 6–7 months after GBR. All implants (#3, #4, #13, #14, #19, #20, #29, #30) were restored with implant-supported fixed restorations after the adequate time for osseointegration (3–5 months).

Treatment

After periodontal therapy, the patient presented for maxillary left sinus augmentation with lateral window technique (Figure 4).

Local anesthetics were used for infiltration over the surgical site to obtain profound anesthesia. A horizontal midcrestal incision using a #15 blade was made on the distal surface of #12 and extended distally and diverged facially as an oblique incision. One vertical incision was made at the #12 mesiobuccal line angle and extended beyond the mucogingival junction. A full-thickness flap was reflected using a periosteal elevator to expose bone (Figure 5).

The design of a bony window was outlined and the osteotomy was performed using a round diamond bur. The coronal horizontal outline of the window was made 3 mm from the floor of the sinus. Subsequently, the mesial vertical incision was made following the slope of the anterior wall. The line was connected to make a trapezoidal/ovoid shape with a height of 7–9 mm. After reaching the Schneiderian membrane, a piezosurgery tip was inserted into the frame of the window to avoid perforation of the membrane during initial separation of the bony window (Figure 6). The Schneiderian membrane was then carefully elevated using a membrane elevator, starting from the apical aspect followed by the mesial and distal aspects

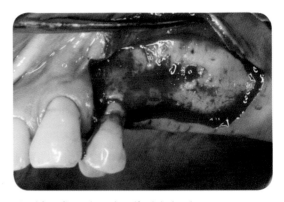

Figure 5: After flap elevation (facial view).

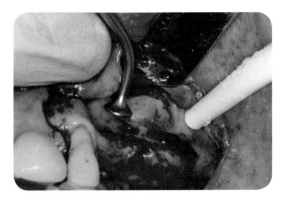

Figure 6 Lateral window (facial view).

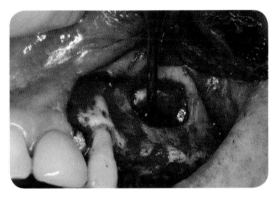

Figure 7: Elevation of the Schneiderian membrane (facial view).

(Figure 7). Xenograft (deproteinized bovine bone mineral, DBBM) (4 cm^3) was saturated in sterilized 0.9% normal saline. The bone grafts were filled and packed in the sinus cavity (Figure 8). A collagen membrane was trimmed and shaped to cover approximately 2–3 mm beyond the border of the window (Figure 9). The flap was closed with several simple interrupted sutures. A postoperative panoramic radiograph indicated a successful augmentation of the left maxillary sinus (Figure 10). Sutures were removed 2 weeks after surgery. Postoperative complications were not observed during

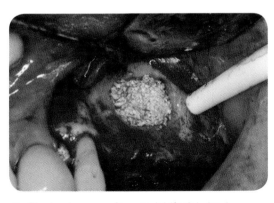

Figure 8: Placing bone graft material (facial view).

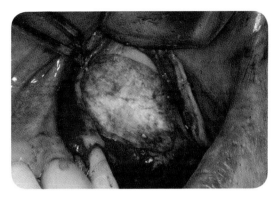

Figure 9: Placement of a membrane over the window (facial view).

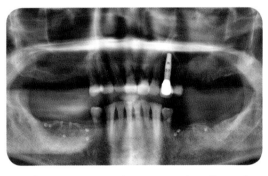

Figure 10: Post-op presentation panoramic radiograph following lateral window.

the healing time. Implants on #13 and #14 were placed 6 months postoperatively with good primary stability and restored 5 months after placement (Figure 11).

Maxillary right sinus augmentation with the lateral window technique was performed in the same manner as the left side. It was followed by implant surgery on #3 and #4 after a 6-month healing period.

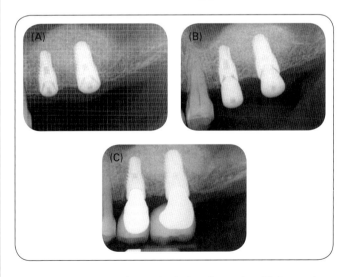

Figure 11: Postoperative periapical radiographs: (A) 3 months postimplant surgery; (B) 5 months postimplant surgery; (C) 2.5 years after prosthetic rehabilitation.

Discussion

Sinus augmentation with the lateral window technique has been studied extensively and considered to be a highly predictable bone augmentation procedure for increasing alveolar bone height in maxillary posterior regions to allow oral rehabilitation with dental implants in an atrophic maxilla. In this case, an atrophic maxilla with pneumatization of the left and right maxillary sinus was noted during the initial implant treatment planning phase. The alveolar bone height from the crest of the ridge to the floor of the sinus was 3–5 mm in the proposed implant locations, as indicated by a surgical stent in a preoperative panoramic radiograph. Maxillary sinus augmentation with the lateral window technique was selected to increase the alveolar bone height to allow for properly sized dental implants. The augmentation of 7–10 mm ridge height was planned prior to the implant placement.

The facial oblique incision was designed as a continuation of a midcrestal incision to have good vision and access to the bone that facilitated the procedure. The location and shape of the window were designed based on the anatomy of the maxillary sinus from the preoperative panoramic radiograph. The incision of the window was made 3 mm from the floor of the sinus and the sloping anterior wall to get good access during the membrane elevation (Figure 12). Perforation of Schneiderian membrane is the most frequent surgical complication of the lateral window technique. Caution should be taken not to perforate the membrane accidentally, but to keep the membrane intact. Perforation often occurs during osteotomy with burs or manual sinus elevators. A special piezoelectric tip was used in this case to reduce the risk of perforation during the initial membrane elevation. A sinus elevator is used to detach the membrane along the floor of the sinus, followed by the anterior and medial walls. The elevator must be on bone surface at all times to avoid inadvertent perforation of the membrane. Additionally, the angulation of the elevator must be changed during the elevation as dictated by the anatomy.

Particulate grafts are commonly used for this procedure; xenograft (deproteinized bovine bone mineral) was used in this case. The graft material was packed inside the sinus cavity without excessive pressure to avoid membrane perforation.

The patient's systemic factors are to be reviewed carefully before the sinus augmentation procedure because the presence of a systemic or preexisting sinus disease can affect the development of postoperative complications, resulting in a compromised surgical outcome. The patient reported no history of past sinusitis, and his diabetic condition and hypertension were well controlled. Also, the absence of periodontal disease or endodontic problems in the patient was confirmed prior to the sinus augmentation procedure to avoid postoperative infection. The patient was cooperative and his oral hygiene was good throughout the treatment, which is one of the most important factors to ensure a successful outcome.

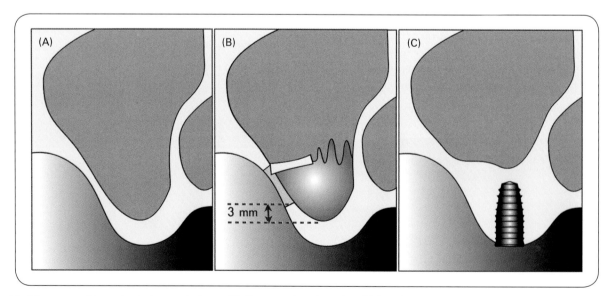

Figure 12: Diagrams of lateral window technique. (A) Preoperative view. Insufficient bone height to place a dental implant. (B) The coronal horizontal outline of the window is made 3 mm from the floor of sinus. (C) After healing period, an implant is placed.

Self-Study Questions

(Answers located at the end of the case)

A. What is sinus augmentation?

B. What are the techniques available for sinus augmentation?

C. What are the indications and contraindications for the lateral window approach?

D. What are the basic surgical steps when performing the lateral window technique?

E. What are the anatomical structures to consider before performing the lateral window technique?

F. What are the commonly used graft materials for the lateral window technique?

G. Is it possible to place implants simultaneously with sinus augmentation?

H. What is the success rate of the implants placed in sites where the lateral window technique was performed?

I. How does one assess the success of the sinus augmentation procedure?

J. What are the prescriptions usually recommended after sinus augmentation with the lateral window approach?

K. What are the common intraoperative complications during the lateral window sinus augmentation and how are they managed?

L. What are the common postoperative complications after lateral window sinus augmentation?

References

1. Tatum Jr H. Maxillary and sinus implant reconstructions. Dent Clin North Am 1986;30(2):207–229.
2. Stern A, Green J. Sinus lift procedures: an overview of current techniques. Dent Clin North Am 2012;56(1):219–233.
3. Boyne PJ, James RA. Grafting of the maxillary sinus floor with autogenous marrow and bone. J Oral Surg 1980;38(8):613–616.
4. Summers RB. A new concept in maxillary implant surgery: the osteotome technique. Compendium 1994;15(2):152, 154–156, 158
5. Davarpanah M, Martinez H, Tecucianu JF, et al. The modified osteotome technique. Int J Periodontics Restorative Dent 2001;21(6):599–607.
6. Garg AK. Augmentation grafting of the maxillary sinus for placement of dental implants: anatomy, physiology, and procedures. Implant Dent 1999;8(1):36–46.
7. Toscano NJ, Holtzclaw D, Rosen PS. The effect of piezoelectric use on open sinus lift perforation: a retrospective evaluation of 56 consecutively treated cases from private practices. J Periodontol 2010;81(1):167–171.
8. Chanavaz M. Maxillary sinus: anatomy, physiology, surgery, and bone grafting related to implantology – eleven years of surgical experience (1979–1990). J Oral Implantol 1990;16(3):199–209.
9. Harris D, Horner K, Gröndahl K, et al. E.A.O. guidelines for the use of diagnostic imaging in implant dentistry 2011. A consensus workshop organized by the European Association for Osseointegration at the Medical University of Warsaw. Clin Oral Implants Res 2012;23(11):1243–1253.
10. Jensen OT, Shulman LB, Block MS, Iacono VJ. Report of the sinus consensus conference of 1996. Int J Oral Maxillofac Implants 1998;13(Suppl):11–45.
11. Chanavaz M. Sinus graft procedures and implant dentistry: a review of 21 years of surgical experience (1979–2000) Implant Dent 2000;9(3):197–206.
12. Tarnow DP, Wallace SS, Froum SJ, et al. Histologic and clinical comparison of bilateral sinus floor elevations with and without barrier membrane placement in 12 patients: Part 3 of an ongoing prospective study. Int J Periodontics Restorative Dent 2000;20(2):117–125.
13. Wallace SS, Froum SJ. Effect of maxillary sinus augmentation on the survival of endosseous dental implants. A systematic review. Ann Periodontol 2003;8(1):328–343.
14. Del Fabbro M, Testori T, Francetti L, Weinstein R. Systematic review of survival rates for implants placed in the grafted maxillary sinus. Int J Periodontics Restorative Dent 2004;24(6):565–577.
15. Hatano N, Shimizu Y, Ooya K. A clinical long-term radiographic evaluation of graft height changes after maxillary sinus floor augmentation with a 2:1 autogenous bone/xenograft mixture and simultaneous placement of dental implants. Clin Oral Implants Res 2004;15(3):339–345.

16. Froum SJ, Tarnow DP, Wallace SS, et al. Sinus
    floor elevation using anorganic bovine bone matrix
    (OsteoGraf/N) with and without autogenous bone: a
    clinical, histologic, radiographic, and histomorphometric
    analysis – part 2 of an ongoing prospective study. Int J
    Periodontics Restorative Dent 1998;18(6):528–543.
17. Batal, H. Norris O. Lateral antrostomy technique
    for maxillary sinus augmentation. Implants
    2013;(1):12–20.
18. Tan WC, Lang NP, Zwahlen M, Pjetursson BE. A
    systematic review of the success of sinus floor elevation
    and survival of implants inserted in combination with
    sinus floor elevation. Part II: transalveolar technique.
    J Clin Periodontol 2008;35(8 Suppl):241–254.
19. Peleg M, Garg AK, Mazor Z. Predictability of simultaneous
    implant placement in the severely atrophic posterior
    maxilla: a 9-year longitudinal experience study of 2132
    implants placed into 731 human sinus grafts. Int J Oral
    Maxillofac Implants 2006;21(1):94–102.
20. Esposito M, Grusovin MG, Loli V, et al. Does antibiotic
    prophylaxis at implant placement decrease early implant
    failures? A Cochrane systematic review. Eur J Oral
    Implantol 2010;3(2):101–110.
21. Misch CM. The pharmacologic management of
    maxillary sinus elevation surgery. J Oral Implantol
    1992;18(1):15–23.
22. Jensen J, Sindet-Pedersen S, Oliver AJ. Varying treatment
    strategies for reconstruction of maxillary atrophy with
    implants: results in 98 patients. J Oral Maxillofac Surg
    1994;52:210–216.
23. Timmenga NM, Raghoebar GM, Boering G, van
    Weissenbruch R. Maxillary sinus function after sinus lifts
    for the insertion of dental implants. J Oral Maxillofac Surg
    1997;55(9):936–939.
24. Misch CE. The maxillary sinus lift and sinus graft surgery.
    In: MischCE (ed.), Contemporary Implant Dentistry.
    Chicago, IL: Mosby; 1999, pp 469–495.
25. Pikos MA. Maxillary sinus membrane repair: report
    of a technique for large perforations. Implant Dent
    1999;8:29–34.
26. Van den Bergh JP, ten Bruggenkate CM, Disch FJ, Tuinzing
    DB. Anatomical aspects of sinus floor elevations. Clin Oral
    Implants Res 2000;11(3):256–265.
27. Pikos MA. Complications of maxillary sinus
    augmentation. In: The Sinus Bone Graft, vol. 9, 2nd edn.
    Hanover Park, IL: Quintessence; 2006, pp 103–125.
28. Proussaefs P, Lozada J, Kim J, Rohrer MD. Repair of the
    perforated sinus membrane with a resorbable collagen
    membrane: a human study. Int J Oral Maxillofac Implants
    2004;19(3):413–420.
29. Zijderveld SA, van den Bergh JP, Schulten EA, ten
    Bruggenkate CM. Anatomical and surgical findings
    and complications in 100 consecutive maxillary sinus
    floor elevation procedures. J Oral Maxillofac Surg
    2008;66(7):1426–1438.
30. Greenstein G, Cavallaro J, Romanos G, Tarnow D. Clinical
    recommendations for avoiding and managing surgical
    complications associated with implant dentistry: a review.
    J Periodontol 2008;79(8):1317–1329.
31. Hernández-Alfaro F, Torradeflot MM, Marti C. Prevalence
    and management of Schneiderian membrane perforations
    during sinus-lift procedures. Clin Oral Implants Res
    2007;19(1):91–98.
32. Proussaefs P, Lozada J. The "Loma Linda pouch": a
    technique for repairing the perforated sinus membrane.
    Int J Periodontics Restorative Dent 2003;23(6):593–597.
33. Fuggazzoto PA, Vlassis J. A simplified classification
    and repair system for sinus membrane perforations.
    J Periodontol 2003;74(10):1534–1541.
34. Pjetursson BE, Tan WC, Zwahlen M, Lang NP. A
    systematic review of the success of sinus floor
    elevation and survival of implants inserted in
    combination with sinus floor elevation. J Clin Periodontol
    2008;35(8 Suppl):216–240.
35. Testori T, Drago L, Wallace SS, et al. Prevention and
    treatment of postoperative infections after sinus elevation
    surgery: clinical consensus and recommendations. Int J
    Dent 2012;2012:365809.
36. Timmenga NM, Raghoebar GM, Liem RS, et al. Effects of
    maxillary sinus floor elevation surgery on maxillary sinus
    physiology. Eur J Oral Sci. 2003;111(3):189–197.
37. Froum SJ. Dental Implant Complications: Etiology,
    Prevention, and Treatment. Wiley-Blackwell; 2010.
38. Misch CE, Moore P. Steroids and the reduction of pain,
    edema and dysfunction in implant dentistry. Int J Oral
    Implantol 1989;6(1):27–31.
39. Galindo-Moreno P, Padial-Molina M, Sánchez-Fernández E,
    et al. Dental implant migration in grafted maxillary sinus.
    Implant Dent 2011;20(6):400–405.

Answers to Self-Study Questions

A. Sinus augmentation is a surgical procedure to provide additional bone height for placing properly sized dental implants in areas of inadequate bone volume in the edentulous posterior maxilla. This procedure involves elevating the Schneiderian membrane and placing bone graft material into the sinus cavity that will create adequate height for a dental implant [1,2].

B. There are two common techniques used for sinus augmentation: the lateral window technique and the internal sinus lift technique.
- *Lateral window technique.* This technique is also known as the external sinus lift technique. In this technique, the lateral wall of the sinus anterior to the zygomatic buttress will be accessed after full-thickness flap elevation. An osteotomy will then be created using a round diamond or carbide bur [3].
- *Internal sinus lift technique.* This technique is also referred to as the transalveolar technique. With this technique, the maxillary bone crest may be accessed with osteotomes of increasing diameter, in order to create a suitable implant site [4,5].

The main difference between these two techniques is the area of access for the elevation of the Schneiderian membrane. The choice of the approach, either lateral window technique or internal sinus lift technique, mainly depends on the vertical height of residual alveolar bone between the alveolar crest and the maxillary sinus floor and the quality of the bone.

C. The contraindications for lateral window technique are classified as medical and local factors.

Medical contraindications
- History of chemotherapy or radiotherapy of the head and neck area at the time of sinus floor elevation or in the preceding 6 months.
- Intravenous administration of bisphosphonate.
- Immunocompromised patients.
- Medical conditions affecting bone metabolism.
- Uncontrolled diabetes.
- Drug/alcohol abuse.
- Noncompliance or psychiatric conditions.

Local contraindications
The presence or history of sinus pathology, which includes acute sinusitis, allergic rhinitis, chronic recurrent sinusitis, scarred and hypofunctional mucosae, and local aggressive benign tumors and malignant tumors [6].

D.
- For local anesthesia, it is recommended to use local anesthetics that contain epinephrine if no medical contraindications are present, because a considerable amount of bleeding is expected during the procedure and the epinephrine will facilitate visibility.
- A midcrestal incision on the edentulous area and a vertical incision are the commonly used incision designs. A minimum of 5 mm distance is required from the bony window to the incision lines. Then, a full-thickness flap elevation will be performed using a periosteal elevator [3,5].
- The design of the bony window follows the outline of the maxillary sinus and the adjacent anatomical structures. Generally, there are two techniques to create a window: "trap-door technique" or "open-window technique." In the former technique, the bony window is lifted into the sinus cavity. Rotary instruments such as a diamond or carbide round bur are used under copious water irrigation (Figure 13) and the bony window can be lifted and left in the sinus cavity. In contrast, in the open-window technique the bony window will be removed by

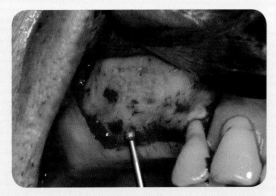

Figure 13: The use of a diamond round bur to design a window.

thinning of the bone. During the procedure, the bluish color of the Schneiderian membrane can be observed [2].

- When available, a piezoelectric device can be used either alone or together with rotary instruments to finalize the contour of the window and gently lift the bony window. Subsequently, the elevation of the Schneiderian membrane can be initiated using piezo tips and hand instruments [7].
- After completing the elevation of the Schneiderian membrane, it is important to confirm the absence of any perforation by using the nose-blowing test (Valsalva test). In the presence of a membrane perforation, the repair technique, depending on the size of the perforation, will be applied.
- Bone graft material will be packed gently into the sinus cavity and a bioabsorbable collagen membrane will be placed over the bony window.
- Before repositioning the flap with suturing, periosteal releasing incisions are often required to assure tension-free primary closure [2,6].

E. Although radiographic examination can be performed with a panoramic radiograph, there is a high distortion of the image and clear visualization of the anatomical structures may not be possible. The use of cone beam computed tomography (CBCT) is recommended to evaluate the anatomy of the maxillary sinus and adjacent vital structures (bone septa, size and pathology of the sinus, sinus compartments, bone height between the sinus floor and the crest of the ridge) prior to the procedure. CBCT provides information that helps clinicians to identify the location of the posterior superior alveolar branch of the maxillary artery, which may anastomose with the infraorbital artery in the lateral bony wall, the thickness of the Schneiderian membrane, the anatomy of the lateral and anterior wall, the presence and location of septa, ostium entrance, and the location of the infraorbital nerve. All of these factors impact the design of the bony window. For example, septae must be taken into consideration when designing the osteotomy and may complicate membrane reflection [8,9]. When a sinus pathology (infective rhinosinusitis, odontogenic/foreign body sinusitis, mucoceles, cysts and tumors) is suspected using these imaging techniques, the patient should be referred to an ear,

nose, and throat (ENT) specialist. These conditions must be diagnosed and addressed prior to the surgical procedure.

F. Many types of bone graft materials can be used for sinus augmentation. Autogenous bone is still considered to be the gold standard of grafting materials owing to the high content of bone morphogenic proteins (BMPs) and the capability of inducing cells to differentiate into bone cells from the surrounding tissues. However, clinical studies have shown successful outcomes with allografts, xenografts, and alloplasts [3,8,10–15]. The different characteristic of these grafting materials is that they provide slower resoprtion when compared with autogenous bone.

A study showed that when a small quantity of autogenous bone was added to xenograft, there was an increase in vital bone formation [16]. Evidence in the literature seems to suggest that the best grafting protocol includes a mixture of autogenous particulate bone and demineralized bovine bone mineral or demineralized freeze-dried bone allograft. The survival rate of rough-surface implants with this grafting protocol is approximately 96.8–99.8% [17].

Current evidence also suggests that there is a better outcome with particulate grafts than block grafts. Wallace and Froum reported an 80.40% success rate of rough-surface implants placed in block grafts compared with 94.83% for particulate bone grafts [13]. Additionally, recombinant human BMP-2 and -7 may improve the final outcome by increasing the amount of bone formed due to their osteoinductive properties [17] (Figure 14).

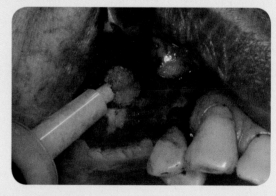

Figure 14: The use of graft material that contains BMPs and growth factors.

G. If the amount of residual bone height and bone quality provides an adequate primary stability for the dental implant, simultaneous implant placement is possible with sinus augmentation. It is referred to as a one-stage approach [6]. When there is insufficient bone height, it may be difficult to achieve primary stability of implants and a two-stage approach (staged approach) is required. As a general rule, a minimum of 3–5 mm height of the alveolar crest is necessary to provide implant primary stability, but the current evidence in the literature is controversial. The recommendations of the 1996 Sinus Consensus Conference are as follows. If the residual bone height is 7–9 mm, an osteotome technique is warranted and implants may be placed simultaneously [10] (Figure 15). If the residual bone height is 4–6 mm, the lateral window approach with delayed or simultaneous implant insertion is recommended. Finally, if the residual bone height is 1–3 mm, a lateral approach with grafting material and delayed implant positioning is the best treatment option.

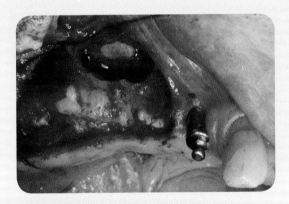

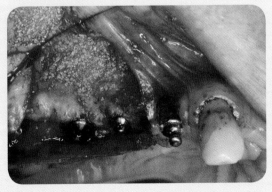

Figure 15: Simultaneous implant placement with the lateral window technique.

H. According to different meta-analyses available in the literature, the 3-year implant survival rate can range from 90% to 98%, based on implant level [13,18]. Many factors can affect the success of the implants placed in augmented sinuses; for example, the residual bone height before the procedure, the implant surface characteristics, and the long-term stability of the bone graft must also be considered. The 3-year survival rate for rough-surface implants (96.5%) seems to be higher than machined-surface implants, whose 3-year success rate is 81.4 % [17]. The residual bone height also seems to play a role: implant success rate with less than 5 mm residual bone height is approximately 85.7%, but when the residual bone height is more than 5 mm the rate is 96%. Many authors have analyzed the survival of implants in grafted sinuses, reporting very high success rates, ranging between 90% and 93% [7,14].

I. Several factors contribute to the success of the procedure, such as the amount of bone height achieved, no complications present during the surgical procedure, and no complications/adverse events after the surgery was performed. Because the goal of the surgery is to provide adequate height for a potential implant placement, the osseointegration of the implant placed in that particular site is the final outcome that will establish if the procedure is successful or not [10,19].

J. Sparse information is available regarding the prescriptions usually recommended, but a Cochrane systematic review indicated the use of antibiotics for this particular procedure – 2 g amoxicillin 1 h prior to the surgery or 1 g 1 h prior and qid for 2 days afterwards [20]. Misch recommends 500 mg amoxicillin 1 h prior to the procedure and 500 mg tid for the following 7–10 days after the procedure [21]. The antibiotic may also be mixed together with the grafting particles for a local effect. Owing to the risk of infection linked to sinus elevation, it is best to use Augmentin (amoxicillin with clavulanic acid), because the clavulanic acid component will destroy the beta-lactamic bacteria and ensure a greater efficacy of the antibiotic agent.

K. Common intraoperative complications are membrane perforation and excessive bleeding.

Perforation of the Schneiderian membrane

The perforation of the sinus membrane is the most common intraoperative complication in the lateral sinus lift procedure with reported rates ranging from 10 to 56% [16] (Figure 16). Evidence in the literature has shown that there is significantly less bone formation (14.58%) in the presence of a membrane perforation, compared with a nonperforated site (33.58%) [28].

- A very small perforation (<2 mm) may not require specific treatment and may resolve simply by membrane fold-over or coagulum formation. Some authors, however, still prefer the use of a resorbable collagen membrane to repair the laceration [29].
- Large perforations must be addressed with specific measures [30,31].
  - The perforated sinus membrane (≥2 mm) can be sealed and repaired with a resorbable collagen membrane.
  - The Loma Linda pouch technique: a large resorbable membrane is used to cover the entire internal aspect of the maxillary sinus, and its borders should extend beyond the osteotomy. A resorbable membrane is placed onto the lateral aspect to seal off the pouch and provide optimal protection of the graft particles [32]. Pins can be used to stabilize a resorbable membrane in the presence of perforation with this technique [33].

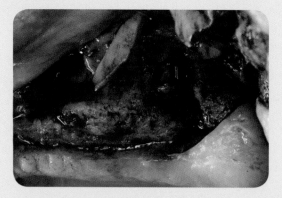

Figure 16: Schneiderian membrane perforation.

- Very large perforation: It may be best to abort the surgical procedure and reenter after 3–4 months to allow for the healing of the perforation.

Excessive bleeding

If excessive bleeding occurs during the procedure, direct pressure should be applied on the bleeding point. A localized vasoconstrictor may be administered. For example, leaving a gauze strip soaked in 2% xylocaine with 1:50,000 epinephrine in the sinus space can be used to control the bleeding and help with visualization. If the hemorrhage is intraosseous, bone wax may be used. If the bleeding point is identified, the vessel may be sutured proximal to the bleeding point. Electrocautery is also considered as a possible option [30,34].

Careful and adequate preoperative planning of the procedure will generally reduce the incidence of this type of complication. The use of CBCT will, for instance, help to correctly identify the vessels in the adjacent area so that they may be avoided throughout the procedure.

L. Major postoperative complications after a lateral window procedure are relatively uncommon. They include infection of grafted sinuses, postoperative maxillary sinusitis, pain, and wound dehiscence.

- *Infection of grafted sinuses.* A mean incidence of 2.9% was reported in a systematic review [34]. The risk of infection was observed more frequently when membrane perforation occurred surgically. The infection of the graft is usually noticed 3–7 days postoperatively. Sinus graft infection is a potentially dangerous event because the infection could potentially spread to other areas, such as the orbit or even the brain. The management of this complication is through antibiotic therapy. Testori et al. recommended a combination of Augmentin and metronidazole or levofloxacin [35]. In certain cases, drainage may be necessary, with antibiotic therapy, surgical debridement, or removal of the graft. For prevention of infections, prophylactic and postoperative antibiotics are recommended. Augmentin (amoxicillin/clavulanate) is the drug of choice. Combination of metronidazole and clarithromycin is recommended as an alternative for penicillin-allergic patients [35].

- *Postoperative maxillary sinusitis.* This event has also been reported with 1% incidence [29]. A study by Timmenga et al. revealed that postoperative sinusitis occurred in patients with septal deviation or oversized turbinates [36]. Mild sinusitis will respond to nasal decongestants such as oxymetazoline. If the etiology is a combination of inflammation and infection, antibiotics and anti-inflammatory therapy can be effective [37].
- *Excessive pain.* The dosage of analgesics may be increased. Ibuprofen 400–800 mg (tid or PRN) or acetaminophen with codeine #3 (q6h or PRN) are commonly prescribed [38].
- *Wound dehiscence.* This is also a rare complication (3%) [29]. It is typically associated with an incision that is too palatal, resulting in the reduction of blood supply to the flap.
- *Implant migration into sinus.* An incidence of 4% was reported [29]. Inadequate stability at implant placement or early loss of primary stability is considered to be the main etiologic factor. A case series addressing potential causes of this complication found that this may include excessive occlusal forces or premature implant insertion, lack of graft consolidation or premature graft resorption, or even be linked to sinus membrane perforation [39]. In fact, the implant may be pulled into the sinus through the perforation due to the negative intrasinus pressure.

Case 2

Internal Sinus Lift: Osteotome

CASE STORY

A 42-year-old Caucasian man who was referred by his general practitioner to our dental clinic for sinus lift and dental implant consultation. He has lost tooth #14 due to decay (Figure 1) and presents with a low sinus floor.

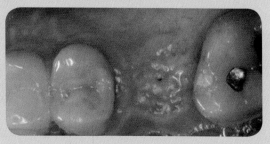

Figure 1: Clinical view of edentulous site #14 in which we can appreciate buccal bone loss.

LEARNING GOALS AND OBJECTIVES

- To understand the indications/contraindications for the crestal/internal approach by having the correct diagnostics tools
- To understand the advantages and disadvantages associated with this technique, and understand the protocol to lead to a successful sinus lift
- To understand the advantages/disadvantages of the osteotome technique
- To learn how to achieve good initial/mechanical stability when placing a dental implant simultaneously after performing sinus bone grafting surgery
- To manage chronic sinusitis before performing a sinus lift

Medical History

The patient is in good health and has regular medical examinations done. He presents with a history of chronic sinusitis.

Family History

Both parents are still alive and in good health condition.

Review of Systems

- Vital signs
  - Blood pressure: 150/90 mmHg and is ASA I
  - Pulse rate: 75 beats/min (regular in males)
- Height: 5'7" (1.70 m)
- Weight: 210 lbs (~95 kg)
- He does not have high cholesterol.
  The patient is not taking any medications that may interfere with the surgical procedure. Nor does he have any complications due to prolonged bleeding or easy bruising, endocrine abnormalities, or malignancy.

Social History

The patient does not drink alcohol, and neither does he smoke or take recreational drugs. These factors are an important aspect that we must consider when performing a dental implant placement, because either one may increase complications in our dental implants site causing an infection (peri-implantitis).

Extraoral Examination

The patient's overall general appearance is good. No skeletal and development discrepancies are observed.
The patient has no masses or swelling. No palpable lymphadenopathy was observed and the temporomandibular joint (TMJ) is within normal limits.

Intraoral Examination

Periodontal Examination

Gingiva color is generalized coral pink.

Consistency of the gingiva is firm and resilient; the generalized form is pyramidal, with knife-edge papilla, well adapted against teeth; however, localized areas of blunted papilla are present. The probing depths are relatively shallow (Figure 2).

- No mobility is present.
- Fremitus: none noted.
- The soft tissues of the mouth, including the tongue, appear to be normal.
- The gingival examination reveals moderate gingivitis.
- Color, shape, and form of patient's teeth are within normal limits.
- Oral hygiene: fair.
- Soft tissue examination is done in which there is no clinical sign of exostoses (tori or mandibular tori).

The edentulous ridge in the maxillary upper left quadrant has slight deformities in the buccolingual dimension.

Prosthodontic Examination

- Diastemas: none.
- Restorative hopeless teeth: none.
- Midline deviation: within normal limits.
- Inter-arch space concerns: none.
- Dental appearance concerns: none.
- Unacceptable crown/root ratios: none.

Occlusion

Lack of upper left posterior support, unprotected occlusion and group function is noted.

- Angle's classification class 1.
- Lateral excursive guidance: group function.
- Anterior protrusive guidance: group function.

- Cross-bite: none.
- Overbite 2 mm and overjet 1 mm.

Temporomandibular Joint Disorders

- Bruxism: potential (recommendation to the patient is to wear a night guard.)
- Trauma from occlusion: none.
- Myalgias: none.
- Muscles of mastication (tenderness on palpation): within normal limits.
- Condyle/disc displacement with of without reduction (clicking): bilateral asymptomatic click.
- Capsulitis (pain upon pressure of TMJ): within normal limits.

Radiographic Examination

A panoramic radiograph shows thickening of the sinus membrane. Cross-sectional computed tomography (CT) shows a low and wide sinus floor which is <6 mm × >12 mm (Figure 3).

Good patency of the natural ostium of the maxillary sinus is observed. If the opening of the ostium is obliterated, sinusitis will most likely develop and result in symptoms such as "pressure in the sinus."

The CT scan shows that the sinus membrane is thickened, which is indicative of asymptomatic chronic sinusitis (Figure 3).

When taking the CT scan we must consider:

- patency of natural ostium
- thickness of Schneiderian membrane
- absence of mucocele presence
- absence of polyp presence
- location of intraosseous anastomosis of PSA artery
- thickness of lateral wall, buccal, lingual anatomy/ dimension
- presence of septum.

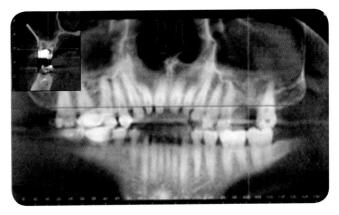

Figure 3: CT scan demonstrating a thickened sinus membrane (indicative of infection). Also of note is the bone height, patency of ostium, and the posterior superior alveolar artery.

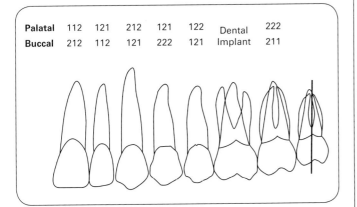

Palatal	112	121	212	121	122	Dental	222
Buccal	212	112	121	222	121	Implant	211

Figure 2: Probing depths.

Endodontic Examination

There are no relevant clinical and radiographic findings.

Treatment

A complete treatment plan has been presented to the patient, which he has agreed on. It will consist of:
1. Intravenous sedation, because the patient expresses dental fear.
2. Crestal/internal approach to the sinus floor.
3. Osteotome technique.
4. Crestal sinus lift.
5. Sinus bone grafting.
6. Placement of dental implant.

Preoperative Consultation

The patient's medical history was reviewed. Proper consent forms associated with the procedure were agreed upon and signed by the doctor and patient.

Emergency phase: immediate treatment is not needed.

Systemic phase: owing to history of chronic sinusitis, we consulted his doctor for medical clearance. We also placed the patient on Augmentin 875 mg bid 1 week prior to the surgery.

Sinus Elevation Procedure

A superior alveolar nerve block, greater palatine nerve block, and local infiltrations were utilized with two carpules of Septocaine 4% with epinephrine 1 : 100,000.

If we were to make this incision again we would make a midcrestal flap (see Figure 4) to avoid having the risk of tissue necrosis. Whenever, the flap is too narrow, there is risk of tissue necrosis during healing. In this case we will use osteotomes in order to achieve a sinus lift.

A full-thickness papilla sparing palatal flap (see Figure 5) was elevated in the maxillary upper left posterior quadrant to expose the crestal ridge of #14 site.

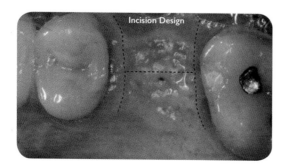

Figure 4: Incision design, which is an envelope flap.

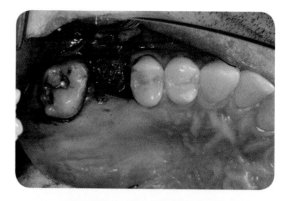

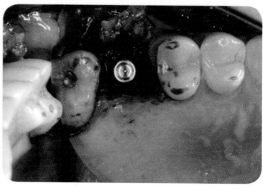

Figure 5: Incision and dental implant position, in which we recommend a minimum of 2 mm or more of autogenous bone around the dental implant.

In order to perform a sinus lift using the osteotomes we recommend following these steps:
1. A crestal incision must be made (for optimum blood supply to flaps), and full-thickness flap elevation must be done.
2. Perform osteotomy greater than 3.5 mm in diameter. In the authors' clinical opinion, a larger size of osteotome is less likely to perforate the membrane.
3. Stop osteotomy 1 mm short of the sinus floor (Figure 6). Multiple radiographs may be taken to ensure that osteotomy is 1 mm short of the sinus floor.
4. Have the osteotome to infracture the sinus floor (Figure 7). This force should be gentle, because we may cause benign positional vertigo. If the patient has anterior teeth, an assistant or operator should hold the maxillary incisor to distribute forces away from the ear canal.
5. Pack bone graft into the osteotome using the osteotime. Typically it requires 1 cm³ of allograft to elevate 4–5 mm of sinus.

Placement of a 4.5 mm × 10 mm dental implant (EZ PLUS) was made with simultaneous placement of healing abutment 603, and suturing was done with 5-0 silk (Figure 8).

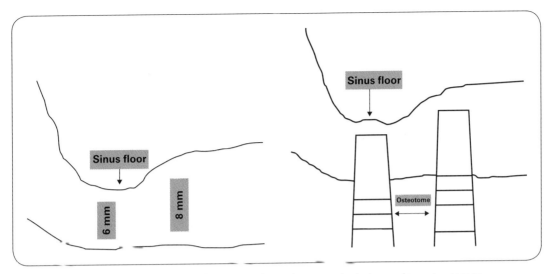

Figure 6: Demonstration of adequate bone height in order to form the crestal window using osteotomes.

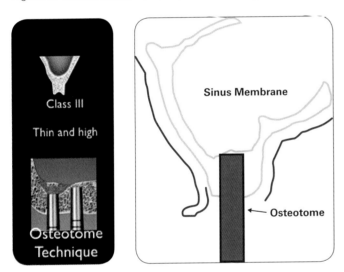

Figure 7: Demonstration of osteotome use to lift the sinus membrane.

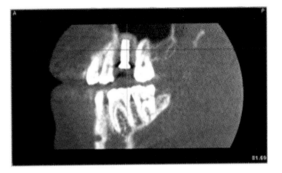

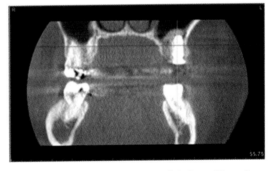

Figure 8: CT scan showing successful sinus lift and good placement of bone graft.

Discussion

Most crestal approaches including this technique are considered a "blind technique." Therefore, visualization of the Schneiderian membrane is impossible with these crestal approaches [1–3]. In contrast, there is another technique called the "crestal window technique" – which was discussed in Chapter 7 in *Clinical Cases in Periodontics* [4] – in which we can create a crestal window and the membrane can be visualized (Figure 9), thus allowing manual elevation of the sinus membrane in a more controlled manner.

In this case, we have used Summer's osteotome technique to achieve sinus bone grafting. However, improper use of forceful use of a mallet can lead to benign positional vertigo, and it may lead to litigation

[1–3,5]. Owing to discomfort from using the mallet, we highly recommend intravenous sedation for this procedure, which will allow better management of pain and anxiety. The most common drug for moderate sedation is midazolam. Typically, 1–10 mg of Versed achieves excellent sedation and amnesia; it should be administered before the induction of anesthesia. The contraindications we must consider are: hypersensitivity to benzodiazepines, and severe respiratory failure or acute respiratory depression. The initial dose recommended is as little as 1 mg, but we must not exceed 10 mg for a healthy adult. But lower doses must

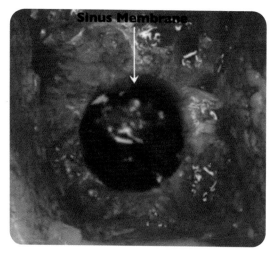

Figure 9: Schneiderian membrane can be observed by utilizing the crestal window sinus grafting technique.

be considered for patients >60 years and debilitated patients. Furthermore, we recommend that the clinician must warn their patient prior to receiving midazolam not to drive a vehicle or operate machinery until they have completely recovered. The patient should be discharged with a family member as there will be an amnesic effect.

Owing to the amnesic property of Versed, the patient did not remember any negative experiences when we interviewed them 1 week later. If intravenous sedation

is not available, we recommend using the crestal window technique with trephine burs, as this technique does not require the use of any mallet. This enhances both the patient's comfort and the clinician's confidence [5–7].

One of the main limitations of conventional crestal approaches (osteotome) is that they require a minimum bone height of 5 mm. In contrast, the crestal window technique is easier if the initial bone height is <5 mm [1–3,6]. The reason why less bone height is easier is due to increased visibility and access inside the sinus. This is why we recommend the crestal window technique in these kinds of cases, because of the morbidity and the "blind" nature of this technique associated with the osteotome technique.

Another important factor when performing implant surgery is to leave a sufficient amount of attached gingival around the dental implant [1–3]. A minimum of 2 mm is recommended [8]. We recommend use of the healing abutment (one-stage approach) to aid in gaining keratinized tissue. However, if we do not gain a good initial stability (<20 N cm), we recommend two-stage surgery to prevent the movement of the dental implant during the healing phase (4–6 months). At the same time, too much torque on a dental implant is not recommended. Too much torque can lead to pressure necrosis, because it may limit blood supply to the cortical bone.

Self-Study Questions

(Answers located at the end of the case)

A. What is the minimum bone height for a conventional crestal/internal approach?

B. Why do we recommend placing a healing abutment?

C. If we apply too much torque on our dental implant, what may happen?

D. What is a common side effect of improper use of the osteotome in this particular technique?

E. How much bone graft material is recommend to elevate the sinus membrane (4–5 mm) in the osteotome technique?

F. What is the measurement of the osteotomy in the osteotome technique?

References

1. Misch C. Maxillary sinus augmentation for endosteal implants: organized treatment plans. Int J.Oral Implantol 1987;4:49–58.
2. Summers R. The osteotome technique part 3 – less invasive methods of the elevation of the sinus floor. Compendium 1994;15:698–704.
3. Lee S, Lee GK, Park K, Han T. Redefining perioplastic surgery. J Implant Adv Clin Dent 2009;1(1):76–88.
4. Lee SS, Karimbux N. Sinus grafting: crestal. In: KarimbuxN (ed.), Clinical Cases in Periodontics. Chchester: Wiley Blackwell; 2012, pp 255–262.
5. Summers R. A new concept in maxillary implant surgery: the osteotome technique. Compendium 1994;15:152–158.
6. Tatum Jr H. Maxillary and sinus implant reconstruction. Dent Clin North Am 1986;30(2):207–229.
7. Boyne P, James R. Grafting of the maxillary sinus floor with autogenous marrow and bone. J Oral Surg 1980;38:613–616.
8. Schrott AR, Jimenez M, Hwang JW, et al. Five-year evaluation of the influence of keratinized mucosa on peri-implant soft-tissue health and stability around implants supporting full-arch mandibular fixed prostheses. Clin Oral Implants Res 2009;20:1170–1177.

Answers to Self-Study Questions

A. Minimum bone height of 5 mm.

B. To aid in gaining keratinized tissue in one-stage-surgery.

C. Pressure necrosis.

D. Benign positional vertigo.

E. 1 cm^3 of bone graft material.

F. Greater than 3.5 mm in diameter.

Case 3

Internal Sinus Lift: Other Techniques

CASE STORY

The patient is a 32-year-old female; she came to our dental clinic for consultation of dental implant treatment for tooth #3. She has had a dental implant and an implant crown on tooth #2, which was performed in a different clinic (Figures 1, 2, and 3).

Chief Complaint

"I have tooth sensitivity on the upper right side and extrusion of tooth #3."

History of Chief Complaint

- She thinks she has had root exposure for 2 years.
- She has had tooth sensitivity for a couple of months, but has not had time to restore due to work issues.

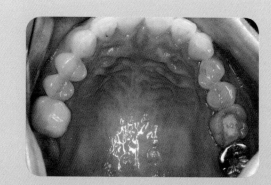

Figure 2: Maxilla (occlusal view). Note decay on #3.

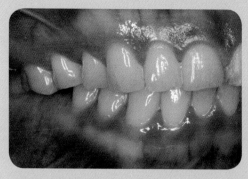

Figure 3: Buccal aspect of #3 and ridge overgrowth due to major guided bone regeneration treatment.

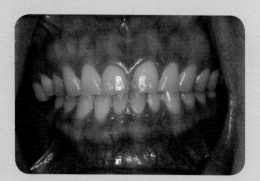

Figure 1: Maxilla (facial view).

LEARNING GOALS AND OBJECTIVES

- To know the different kinds of techniques that can be applied in order to achieve a successful sinus bone grafting
- To understand the indications/contraindications for the crestal approach and the diagnostic information needed to make this decision
- To understand the advantages and disadvantages of the crestal/internal approach, including the sequence of the treatment subprocedures (internal sinus lift/graft/implant all at the same time)
- To learn how to achieve good initial stability in situations with limited amount of bone of poor quality
- To estimate the correct time to load a dental implant, and how to appropriately measure the implant stability quotient (ISQ).
- To understand the advantages and disadvantages of the crestal window created with the "sinus express burs"
- To understand the advantages and disadvantages of the new technique "aqua sinus lift" to lift the sinus membrane

Medical History

The patient was in good health and she has had regular physical examinations. She did not have any medical factors that will interfere with extraction of tooth #3 and the performance of the dental implant surgery and sinus lift surgery.

Review of Systems

- Vital signs
  - Blood pressure: 115/70 mmHg (ASA type I)
  - Pulse rate: 62 beats/min (regular)
- Normal cholesterol levels
- Patient is not taking any medications at the moment
- Patient denies a history of any allergies, fever, heart disease, or immunocompromising diseases (e.g., hepatitis, HIV)
- No prolonged bleeding or easy bruising
- No endocrine abnormalities

Social History

The patient is currently a physician at Johns Hopkins Hospital. She does not drink alcohol and does not smoke, which is considered ideal when performing oral surgery. She is married, and her hobbies include reading and walking.

Family History

Both parents are still alive and in good health.

Extraoral Examination

A full extraoral examination was completed.

Overall general appearance appears to be normal. Chronological–physiological age match is in proportion; size and skeletal discrepancies and development are within normal limits.

No asymmetries were observed in the head and neck examination; the submandibular, submental, and anterior/posterior lymph nodes were palpated and no swelling or masses were detected.

A temporomandibular joint examination was done; the patient expresses no pain but slight deviation to the right is detected. The patient is a potential bruxist. We recommended wearing a night guard and the use of a metal occlusal surface to avoid a fracture of the porcelain.

Intraoral Examination

A full intraoral examination was completed.
- Miller class 1 recession on tooth #3.
- Probing depths were measured and recorded (Figure 4).
- There is no furcation involvement in any tooth.
- Edentulous spaces are present in lower right posterior quadrant.
- Soft tissue examination was done; lips and labial and vestibular mucosa are within normal limits.
- There is a supereruption of tooth #3, so crown lengthening has been treatment-planned simultaneously with immediate implant and sinus bone grafting.

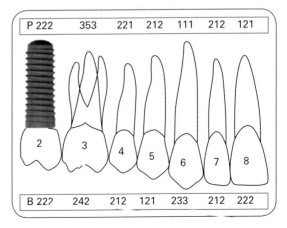

Figure 4: Periodontal probing depths.

- During the periodontal examination, we observed generalized coral pink – consistency is firm and resilient.
- The form of the gingiva is generalized pyramidal and knife-edge papilla that is well adapted against teeth.

Occlusion

- Angle's class 1 occlusion.
- Lack of right posterior teeth.
- Loss of vertical dimension.
- Extrusion of tooth #3 due to no contact with antagonist tooth. In consequence, the ridge has also been extruded, which will be corrected with crown lengthening procedure.

Radiographic Examination

The preoperative computed tomography (CT) scan shows healthy sinus despite the perforation of the Schneiderian membrane by a previously placed dental implant on #2 site (Figure 5).

The CT scan demonstrates a high and thin sinus floor, which is considered to be a class III according to Lee et al. [1] with measurements of >6 mm × <12 mm.

The CT scan shows adequate height in order to use the transalveolar technique with the "sinus express burs."

Good patency of the natural ostium of the maxillary sinus is observed on cross-section of the CT scan. This is a very important factor to consider because if the ostium opening is obliterated, sinusitis will develop with the patient having symptoms of "pressure in the sinus."

The CT scan shows no sign of a thickened sinus membrane and no mucocele, which is characteristic of a healthy sinus.

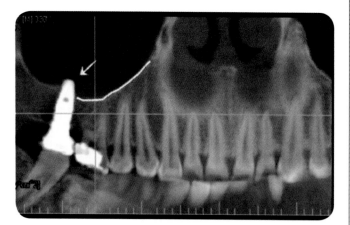

Figure 5: CT scan showing dental implant #2 appears to be inside the sinus. In addition, note decay of #3 and root resorption.

Treatment

A comprehensive treatment was presented to the patient to address all issues regarding her oral health. The treatment plan consisted of:

- atraumatic (preservation of buccal plate) extraction of tooth #3;
- degranulation of the socket using a Lucas curette;
- crown lengthening due to extrusion of tooth #3 and limited interocclusal space;
- internal/crestal approach to the sinus floor with the use of the "sinus express burs";
- internal/crestal sinus lift achieved with hydraulic pressure "Aqua-Sinus Lift";
- internal/crestal sinus grafting;
- placement of immediate dental implant;
- accurate measurement of dental implant stability using ISQ values;
- placement of healing abutment;
- appropriate suture technique.

The patient received oral hygiene instructions and prophylaxis and scaling/root planing were done prior to the surgery. She was premedicated one day before dental implant surgery with anti-inflammatory/pain killers (ibuprofen 600 mg q6h prn for pain), antibiotic (amoxicillin 875 mg BID) and long-lasting Sudafed.

Preoperative Consultation

Preoperative and postoperative instructions were given to the patient before any surgery was performed.

The patient medical history was reviewed. Appropriate consent forms with the explanations for surgical, anesthetic and intravenous sedation were signed by the patient and the doctor.

The patient was concerned about postoperative discomfort, and because of this we pursued the internal/crestal approach since the literature states that it reduces patient morbidity and swelling.

In this case, we opted to extract tooth #3, perform crown lengthening due to supereruption of tooth #3, and simultaneously graft bone in the sinus and place dental implant and accurate measurement of dental implant stability (ISQ) (Figure 6).

Sinus Elevation Procedure

Local infiltrations were given with two carpules of 4% Septocaine (articaine) with 1:100,000 epinephrine.

A sulcular incision is made with a #15c blade. An elevator was used to separate the gingiva from the tooth. Owing to the extrusion of tooth #3, crown lengthening was planned. Osteotomy was initiated with a lance drill at 1000 rpm 1 mm short of the

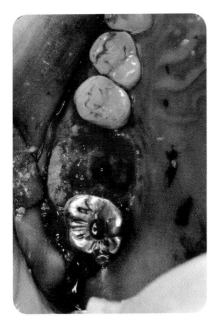

Figure 6: Atraumatic extraction used to conserve the four walls (buccal, lingual, mesial, and distal) because at least 2 mm of autogenous bone needed to surround the dental implant. Note the crown lengthening and the osteotomy at the center of the septum.

sinus floor with the aid of a surgical guide and saline solution (NaCl) irrigation. Twist drills of diameters 2.0, 2.9, 3.3, and 3.8 mm were used to further widen the osteotomy 1 mm short of the sinus floor. A sinus express bur was used to penetrate the sinus floor at 50 rpm 1 mm beyond the sinus floor with the aid of an adjustable stopper (Figures 7 and 8). A sinus reamer with a hollow shank (4.0 mm outer diameter) was used to deliver controlled water pressure, which elevates the Schneiderian membrane. In order to accelerate healing and congeal bone grafts, blood was drawn and centrifuged to make platelet-rich fibrin and concentrated growth factor. Autogenous bone from the drill used during osteotomy was mixed with EnCore® and mixed with metronidazole 250 mg/mL solution and concentrated growth factor. Membrane was made from platelet-rich fibrin and inserted into the maxillary sinus.

A dental implant (size 5 mm diameter, 11.5 mm height) was placed at the implant site #3 with a torque of 70 N cm (Any Ridge Implant Fixture® with XSpeed Surface by Megagen).

A smart peg was utilized to measure the ISQ. A common mistake made by many doctors is finger-tightening; this leads to inadequate ISQ readings. The smart peg must be tightened down with an osteo-peg mount. Depending on the ISQ value, the clinician can make an appropriate judgment (Figure 9). For

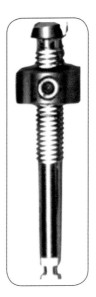

Figure 7: Adjustable stopper.

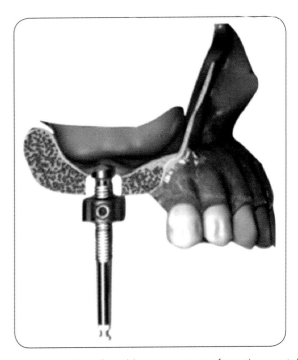

Figure 8: Using the adjustable stopper to perform the crestal/internal approach.

example, if the value is greater than 70, loading is indicated. If it is less than 70, then waiting 4–6 months is recommended. For values lower than 60 we recommend placing a wider dental implant.

However, we should not take this indication as an imperative. In actuality, longer healing time may be required because multiple surgeries were done (extraction, crestal sinus lift, and placement of dental implant). The manufacturer recommends submerging 0.5 mm below the crest to optimize healing.

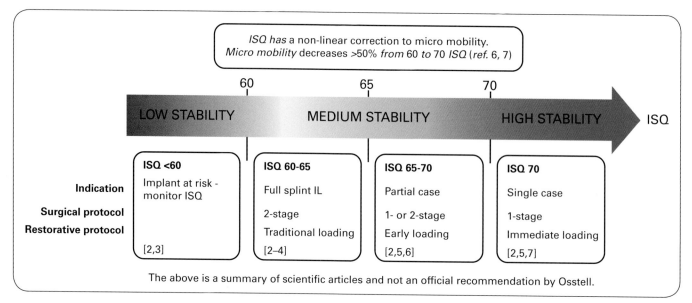

ISQ has a non-linear correction to micro mobility.
Micro mobility decreases >50% from 60 to 70 ISQ (ref. 6, 7)

	60	**65**	**70**	
	LOW STABILITY	MEDIUM STABILITY	HIGH STABILITY	ISQ

	ISQ <60	**ISQ 60-65**	**ISQ 65-70**	**ISQ 70**
Indication	Implant at risk - monitor ISQ	Full splint IL	Partial case	Single case
Surgical protocol		2-stage	1- or 2-stage	1-stage
Restorative protocol		Traditional loading	Early loading	Immediate loading
	[2,3]	[2–4]	[2,5,6]	[2,5,7]

The above is a summary of scientific articles and not an official recommendation by Osstell.

Figure 9: Summary of recommendations from the scientific literature. *Source:* Osstell.

This device will, however, give us an estimation of proper and predictable time to load the dental implant. After proper reading (ISQ) of dental implant stability, a healing abutment of 7 diameter × 4 mm of gum height was placed on dental implant #3 to seal the socket.

A 2-month follow-up showed good healing in soft tissue, and good stability was obtained on dental implant site #3, with (Osstell) ISQ measurements readings of 77, 77, 81, and 81 being obtained on buccal, lingual, mesial, and distal walls respectively. These readings in general are considered to indicate high stability.

Removal of the healing abutment was done and the impression was taken for #3 and #30.

In addition, one of the most common problems when loading a dental implant is that we can cause crestal bone loss, which means we will have a decreased amount of hard tissue (bone) around our dental implant, which can lead to a peri-implantitis, which is a dental implant complication.

Discussion

We may reduce morbidity to our patients by combining multiple surgeries into one and by choosing a minimally invasive approach. For example, we have chosen the crestal approach, which consists of a flapless surgery, hydraulic sinus lift, and immediate implant therapy at the same time.

Most of the crestal/internal approaches to the sinus are "blind techniques." However, the internal/crestal sinus lift is very popular nowadays for reducing patient morbidity. The osteotome was a commonly used instrument to carry out the crestal sinus lift; however,

this technique can lead to benign positional vertigo. Therefore, it is safer not to mallet when employing the crestal approach. In this case, we have used specialized "sinus express" surgical burs. This technology allows us to remove sinus floor without tearing the Schneiderian membrane. Therefore, the treatment is simpler and predictable [1,8].

Immediate implant surgery is beneficial because it decreases treatment time and minimizes the number of surgeries for the patient. Furthermore, this procedure has been shown to be predictable and successful [9]. However, some studies have shown that the residual alveolar ridge remodels regardless of dental implant placement. Therefore, many clinicians fear performing immediate implant placement. There is a misconception present in the general population of clinicians due to the Araújo et al. animal study in 2005 [10]. In the 2005 paper, the Araújo group's implant was too wide (4.1 mm) in the p3 and p4 extraction sockets (3.3 mm, 3.6 mm). However, later in 2011, Araújo's group published a similar study with 3.3 mm implant and xenograft successfully placed in an extraction site. Therefore, the appropriate dental implant diameter should be chosen to reserve enough buccal bone space for bone graft for a successful outcome [11]. Author recommends careful bone evaluation, atraumatic extraction, and clinical judgment for a successful outcome.

What is the ideal location for immediate dental implant on a molar site? In this particular case, the dental implant was placed on the center of the septum, because it was thought that the dental implant should be placed in native bone as much as possible while considering location of occlusal force and crown dimension. Furthermore, to achieve this, the dental implant must exit on the functional cusp of the lower molar. Many literature studies state than on maxillary teeth many surgeons have placed the dental implant on the palatal root, but studies have shown that we can cause a crossbite relationship [11,12].

When is the appropriate time to load, to put the healing abutment, or to submerge the implant? How can we accurately determine the stability of an implant? Stability of a dental implant can be obtained from an Osstell device, in which we have obtained an average reading of 75 [13]. Obtaining the dental ISQ is an important clinical measurement to minimize the risk of losing the dental implant. We recommend measuring ISQ right after the dental implant placement (as a

baseline), and subsequently comparing it with that obtained upon healing (2–6 months later) to evaluate the formation of secondary stability. For example, if the ISQ obtained is 70, it means we have a good initial or mechanical stability and we recommend performing an immediate loading (Figure 9). If the ISQ is 65–70, we recommend a two-stage approach. If it is less than 60, then a wider diameter implant should be used to regain initial stability. But, the main reason we did not incorporate immediate loading in this particular case (although it was above 70) was due to the simultaneous sinus bone grafting procedure and immediate placement of the dental implant. When native bone is less than ideal, we recommend to wait even if the ISQ is more than 70 [5,7].

Self-Study Questions

(Answers located at the end of the case)

A. What are the advantages of performing the crestal approach with the "specialized sinus drills" (sinus express burs)?

B. What anatomical structures must be considered when performing this surgical procedure?

C. What is the most important factor that we must consider when performing an extraction?

D. Why is it important to know the ISQ readings of our dental implant?

E. How can we achieve good initial/mechanical stability?

F. When the CT scan shows signs of thickened membrane, what does this mean?

G. What anatomical structures should be evaluated in a CT scan?

References

1. Lee S, Lee GK, Park K, Han T. Redefining perioplastic surgery. J Implant Adv Clin Dent 2009;1(1):76–88.
2. Sennerby L. 20 Jahre Erfahrung mit der Resonanzfrequenzanalyse. Implantologie 2013;21(1):21–33.
3. Rodrigo D, Aracil L, Martin C, Sanz M. Diagnosis of implant stability and its impact on implant survival: a prospective case series study. Clin Oral Implants Res 2010;21:255–261.
4. Östman P-O. Direct loading of implants. Clin Implant Dent Relat Res 2005;7(Suppl 1):paper IV.
5. Bornstein MM, Hart CN, Halbritter SA, et al. Early loading of nonsubmerged titanium implants with a chemically modified sand-blasted and acid-etched surface: 6-month results of a prospective case series study in the posterior mandible focusing on peri-implant crestal bone changes and implant stability quotient (ISQ) values. Clin Implant Dent Relat Res 2009;11(4):338–347.
6. Baltayan S, Mardirosian M, El-Ghareeb M, et al. The predictive value of resonance frequency analysis in the surgical placement and loading of endosseus implants. AAID Poster 2011.
7. Kokovic V, Jung R, Feloutzis A, et al. Immediate vs. early loading of SLA implants in the posterior mandible: 5-year results of randomized controlled clinical trial. Clin Oral Implants Res 2014;25(2):e114–e119.
8. Tatum Jr H. (1986) Maxillary and sinus implant reconstruction. Den Clin North Am 1986;30:207–229.
9. Lang NP, Pun L, Lau KY, et al. A systematic review on survival and success rates of implants placed immediately into fresh extraction sockets after at least 1 year. Clin Oral Implants Res 2012;23(Suppl 5):39–66.

10. Araújo MG, Sukekava F, Wennström JL, Lindhe J. Ridge alterations following implant placement in fresh extraction sockets: an experimental study in the dog. J Clin Periodontol 2005;32:645–652.

11. Becker CM, Wilson Jr T, Jensen OT. Minimum criteria for immediate provisionalization of single-tooth dental implants in extraction sites: a 1 year retrospective study of 100 consecutive cases. J Oral Maxillofac Surg 2011;69(2):491–497.

12. Rodriguez-Tizcareño MH, Bravo Flores C. Anatomically guided implant site preparation technique at molar sites. Implant Dent 2009;18(5):393–401.

13. Boyne P, James R. Grafting of the maxillary sinus floor with autogenous marrow and bone. J Oral Surg 1980;38:613–616.

14. Vernamonte S, Mauro V, Vernamonte S, Meissina AM. An unusual complication of osteotome sinus floor elevation: benign paroxysmal positional vertigo. Int J Oral Maxillofac Surg 2011;40(2):216–218.

15. Liang L, Liu HG, He CY. Morphological study of thick basement membrane-like layer in chronic rhinosinusitis. Zhonghua Er Bi Yan Hou Tou Jing Wai Ke Za Zhi. 2006;41(1):31–34 (in Chinese).

16. Elian N, Wallace S, Cho SC, et al. Distribution of the maxillary artery as it relates to sinus floor augmentation. Int J Oral Maxillofac Implants 2005;20(5):784–787.

Answers to Self-Study Questions

A. Unlike the osteotome, there is no hammering with a mallet. This eliminates complications such as benign vertigo and decreases intraoperative dental fear [14]. In addition, the "sinus express bur" is proven to be safe on sinus membrane in numerous clinical cases [1]. This bur has a flat-ended tip, which grinds the bone while not tearing the Schneiderian membrane.

B. The thickness of the sinus membrane, posterior superior alveolar (PSA) artery, sinus ostium, and presence of mucocele. Sinus membranes thicker than 3 mm are considered chronic sinusitis [15]. The PSA artery is often found 16.4 mm from the crest according to Elian et al. [16]. Without patency of the sinus ostium there is a greater chance of sinusitis after surgery. A mucocele can obliterate the ostium after a sinus lift procedure.

C. Preservation of the four bony walls (bucal, palatal, mesial, and distal) of the socket is most important in an extraction technique. Blood supply to graft and implant fixtures comes from bony walls. With a compromised buccal plate, it loses critical blood supply to the grafts. Epithelial invagination will occur, and the graft will eventually be expelled. Therefore, it is crucial to preserve all four walls, especially the buccal plate as it is thinnest and it is made out of bundle bone. A periotome, sectioning of a tooth, and piezosurgical tips are commonly used to preserve the buccal plate during extraction.

D. Radiographs do not have a high sensitivity in detecting failing/ailing implants. On the other hand, the ISQ measures the stability of the implant by magnetic resistance. Therefore, it has a higher sensitivity in measuring implant success. The ISQ is used to obtain a quantitative value to estimate the appropriate time for loading our dental implant. It is recommended to measure the ISQ right after the dental implant placement (as a baseline), and subsequently comparing it with that obtained upon healing (2–6 months later) to evaluate formation of secondary stability. For example, if the ISQ obtained is 70, it means we have a good initial or mechanical stability and we recommend performing an immediate loading. If the ISQ is 65–70 we recommend a two-stage approach. If it is less than 60, then a wider diameter implant should be used to regain initial stability.

E. By making the osteotomy slightly narrower we can achieve better initial stability in D3 or D4 bone (skipping last drill recommended by the manufacturer). There are four types of bone quality: D1 is completely cortical and is found in cavarium. D2 is mostly cortical and is found around mandibular anteriors, and sometimes in posterior mandible. D3 bone has thinner cortical bone surrounded by mostly medullary bone. These types of bone are found in posterior mandible and anterior maxilla. D4 bone is mostly medullary in nature and is found around posterior maxilla. D3 and D4 bone are prone to poor initial stability, and it is crucial for the surgeon to underprepare the osteotomy or use a tapered aggressively threaded implant to achieve more than 35 N cm or an ISQ of 65 and above.

F. A thickened membrane usually hints at the presence of sinusitis, an infection in the sinus [15]. We must delay performing the sinus lift surgery until proper medical care is taken. If thickness is more than 3 mm, then referral to ear, nose, and throat is recommended as it is defined as chronic sinusitis.

G. When taking a CT scan, we must consider:
• patency of natural ostium
• thickness of the Schneiderian membrane
• mucocele presence
• polyp presence
• location of intraosseus anastomosis of PSA artery
• thickness of lateral wall, buccal, lingual anatomy/ dimension
• septum presence.

Conclusion

This case presented here is a unique sinus bone grafting technique with simultaneous immediate implant placement in the upper molar site. This technique simplified surgical challenges and reduced treatment time and morbidity to our patients. Although sinus bone grafting is considered a highly predictable procedure, a long-term study with a large sample size is recommended for future studies.

7

Implant Placement

Clinical Cases in Implant Dentistry, First Edition. Edited by Nadeem Karimbux and Hans-Peter Weber.
© 2017 John Wiley & Sons, Inc. Published 2017 by John Wiley & Sons, Inc.

Case 1

One-Stage/Two-Stage Placement

CASE STORY

A 31-year-old Caucasian female presented with a chief complaint of "I need an implant for my missing tooth." Tooth #12 had been extracted 6 months prior to her initial visit, due to failed endodontic treatment. Prior to the extraction the patient was complaining about severe pain. Endodontic therapy had been initiated several years previously. Two attempts were made to retreat the tooth, but due to calcified roots the treatment was unsuccessful. The prognosis was hopeless. At the time of extraction of #12, ridge preservation with freeze-dried bone allograft (FDBA, Mineross®) and a resorbable collagen membrane (Dynamatrix®) was performed. An Essix appliance was delivered to replace the missing #12. The patient presented for implant placement 6 months later (Figures 1 and 2). The patient reported that she had visited her dentist regularly for uninterrupted dental care and reported that she brushed twice per day, flossed once a day, and used a mouthrinse twice per day. She had several amalgam and composite restorations, mainly in her posterior teeth.

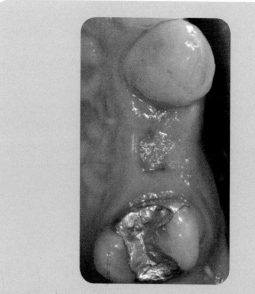

Figure 2: Pre-op presentation (occlusal view).

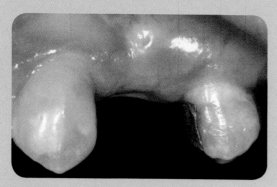

Figure 1: Pre-op presentation (facial view).

LEARNING GOALS AND OBJECTIVES

- To understand the concept of one-stage implant placement
- To understand the indications for one-stage implant placement
- To understand the technique of one-stage implant placement
- To understand and determine the differences between one-stage and two-stage implant placement
- To understand that one-stage implant placement procedure is successful
- To understand the factors affecting the outcome of one stage implant placement procedures

Medical History

The patient presented without any medical conditions that would impact therapy. The patient was taking fish oil as a supplement. The patient reported that she had no known drug allergies.

Review of Systems

- Vital signs
  - Blood pressure: 100/70 mmHg
  - Pulse rate: 52 beats/min (regular)
  - Respiration: 15 breaths/min

Social History

The patient had no history of smoking or alcohol consumption at the time of treatment.

Extraoral Examination

The extraoral examination showed absence of any clinical pathology. The temporomandibular joints were stable, functional, with no pain reported during movements. There was no facial asymmetry or lymphadenopathy noted.

Intraoral Examination

- Oral cancer screening was negative.
- Soft tissue exam, including her tongue and floor of the mouth and fauces, showed no clinical pathology.
- Periodontal examination revealed pocket depths in the range 1–3 mm (Figure 3).
- Localized areas of slight gingival inflammation and bleeding on probing were noted.
- The color, size, shape, and consistency of the gingiva were normal. The keratinized tissue was firm and stippled.
- An aberrant mandibular right labial frenum was noted, which was acting as a contributing factor for the recession on the buccal side of #28.
- Localized plaque was found around the teeth, resulting in a plaque-free index of 85%
- Evaluation of the alveolar ridges showed slight horizontal bone resorption (Seibert class I) in the areas of #12 and #14. The patient lost #14 4 years ago due to a vertical fracture. Teeth #13 and #15 were rotated and tilted towards the edentulous space.

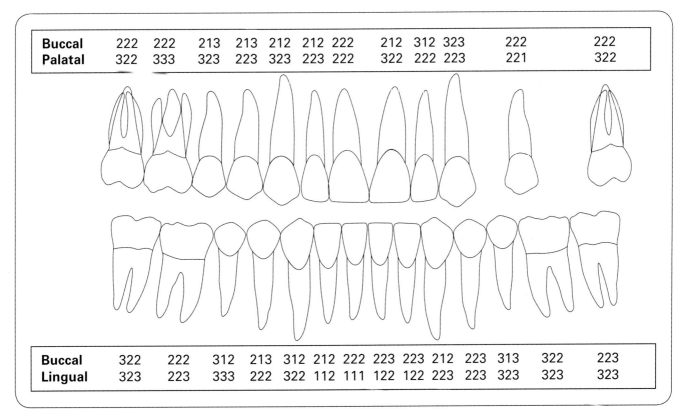

Buccal	222	222	213	213	212	212	222	212	312	323		222		222
Palatal	322	333	323	223	323	223	222	322	222	223		221		322

Buccal	322	222	312	213	312	212	222	223	223	212	223	313	322	223
Lingual	323	223	333	222	322	112	111	122	122	223	223	323	323	323

Figure 3: Probing pocket depth measurements during the initial visit.

The patient was not interested in having orthodontic treatment to create adequate space for possible implant placement in the area of #14.

- Extensive amalgam and composite restorations in the posterior teeth were also noted.

Occlusion

There was a crossbite #13–#19 and #7–#27. Signs of occlusal traumatism (worn dentition) were noted.

Radiographic Examination

A full mouth radiographic series was ordered (see Figure 4 for patient's periapical radiograph of the area of interest). Radiographic examination revealed normal bone levels. No other pathology was noted. No loss of bone was noted in the crestal bone height at #12 site. There was adequate mesiodistal space for placement of a 4.3 mm diameter implant (Nobel, Replace Select®).

Diagnosis

An American Academy of Periodontology diagnosis of localized slight plaque-induced gingivitis with mucogingival deformities and conditions around teeth (presented as recession, lack of keratinized gingiva, and an aberrant frenum #28), mucogingival deformities and conditions on the edentulous ridges (horizontal ridge deficiency #12, #14), and occlusal trauma was made. Additional diagnosis of partial edentulism was made.

Treatment Plan

The treatment plan for this patient consisted of initial-phase therapy that included oral prophylaxis

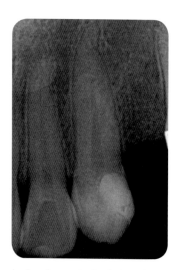

Figure 4: Periapical radiograph depicting the crestal bone levels at site #12.

and oral hygiene instructions to address the gingival inflammation. This was followed by a single-stage implant placement procedure for #12. The implant was restored after adequate time for osseointegration (4 months).

Treatment

After the initial phase of therapy, the patient presented for implant placement of #12. Having obtained profound anesthesia at the surgical site using local anesthetic (Septocaine), full-thickness buccal and palatal flaps were reflected. The incision was midcrestal at site #12 with a semilunar shape, which extended to the adjacent teeth #11 and #13 with intrasulcular incisions (Figure 5A). Using the roll-flap procedure, the underlying and de-epithelialized connective tissue was used as a pedicle graft, which was subsequently placed in a subepithelial pouch buccally (Figure 5B). The ideal location of the implant was verified using guide pins, and the osteotomy was extended to the final length of 10 mm and diameter of 4.3 mm (according to manufacturer's instructions) (Figure 5C). A regular platform implant with a healing abutment was placed. There was no need for any additional grafting (Figure 5D and G). The palatal and buccal flaps were sutured around the healing abutment with two simple interrupted vicryl sutures (Figure 5E and F).

The sutures were removed after 2 weeks and the area was swabbed with chlorhexidine 0.12%. The adjacent teeth were debrided gently using hand instrumentation and were polished with a rubber cup as well. At 4 months, on completion of healing without complications and radiographic verification, final impressions were made and the implant was restored with a porcelain-fused cemental crown (Figure 6).

Discussion

In this case, different factors have been evaluated to select the one-stage implant placement approach. The edentulous area was healed completely after extraction of tooth #12 and preservation of the site. Hard and soft tissue were adequately mature at the time of implant placement. Minimal horizontal resorption was noted at the edentulous area, which could be retrieved with suitable soft tissue manipulation (roll-flap procedure) during the implant placement.

Traditionally, to minimize implant failures, dental implants were inserted following a two-stage protocol. Some workers developed dental implants

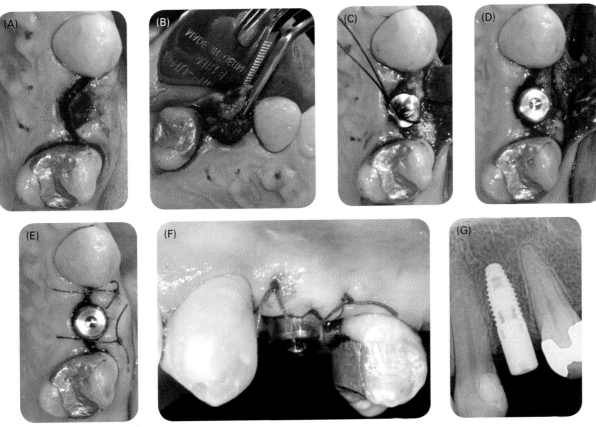

Figure 5: (A) Incision design for implant placement #12; (B) full-thickness flap elevation, roll-flap technique; (C) guiding pin; (D) implant in place. (E, F) Flaps were approximated and sutured. (G) Postoperative radiograph.

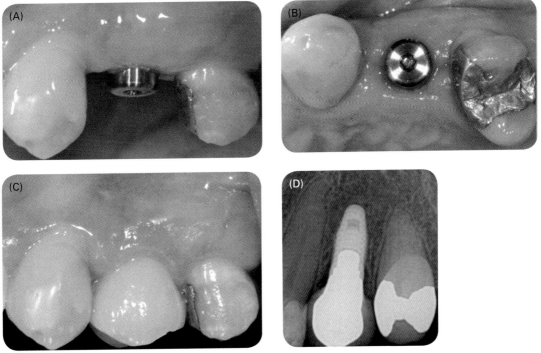

Figure 6: (A, B) Four months post-op after implant placement #12. (C) Restored implant. (D) Periapical radiograph showing the restored implant.

to be used with a one-stage procedure (refer to answers of self-study questions A and B). One-stage implant placement appears to provide predictable results in partially edentulous patients, avoiding one surgical intervention, shortening treatment time, and decreasing patient morbidity (refer to answer of self-study question C). When a clinician is faced with the dilemma of submerging the implants or not, some considerations should be made. In the case of poor implant stability, a submerged technique may be preferable. In the case of excellent implant stability (implants placed with insertion torque >32 N cm), implants can be left healing according to a one-stage procedure, and a possible immediate loading technique could also be considered (refer to answer of self-study question D). There is a limited amount of evidence available, but it has been shown that there might be

a potential increased risk for early implant failures and complications when using one-stage implants in edentulous arches. Additionally, in cases where it is expected that a provisional prosthesis could transmit excessive forces on the healing implants, it might be preferable to opt for a more conservative two-stage procedure (refer to answers of self-study questions E and F). Therefore, proper patient and site selection are important to increase the likelihood of success. The patient in this case had proper site preparation prior to implant placement, achieving an almost optimal hard and soft tissue profile. Additionally, the patient's esthetic demands were not high during the healing period, which indicated that the implant would not be loaded with any provisional prosthesis and therefore the risk of excessive forces transmitted on the healing implant would be zero.

Self-Study Questions

(Answers located at the end of the case)

A. What is one-stage implant placement?

B. What is the difference between one-stage and two-stage implant placement?

C. What are the advantages of a one-stage implant placement procedure?

D. What are the indications for one-stage implant placement?

E. Is there a better long-term prognosis with one-stage or two-stage implant placement?

F. What are the factors that influence one-stage implant prognosis?

References

1. Brånemark P-I, Hansson BO, Adell R, et al. Osseointegrated Implants in the Treatment of the Edentulous Jaw. Experience from a 10-Year Period. Scandinavian Journal of Plastic and Reconstructive Surgery, Supplementum 16. Stockholm: Almqvist & Wiksell International; 1977.
2. Albrektsson T, Brånemark P-I, Hansson H-A, Lindström J. Osseointegrated titanium implants. Requirements for ensuring a long-lasting, direct bone-to-implant anchorage in man. Acta Orthop Scand 1981;52:155–170.
3. Brunski JB, Moccia AFJ, Pollack SR, et al. The influence of functional use of endosseous dental implants on the tissue–implant interface. I. Histological aspects. J Dent Res 1979;58:1953–1969.
4. Schroeder A, Pohler O, Sutter E. Gewebsreaktion auf ein Titan-Hohlzylinderimplantat mit Titan-Spritzschichtoberflache [Tissue reaction to an implant of a titanium hollow cylinder with a titanium surface spray layer]. SSO Schweiz Monatsschr Zahnheilkd 1976;86:713–727.
5. Schroeder A, Stich H, Straumann F, Sutter E. Ueber die Anlagerung von Osteozement an einen belasteten Implantatkorper. SSO Schweiz Monatsschr Zahnheilkd 1978;88:105–1057.
6. Schroeder A, van der Zypen E, Stich H, Sutter F. The reaction of bone, connective tissue and epithelium to endosteal implants with sprayed titanium surfaces. J Maxillofac Surg 1981;9:15–25
7. Buser D, Belser UC, Lang NP. The original one-stage dental implant system and its clinical application. Periodontol 2000 1998;17:106–118.
8. Buser D, Weber HF, Donath K, et al. Soft tissue reactions to non-submerged unloaded titanium implants in beagle dogs. J Periodontol 1992;63:225–235.
9. Cochran DL, Hermann JS, Schenk RK, et al. Biologic width around titanium implants: a histometric analysis of the implanto-gingival junction around unloaded and loaded nonsubmerged implants in the canine mandible. J Periodontol 1997;68:186–198.

10. Listgarten MA, Buser D, Steinemann SG, et al. Light and transmission electron microscopy of the intact interfaces between non-submerged titanium-coated epoxy resin implants and bone or gingiva. J Dent Res 1992;71:364–371.

11. Weber HP, Buser D, Donath K, et al. Comparison of healed tissues adjacent to submerged and non-submerged unloaded titanium dental implants. A histometric study in beagle dogs. Clin Oral Implants Res 1996;7:11–19.

12. Buser D, Weber HP, Lang NP. Tissue integration of nonsubmerged implants. 1-year results of a prospective study with 100 ITI hollow-cylinder and hollow-screw implants. Clin Oral Implants Res 1990;1:33–40.

13. Buser D, Mericske-Stern R, Bernard JP, et al. Long-term evaluation of non-submerged ITI implants. Part 1: 8-year life table analysis of prospective multicenter study with 2359 implants. Clin Oral Implants Res 1997;8:161–172.

14. Esposito M, Grusovin MG, Chew YS, et al. One-stage versus two-stage implant placement. A Cochrane systematic review of randomised controlled clinical trials. Eur J Oral Implantol 2009;2(2):91–99.

15. Brunski JB, Moccia AFJ, Pollack SR, et al. The influence of functional use of endosseous dental implants on the tissue–implant interface. I. Histological aspects. J Dent Res 1979;58:1953–1969.

16. Collaert B, De Bruyn H. Comparison of Brånemark fixture integration and short-term survival using one-stage or two-stage surgery in completely and partially edentulous mandibles. Clin Oral Implants Res 1998;9:131–135.

17. Ericsson I, Randow K, Nilner K, Petersson A. Some clinical and radiographical features of submerged and non-submerged titanium implants. A 5-year follow-up study. Clin Oral Implants Res 1997;8:422–426.

18. Ericsson I, Randow K, Glantz PO, et al. Clinical and radiographical features of submerged and nonsubmerged titanium implants. Clin Oral Implants Res 1994;5:185–189.

19. Ericsson I, Nilner K, Klinge, B, Glantz PO. Radiographical and histological characteristics of submerged and nonsubmerged titanium implants. An experimental study in the Labrador dog. Clin Oral Implants Res 1996;7:20–26.

20. Becker W, Becker BE, Israelson H, et al. One-step surgical placement of Brånemark implants. A prospective multicenter clinical study. Int J Oral Maxillofac Implants 1997;12:454–462.

21. Becktor JP, Isaksson S, Billstrom C. A prospective multicenter study using two different surgical approaches in the mandible with turned Brånemark implants: conventional loading using fixed prostheses. Clin Implant Dent Relat Res 2007;9:179–185.

22. Esposito M, Murray-Curtis L, Grusovin MG, et al. Interventions for replacing missing teeth: different types of dental implants. Cochrane Database Syst Rev 2007;(4):CD003815.

23. Cordaro L, Torsello F, Roccuzzo M. Clinical outcome of submerged versus non-submerged implants placed in fresh extraction sockets. Clin Oral Implants Res 2009;20(12):1307–1313.

Answers to Self-Study Questions

A. There is no question that endosseous dental implants have revolutionized tooth replacement therapies. During the past decades implant therapy has developed into a successful treatment for partial and complete edentulism. Traditionally, to minimize implant failures, osseointegrated dental implants were inserted following a two-stage protocol [1]. Implants were completely submerged under the soft tissues and left to heal for a period of 3–4 months in mandibles and 6–8 months in maxilla [2]. Primary implant stability and lack of micromovements are considered to be two of the main factors necessary to achieve a predictably high success rate of osseointegrated dental implants [2,3].

The development of the original one-stage dental implant system utilizing nonsubmerged implants was initiated in the early 1970s, based on the principle of osseointegration as described by Schroeder and coworkers [4–6]. These histological studies in monkeys showed that nonsubmerged titanium implants achieve ankylotic anchorage in bone characterized by direct bone-to-implant contact. Since then, different materials and surfaces have been tested in an attempt to improve physical and biomechanical properties, biologic principles, and finally clinical applications, with promising short- and long-term results [7]. In the past years, these observations with nonsubmerged implants have been confirmed by numerous experimental studies [8–11]. Longitudinal follow-up studies have also suggested that high early success rates could also be achieved using a one-stage approach [12,13]. With this approach, flaps are sutured around the polished neck of the implants, after their placement, avoiding the need for a second surgical intervention.

B. With a two-stage approach, the implants are completely submerged under the soft tissues after their placement and they are left to heal for a period of 2–6 months. Utilizing this approach, the implants are load free during the healing period. Two-stage implant placement is used to minimize the micromovements during healing and the risk of transmitting unwanted loading forces to the healing bone at the implant interface (which may lead to soft tissue encapsulation), and therefore to increase the possibility of successful osseointegration [14,15]. However, a second surgical intervention (usually a minor one, unless soft tissue augmentation is necessary) is needed to connect the implants to the abutments holding the future prosthesis. In addition, after the second intervention, some weeks of healing are needed for the soft tissues to stabilize around the penetrating abutment(s) to allow for a predictable esthetic outcome [14].

When one-stage approach is used, the flaps are sutured around the polished neck of the implants, avoiding the need for a second surgical intervention. Alternatively, a one-stage technique can be achieved by immediate connection of a temporary healing abutment to a two-piece implant that protrudes through the soft tissue in much the same way as a one-piece implant. Different controlled clinical trials comparing implants placed according to a one-versus two-stage procedure suggest that implants placed with a one-stage approach may achieve a high degree of success rate as well [14–17].

C. One-stage implant placement procedure offers several clinical advantages, such as the avoidance of second-stage surgery, an overall shorter treatment and healing period with reduced costs to the patient, a more favorable crown-to-root ratio, and direct access to the implant shoulder at the soft tissue level, allowing for a simple prosthetic approach with either cemented or screw-retained implant restorations [7,14].

Several investigators have studied the marginal peri-implant tissues at nonsubmerged and submerged implant systems and demonstrated that, irrespective of surgical installation protocol (one or two stages), implants exhibited only small amount of radiographic marginal bone loss, which does not also differ between the two protocols [11,17–19]. Additionally, the marginal bone level following rehabilitation appears to remain stable irrespective

of whether the implants had been placed according to a one- or two-stage surgical protocol [17–19]. These observations led to the conclusion that the surgical protocol does not influence the outcome of implant therapy and that there is no significant difference of peri-implant bone level changes between the two surgical protocols.

D. A recent systematic review of randomized controlled clinical trials concluded that the one-stage approach might be preferable in partially edentulous patients, since it avoids one surgical intervention and shortens treatment time, while a two-stage submerged approach could be indicated when an implant has not obtained an optimal primary stability, when barriers are used for guided tissue regeneration or when it is expected that removable temporary prostheses could transmit excessive forces on the penetrating abutments, especially in fully edentulous patients [14]. Additionally, submerged implants are commonly more often utilized particularly in esthetic sites in the anterior maxilla, where specific esthetic demands and the patient's expectations are increased [7].

E. Several experimental and clinical studies have demonstrated that nonsubmerged titanium implants achieve successful tissue integration as predictably as submerged implants [11,12,18–20].

In a 2009 systematic review the authors concluded, though, that the number of patients included in the evaluated clinical trials was too small to draw definitive conclusions about effectiveness, long-term prognosis, and any clinically significant difference among implants placed according to one-stage (nonsubmerged) versus two-stage (submerged) procedures. In addition, the risk of bias in the majority of the studies was high and therefore the evidence was not sufficient to draw reliable conclusions [14].

Different trials evaluated peri-implant marginal bone level changes among implants placed with either a one-stage or two-stage approach, but meta-analysis of those did not show any significant difference in bone loss between the two procedures [14].

That same systematic review concluded that, taking the results of all trials into consideration, it might be implied that no major clinical differences exist between the two procedures, though these preliminary findings needed to be confirmed by more robust trials [14].

F. There are no clear-cut factors that may influence one-stage implant prognosis. Several factors may play a role, as revealed in different randomized clinical trials.

In one clinical trial [21], comparing four to six implants in edentulous mandibles, more failures of implants placed with one-stage procedure occurred. A likely explanation for increased failure rates in edentulous patients when placing implants according to a one-stage protocol could be that dentures may transmit excessive loading on the healing abutments while the osseointegration process is taking place [21].

Another clinical trial [22] mentioned that a possible contributing factor could be the surface characteristics of the implants used (machined or turned implant surface). It has been hypothesized that implants with a turned surface may be at higher risk for early implant failures, and this risk could be further increased if these implants are loaded during the bone healing period [22].

Some clinical trials have also evaluated complications occurring after one-stage and two-stage implant placement procedures. A multicenter trial included patients with edentulous mandibles and evaluated the complications that happened using either of the two approaches. The impression was that there were many more complications up to abutment connection in the one-stage group, in terms of soft tissue reactions and pain [21].

Esthetic outcomes were reported only in one trial [23]. There were no differences in soft tissue recession around postextractive single implants when using a submerged or nonsubmerged technique. Using either one-stage or two-stage implant placement procedure, 1 mm of mean soft tissue recession is seen after 1 year when compared with the pre-extraction situation. Changes in keratinized tissue height were also evaluated in the same trial and it was found that, at the 1-year follow-up, there was statistically significant less keratinized tissue (1.1 mm) around implants placed according to a two-stage technique. While this finding applies to postextractive sites (since flaps have to be mobilized to close the socket, thus moving the mucosal junction coronally), it is unlikely to apply in sites without extraction, when no tissues have to be mobilized [23].

Conclusion

More randomized controlled trials with a larger number of patients are needed to confirm these preliminary findings. Possible complications should also be thoroughly reported, and esthetic outcomes could also be evaluated to see whether one of the procedures offers some advantages over the other.

Case 2

Immediate Placement

CASE STORY

A 76-year-old woman was referred due to fractured crown of the maxillary left central incisor with a chief complaint of "My dentist told me that tooth couldn't be saved." Tooth #9 had previous root canal therapy and was restored with a post and full-coverage porcelain-fused-to-metal crown. The crown came loose several times, a horizontal root fracture was noticed by the referring prosthodontist and it was deemed nonrestorable (Figures 1 and 2). The patient brushes her teeth twice a day and she flosses once a week.

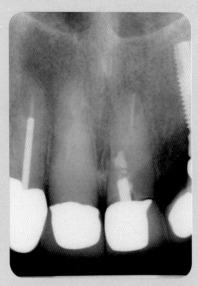

Figure 1: Preoperative periapical radiograph of tooth #9.

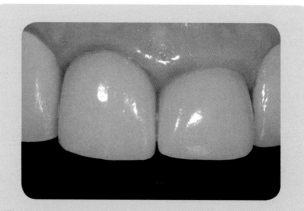

Figure 2: Preoperative buccal view of tooth #9.

LEARNING GOALS AND OBJECTIVES

■ To understand the concept of immediate implant placement into extraction sockets
■ To understand the technique and materials used in immediate implant placement
■ To understand the indication of immediate implant placement

Medical History

The patient is a former smoker, has asthma and takes two puffs of albuterol every 6 h. She is allergic to dairy products and takes 81 mg of aspirin every day.

Review of Systems

• Vital signs
  ○ Blood pressure: 132/73 mmHg
  ○ Pulse rate: 70 beats/min

Social History

The patient typically drinks two glasses of wine per week.

Extraoral Examination

There are no significant findings. There are no masses or swelling and the temporomandibular joint is within normal limits.

Intraoral Examination

- The oral cancer screening was negative.
- A four-unit fixed partial denture supported with two implants and mesial cantilever was present in the maxillary left quadrant.
- An intrabony defect with a probing depth of 7 mm was observed around the mandibular left canine.
- The patient has a low smile line.

Occlusion

The patient presents with a normal molar and canine relationship.

Radiographic Examination

An examination of a full-mouth series of radiographs revealed inadequate endodontic treatment of #9 with a possible root perforation. Tooth #9 also presented with a short post and a radiolucency between the porcelain-fused-to-metal crown and root. Bone resorption was observed around teeth #22 and #31 (which was mesially tilted).

Diagnosis

The patient has a localized severe chronic periodontitis.

Treatment Plan

The treatment plan for this patient includes an initial phase of scaling and root planing with oral hygiene instructions, guided-tissue regeneration (GTR) of tooth #22, and extraction of tooth #9 with an immediate implant placement with bone graft.

Treatment

After the initial consult and the diagnostic phase, the patient received initial therapy of scaling and root planing. Tooth #22 was treated with the GTR technique. Tooth #9 was deemed nonrestorable; therefore, extraction and immediate implant placement was planned.

At the time of the surgery, local infiltrative anesthesia was administered (lidocaine 2%, epinephrine 1 : 100,000). The crown was removed and a #15 blade was used to excise fibers in the sulcus. A minimally invasive extraction technique was used for

maximum preservation of socket wall (Figure 3). The buccal plate was located approximately 4 mm apical from the marginal gingiva (Figure 4). The implant was immediately placed in the socket following sequential drills according to the manufacturer's recommendation (4.1 mm × 12 mm Bone Level, Straumann, MA) (Figure 5). The implant had a good primary stability and the gap between the implant and extraction socket was grafted with xenograft (Bio-Oss Collagen, Geistlich Pharma North America, Princeton, NJ) (Figure 6). The gingival flaps were sutured with chromic gut and an interim partial denture was delivered (Figures 7 and 8).

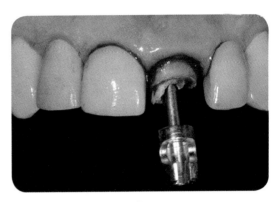

Figure 3: Flapless extraction of tooth #9.

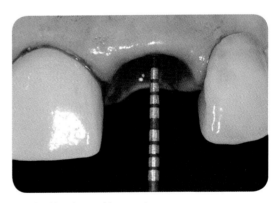

Figure 4: Probing buccal bone plate.

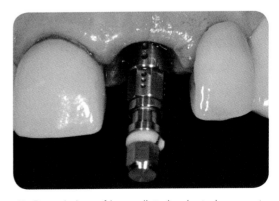

Figure 5: Buccal view of immediate implant placement.

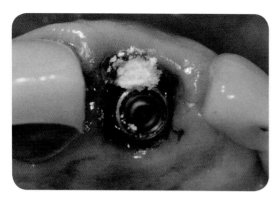

Figure 6: Occlusal view of immediate implant and bone graft (Bio-Oss Collagen).

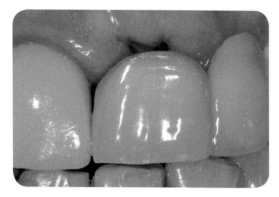

Figure 7: Buccal view of interim removable partial denture.

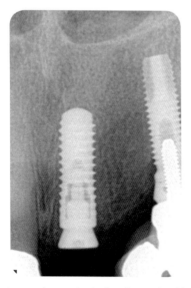

Figure 8: Postoperative periapical radiograph of implant (immediately after placement).

The patient returned for a 2-week follow-up visit and reported minimum discomfort.

A temporary abutment/crown was delivered after a 4-month healing period (Figure 9A). A final implant-supported crown with custom abutment was delivered 3 months later (Figures 9B and 10).

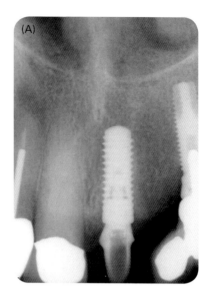

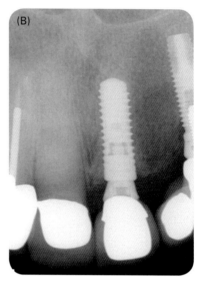

Figure 9: (A) Seven-month postoperative periapical radiograph; (B) 18-month postoperative periapical radiograph.

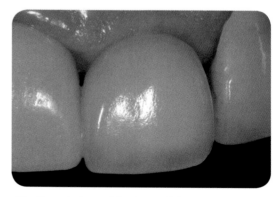

Figure 10: Buccal view of final porcelain crown and gingival margin healing after 18 months.

Discussion

A successful implant treatment should be without any biological, technical, or esthetic complication [1]. Long-term stability and survival of both implant and its restoration are the ultimate goal of each treatment. In this case, we describe a clinical case where an implant was placed immediately after an extraction in the anterior maxillary region.

Over the years, the technique of placing implants immediately after an extraction has become an attractive option. In fact, Schulte et al. [2] first reported a case that in the same appointment an implant was placed into the fresh socket, reducing the dental appointments, the time of surgeries, and total treatment length. The initial implant stability is achieved by engaging the residual bony walls, and primary stability is mostly achieved at the apical region. It has been shown that spontaneous bone fill in animal models [3] and in human studies [4,5] occurs after 3–4 months.

Immediate implant placement immediately after extraction has been recognized to be a highly predictive treatment for fully and partially edentulous cases [6]. According to a longitudinal study, 5-year survival rate of implants is approximately 95%, and the 10-year survival rate is 89% [7]. The Cochrane systematic review demonstrated no statistical significant difference between success, complications, esthetics, and patient satisfaction among different timing of implant placement after tooth extraction [6]. According to one study, a 9.9-out-of-10 satisfaction rate was found after 1-year follow-up after immediate implant placement [8]. While the previous implant success criteria [9] have not considered esthetic complications, this has become an important factor to be considered.

However, immediate implant placement cannot prevent intra- and extraalveolar modeling and remodeling, which lead to vertical and horizontal reductions of bone walls. Such tissue changes imply increased risk of facial bone wall resorption, marginal mucosa instability, and, consequently, influencing esthetic outcomes and implant survival. In fact, the presence of active infection factors has been listed in the development of mucosal recession, such as smoking, presence of a thin buccal bone plate, presence of a thin tissue biotype, and facial implant position. Thus, the need for soft tissue graft and bone substitutes in the clinical armamentarium is imperative to prevent complications and to favor an optimal healing response.

The main purposes of using grafting materials were to fill the marginal gaps between implants and socket walls and to cover bony dehiscences and/or fenestrations. Recent studies have clearly shown that the facial bone in the anterior maxilla is usually very thin ($\leq$1 mm) [10], and experimental and clinical studies have demonstrated that thin buccal bone will be quickly resorbed within 4–8 weeks following tooth extraction, leading to a reduction in bone height [3,11,12]. Demineralized bovine bone matrix, freeze-dried bone allograft, and demineralized freeze-dried bone allograft are commonly used bone substitute graft materials.

Overall, implants placed in the anterior region showed slightly lower failure rate when compared with a posterior position. The implants placed in the maxilla had a higher estimated annual failure rate (0.73%) than implants placed in the mandible (0.50%). The estimated annual failure rate of the conventional loading group was lower than that of the immediate loading group (0.75% versus 0.89%) [1]. Thus, immediate placement implant techniques may be a predictable treatment option when biological, esthetic, and clinical concepts described here are properly respected.

Self-Study Questions

(Answers located at the end of the case)

A. What is an immediate implant placement?

B. What is the predictability of immediately placed implants?

C. What are the factors influencing the final esthetic outcome?

D. What other adjunct procedures might improve the outcome of immediate implant placement?

E. What are the indications of immediate implant placement?

F. What are the advantages and disadvantages of immediate implant placement?

G. Where is the ideal implant position?

References

1. Lang NP, Pun L, Lau KY, et al. A systematic review on survival and success rates of implants placed immediately into fresh extraction sockets after at least 1 year. Clin Oral Implants Res 2012;23(Suppl 5):39–66.
2. Schulte W, Kleineikenscheidt H, Lindner K, Schareyka R. The Tubingen immediate implant in clinical studies. Dtsch Zahnarztl Z 1978;33(5):348–359 (in German).
3. Araujo MG, Sukekava F, Wennstrom JL, Lindhe J. Ridge alterations following implant placement in fresh extraction sockets: an experimental study in the dog. J Clin Periodontol 2005;32(6):645–652.
4. Cornelini R, Cangini F, Covani U, Wilson Jr TJ. Immediate restoration of implants placed into fresh extraction sockets for single-tooth replacement: a prospective clinical study. Int J Periodontics Restorative Dent 2005;25(5):439–447.
5. Covani U, Chiappe G, Bosco M, et al. A 10-year evaluation of implants placed in fresh extraction sockets: a prospective cohort study. J Periodontol 2012;83(10):1226–1234.
6. Esposito M, Grusovin MG, Polyzos IP, et al. Timing of implant placement after tooth extraction: immediate, immediate-delayed or delayed implants? A Cochrane systematic review. Eur J Oral Implantol 2010;3(3):189–205.
7. Pjetursson BE, Tan K, Lang NP, et al. A systematic review of the survival and complication rates of fixed partial dentures (FPDs) after an observation period of at least 5 years. Clin Oral Implants Res 2004;15(6):625–642.
8. Kan JY, Rungcharassaeng K, Lozada J. Immediate placement and provisionalization of maxillary anterior single implants: 1-year prospective study. Int J Oral Maxillofac Implants 2003;18(1):31–39.
9. Albrektsson T, Zarb G, Worthington P, Eriksson AR. The long-term efficacy of currently used dental implants: a review and proposed criteria of success. Int J Oral Maxillofac Implants 1986;1(1):11–25.
10. Januario AL, Duarte WR, Barriviera M, et al. Dimension of the facial bone wall in the anterior maxilla: a cone-beam computed tomography study. Clin Oral Implants Res 2011;22(10):1168–1171.
11. Schropp L, Kostopoulos L, Wenzel A. Bone healing following immediate versus delayed placement of titanium implants into extraction sockets: a prospective clinical study. Int J Oral Maxillofac Implants 2003;18(2):189–199.
12. Schropp L, Isidor F. Timing of implant placement relative to tooth extraction. J Oral Rehabil 2008;35(Suppl 1):33–43.
13. Hämmerle CH, Chen ST, Wilson Jr TG. Consensus statements and recommended clinical procedures regarding the placement of implants in extraction sockets. Int J Oral Maxillofac Implants 2004;19(Suppl):26–28.
14. Chen ST, Darby IB, Reynolds EC. A prospective clinical study of non-submerged immediate implants: clinical outcomes and esthetic results. Clin Oral Implants Res 2007;18:552–562.
15. Chen ST, Darby IB, Reynolds EC, Clement JG. Immediate implant placement post extraction without flap elevation. J Periodontol 2009;80:163–172.
16. DeRouck T, Collys K, Cosyn J. Immediate single-tooth implants in the anterior maxilla: a 1-year case cohort study on hard and soft tissue response. J Clin Periodontol 2008;35:649–657.
17. De Rouck T, Collys K, Wyn I, Cosyn J. Instant provisionalization of immediate single-tooth implants is essential to optimize esthetic treatment outcome. Clin Oral Implants Res 2009;20:566–570.
18. Kan JY, Rungcharassaeng K, Lozada JL, Zimmerman G. Facial gingival tissue stability following immediate placement and provisionalization of maxillary anterior single implants: a 2- to 8-year follow-up. Int J Oral Maxillofac Implants 2011;26:179–187.
19. Kan JY, Rungcharassaeng K, Sclar A, Lozada JL. Effects of the facial osseous defect morphology on gingival dynamics after immediate tooth replacement and guided bone regeneration: 1-year results. J Oral Maxillofac Surg 2007;65(7, Suppl 1):13–19.

20. Ferrus J, Cecchinato D, Pjetursson EB, et al. Factors influencing ridge alterations following immediate implant placement into extraction sockets. Clin Oral Implants Res 2010;21:22–29.
21. Koh RU, Oh TJ, Rudek I, et al. Hard and soft tissue changes after crestal and subcrestal immediate implant placement. J Periodontol 2011;82:1112–1120.
22. Evans CD, Chen ST. Esthetic outcomes of immediate implant placements. Clin Oral Implants Res 2008;19:73–80.
23. Seibert J, Lindhe J. Esthetics and periodontal therapy. In: Lindhe J (ed.), Textbook of Clinical Periodontology, 2nd edn. Copenhagen: Munksgaard; 1989, pp 477–514.
24. Crespi R, Cappare P, Gherlone E. A 4-year evaluation of the peri-implant parameters of immediately loaded implants placed in fresh extraction sockets. J Periodontol 2010;81:1629-1634.
25. Fu JH, Lee A, Wang HL. Influence of tissue biotype on implant esthetics. Int J Oral Maxillofac Implants 2011;26:499–508.
26. Kupershmidt I, Levin L, Schwartz-Arad D. Inter-implant bone height changes in anterior maxillary immediate and non-immediate adjacent dental implants. J Periodontol 2007;78:991–996.
27. Levin L, Pathael S, Dolev E, Schwartz-Arad D. Aesthetic versus surgical success of single dental implants: 1- to 9-year follow-up. Pract Proced Aesthet Dent 2005;17:533–538; quiz 540, 566.
28. Tomasi C, Sanz M, Cecchinato D, et al. Bone dimensional variations at implants placed in fresh extraction sockets: a multilevel multivariate analysis. Clin Oral Implants Res 2010;21:30–36.
29. Kan JY, Roe P, Rungcharassaeng K, et al. Classification of sagittal root position in relation to the anterior maxillary osseous housing for immediate implant placement: a cone beam computed tomography study. Int J Oral Maxillofac Implants 2011;26:873–876.
30. Chen ST, Buser D. Clinical and esthetic outcomes of implants placed in post extraction sites. Int J Oral Maxillofac Implants 2009;24(Suppl):186–217.
31. Koticha T, Fu JH, Chan HL, Wang HL. Influence of thread design on implant positioning in immediate implant placement. J Periodontol 2012;83:1420–1424.
32. Botticelli D, Berglundh T, Lindhe J. Resolution of bone defects of varying dimension and configuration in the marginal portion of the peri-implant bone. An experimental study in the dog. J Clin Periodontol 2004;31:309–317.
33. Schwartz-Arad D, Chaushu G. Immediate implant placement: a procedure without incisions. J Periodontol 1998;69:743–750.
34. Groisman M, Frossard WM, Ferreira HM, et al. Single-tooth implants in the maxillary incisor region with immediate provisionalization: 2-year prospective study. Pract Proced Aesthet Dent 2003;15:115–122, 124; quiz 126.
35. Canullo L, Rasperini G. Preservation of peri-implant soft and hard tissues using platform switching of implants placed in immediate extraction sockets: a proof-of-concept study with 12- to 36-month follow-up. Int J Oral Maxillofac Implants 2007;22:995–1000
36. Salama H, Salama M. The role of orthodontic extrusive remodeling in the enhancement of soft and hard tissue profile prior to implant placement: a systemic approach to the management of extraction site defects. Int Periodontics Restorative Dent 1993;13:312–333.
37. Hammerle CH, Araujo MG, Simion M. Evidence-based knowledge on the biology and treatment of extraction sockets. Clin Oral Implants Res 2012;23(Suppl 5):80–82.
38. Koh RU, Rudek I, Wang HL. Immediate implant placement: positives and negatives. Implant Dent 2010;19(2):98–108.
39. Lazzara RJ. Immediate implant placement into extraction sites: surgical and restorative advantages. Int Periodontics Restorative Dent 1989;9:332–343.
40. Saadoun AP, Le Galle M, Touati B. Selection and ideal tridimensional implant position for the soft tissue aesthetics. Pract Periodontics Aesthetic Dent 1999;11:1063–1072.
41. Tarnow DP, Cho SC, Wallace SS. The effect of inter-implant distance on the height of inter-implant bone crest. J Periodontol 2000;71:546–549.

Answers to Self-Study Questions

A. The timing of extraction and implant placement is classified as follows:
- type 1, immediate implant placement;
- type 2, early implant placement – 6–8 weeks after extraction to allow soft tissue healing over the extraction socket;
- type 3, delayed implant placement – 3–4 months after extraction;
- type 4, matured extraction site – typically more than 4 months of healing after extraction.

Immediate implant placement is defined as the placement of an implant immediately following tooth extraction and as part of the same surgical procedure [13].

A tooth assigned for extraction and subsequent immediate implant placement is generally diagnosed as nonsalvageable for at least one of the following reasons: endodontic failure, internal and/or external root resorption, root fracture, or subcrestal extensive caries. A tooth targeted for immediate implant placement should not present with any osseous defect. But, in practice, a tooth with a nonsalvageable diagnosis often will be associated with a compromised osseous anatomy. A careful examination of the targeted tooth is very important to ensure that immediate implant placement is indicated.

B. The immediate placement of implants has been well documented, and the predictability is generally similar to traditional staged implant placement [14–19].

When reviewing the literature and in clinical practice, however, it is important to keep in mind that implant survival and esthetic outcomes of immediate implant placement in the esthetic zone should be evaluated separately.

Incorrect implant selection, incorrect three-dimensional implant positioning, an unfavorable extraction socket anatomy and surrounding soft tissue profile, and unpredicted hard and soft tissue remodeling/resorption could result in esthetic complications [14–18,20–29].

C. Thin biotype and/or buccal plate bony defects are associated with a higher chance of poor esthetic outcomes with immediate implant placement [30]. There is a natural tendency for surgical drills and implants to shift buccally during the surgery, which leads to a more buccally inclined implant position and a smaller gap between the buccal bony wall and the implant [31]. A staged, delayed approach is warranted for some cases.

D. Buccal bone remodeling/resorption after tooth extraction is very unpredictable. And immediate implant placement into an extraction socket has little or no effect on buccal bone remodeling/resorption [32]. The literature contains reports of buccal tissue volume loss, mid facial recession, and papillae height loss after immediate implant placement [14–18].

Bone grafting into the gap between the implant body and the buccal bone wall of the extraction socket has been shown to significantly reduce horizontal buccal bone resorption [14,16,17,19,21]. Many different grafting materials were studied, including autogenous bone grafts [33,34], allografts

[21], and xenografts [14,16,17,19], and all showed positive outcomes.

Use of a connective tissue graft also has been shown to have a positive effect by increasing the soft tissue thickness and the soft tissue level gain [15,19]. A flapless approach is a less invasive and less traumatic option for an immediate implant placement [8,15,18]. Platform switching [35] and immediate provisionalization [16,19,24] also have some positive effects on final esthetic outcomes by reducing buccal tissue volume loss, mid facial recession, and papillae height loss. Orthodontic extrusion prior to immediate implant placement could potentially improve esthetic outcomes [36]. Potential benefits of orthodontic extrusion are the following:

- it augments the crestal bone height and width and the overlaying gingival tissue, decreasing the negative impact of postextraction alveolar resorption and recession;
- it decreases or minimizes the gap between the implant and the extraction socket;
- it helps to enhance primary stability on the implant by developing the alveolar bone beyond the root apex; and
- it helps to facilitate extraction by loosening the tooth.

E. According to the Osteology Consensus Report implant placement leads to high survival rates [37]. Indications regarding sites for single tooth implants include molar sites with limited indications due to anatomical reasons and premolars as the most favorable sites due to anatomical situation and low esthetic demands. In addition, critical evaluation of the gingival and bone architecture, hard and soft tissue, and smile line are essential for implant esthetics.

A list of clinical indications and absolute/relative contraindications for immediate implant placement has been described [21,38]. For indications, many factors that relate to local and systemic health of the patient are included: (1) systemically healthy patients, (2) adequate soft tissue, (3) adequate hard tissue, (4) intact facial plate, and (5) thick tissue biotype. Absolute contraindications include (1) compromised systemic diseases, (2) maxillary sinus involvement, (3) history of bisphosphonates, (4) history of periodontal disease, (5) absence of intact labial bone, and (6) presence of active infection. Heavy smokers are relatively contraindicated for immediate implant placement.

F.
Advantages
- Preservation of the soft tissue drape and the bone architecture.
- Reduce the number of dental appointments [39].
- Reduce the number of surgical procedures.
- Fast rehabilitation of the area.
- Avoid raising a flap.
- Utilizes all available existing bone.

Disadvantages
- Technique sensitive for ideal three-dimensional implant positioning [40].
- Increased risk for infection and associated failures.
- Primary closure is more difficult to achieve.
- The discrepancy of morphology of implant and socket preservation may influence primary stability.

- Primary stability is mostly done in the apical region.
- Optimum esthetic outcome in a patient with thin biotype may not be predictable [14].

G. An ideally placed immediate implant in the esthetic zone should engage the palatal wall of the extraction socket and leave a gap between the buccal bone of the extraction socket and the implant body of at least 2 mm or more [14,32].

The implant platform should be positioned 2–4 mm apical to the mid-facial aspect of the free gingival margin of the final restoration [40]. The implant angulation has been suggested in the following angulations: (1) the facial angulation to mimic the emergence profile of the adjacent tooth; (2) under the incisal edge of the final restoration; (3) within the cingulum position of the implant crown. Care must be taken to assure that the distance to the adjacent tooth is at least 1.5 mm [41]. Crestal bone should be at least 1 mm wider than the implant on the facial and the palatal aspects.

Case 3

Delayed Placement: Site Development

CASE STORY

A 73-year-old Caucasian man presented to the clinic with the chief concern of wanting implants on his lower right jaw. The patient's dental history revealed that he had a four-unit fixed partial bridge from teeth #27 to #30 with pontics on teeth #28 and #29 (Figure 1). Tooth #30 was diagnosed with a vertical fracture and had to be extracted. At the time of extraction of tooth #30, the bridge was sectioned between pontic #28 and the abutment of tooth #27. An atraumatic extraction of tooth #30 (11-16-2012) was performed, showing adequate buccal plate thickness. A collagen wound dressing (Helicote®) was applied in the socket, and an X-suture with 5/0 Vicryl® was used.

When the patient presented to the clinic he had single-unit crowns on teeth #27 and #31 with an edentulous space from teeth #28 to #30 (Figure 2). The patient stated that his last professional debridement or prophylaxis had taken place 9 months earlier. He reports brushing with a manual toothbrush twice a day and flossing daily. He occasionally uses an interproximal toothbrush.

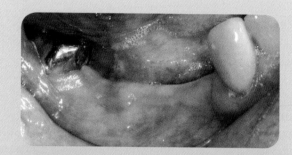

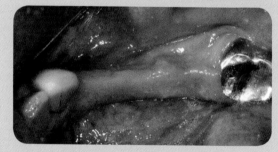

Figure 2: Initial clinical situation.

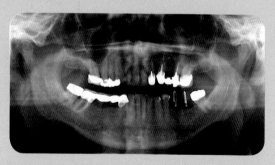

Figure 1: Panoramic showing the four-unit bridge from #27 to #30.

LEARNING GOALS AND OBJECTIVES

- To understand when to utilize horizontal ridge augmentation
- To understand the various materials utilized in guided bone regeneration (GBR)
- To understand the surgical technique employed in GBR
- To understand how to evaluate the treatment outcome

Medical History

At the time of the initial visit the patient presented with a history of glaucoma that was controlled with timolol and Xalatan® eyedrops. The patient also has hypercholesterolemia that is controlled with lovastatin. He also reports having heartburn that is controlled with famotidine. He was also taking low-dose aspirin (81 mg/day) and a multivitamin complex prophylactically. He did not report any drug allergy.

Review of Systems

- Vital signs:
  - Blood pressure: 132/79 mmHg
  - Pulse: 62 beats/min
  - Respiration: 16 breaths/min

Social History

The patient is a former smoker who smoked a pack a day for 28 years. He quit smoking in 1983.

Extraoral Examination

No significant findings were noted. The patient exhibited no masses or swelling, and the temporomandibular joint was within normal limits, with no clicking, popping, or deviation of the mandible upon opening. There was no noticeable facial asymmetry, and his lymph nodes appeared normal on palpation.

Intraoral Examination

The oral cancer screening was negative. The soft tissue exam, including the tongue, cheeks, throat, and floor of the mouth, were within normal limits.

Once the medical history was reviewed, clinical reports were taken. This included the following:

- complete mouth periapical series and panoramic radiographs;
- study casts;
- intra- and extraoral photographs;
- periodontal charting (e.g., bleeding on probing, probing depth, clinical attachment loss, recession, mucogingival defects, mobility, and suppuration)
- dental examination evaluating fremitus, centric relation prematurities, working and nonworking side contacts, occlusal wear, open interproximal contacts, and caries.

The periodontal examination revealed localized >3 mm probing depths (see Figure 3) – 4 mm: #3, #5, #14, #18, #20, and #31.

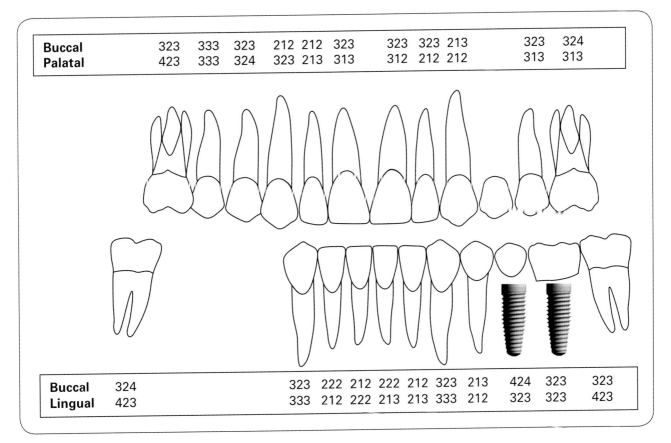

Figure 3: Periodontal chart.

There was localized marginal erythema noted on the marginal gingiva and the interdental papilla. There was a localized presence of plaque and a localized slight calculus accumulation. On probing, localized bleeding on probing was also found.

Occlusion

No occlusal discrepancies or interferences were noted. However, there was evidence of parafunctional habits with slight generalized attrition.

Radiographic Examination

A full mouth radiographic series was exposed (Figure 4). The radiographic examination revealed a generalized mild to moderate horizontal bone loss pattern with absence of crestal lamina dura. There was a defective restoration on tooth #13D.

Diagnosis

- Partial edentulism
- Caries on tooth #15
- Defective restorations
- Generalized slight–moderate chronic periodontitis (based on Armitage's classification [1])

- Developmental or acquired deformities and conditions
  - Mucogingival deformities and conditions around teeth:
    - soft tissue recession
    - lack of keratinized gingiva
  - Mucogingival deformities and conditions on edentulous ridges:
    - vertical and horizontal ridge deficiency (Seibert class III)
    - abnormal color
  - Peri-implant mucositis associated with implants in the area of tooth #20 (based on Zitzmann and Berglundh's definition [2])

Treatment Plan

The treatment plan for this patient consisted of four phases that included the following.

Phase I

- patient motivation;
- instruction in appropriate oral hygiene technique;
- full mouth debridement (prophylaxis);
- caries control;

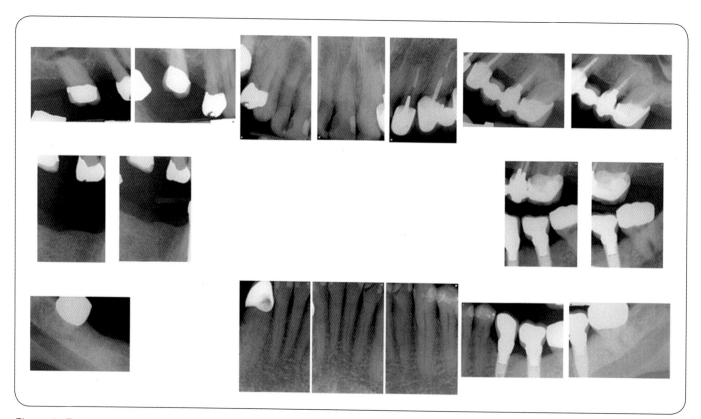

Figure 4: Full-mouth radiographs

- cone beam computed tomography (CBCT) scan of mandibular right quadrant;
- reevaluation of initial phase after 4–6 weeks.

Phase II
- pre-implant GBR of area around teeth #28–#30;
- implant placement on teeth #28–#30, occurring 6 months after GBR.

Phase III
- three-unit implant-supported fixed partial denture.

Phase IV
- night guard;
- maintenance every 3 months;
- complete periodontal evaluation every 12 months, periapical radiographs and bitewings at 6 months after prosthesis installation and every 1–2 years thereafter.

Treatment
After the initial-phase therapy, the patient presented for a horizontal ridge augmentation procedure. After clinical inspection, the area presented with a severe horizontal and slight vertical ridge deficiency (Seibert class III). There was inadequate buccolingual width to assure

ideal implant placement. Following profound anesthesia at the surgical site using local anesthetic (Marcaine® 0.5% and Septocaine® 4%), a midcrestal incision was performed on the edentulous area #28–#30 that extended to the adjacent teeth #27 and #31 (Figure 5A). Buccal and lingual mucoperiosteal flaps were reflected beyond the mucogingival junction. A severe concavity was observed on the buccal aspect of teeth #28 and #29 (Figure 5B). The osseous crest was decorticated with a #1/2 round carbide bur to allow entry of cells to the bone graft scaffold (Figure 5C and D). A periosteal fenestration was performed on the buccal flap to allow adequate flap release and a tension-free primary closure. A 30 mm × 40 mm resorbable collagen membrane (RCM6 – ACE®) was positioned over the defect, extending at least 3 mm over the defect in all directions (Figure 5E).

A bovine-derived xenograft (Bio-Oss®) was hydrated with sterile saline and packed into the defect (Figure 5E). The resorbable membrane was adapted over the bone graft. The flaps were repositioned over the membrane, and sutured with 5/0 Vicryl as simple interrupted sutures (Figure 5F). This helped achieve

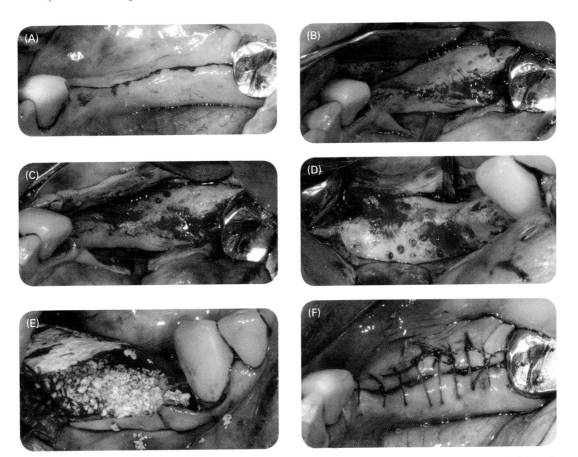

Figure 5: GBR: (A) incision; (B) defect morphology; (C, D) crestal bone decortication; (E) xenograft plus resorbable collagen membrane placed over the defect; (F) suture.

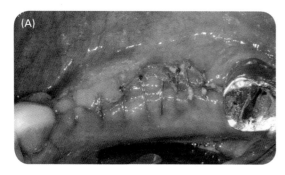 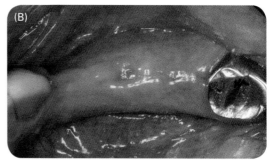

Figure 6: (A) Two weeks post-op. (B) Eight weeks post-op.

primary flap closure. An ice pack was given to the patient following the surgery. The patient was instructed to take 600 mg of ibuprofen three times a day for the first 2 days and then as needed. Chlorhexidine 0.12% mouthwash was prescribed to be used twice a day for 14 days postoperatively. In addition, 500 mg of amoxicillin was prescribed to be taken orally every 8 h for 7 days. After 2 weeks, the sutures were removed, and the area was debrided with chlorhexidine (Figure 6). The adjacent teeth were gently debrided using hand instruments.

Following 6 months of healing, a CBCT scan was exposed, noting significant buccal bone gain (Figure 7). With the tri-dimensional information, the inferior

alveolar canal, mental foramen, and a possible lingual concavity were identified. Two implants – 10 mm regular platform for #28 and 10 mm wide platform for #30 (Nobel® Replace Select)– were placed according to the manufacturer's instructions (Figure 8). The implants were restored 3 months following their placement.

Discussion

Several surgical techniques have been used to correct ridge deformities and to create an adequate bony housing for dental implants. GBR is a procedure that uses occlusive barrier membranes to protect osseous defects from the ingrowth of soft tissue cells and encourages the development of new bone [3].

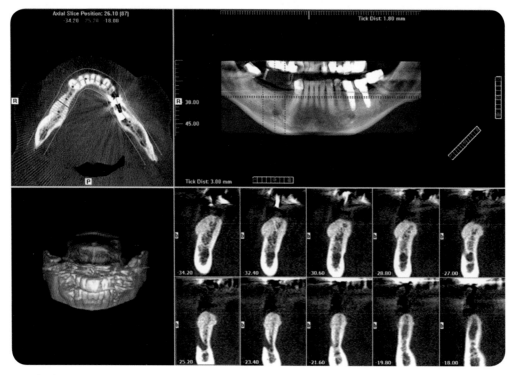

Figure 7: Pre-implant CBCT scan.

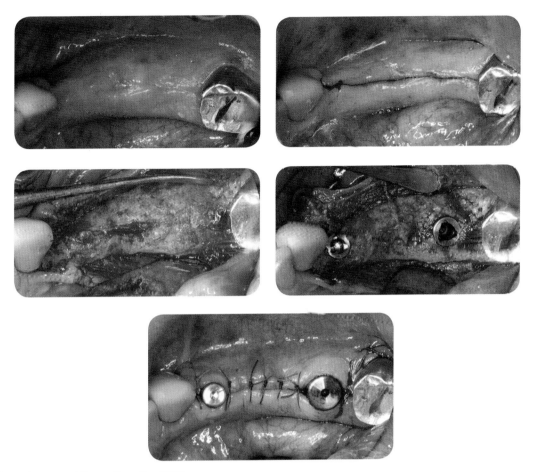

Figure 8: Implant placement 6 months after GBR.

The concept of GBR is derived from the application of the guided tissue regeneration (GTR) principle, in which vertical bone defects around teeth were regenerated through the use of barrier membranes that excluded the ingrowth of gingival epithelial and connective tissue and allowed the repopulation of the root surface with cells originating from the periodontal ligament [4]. With this concept, Dahlin et al. [5] investigated bone regeneration in an animal study using expanded polytetrafluoroethylene (ePTFE) membranes. By this means, a secluded space was created between the inner surface of the membrane and the bone defect, which would keep the nonosteogenic extraskeletal connective tissue from proliferating into the defect [6].

The three most common applications of GBR are [7]:

1. for ridge augmentation and subsequent placement of dental implants;
2. in conjunction with implant placement;
3. to cover an already installed implant with a peri-implant bone defect.

Wang and Boyapati [8] underlined the four major principles for successful GBR, which are referred to as PASS:

1. primary wound closure;
2. angiogenesis;
3. space creation/maintenance;
4. stability of initial blood clot and implant fixture.

The principal materials for GBR are barrier membranes. They can be divided into resorbable and nonresorbable membranes.

- Resorbable:
  - natural – porcine or bovine collagen
  - synthetic – polylactic acid, copolymers of polylactic acid, or polyglycolic acid.
- Nonresorbable – polytetrafluoroethylene (PTFE), ePTFE, or titanium mesh.

The other components of GBR are agents and biomaterials that are placed under the membrane to preserve the space to be regenerated. They might be applied by themselves or in combination with one another. The most widely used are the following [3].

- Autogenous bone grafts are taken from other sites in the same patient.
- Allografts come from cadavers of the same species as the recipient. The most widely used are demineralized, freeze-dried bone allograft (DFDBA) or freeze-dried bone allograft (FDBA). Both are resorbable; the only difference is in the rate of resorption. Whereas DFDBA can be resorbed in a few months, FDBA will be resorbed more slowly and, as a result, will maintain the space for a longer period [9].

- Xenografts are derived from a species different from the recipient's, such as a cow or horse. The most commonly used source is bovine bone, once its organic component has been removed. Its rate of resorption is slower than that of allografts, and in some instances it is never resorbed [10–12].
- Alloplastic graft materials are synthetic bone substitutes that include bioactive glasses and calcium phosphates.

Self-Study Questions

(Answers located at the end of the case)

A. When is horizontal ridge augmentation employed?

B. What are the available techniques for horizontal ridge augmentation?

C. What is the difference between osteogenic, osteoconductive, and osteoinductive bone graft material?

D. What is the role of barrier membranes in GBR?

E. What are the different types of bone graft materials?

F. How long should nonresorbable membranes stay submerged to avoid complications during healing?

G. What are the potential surgical complications that result in unfavorable surgical outcomes?

H. What are the potential healing complications that negatively affect the surgical outcome?

References

1. Armitage GC. Development of a classification system for periodontal diseases and conditions. Ann Periodontol 1999;4(1):1–6.
2. Zitzmann NU, Berglundh T. Definition and prevalence of peri-implant diseases. J Clin Periodontol 2008;35(8 Suppl):286–291.
3. Esposito M, Grusovin MG, Felice P, et al. Interventions for replacing missing teeth: horizontal and vertical bone augmentation techniques for dental implant treatment. Cochrane Database Syst Rev 2009;(4):CD003607.
4. Gottlow J, Nyman S, Karring T, Lindhe J. New attachment formation as the result of controlled tissue regeneration. J Clin Periodontol 1984;11(8):494–503.
5. Dahlin C, Linde A, Gottlow J, Nyman S. Healing of bone defects by guided tissue regeneration. Plast Reconstr Surg 1988;81(5):672–676.
6. Seibert J, Nyman S. Localized ridge augmentation in dogs: a pilot study using membranes and hydroxyapatite. J Periodontol 1990;61(3):157–165.
7. Buser D, Brägger U, Lang NP, Nyman S. Regeneration and enlargement of jaw bone using guided tissue regeneration. Clin Oral Implants Res 1990;1(1):22–32.
8. Wang HL, Boyapati L. "PASS" principles for predictable bone regeneration. Implant Dent 2006;15(1):8–17.
9. Wood RA, Mealey BL. Histologic comparison of healing after tooth extraction with ridge preservation using mineralized versus demineralized freeze-dried bone allograft. J Periodontol 2012;83(3):329–336.
10. Galindo-Moreno P, Hernández-Cortés P, Mesa F, et al. Slow resorption of anorganic bovine bone by osteoclasts in maxillary sinus augmentation. Clin Implant Dent Relat Res 2013;15(6):858–866.
11. Sartori S, Silvestri M, Forni F, et al. Ten-year follow-up in a maxillary sinus augmentation using anorganic bovine bone (Bio-Oss). A case report with histomorphometric evaluation. Clin Oral Implants Res 2003;14(3):369–372.
12. Skoglund A, Hising P, Young C. A clinical and histologic examination in humans of the osseous response to implanted natural bone mineral. Int J Oral Maxillofac Implants 1997;12(2):194–199.
13. Schropp L, Wenzel A, Kostopoulos L, Karring T. Bone healing and soft tissue contour changes following single-tooth extraction: a clinical and radiographic 12-month prospective study. Int J Periodontics Restorative Dent 2003;23(4):313–323.

14. Iasella JM, Greenwell H, Miller RL, et al. Ridge preservation with freeze-dried bone allograft and a collagen membrane compared to extraction alone for implant site development: a clinical and histologic study in humans. J Periodontol 2003;74(7):990–999.
15. Cardaropoli G, Araújo M, Lindhe J. Dynamics of bone tissue formation in tooth extraction sites. An experimental study in dogs. J Clin Periodontol 2003;30(9):809–818.
16. Araújo MG, Lindhe J. Dimensional ridge alterations following tooth extraction. An experimental study in the dog. J Clin Periodontol 2005;32(2):212–218.
17. Nevins M, Camelo M, De Paoli S, et al. A study of the fate of the buccal wall of extraction sockets of teeth with prominent roots. Int J Periodontics Restorative Dent 2006;26(1):19–29.
18. Becker W, Becker BE. Guided tissue regeneration for implants placed into extraction sockets and for implant dehiscences: surgical techniques and case report. Int J Periodontics Restorative Dent 1990;10(5):376–391.
19. Becker W, Becker BE, Handlesman M, et al. Bone formation at dehisced dental implant sites treated with implant augmentation material: a pilot study in dogs. Int J Periodontics Restorative Dent 1990;10(2):92–101.
20. Becker W, Dahlin C, Becker B, et al. The use of e-PTFE barrier membranes for bone promotion around titanium implants placed into extraction sockets: a prospective multicenter study. Int J Oral Maxillofac Implants 1994;9(1):31–40.
21. Villar CC, Cochran DL. Regeneration of periodontal tissues: guided tissue regeneration. Dent Clin North Am 2010;54(1):73–92.

Answers to Self-Study Questions

A. Buccolingual bone resorption is one of the common sequelae following tooth extraction [13–16]. The extent of this defect can be severe following extraction of teeth with advanced periodontal disease or periapical lesions. This severe defect leads to complications during the implant placement, such as failure to place an implant in an ideal position and thread exposures [17]. Horizontal ridge augmentation can be utilized to generate hard tissue over the existing ridge buccolingually to overcome this challenge. Horizontal ridge augmentation can be performed either prior to implant placement in a separate surgery or at the time of implant placement.

B.
• Particulate bone graft with/without growth factors and barrier membrane (Figure 5).
• Autogenous block graft (e.g., chin graft, ramus graft) with or without membrane.
• Block allograft (freeze-dried bone) with or without membrane.
• Ridge-splitting technique.

C.
• Osteogenic: any "live-autograft" tissue or substance with the potential to induce growth or repair of bone.

• Osteoconductive: graft material that provides a matrix for cell migration (e.g., FDBA).
• Osteoinductive: bone formation stimulated in the surrounding tissue by the presence of the graft material that has the ability to "induce" tissue formation – typically growth factor is present (e.g., demineralized bone matrix).

D. Membranes act as physical barriers if they are adapted over bone grafts, preventing the ingrowth of nonosteogenic cells into the membrane-protected space (Figure 5E). Membranes also allow the ingrowth of osteogenic cells to populate [7]. Secondary-wound/graft stabiliztion.

E.
• Autogenous: bone taken from one area of the patient and transplanted to another area in the same patient.
• Allograft: bone from same species, different donor. Bone from a tissue bank (i.e., cadaver bone).
• Xenograft: bone from another species (Figure 5E).
• Synthetic: material used as a bone graft substitute (i.e., alloplast).

F. Studies have shown that nonresorbable ePTFE membranes should remain submerged completely for 6–9 months to allow for uneventful healing and bone growth [18–20].

G.

- *Flap damage.* Excessive thinning of the flap and a deep periosteal incision should be avoided. Flap damage will result in improper soft tissue healing and jeopardize vascular supply.
- *Neurovascular complications.* The locations of critical anatomical structures, such as the mental nerve, infraorbital nerve, lingual nerve, sublingual artery, and mylohyoideus artery, need to be studied carefully during the presurgical phase. Care should be taken during the surgery not to induce direct trauma to these structures.

H.

- *Premature exposure of the membrane to the oral environment.* Clinicians should manage membrane exposure by considering the extent of the exposure, presence or absence of purulent exudate, and patient compliance with a strict hygiene regimen. The patient should be seen weekly and instructed to use chlorhexidine. The membrane may need to be removed if the exposure is increasing.
- *Infection of the graft or the surgical wound.* Patient factors, such as systemic conditions and smoking, or surgical-technique-related factors may predispose a patient to a postsurgical infection. The patient should take antibiotics and rinse with 0.12% chlorhexidine postoperatively [21].
- *Premature loss of the bone graft.* Premature disintegration of graft material may be followed by premature membrane exposure.

Conclusions

GBR is a critical and complex surgical technique of capital importance prior to or during implant placement. Each clinician should utilize the materials or techniques according to their preferences, experience, and the needs of the patient. Therefore, there is no single path to optimal clinical outcomes. The most important step in GBR is the diagnosis of the initial situation and the awareness of the final implant's outcome.

Case 4

Submerged Implant Placement and Provisional Restorations

CASE STORY

A 26-year-old Caucasian female presented with the following chief complaint: "I have been missing my lateral incisors forever and have Maryland bridges, which had to be re-glued a couple of times recently. I hope the missing teeth can be replaced with implants and crowns. I also had a bike accident as a child and chipped my central incisors. They were repaired with tooth-colored fillings. I hope for pretty front teeth with a better color match than now."

LEARNING GOALS AND OBJECTIVES

- To recognize the specific clinical indications for submerged implant placement and its advantages
- To understand the concept and importance of contour augmentation at time of implant placement
- To outline the treatment steps and sequence involved with submerged implant placement in the esthetic zone
- To describe options for temporary restoration prior to implant placement, during submerged implant healing, and after second-stage surgery

Medical History

The patient had an unremarkable medical history without any contraindications for dental treatment, including surgical procedures. She was not taking any medications and had no known drug, food, and/or material allergies.

Review of Systems

- Vital signs
  - Average blood pressure: 117/70 mmHg
  - Average respiration rate: 16 breaths/min
  - Average pulse rate: 70 beats/min

Dental History and Patient Compliance

The patient presented with absent teeth #7 and #10 (FDI #12 and #22) (congenitally missing). They had been replaced with a metal-ceramic resin-bonded fixed prosthesis (Figure 1), which in recent months had to be rebonded twice. Partial fractures of teeth #8 and #9 (FDI #11 and #21) caused by a childhood dental trauma were restored with composite restorations. She brushes and flosses daily and follows regular visits with her hygienist and general dentist every 6 months. The patient did not have any orthodontic treatment and was not aware of any bruxism or clenching.

Social History

The patient revealed no history of smoking or use of tobacco-containing products. She does occasionally drink alcohol socially. She works full time in the

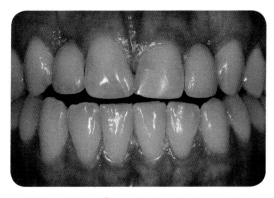

Figure 1: Efrontal view. Congenitally missing teeth #7 and #10 (FDI #12 and #22) replaced with resin-bonded fixed dental prosthesis; composite repair of tooth fracture #9 (FDI #21).

administration of a large dental laboratory and has limited insurance coverage for implants and related prosthodontic procedures.

Extraoral Examination

There were no significant findings. No masses or lesions were noted, and lymph nodes of the head and neck were within normal limits. Temporomandibular joints and muscles of the head and neck were without symptoms upon palpation. Mandibular range of motion was excellent.

Esthetic Risk Assessment

The patient's lip line was low (Figure 2). She did not reveal any of the gingival marginal areas of her anterior teeth in her smile and speech, and the noted difference in gingival marginal height between her two central incisors was not at all a concern to her. The correction of the notable color mismatch in her upper anterior teeth did not present a major problem in terms of restorative management. Her expectations in regard to the esthetic outcome were reasonable and appeared fully achievable.

Intraoral Examination

Floor of the mouth, tongue, cheek, palate, and oropharynx were all within normal limits. No masses or lesions were detected. Salivary flow was normal.

Except for teeth #7 and #10 (FDI #12 and #22) and the third molars, all teeth were present, vital, and free of caries. Teeth #8 and #9 showed extended composite restorations. Intact amalgam restorations were present on the upper first premolars (class 2), as well as the upper second premolars and upper molars (class 1). The missing upper lateral incisors had been replaced with a one-piece, acid-etched fixed prosthesis based on a metal retainer extending along the lingual surfaces from teeth #6 to #11 (FDI #13–#11 and #21–#23) (Figure 3). Metallic shine through caused by the lingual retainer portion of the resin-bonded bridge was noted especially on tooth #8. Multiple white spots due to fluorosis were

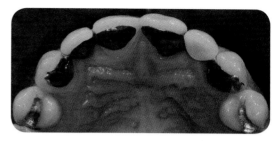

Figure 3: Occlusal view of resin-bonded prosthesis #6–#8 (FDI #13–#11) and #9–#11 (FDI #21–#23). Class 2 amalgam restorations #5 and #12 (FDI #14 and 24).

noted on her upper anterior teeth. In addition, mild to moderate chipping and wear of the lower incisors and canines was recorded. The interdental space between canines and central incisors was ≥6 mm for both sites #7 and #10. The edentulous areas showed mild to moderate horizontal bone deficiencies (Seibert class I) [1,2] (Figure 4). Soft tissues in the edentulous sites were well keratinized and attached. Her gingival biotype was defined as moderately thin [3].

The periodontal examination showed healthy gingivae with absence of bleeding. Probing depths were within 1–2 mm for all teeth.

Occlusal Analysis

The molar and canine occlusal relationship was class 1. No occlusal discrepancies or interferences were noted. The mentioned mild to moderate incisal/cuspal chipping and/or wear of the lower incisors and canines did not seem to be caused by bruxism according to the patient's opinion.

Radiographic Examination

Since the patient was in regular dental care with her family dentist and revealed clinically healthy oral and dental conditions, new radiographic studies were only obtained for the maxillary anterior areas requiring treatment. Periapical radiographs showed overall

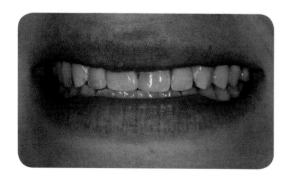

Figure 2: Smile line.

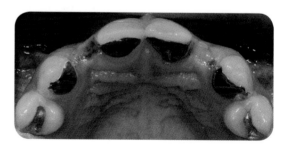

Figure 4: Occlusal view of anterior maxillary area after removal of pontics #7 and #10. Note areas of localized inflammation of alveolar ridge mucosa caused by the pontics #7 and #10.

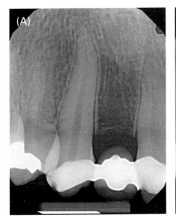
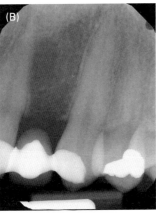

Figure 5: Periapical radiographs of (A) edentulous site #7 and adjacent teeth #6 and #8, and (B) edentulous site #10 and adjacent teeth #9 and #11.

healthy conditions with normal bone levels in the area of teeth #6–#11 (FDI #13–#11, #21–#23) (Figure 5). Roots adjacent to the edentulous sites were parallel and in sufficient distance from each other for safe implant placement. An idiopathic radiolucency was observed in site #10 distal to the apical portion of tooth #9.

Cone beam computer tomograms were ordered, which revealed labial concavities in the alveolar ridge of sites #7 and #10 that would require contour augmentation via simultaneous bone grafting at the time of implant placement (Figure 6).

Diagnosis

The oral–dental diagnoses were as follows: partial edentulism due to congenitally missing maxillary lateral incisors. Failing resin-bonded fixed dental prosthesis in the maxillary anterior. Incisal fractures of teeth #8 and #9 restored with composite. Occlusal wear on lower front teeth most likely caused by excursive occlusal contacts on the metal retainer portion of the resin-bonded prosthesis.

Treatment Plan

The treatment plan for this patient included the removal of the resin-bonded prosthesis and its replacement with an interim partial denture, followed by implant placement in sites #7 and #10 combined with labial bone grafting using xenografts and absorbable membranes for contour augmentation; 6–8 weeks after implant placement, second-stage surgery with impressions for temporary implant restorations for the purpose of soft tissue contouring; 2–3 months after delivery of the implant provisionals, preparation of teeth #8 and #9 for veneers and impressions for the final restorations (implants #7 and #10: zirconia custom abutments and cemented full ceramic crowns; teeth #8 and #9 labial ceramic veneers).

Both surgical and restorative risk assessments were performed based on the clinical esthetic risk assessment outline above and the digital implant plan (Figure 6).

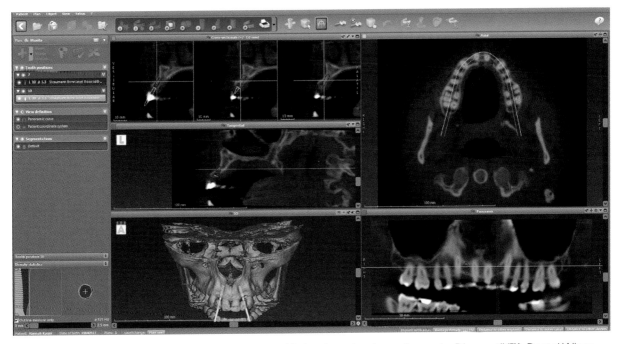

Figure 6: Cone beam computer tomographic images viewed in implant planning software (coDiagnostiX™, Dental Wings, Montreal, Canada) including implant plans for sites #7 and #10.

Using the SAC classification [4], surgical and restorative levels of difficulty were determined as being *advanced*.

Treatment

Surgical

Upon completion of diagnosis, treatment planning, and fabrication of a surgical template and an interim removable partial denture to replace #7 and #10 postoperatively, the patient presented for implant surgery. She had been prescribed a perioperative antibiotic regimen of amoxicillin 875 mg twice daily for 5 days starting with breakfast on the morning of the surgery appointment. First, the acid-etched interim fixed dental prosthesis was removed by cutting the metal frame in the connector areas adjacent to each tooth involved. The lingual retainer units on each tooth could not easily be removed and were left in place for the time being to not extend the appointment duration unnecessarily. The mouth was carefully washed to remove all debris and the implant areas, which were now fully visible after removal of the resin-bonded prosthesis, were inspected (Figure 4). Localized erythema of the underlying mucosa caused by the pontics was observed in both sites. The interim partial denture was tried in for fit, retention, and proper occlusion. Adjustments were made as needed. The patient then was asked to rinse with chlorhexidine gluconate 0.12% for 30 s. Local anesthesia for each site was achieved via local infiltration of 1.8 mL articaine 4%, 1 : 100,000 epinephrine, per site. Site #7 was treated first, followed by site #10. Crestal incisions lingual to the height of each papilla involved were made, followed by intrasulcular incisions that extended to the distal or mesial aspects of each tooth neighboring the implant sites. No vertical relieving incisions were placed (Figure 7).

Full-thickness flaps were gently elevated, and the implant sites prepared according to the manufacturer's guidelines with the help of a conventional surgical guide

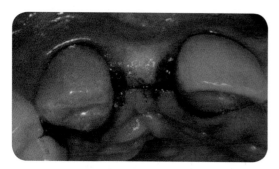

Figure 7: Incision design (image from different patient with similar indication and treatment plan).

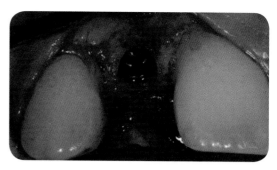

Figure 8: Implant inserted to appropriate depth after localized flap elevation and implant site preparation.

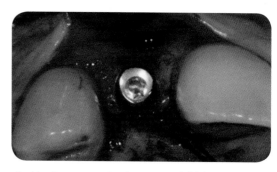

Figure 9: Healing screw in place; note labial ridge concavity.

obtained from the prosthodontic plan. In each site, a 3.3 mm diameter, 10 mm long Bone Level Narrow Crossfit implant (BL NC), TiZr, SLActive (Straumann USA, Andover, MA) was inserted. Implants were placed to a cervical depth about 3 mm apical to the cement–enamel junction of the adjacent central incisors (Figure 8).

Confirmation of primary stability was assessed with the insertion torque instrument and was found to be >30 N cm for each implant. A cover screw for BL NC implants with 0.5 mm height (Straumann USA, Andover, MA) was placed onto each implant (Figure 9).

Labial contour augmentation was performed by placing a layer of autogenous bone retrieved from the implant drill flutes directly onto the implant surfaces, followed by adding the necessary bulk with anorganic bovine bone (Figure 10), which was covered with a layer

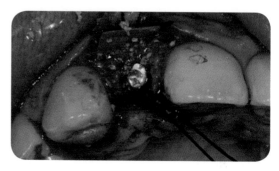

Figure 10: Contour augmentation with anorganic bovine bone.

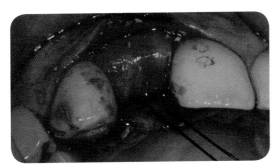

Figure 11: Bone graft coverage with absorbable collagen membrane.

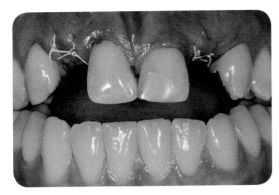

Figure 12: Primary flap closure with interrupted Teflon sutures.

of a resorbable collagen membrane (Bio-Oss and Bio-Gide, Geistlich Pharma North America, Inc., Princeton, NJ) (Figure 11).

Each flap was then closed tension free using three interrupted Teflon sutures (GoreTex, W.L. & Associates, Flagstaff, AZ), leaving the implants with cover screws submerged under the local oral mucosa (Figure 12).

The cervical aspects of teeth #7 and #10 in the interim partial denture were shortened to assure the absence of any pressure to the surgical sites (Figure 13). The patient was dismissed after she was given instructions for postoperative care, verbally and in writing.

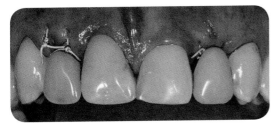

Figure 13: Denture teeth #7 and #10 in interim removable partial denture adjusted to avoid direct contact to underlying tissues.

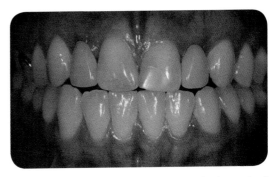

Figure 14: Follow-up at 2 weeks postoperatively; esthetic adjustment to interim partial denture teeth #7 and #10 by adding acrylic to extend tooth length cervically.

Postoperative Care

As mentioned earlier, the patient was prescribed a 5-day perioperative regimen of amoxicillin 875 mg q 12 h starting with breakfast on the day of surgery. Additionally, ibuprofen 600 mg q 6 h as needed for pain control and a 7-day regimen of 0.12% chlorhexidine gluconate mouthwash were prescribed. The patient was seen 1 week after surgery for a follow-up, and 2 weeks postoperatively for suture removal. At the 2-week postoperative visit, the incision areas in both sites were firmly closed, which allowed the addition of acrylic resin to extend the cervical length of the denture teeth over the implant sites to improve esthetics (Figure 14).

Second-Stage Surgery and Impression for Provisional Restorations

The implant sites were allowed to heal for 8 weeks, at which time second-stage surgery combined with impressions for provisional implant restorations were preformed. Second-stage surgery included a small amount of local infiltration anesthetic (0.9 mL lidocaine 2%, 1 : 100,000 epinephrine per site). Since a wide band of keratinized mucosa was present over both sites (Figure 15), access to the cover screws was obtained with a 3 mm diameter disposable punch (ACE Surgical Supply Inc., Brockton, MA) (Figure 16).

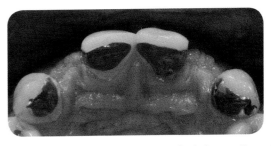

Figure 15: Occlusal view of healed surgical sites at 8 weeks postoperatively.

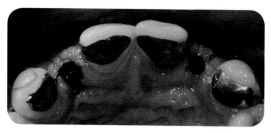

Figure 16: Punch access to top of implant healing screws using a 3 mm diameter tissue punch. Note presence of wide band of well-keratinized attached mucosa.

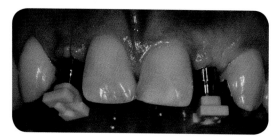

Figure 17: Closed-tray impression posts inserted after removal of healing screws.

After removal of the cover screws, closed-tray impression posts (Narrow Crossfit, Straumann USA, Andover, MA) were placed (Figure 17) and a polyether impression (Impregum, 3M ESPE, St. Paul, MN) obtained. Impression posts were removed and transmucosal healing abutments placed (NC Healing Abutments, height 5 mm, diameter 3.5 mm, Straumann USA, Andover, MA). A mandibular full-arch alginate opposing impression was taken as well, and the shade obtained for manufacture of laboratory-processed provisional crowns.

Provisional Restoration and Tissue Shaping

Owing to the fact that both implants could not be placed in an axis that allowed screw-retained temporary crowns, customized provisional abutments were made using poly(methyl methacrylate) (PMMA) temporary abutments (NC Temporary Abutment VITA CAD-Temp®, height 11 mm, diameter mm, PMMA, TAN; Straumann USA, Andover, MA). They were completed with heat-cured acrylic provisional crowns (Figure 18). The provisional abutments and crowns were designed with the proper emergence contours for the respective teeth to be replaced with the goal to optimally shape and mature the peri-implant soft tissues in sites #7 and #10 prior to final prosthodontics treatment in the area.

Temporary abutments and crowns were delivered 2 weeks after second-stage surgery and impression. A small amount of local anesthetic was again applied

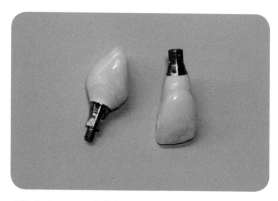

Figure 18: Laboratory-fabricated provisional implant restorations #7 and #10. Customizable polymer abutments with a titanium base for Bone Level Narrow Crossfit implants (Institut Straumann AG, Basel, Switzerland, http://www.straumann.com/) were used. Provisional crowns were made from heat-cured acrylic. Note the emergence contours of the transmucosal portion of the customized abutments and the scalloped finishing line for the cementable provisional crowns.

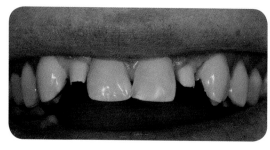

Figure 19: Temporary custom abutments inserted. Note blenching of surrounding mucosa.

to both sites, the healing screws removed, and the abutments inserted with 35 N cm according to manufacturer's specifications (Figure 19). The noted tissue blanching is caused by the transmucosal emergence shape of the abutments and generally disappears within a few minutes following abutment insertion. Screw-access holes were obturated with Teflon tape to cover the screw-heads and a soft composite (Fermit, 3M Espe, St. Paul, MN). The provisional crowns were subsequently cemented with Temp-Bond NE (Kerr Corporation, Orange, CA) making sure that a minimal amount of cement was used and overflow carefully removed after setting (Figure 20).

Final Prosthodontic Treatment

After about 10 weeks of peri-implant soft tissue maturation with the provisional restorations, the final prosthodontic restorations were initiated. Temporary restorations were removed, and tooth preparations for the ceramic veneers on teeth #8 and #9 (FDI #11 and

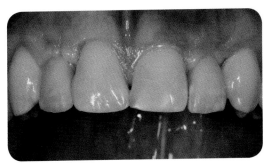

Figure 20: Provisional crowns #7 and #10 inserted with temporary cement.

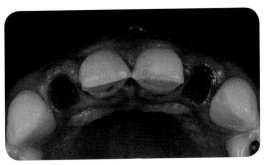

Figure 21: Occlusal view of treatment area in maxillary anterior 10 weeks after delivery of provisional restoration. Note the favorable and matured soft tissue contours of the implant sites. Lingual brackets of the former resin-bonded fixed provisional prostheses removed and areas polished. Teeth #8 and #9 prepared for ceramic veneers.

#21) performed. At this time, the four lingual retainer pieces were removed with a football-shaped diamond burr and the lingual tooth surfaces polished (Figure 21).

A closed-tray impression with customized impression copings to accurately record the created emergence contours of the peri-implant soft tissues was obtained (Figure 22), and the implant provisionals

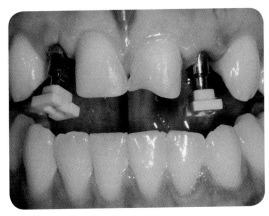

Figure 22: Closed-tray impression posts inserted for final impression.

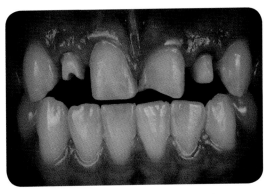

Figure 23: Final Zr custom abutments inserted.

reinserted. Temporary composite resin veneers were made chairside using the spot etching technique. Final restorations were then manufactured and delivered after try-in and completion by the dental technician. The custom CAD/CAM Zr abutments (CARES®, Straumann USA, Andover, MA) were inserted to the implants #7 and #10 with 35 N cm torque (Figure 23).

The screw-access-holes were again obturated with Teflon tape directly over the screw heads followed by Fermit® resin temporary material (3M Espe, St. Paul, MN). Pressed/layered lithium disilicate crowns (e.max press, Ivoclar Vivadent, Schaan, Liechtenstein) were then placed with Temp-Bond NE (Kerr Corporation, Orange, CA). The ceramic veneers on teeth #8 and #9 were bonded with Variolink II resin cement according to manufacturer's guidelines (Ivoclar Vivadent, Schaan, Liechtenstein) (Figure 24).

The patient was extremely pleased with the esthetic appearance of her "new teeth" at time of insertion as well as at the 1-year follow-up visit (Figures 25 and 26).

The radiographic controls showed stable peri-implant bone levels and absence of any peri-implant pathology (Figure 27).

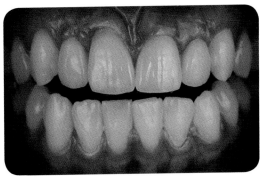

Figure 24: Final restorations at time of delivery: lithium disilicate crowns (e.max pressed) on implants #7 and #10; veneers #8 and #9.

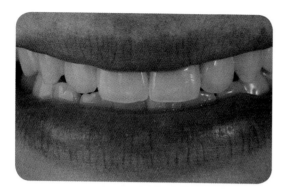

Figure 25: Frontal view of new smile.

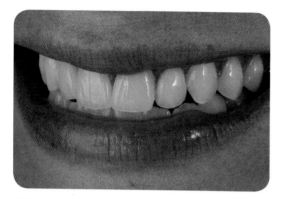

Figure 26: Lateral view of new smile.

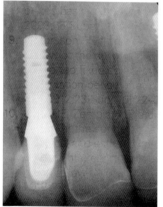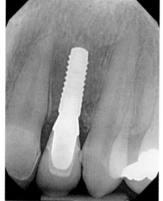

Figure 27: Radiographic views of restored area.

Discussion

This case scenario describes the replacement of two congenitally missing lateral incisors with implant restorations using a submerged (two-stage) implant placement protocol. While one-stage surgical placement of dental implants has been shown to work predictably [5] and facilitates treatment for patient and clinician by reducing the number of surgical interventions and overall treatment time, the submerged technique originally recommended by Brånemark et al. [6] still

finds its place in many indications. In particular, when bone grafting is required combined with implant placement the submerging of implant and bone graft enhances the predictability of optimal healing, as demonstrated in this case.

Provisional restorations are an important and often challenging part of implant dentistry [7]. Besides the fact that they need to maintain an acceptable function and esthetic appearance until a permanent restoration can be placed, they serve as placeholders to avoid migration of neighboring teeth and extrusion of opposing teeth. They are also important for determining the best restorative design for the given scenario and providing a template for soft tissue contouring and maturing.

Provisionalization in an area of esthetic visibility can be divided into three phases. The first phase involves provisional restorations immediately after tooth extraction and prior to implant placement; the second phase entails provisionalization after implant placement but prior to attaching a temporary restoration to an implant; and the third phase is the actual implant-supported provisional restoration. In the third phase, the implant-supported provisional restoration ultimately loads the implant and develops optimal contours of the peri-implant mucosa prior to fabricating the final restoration.

Provisional Restorations During Healing After Implant Surgery

Esthetically, provisional restorations after tooth extraction and prior to implant placement or during implant healing can be especially challenging. Combining the demands for an acceptable esthetic appearance with those of undisturbed tissue healing often requires a compromise agreed upon by patient and dentist. Several options for provisional restorations during the healing period after tooth extraction and/ or implant placement are available. These include removable and fixed alternatives. While removable interim partial dentures are the go-to option in most cases, special attention has to be given to their design in the areas of implant surgery. After implant placement, especially when combined with bone augmentation procedures, pressure may inadvertently be applied to the healing site. This pressure, defined as "transmucosal loading," may be detrimental to bone graft healing and implant survival [1]. It may also alter the surrounding soft tissue contours unfavorably. Therefore, interim removable partial dentures have to be designed carefully and checked for stability in function to avoid any contact and pressure to the underlying tissues.

As the healing progresses, the provisional partial denture teeth can be extended in their tissue-facing cervical area by adding acrylic resin for improved esthetics.

If tissue contact with the temporary partial denture teeth during the early healing phase is being avoided (e.g., because of insufficient vertical space), an interim removable partial is not the adequate choice. Alternatives are Essix retainers, resin-bonded fixed prostheses, or fixed "bridge" provisionals in cases with adjacent teeth that need to be crowned.

An overview and description of the options mentioned along with indications, advantages, and disadvantages are summarized in Table 1.

Implant-Supported Provisional Restorations

Early loading of dental implants 6–8 weeks after placement has been shown to be equally as predictable as conventional loading of 3–6 months when assessing treatment success [8].

Conventional loading after 3–6 months of healing remains the choice if the primary implant is considered inadequate for early or immediate loading, and if specific clinical conditions exist, such as a compromised host and/or implant site, the presence of parafunctions, or the need for extensive bone augmentation [9].

Implant-Supported Provisional Restorations and Soft Tissue Conditioning

An esthetic implant rehabilitation depends on both biologically and prosthodontically driven implant placement [2,10], a visually pleasing prosthesis [11], and an intact surrounding peri-implant mucosa [12]. The peri-implant tissue architecture is the essence of implant esthetics [13], and the presence of a proportionally pleasing papilla is an important part of implant esthetics [14]. Patient perceptions on the presence of interdental papillae are subjective and dependent upon individual interpretation [15], although the lack of a papilla, resulting in an open embrasure, can affect the patient's smile negatively. Kokich et al. [16] showed that the threshold for an open gingival embrasure, defined as the tip of the interdental papilla to the interproximal contact point, was 3 mm when assessed by general dentists and lay people.

The form of an endosseous implant differs from a natural tooth root in various ways. This is of primary significance in the transmucosal region. Natural anterior teeth have a triangular shape when viewed in a cross-section at the mucosa level. In contrast, the cross-section of an implant is round. To create the proper illusion of an implant restoration emerging through the surrounding mucosa like a natural tooth crown, the mucosa has to be shaped and matured in that manner. This can be done with the help of a customized healing abutment or, preferably, with the provisional restoration. Hence, an impression including the implants is obtained using implant-specific impression posts.

Laboratory-processed, screw-retained provisional restorations are our first choice. In the resulting master cast, which contains the implant analog(s), a wax-up is performed and indexed. Subsequently, the peri-implant areas in the stone cast are carved according to the desirable emergence contours of the restoration. The provisional is usually made from heat-polymerized PMMA on the basis of a provisional titanium abutment. The material is contoured and highly polished to minimize plaque accumulation and tissue irritation.

If implant axis correction is necessary, customizable temporary polymer abutments (polyether ether ketone) with a titanium base are used. They are contoured in their transmucosal portion according to the desirable emergence profile. The cervical shoulders are prepared to follow the soft tissue margins. Deep subgingival preparation is contraindicated due to risk of cement impaction into the peri-implant soft tissue.

There is little evidence in the current literature in regard to the best techniques for peri-implant soft tissue conditioning. We recommend the dynamic compression method [17]. In the initial phase of tissue shaping, it is important to create some pressure on the peri-implant mucosa. Care needs to be taken to not overcontour the restoration in the interproximal area. Otherwise, there will not be space for papillary tissues to fill in. The method relies on creating initial pressure by adding material and subsequent periodic reduction in the interproximal area to create space for the papilla. Reducing the contours of the provisional restoration can be performed intraorally with fine diamond burs followed by polishing with fine stones or rubber tips of different abrasiveness. Additive or subtractive modifications of the provisional can be done in steps over several appointments if needed.

The implant-supported provisional restoration is designed to:
- establish an adequate restorative emergence profile in the peri-implant mucosa;
- define the correct proximal contact location of the implant restoration to the adjacent teeth;
- regenerate adequate papillae in height and width;
- establish peri-implant mucosa margins in harmony with the gingival contours of the adjacent teeth.

Table 1: Overview of Provisional Restorations for Dental Implants in the Esthetic Zone

	Description	Indication	Advantages	Disadvantages	Caution
Removable provisional options					
Essix retainer	• clear thermoplastic appliance with integrated denture teeth or filled acrylic to replace teeth • should cover all remaining teeth	• provisionalization after tooth extraction and/or implant placement • short term only	• no transmucosal loading on the healing site • low costs • good esthetics in low lip-line cases • psychological advantage of not wearing a denture • easy to modify pre- and postsurgery • soft tissue conditioning possible	• esthetically compromised if patient has high smile line • occlusal interference • low durability • plaque accumulation • difficulty in mastication (?)	• high lip line • patient has to be compliant with good oral hygiene
Provisional partial denture	• PMMA-based interim removable denture with or without wrought wire clasps and denture teeth to replace missing teeth	• provisionalization after tooth extraction and/or implant placement • use as short- or long-term provisional	• easy to fabricate, reline and modify • stable if extended sufficiently for palatal support and wire clasps around molars • low cost	• not esthetic if clasps are used, especially in high lip-line cases • a partial denture, unless it can be completely relieved of the mucosa during healing, is not recommended for cases with the use of guided bone regeneration because of transmucosal loading • potential gag reflex issues • can interfere with speech • psychologically difficult for patients who have never worn dentures, and especially young patients	• deep overbite: provisional partial denture, unless it can be completely relieved of the mucosa during healing, is not recommended after implant placement (transmucosal loading) • transmucosal loading possible
Valplast/Flex	• PMMA-based interim removable prosthesis without metal clasps, softer material	• provisionalization after tooth extraction • short-term use only	• softer material gives comfort for the patient • no metal claps • good esthetic outcome	• not very stable • difficult to modify after surgical procedures • risk of impinging on marginal gingivae during healing	• not indicated after implant placement
Fixed provisional options					

Resin-bonded fixed bridge	• variations:
	  ○ all-acrylic resin
	  ○ metal base with acrylic-resin tooth
	  ○ zirconia or lithium disilicate frame and tooth
		• patients, who do not accept a removable device
		• long-term provisional prior to implant placement if patient is too young for implant placement
			• fixed, stable
			• no transmucosal loading on healing site
			• favorable esthetics
				• weak if all acrylic
				• requires metal or ceramic frame if provisional is needed for longer time period
				• cost high if metal or ceramic frame is needed
				• needs to be destroyed for access to implant site for surgical or prosthodontics treatment steps
					• retention with bonding to one adjacent tooth often more stable than bonding to both adjacent teeth

Tooth-supported bridge	• acrylic-based long-term provisional bridge reinforcement with gold mesh, cast metal, or glass fiber possible to increase stability	• provisionalization after tooth extraction and/or implant placement • long-term provisional	• fixed, stable • no transmucosal loading on healing site • favorable esthetics • easy to modify/reline • good diagnostic tool to perform esthetic analysis	• case selective, only indicated if neighboring teeth are already restored • contraindicated on natural unrestored neighboring teeth	• trauma due to the preparation of the abutment teeth, especially with long-term use

As mentioned earlier, the provisional restoration also serves as a communication tool for patient, dentist, and dental technician to optimize the design of the final restoration.

After completion of the soft tissue conditioning and maturing phase, which can take several weeks or even months, depending on the tissue volumes to be conditioned, it is recommended to transfer the created soft tissue architecture to the master cast by using customized impression copings as described by Elian et al. [18].

Consequently, the identical soft tissue profiles are created in the master cast as established intraorally, facilitating the fabrication of the final implant restoration according to the design tested with the provisional restoration.

Self-Study Questions

(Answers located at the end of the case)

A. What are the possible surgical implant placement modalities?

B. What are the potential advantages and disadvantages of submerged dental implant placement?

C. What are the indications and contraindications for nonsubmerged implant placement?

D. Does submerged implant placement change the treatment plan compared with nonsubmerged placement?

References

1. Seibert JS. Reconstruction of deformed, partially edentulous ridges, using full thickness onlay grafts. Part II. Prosthetic/periodontal interrelationships. Compend Contin Educ Dent 1983;4(6):549–562.
2. Belser UC, Bernard JP, Buser D. Implant-supported restorations in the anterior region: prosthetic considerations. Pract Periodontics Aesthet Dent 1996;8(9):875–883; quiz 884.
3. Cordaro L, Torsello F, Roccuzzo M. Implant loading protocols for the partially edentulous posterior mandible. Int J Oral Maxillofac Implants 2009;24(Suppl):158–168.
4. Chen S, Dawson, A. Esthetic modifiers. In: DawsonA, ChenS (eds), The SAC Classification in Implant Dentistry. Chicago, IL: Quintessence; 2009, pp 15–17.
5. Buser D, Weber HP, Lang NP. Tissue integration of non-submerged implants. 1-year results of a prospective study with 100 ITI hollow-cylinder and hollow-screw implants. Clin Oral Implants Res 1990;1(1):33–40.
6. Brånemark P-I, Hansson BO, Adell R, et al. Osseointegrated Implants in the Treatment of the Edentulous Jaw. Experience from a 10-Year Period. Scandinavian Journal of Plastic and Reconstructive Surgery, Supplementum 16. Stockholm: Almqvist & Wiksell; 1977.
7. Cho SC, Shetty S, Froum S, et al. Fixed and removable provisional options for patients undergoing implant treatment. Compend Contin Educ Dent 2007;28(11):604–608; quiz 609, 624.
8. Buser D, Chappuis V, Bornstein MM, et al. Long-term stability of contour augmentation with early implant placement following single tooth extraction in the esthetic zone: a prospective, cross-sectional study in 41 patients with a 5- to 9-year follow-up. J Periodontol 2013;84(11):1517–1527.
9. Weber HP, Morton D, Gallucci GO, et al. Consensus statements and recommended clinical procedures regarding loading protocols. Int J Oral Maxillofac Implants 2009;24(Suppl):180–183.
10. Buser D, Martin W, Belser UC. Optimizing esthetics for implant restorations in the anterior maxilla: anatomic and surgical considerations. Int J Oral Maxillofac Implants 2004;19(Suppl):43–61.
11. Cooper LF. Objective criteria: guiding and evaluating dental implant esthetics. J Esthet Restor Dent 2008;20(3):195–205.
12. Belser UC, Belser UC, Grütter L, et al. Outcome evaluation of early placed maxillary anterior single-tooth implants using objective esthetic criteria: a cross-sectional, retrospective study in 45 patients with a 2- to 4-year follow-up using pink and white esthetic scores. J Periodontol 2009;80(1):140–151.
13. Kan JY, Rungcharassaeng K, Fillman M, Caruso J. Tissue architecture modification for anterior implant esthetics: an interdisciplinary approach. Eur J Esthet Dent 2009;4(2):104–117.
14. Chu SJ, Tarnow DP, Tan JH, Stappert CF. Papilla proportions in the maxillary anterior dentition. Int J Periodontics Restorative Dent 2009;29(4):385–393.
15. Kan JY, Rungcharassaeng K, Umezu K, Kois JC. Dimensions of peri-implant mucosa: an evaluation of maxillary anterior single implants in humans. J Periodontol 2003;74(4):557–562.
16. Kokich Jr VO, Kiyak HA, Shapiro PA. Comparing the perception of dentists and lay people to altered dental esthetics. J Esthet Dent 1999;11(6):311–324.

17. Wittneben JG, Buser D, Belser U, Brägger U. Peri-implant soft tissue conditioning with provisonal restorations in the esthetic zone: the dynamic compression technique. Int J Periodontics Restorative Dent 2013;33(4):447–455.

18. Elian N, Tabourian G, Jalbout ZN, et al. Accurate transfer of peri-implant soft tissue emergence profile from the provisional crown to the final prosthesis using an emergence profile cast. J Esthet Restor Dent 2007;19(6):306–314; discussion 315.

19. Esposito M, Grusovin MG, Chew YS, et al. Interventions for replacing missing teeth: 1- versus 2-stage implant placement. Cochrane Database Syst Rev 2009;(3):CD006698.

20. Ericsson I, Nilner K, Klinge B, Glantz P-O. Radiographical and histological characteristics of submerged and nonsubmerged titanium implants. An experimental study in the Labrador dog. Clin Oral Implants Res 1996;7:20–26.

21. Ericsson I, Randow K, Nilner K, Petersson A. Some clinical and radiographical features of submerged and non-submerged titanium implants. A 5-year follow-up study. Clinical Oral Implants Res 1997;8:422–426.

22. Collaert B, De Bruyn H. Comparison of Brånemark fixture integration and short-term survival using one-stage or two-stage surgery in completely and partially edentulous mandibles. Clin Oral Implants Res 1998;9:131–135.

23. Cochran DL. The scientific basis for and clinical experiences with Straumann implants including the ITI Dental Implant System: a consensus report. Clin Oral Implants Res 2000;11(Suppl 1):33–58.

24. Abrahamsson I, Berglundh T, Moon I-S, Lindhe J. Peri-implant tissues at submerged and non-submerged titanium implants. J Clin Periodontol 1999;26:600–607.

25. Berglundh T, Lindhe J, Ericsson I, et al. The soft tissue barrier at implants and teeth. Clin Oral Implants Res 1991;2:81–90.

26. Gotfredsen K, Rostrup E, Hjörting-Hansen E, et al. Histological and histometrical evaluation of tissue reactions adjacent to endosteal implants in monkeys. Clin Oral Implants Res 1991;2:30–37.

27. Buser D, Weber HP, Donath K, et al. Soft tissue reactions to non-submerged unloaded titanium implants in beagle dogs. J Periodontol 1992;63:226–236.

28. Abrahamsson I, Berglundh T, Wennström J, Lindhe J. The peri-implant hard and soft tissues at different implant systems. A comparative study in the dog. Clin Oral Implants Res 1996;7:212–219.

29. Berglundh T, Lindhe J. Dimension of the peri-implant mucosa. Biological width revisited. J Clin Periodontol 1996;23:971–973.

30. Cochran DL, Hermann JS, Schenk RK, et al. Biologic width around titanium implants. A histometric analysis of the implanto-gingival junction around unloaded and loaded nonsubmerged implants in the canine mandible. J Periodontol 1997;68:186–198.

31. Cecchinato D, Olsson C, Lindhe J. Submerged or non-submerged healing of endosseous implants to be used in the rehabilitation of partially dentate patients. J Clin Periodontol 2004;31:299–308.

32. Hermann JS, Cochran DL, Nummikoski PV, Buser D. Crestal bone changes around titanium implants. A radiographic evaluation of unloaded nonsubmerged and submerged implants in the canine mandible. J Periodontol 1997;68:1117–1130.

33. Fiorellini JP, Buser D, Paquette DW, et al. A radiographic evaluation of bone healing around submerged and non-submerged dental implants in beagle dogs. J Periodontol 1999;70:248–254.

34. Broggini N, McManus LM, Hermann JS, et al. Persistent acute inflammation at the implant–abutment interface. J Dent Res 2003;82:232–237.

35. Van Winkelhoff AJ, Goene RJ, Benschop C, Folmer T. Early colonization of dental implants by putative periodontal pathogens in partially edentulous patients. Clin Oral Implants Res 2000;11:511–520.

36. Todescan FF, Pustiglioni FE, Imbronito AV, et al. Influence of the microgap in the peri-implant hard and soft tissues: a histomorphometric study in dogs. Int J Oral Maxillofac Implants 2002;17:467–472.

37. Broggini N, McManus LM, Hermann, JS, et al. Peri-implant inflammation defined by the implant–abutment interface. J Dent Res 2006;85:473–478.

38. Piattelli A, Vrespa G, Petrone G, et al. Role of the microgap between implant and abutment: a retrospective histologic evaluation in monkeys. J Periodontol 2003;74:346–352.

39. Enkling N, Jöhren P, Klimberg T, et al. Open or submerged healing of implants with platform switching: a randomized, controlled clinical trial. J Clin Periodontol 2011;4:374–384.

40. Weber HP, Buser D, Donath K, et al. Comparison of healed tissues adjacent to submerged and nonsubmerged unloaded titanium dental implants. A histometric study in beagle dogs. Clin Oral Implants Res 1996;7:11–19.

41. Henry P, Rosenberg I. Single-stage surgery for rehabilitation of the edentulous mandible: preliminary results. Pract Periodontics Aesthet Dent 1994;6:1–8.

42. Bernard J-P, Belser UC, Martinet J-P, Borgis SA. Osseointegration of Brånemark fixtures using a single-step operating technique. A preliminary prospective one year study in the edentulous mandible. Clin Oral Implants Res 1995;6:122–129.

43. Balshi TJ, Wolfinger GJ. Immediate loading of Brånemark implants in edentulous mandibles: a preliminary report. Implant Dent 1997;6:83–88.

44. Becker W, Becker BE, Ricci A, et al. A prospective multicenter clinical trial comparing one- and two-stage titanium screw-shaped fixtures with one-state plasma-sprayed solid-screw fixtures. Clin Implant Dent Relat Res 2000;2:159–165.

45. Tarnow DP, Emtiaz S, Classi A. Immediate loading of threaded implants at stage 1 surgery in edentulous arches: ten consecutive case reports with 1- to 5-year data. Int J Oral Maxillofac Implants 1997;12:319–324.

46. Randow K, Ericsson I, Nilner K, et al. Immediate functional loading of Brånemark dental implants. An 18-month clinical follow-up study. Clin Oral Implants Res 1999;10:8–15.

Answers to Self-Study Questions

A. There are two principal modalities of surgical implant placement in regard to flap repositioning and suturing after implant insertion: (1) the submerged (two-stage) and (2) the nonsubmerged (one-stage) protocol. In the first stage of a two-stage protocol, the implant is inserted in the bone housing and the cover screw is placed. The mucosal flap is then closed with sutures and the implant is completely buried under the soft tissues during the healing phase. After a healing period of about 3 months (mandible) or 6 months (maxilla), abutment connection is performed. The center of a submerged cover screw is identified using the surgical template that has been used at the time of implant placement or with a probe and the fixture is uncovered. A minimal incision or a mucosal punch or laser can be used to remove the covering mucosa. In the one-stage protocol a healing abutment (gingiva former or soft tissue shaper) or the final abutment is installed immediately after implant insertion. The soft-tissue flap is adjusted and sutured around the transgingival portion of the structure (healing screw or abutment). This component is exposed to the oral cavity.

B. A two-stage surgical technique was originally advocated in order to optimize the process of new bone formation and remodeling following implant installation [6]. The predictable outcome of this two-stage surgical technique was verified in several clinical trials that reported high survival and success rates for submerged implants [19].

In subsequent studies, however, it was recognized that proper osseointegration and subsequent good long-term success could also be obtained with nonsubmerged implant placement, either with one-piece implants or two-piece implants placed in a one-stage surgical mode by adding transmucosal healing screws or healing abutments to the implants at the time of implant surgery [20–23].

Results of other prospective experiments disclosed that "correctly performed implant surgery may ensure proper conditions for both soft and hard tissue healing" and that no quantitative or qualitative differences regarding soft- and hard-tissue integration could be observed between initially submerged and nonsubmerged implant systems. Abrahamsson et al. [24] compared the mucosa and bone tissue surrounding implants that had been placed either in a one- (nonsubmerged) or a two-stage (submerged) surgical procedure. It was observed that parameters such as the length of the barrier epithelium of the peri-implant mucosa, the length of the junctional epithelium, and the height and quality of the zone of connective tissue integration, the level of the marginal bone, and the density of bone between threads were almost identical in the two experimental groups at the end of the healing period [24]. These observations are in agreement with findings of other investigations [25–31]. However, other studies demonstrated that the temporal pattern of bone resorption was not the same; the open-healing procedure (nonsubmerged) provoked immediate bone resorption, whereas bone resorption was limited under submerged healing conditions before the reopening operation and accelerated afterwards [32–34]. One possible reason for these differences in the temporal pattern of bone-level alterations between open and submerged healing conditions is bacterial colonization of the microgap between the implant and abutment [35], which is related to the abutment-associated inflammatory cell infiltration close to the crestal bone [20,36–38] and can be minimized by using platform-switched implants [39]. Bacterial contamination of the microgap and subsequent peri-implant mucositis may also be possible during reentry and abutment incorporation if adequate plaque control and cleaning measures are not taken into consideration. Weber et al. [40] reported on the presence of clinically visible inflammation in the mucosa following abutment connection of the initially submerged implants.

Prospective studies and case reports in humans indicate that the marginal bone level remains stable also following rehabilitation irrespective of whether the implants had been placed according to a one- or two-step surgical protocol [20,41–46].

With a two-stage procedure the risk of having unwanted loading onto the implants is minimized, but the need for a second minor surgical intervention and more time prior to starting the prosthetic phase because of the wound-healing period required in relation to the second surgical intervention are sometimes a disadvantage.

C. A two-stage submerged approach may be preferred when:
1. An implant does not have excellent primary stability at implant placement.
2. When bone grafting procedures are combined with implant placement.
3. When vertical space is reduced so that an interim prosthesis cannot be designed without creating contact to the transmucosal implant portion or healing abutment as well as the surrounding surgical site. This is especially the case in edentulous indications, but can also occur in the partially edentulous arch.

D. Choosing a two-stage surgical approach influences the overall treatment plan and sequence in terms of overall treatment time and restorative steps involved.

During the submerged healing period no fixed provisional restoration directly supported by the submerged implants is possible. As described earlier, for these patients an esthetically pleasing interim prosthesis is needed. This can be fixed if either remaining teeth or additional nonsubmerged implants can be used. Otherwise, it will have to be a removable interim prosthesis as described in detail in the Discussion section of this case.

After completion of bone and soft tissue healing, which can range from 6 weeks to 6 months depending on the involvement and extent of accompanying bone grafting procedures, the submerged implants need to be uncovered with a second-stage surgical procedure. An impression can be obtained at the time of the second-stage surgery or a few weeks later. An implant-supported provisional prosthesis is then fabricated and inserted at a subsequent appointment and left in place to (1) establish an adequate restorative emergence profile in the peri-implant mucosa, (2) define the correct proximal contact location of the implant restoration to the adjacent teeth, (3) regenerate adequate papillae in height and width, and (4) establish peri-implant mucosa margins in harmony with the gingival contours of adjacent teeth or implant restorations.

8

Restoration

Case 1

Single-Tooth Implants: Posterior

CASE STORY

A 55-year-old white Caucasian male patient came to the office for a consult and possible treatment to replace the maxillary second premolar, which had been extracted in an emergency clinic after the patient had experienced severe pain and buccal swelling while traveling a few months ago. It had been decided by the emergency dentist that the tooth could not be saved on the basis of the clinical and radiographic findings as well as the history of treatment, which the patient had provided: the tooth had been root canal treated over 30 years ago and had undergone an apico-ectomy about 3 years later because of persisting pain. During the following years, it still caused the patient occasionally mild to moderate discomfort when biting on it. But the tooth would usually calm down within a few days without any specific treatment. This time, pain had persisted and had become severe, so that the patient sought emergency care.

LEARNING GOALS AND OBJECTIVES
- Review the predictability of single-unit implant restorations in the posterior arch as an alternative to conventional fixed dental prostheses
- Review the systemic and local requirements for the replacement of a missing posterior tooth with a single implant-supported restoration
- Discuss the optimal treatment sequence for a failing or failed posterior tooth to be replaced with an implant-supported restoration
- Describe the benefits and risks of cemented implant restorations

Medical History

The patient underwent total replacement of his left hip in 2004 and requires antibiotic prophylaxis prior to dental procedures. Otherwise, he is healthy, has no allergies, and is not taking any medications. He does not smoke or use any tobacco-containing products. He drinks alcohol socially on occasion. He exercises regularly and appears to be very fit for his age.

Review of Systems
- Vital signs
  - Average blood pressure: 118/70 mmHg
  - Average respiration rate: 16 breaths/min
  - Average pulse rate: 72 beats/min

Social History

The patient is a professional in a high-ranking administrative position in a health-care-related business. He is married and has two adult children. He has some insurance coverage for major dental treatment.

Extraoral Examination

The extraoral examination did not reveal any significant findings. No masses or lesions were noted, and lymph nodes of the head and neck were normal. No discomfort, clicking, or crepitus were detected during temporomandibular joint function. Range of motion was not limited, and palpation of the muscles of the head and neck showed no signs of soreness or tenderness.

Intraoral Examination

The patient stated that he sees his dentist and hygienist every 6 months for prophylaxis and periodic exam visits. Floor of the mouth, tongue, cheek, palate, and oropharynx were all within normal limits, and no masses or lesions were found. Salivary flow and consistency were normal. All teeth except third molars were present. Multiple single-unit restorations in the posterior segments of the patient's dentition in the form of gold crowns, inlays, or onlays were identified. Tooth #10 (FDI #22) showed an intact disto-lingual composite restoration. All permanent restorations were over 15 years old at the time of this visit. Teeth #5 (FDI #14), 13 (FDI #25), 14 (FDI #26), 15 (FDI #27), and 30 (FDI #46) tested negative to pulp testing with ice. The patient confirmed that he had to undergo root canal treatments of these teeth many years ago. He also mentioned that apical root resections were performed twice on tooth #13 (FDI #25) because of repeated episodes of substantial discomfort. All other teeth were vital.

In the upper left quadrant, the extraction site of #13 (FDI #25) had completely healed, presented an excellent alveolar ridge volume, and had a wide band of well-keratinized attached mucosa (Figure 1). The interdental space between neighboring teeth was 7 mm, and the interarch space in the area was unrestricted. Tooth #12 (FDI #24) was restored with a class II disto-occlusal gold onlay; it showed mild gingival recession and moderate cervical abrasion. The patient expressed that he would like this tooth to be re-restored with a tooth-colored restoration. Tooth #14 (FDI #26) exhibited an onlay with a temporary occlusal restoration. It had needed root

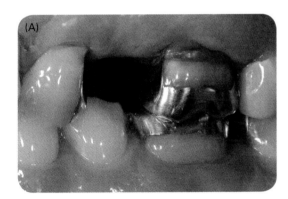

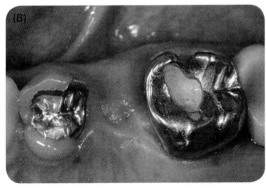

Figure 1: (A) Buccal and (B) occlusal views of upper left quadrant.

canal retreatment (Figure 1B) shortly after the extraction of tooth #13 (FDI #25). Mild gingival recession and an advanced cervical hard tissue defect were found consistent with an abfraction-type lesion. Tooth #15 (FDI #27) was currently restored with a provisional crown provided by the patient's primary dentist after the former gold crown had incurred a perforation due to occlusal wear.

Periodontal Examination

The patient practices an excellent oral hygiene. Small amounts of localized supragingival calculus were found in the lingual–cervical aspect of the lower incisors. Full mouth periodontal charting revealed no probing depths greater than 3 mm, and no bleeding on probing was noted for any sites. On the buccal aspect of tooth #30 (FDI #46), the entrance to the furcation could be probed minimally. Buccal and lingual probing depths of the furcation area were, however, only 1–2 mm, and bleeding on probing was absent.

Occlusal Analysis

The molar and canine occlusal relationships were consistent with an Angle class 1. No occlusal discrepancies or interferences were noted. Lateral and anterior excursions occurred in group function with the posterior antagonists out of contact as the respective movements progressed. The anterior overbite was 3 mm, and his overjet 2 mm. Cuspal wear was noticed on canines and buccal cusps of all premolars, indicative of a potential bruxing. The patient, however, was unaware of any such habit.

Radiographic Examination

A periapical radiograph of the upper left quadrant was brought to the visit by the patient (Figure 2). The image had been obtained at the time when the patient went for emergency care because of the acute pain, which resulted in the extraction of tooth #13 (FDI #25). It confirmed the root canal treatments of teeth #13, #14, and #15 (FDI #25, #26, and #27). Periapical radiolucencies could be found at teeth #13 and #14 (FDI #25 and #26). The image also showed the resected apical root portion of tooth #13 (FDI #25). In addition to the periapical radiolucency in the mesial root area, tooth #14 (FDI #26) also had an apical radiodensity at the apex of the palatal root. The diagnosis for this finding was condensing osteitis. As mentioned before, root canal retreatment had been performed on tooth #14 (FDI #26) in the meantime, and a temporary restoration had been placed on tooth #15 (FDI #27).

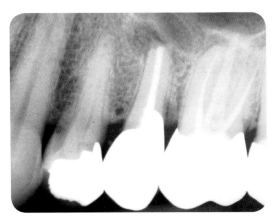

Figure 2: Periapical radiograph of treatment area prior to extraction of tooth #13 (FDI #25). Radiograph provided by patient.

The radiographic bone levels of the teeth imaged in the radiograph were at normal levels. The root length of tooth #13 (FDI #25) was approximately 10 mm. It was planned that additional radiographic information on the status of the patient's dentition would be obtained with the subsequent implant-specific radiographic information.

Diagnosis

Single-tooth partial edentulism in maxillary left quadrant (tooth #13; FDI #25 missing). Defective restorations on teeth #12, #14, and #15 (FDI #24, #26, and #27).

Treatment Plan

The treatment plan established at the patient's initial consult visit was as follows:
1. Obtain diagnostic impressions and prepare a diagnostic template for further radiographic study.
2. Obtain a panoramic radiograph as well as tomographic images of the potential implant site #13 (FDI #25) with the diagnostic template in place.
3. Implant placement and provisional fixed dental prosthesis (FDP) #12–#14 (FDI #24–#26).
4. Implant-supported single crown (SC) to replace tooth #13 (FDI #25); (ceramic) onlay for tooth #12 (FDI #24), and new build-ups and ceramic crowns for teeth #14 and #15 (FDI #26 and #27).

A three-unit FDP #12–#14 (FDI #24–#26) and an SC #15 (FDI #27) were proposed as an alternative treatment plan. The patient was clearly in favor of the implant alternative, assuming that no contraindication for implant treatment would be identified in the further radiographic assessment.

Treatment

Diagnostic Preparations for Implant Surgery

Alginate impressions were made at the initial visit and diagnostic casts subsequently obtained. A diagnostic template was produced on the diagnostic cast using a simple thermoplastic device (Figure 3), which allows the positioning of a metal sleeve in the prosthodontically optimal location and direction (EZ Stent, AD Surgical, Sunnyvale, CA). An instructional video about the use of this surgical template (Figure 4) can be found at http://www.ad-surgical.com/ez-stent_feature#.Vti5M9L2bmE.

The device was tried in the patient (Figure 5), and panoramic as well as lateral tomographic radiographs were obtained with the template inserted. The panoramic radiograph (Figure 6) confirmed the intraoral clinical findings of the overall healthy conditions and intact restorations outlined earlier. A small radiolucent area was found at the entrance of the furcation of the lower right first molar, which had been found to be clinically healthy. The site of the extracted tooth #13 (FDI #25) showed excellent healing. The proposed implant axis, visible on the hand of the metal sleeve in the thermoplastic template, was ideal. The root canal

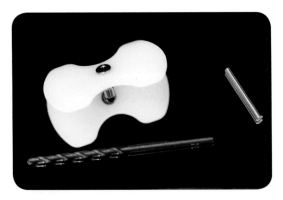

Figure 3: Diagnostic template assembly (EZ Stent, AD Surgical, Sunnyvale, CA).

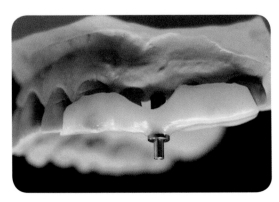

Figure 4: Diagnostic template prepared on diagnostic cast.

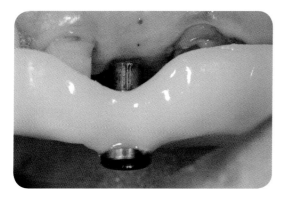

Figure 5: Diagnostic template intraorally.

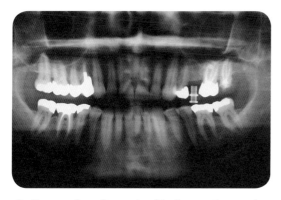

Figure 6: Panoramic radiograph with diagnostic template in situ.

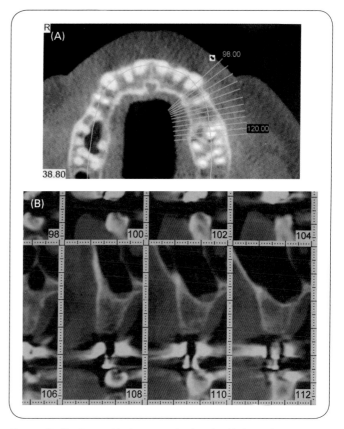

Figure 7: Radiographic images obtained with lateral tomography: (A) occlusal view with cross-section intervals; (B) cross-sectional views including diagnostic template.

retreatment of tooth #14 (FDI #26) showed some apical overfill. However, the periapical lucencies on both #13 and #14 (FDI #25 and #26) had healed. The lateral tomographic images demonstrated excellent bone width for a regular-diameter implant. The available endosseous bone height from alveolar crest to sinus floor was 10 mm (Figure 7).

Based on this positive additional diagnostic information, the final treatment plan was confirmed and foresaw to replace the missing tooth #13 (FDI #25) with an implant-supported full ceramic restoration on a synOcta titanium abutment for cemented restorations and a full ceramic crown. Tooth #12 was to be restored with a ceramic onlay, and teeth #14 and #15 (FDI #26 and #27) with ceramic crowns. A flapless surgery combined with immediate restoration was envisioned for this case, the latter depending on the primary stability of the implant at the time of placement. The patient consented to this treatment plan.

Risk Assessment

Based on the diagnostic information obtained, the proposed implant treatment was considered to be

"straightforward" in the case of restoration after healing (early loading) or "advanced" in the context of immediate restoration at time of surgery according to the ITI SAC Risk Assessment Tool (iti.org).

Surgical and Provisional Prosthodontic Treatment
Surgical Procedure

In a visit prior to the surgical appointment, the gold restorations on teeth #12 and #14 (FDI #24 and #26) had been removed and replaced with a provisional three-unit fixed acrylic prosthesis. The surgical template was inserted and rested stably on the left upper canine and second molar. With the detailed clinical and radiographic information indicating good bone height and width, a wide band of keratinized attached mucosa, as well as the availability of a precise surgical guide, it was decided to use a flapless surgical approach. The patient had taken the prophylactic antibiotics as prescribed (2 g amoxicillin 1 before the implant surgery). Local infiltration anesthesia was administered (1.8 mL lidocaine 2%, 1:100,000 parts epinephrine). A 4 mm diameter soft-tissue punch was used in the planned implant location to create access to the underlying bone. After removal of the soft tissue plug, soft tissue thickness at the buccal entrance of the punch hole was measured to be 2 mm. The buccal soft tissue margin would serve as landmark to verify the drilling depth. As determined from the lateral tomograms, an intraosseous implant length of 10 mm was possible without intruding into the sinus floor. The 2 mm soft tissue thickness was added to the overall drilling depth. A 2.2 mm diameter pilot hole was then drilled with the help of the surgical template (Figure 8) to a depth of 12 mm from the buccal soft tissue margin, following the markings on the drill. The widening of the pilot whole with the 2.8 and 3.5 mm diameter spiral drills was subsequently done freehand. After completion of the implant osteotomy, the presence of the buccal and lingual bone in the implant bed was confirmed with a periodontal probe. The implant bed was rinsed with sterile saline, and the regular neck soft tissue level implant inserted (Straumann SP Implant, RN, diameter 4.1 mm, SLActive, 10 mm; Straumann USA, Andover, MA) using an inserting device and manual torque driver (Figure 9). Excellent primary stability

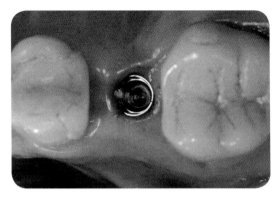

Figure 10: Implant shoulder located slightly below soft tissue level.

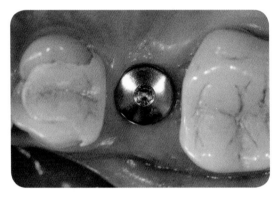

Figure 11: Healing screw inserted.

was obtained and verified with an insertion torque of >35 N cm. The insertion device was removed and the implant site assessed: the implant shoulders were ideally located slightly below the surrounding soft tissue margins (Figure 10). There was no to minimal bleeding of the wound margin, which was firmly adapted to the circumference of the implant shoulder. A 2 mm regular neck (RN) healing screw was subsequently placed (Straumann USA, Andover, MA) (Figure 11).

Provisional Restoration During Healing Phase

The existing three-unit provisional supported by teeth #12 (FDI #24) and #14 (FDI #26) (Figure 12) was relined and adjusted so that the implant-facing surface of pontic #13 (FDI #25) did not have immediate contact with the healing screw. The proximal embrasures were designed for easy access for cleaning with proximal brushes (Figure 13). The provisional was carefully polished and inserted with provisional cement (Temp-Bond NE, Kerr).

Postoperative Treatment and Tissue Contouring Provisional

The patient was instructed to use over-the-counter pain medication as needed and to clean the implant area

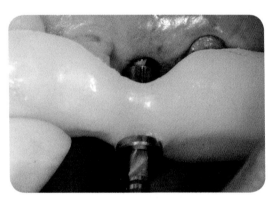

Figure 8: Precise implant site preparation with drill guide.

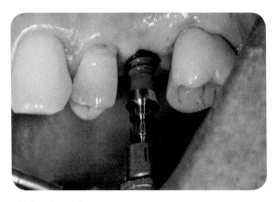

Figure 9: Implant placement.

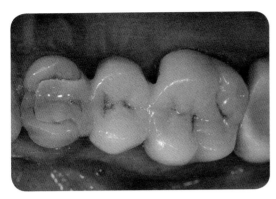

Figure 12: Three-unit provisional FDP prior to reline and adjustments.

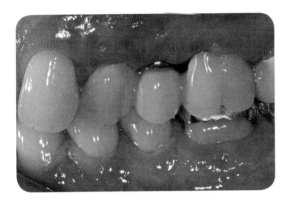

Figure 13 Provisional FDP inserted

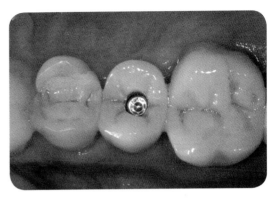

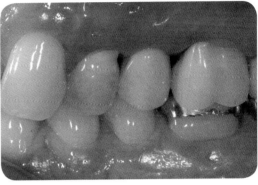

Figure 14: Modified provisional restoration for soft tissue contouring of implant site.

with a soft toothbrush and small interproximal brushes daily. He was also advised not to chew any unusually hard foods on the implant side, and he was also instructed to call the office in case of any discomfort or signs of swelling. He was seen for a re-care visit and postoperative evaluation at 4 weeks following surgery. He stated that he had not incurred any postoperative discomfort or swelling. The peri-implant tissues appeared well healed and healthy.

At this time, the provisional pontic over the implant site was connected to the implant for the purposes of soft tissue contouring of the implant site. The provisional bridge was removed and cleaned, the pontic hollowed out, and an access hole drilled in the center of the occlusal table. The healing screw was removed from the implant, an RN titanium temporary abutment for crowns (Straumann USA, Andover, MA), shortened, and screwed onto the implant. The screw access was obturated with soft wax. Acrylic resin was then filled into the pontic shell and the entire provisional reinserted. After setting of the acrylic, the wax was removed and the provisional unscrewed. The emergence contours of the implant provisional were

smoothened by adding acrylic resin as needed, and the provisional finished and carefully polished. Temporary cement was again applied to both tooth units (Temp-Bond NE, Kerr Corporation, Orange, CA), and the provisional bridge inserted and secured to the implant via the temporary abutment screw using 35 N cm torque (Figure 14).

Final Prosthodontic Treatment

Impressions for the final restorations were obtained 8 weeks after implant surgery using a polyvinyl silicone impression material with a closed-tray technique. Figure 15 shows the resulting master cast with preparations for teeth #12, #14, and #15 (FDI # 24, #26, and #27) and the implant analog in position #13 (FDI #25). The buccal emergence contour created by the implant-supported provisional is visible in the soft tissue modeling material. Lithium disilicate restorations were fabricated for the natural teeth involved. The implant was restored with a cemented full ceramic crown made of a zirconia coping veneered with porcelain (Figure 16). After try-in, adjustments, and polishing with porcelain polishers, the synOcta RN cementable titanium abutment (Straumann USA, Andover, MA) was secured with 35 N cm torque according to the manufacturer's

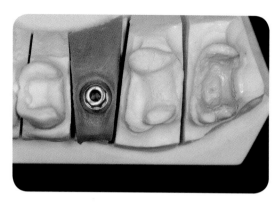

Figure 15: Master cast for fabrication of final restorations.

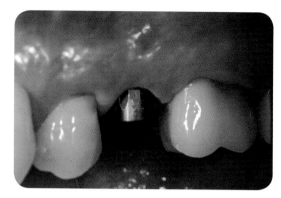

Figure 17: SynOcta RN cementable abutment inserted.

guidelines (Figure 17). All restorations were delivered with resin-based luting cement (Multilink, Ivoclar Vivadent, Schaan, Liechtenstein) (Figure 18). Special care was taken to assure removal of any excess cement with micro-brushes and floss prior to curing, specifically around the implant crown. The periapical radiograph illustrated in Figure19 documents the completion of treatment.

Discussion

This case discusses the replacement of a missing posterior tooth with an implant-supported restoration. The fact that both adjacent teeth required indirect

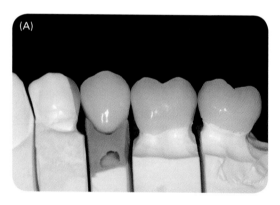

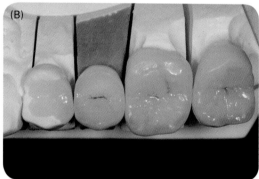

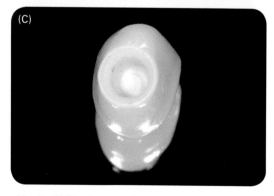

Figure 16: (A, B) Final restorations ready for try-in. (C) Full ceramic, cementable crown for implant #13 (FDI #25)

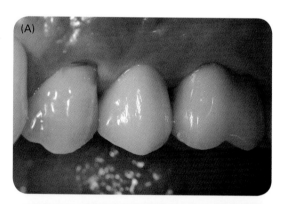

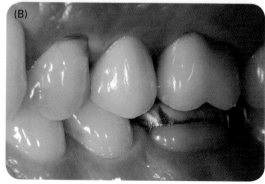

Figure 18: (A, B) Final restorations delivered.

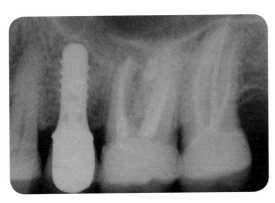

Figure 19: Posttreatment periapical radiograph.

roctorations in the form of an onlay or a crown brings up the question of whether the replacement of the missing second premolar would preferably have been achieved via a three-unit FDP instead of an implant-supported crown. As discussed in more scientific detail later in the answers to the self-study questions, the long-term predictability of single-tooth implant restorations compares favorably with that of FPDs. Hence, in a healthy patient with favorable local conditions and good compliance, both alternatives could be recommended. When considering the impact of a possible biological or technical complication down the road, a single-unit, tooth-independent replacement would appear to have a considerable advantage over a multiunit fixed prosthesis that involves several teeth. In terms of local requirements for an implant, the bone volume (height and width) needs to be adequate for a relatively straightforward implant placement to maintain the balance of this equation on the implant side. In a favorable indication for an implant restoration as documented in this case, both treatment options are presented to the patient and the benefits and risks of both discussed. It is then ultimately the informed patient who will assist in the decision-making process, taking into account that an implant-supported restoration may have higher upfront out-of-pocket costs to the patient than an FDP, depending on their insurance coverage for major restorative work.

Owing to the favorable bone width and height recognized in the cross-sectional radiograph, as well as the presence of a wide band of thick keratinized mucosa at the implant site, a flapless surgery approach could be chosen in combination with the exact drill guide. This makes the implant surgical procedure quick and easy for the surgeon and reduces the level of postoperative discomfort for the patient substantially. Caution is required, however, to limit this surgical approach to those indications where the previously cited conditions are present.

An early loading protocol was applied for the implant restoration presented in this case. Since an easy option for a fixed provisional restoration was available via the illustrated three-unit acrylic temporary supported by the adjacent teeth, the consideration of an immediate restoration protocol was not necessary.

A cemented full-ceramic crown was used to restore the implant in the case presented. Please refer to the following self study questions and answers to this case for an assessment of the cemented versus screw-retained "dilemma." Chapter 3 Case 3 addresses material selection questions for implant restorations.

Self-Study Questions

(Answers located at the end of the case)

A. How predictable are single-unit implant restorations in the posterior arch compared with other fixed replacement options?

B. What are the basic requirements for single implant restorations – systemic and local factors?

C. What are the advantages and disadvantages of cemented versus screw-retained implant restorations?

D. Under which conditions can a flapless surgical approach be chosen?

References

1. Palmqvist S, Swartz B. Artificial crowns and fixed partial dentures 18 to 23 years after placement. Int J Prosthodont 1993;6:279–285.

2. Kerschbaum T, Haastert B, Marinello CP. Risk of debonding in three-unit resin-bonded fixed partial dentures. J Prosthet Dent 1996;75:248–253.

3. Romeo E, Lops D, Margutti E, et al. Long-term survival and success of oral implants in the treatment of full and partial arches: a seven-year prospective study with the ITI dental implant system. Int J Oral Maxillofac Implants 2004;19:247–259.

4. Jung RE, Pjetursson BE, Glauser R, et al. A systematic review of the 5-year survival and complication rates of implant-supported single crowns. Clin Oral Implants Res 2008;19 (2):119–130.

5. Brägger U, Bürgin W, Hämmerle CHF, Lang NP. Associations between clinical parameters assessed around implants and teeth. Clin Oral Implants Res 1997;8:412–421.

6. Krieger O, Matuliene G, Hüsler J, et al. Failures and complications in patients with birth defects restored with fixed dental prostheses and single crowns on teeth and/or implants. Clin Oral Implant Res 2009;20:809–816.

7. Jokstad A, Brägger U, Brunski JB, et al. Quality of dental implants biologic outcome of implant-supported restorations in the treatment of partial edentulism. Part I: a longitudinal clinical evaluation. Int Dent J 2003;53:409–443.

8. Pjetursson BE, Lang NP. Prosthetic treatment planning on the basis of scientific evidence. J Oral Rehabil 2008;35(Suppl 1):72–79.

9. Pjetursson BE, Thoma D, Jung R, et al. A systematic review of the survival and complication rates of implant-supported fixed dental prostheses (FDPs) after a mean observation period of at least 5 years. Clin Oral Implants Res 2012;23(Suppl 6):22–38.

10. Jung RE, Zembic A, Pjetursson BE, et al. Systematic review of the survival rate and the incidence of biological, technical and esthetic complications of single crowns on implants reported in longitudinal studies with a mean follow-up of 5 years. Clin Oral Implants Res 2012;23(Suppl 6):2–21.

11. Wennström J, Palmer R. Consensus report: clinical trials. In: Lang NP, Karring T, Linde J (eds), Proceedings of the 3rd European Workshop on Periodontology. Berlin: Quintessence; 1999, pp 255–259.

12. Pjetursson BE, Tan K, Lang NP, et al. A systematic review of the survival and complication rates of fixed partial dentures (FPDs) after an observation period of at least 5 years. Clin Oral Implants Res 2004;15:625–642.

13. Leempoel PJ, Eschen S, De Haan AF, Van't Hof MA. An evaluation of crowns and bridges in a general dental practice. J Oral Rehabil 1985;12:515–528.

14. Karlsson S. Failures and length of service in fixed prosthodontics after long-term function. A longitudinal clinical study. Swed Dent J 1989;13:185–192.

15. Tan K, Pjetursson BE, Lang NP, Chan ESY. A systematic review of the survival and complication rates of fixed partial dentures (FPDs) after an observation period of at least 5 years. III. Conventional FPDs. Clin Oral Implants Res 2004;15:654–666.

16. Pjetursson BE, Brägger U, Lang NP, Zwahlen M. Comparison of survival and complication rates of tooth-supported fixed dental prostheses (FDPs) and implant-supported FDPs and single crowns (SCs). Clin Oral Implants Res 2007;18(Suppl 3):97–113.

17. Libby G, Arcuri MR, LaVelle WE, Hebl L. Longevity of fixed partial dentures. J Prosthet Dent 1979;78:127–131.

18. Reichen-Graden S, Lang NP. Periodontal and pulpal conditions of abutment teeth. Status after four to eight years following the incorporation of fixed reconstructions. Schweiz Monatsschr Zahnmed 1989;99:1381–1385.

19. Fayyad MA, al-Rafee MA. Failure of dental bridges. II. Prevalence of failure and its relation to place of construction. J Oral Rehabil 1996;23:438–440.

20. Walton TR. An up to 15-year longitudinal study of 515 metal-ceramic FDPs: part 2. Modes of failure and influence of various clinical characteristics. Int J Prosthodont 2003;16:177–182.

21. Bergenholtz G, Nyman S. Endodontic complications following periodontal and prosthetic treatment of patients with advanced periodontal disease. J Periodontol 1984;55:63–68.

22. Brägger U, Karoussis I, Persson R, et al. Technical and biological complications and failures with single crowns and fixed partial dentures on implant of the ITI Dental Implant System: a 10-year prospective cohort study. Clin Oral Implants Res 2005;16:326–334.

23. Pjetursson BE, Karoussis I, Bürgin W, et al. Patients' satisfaction following implant therapy. A 10-year prospective cohort study. Clin Oral Implants Res 2005;16:185–193.

24. Brägger U, Krenander P, Lang NP. Economic aspects of single-tooth replacement. Clin Oral Implants Res 2005;16:335–341.

25. Klinge B, Flemming T, Cosyn J, et al. The patient undergoing implant therapy. Summary and consensus statements. The 4th EAO Consensus Conference 2015. Clin Oral Implants Res 2015;26(Suppl 11):64-67. doi: 10.1111/clr.12675.

26. Weber HP, Kim DM, Ng MW, et al. Peri-implant soft-tissue health surrounding cement- and screw-retained implant restorations: a multi-center, 3-year prospective study. Clin Oral Implants Res 2006;17(4):375–379.

27. Present S, Levine RA. Techniques to control or avoid cement around implant-retained restorations. Compend Contin Educ Dent 2013;34(6):432–437.

28. Zitzmann NY, Berglundh T. Definition and prevalence of peri-implant diseases. J Clin Periodontol 2008;35:286–291.

29. Heitz-Mayfield LJA, Lang NP. Comparative biology of chronic & aggressive periodontitis vs. peri-implantitis. Periodontol 2000 2010;53:167–181.

30. Linkevicius T, Vindasiute E, Puisys A, Peciuliene V. The influence of margin location on the amount of undetected cement excess after delivery of cement-retained implant restorations. Clin Oral Implant Res 2011;22:1379–1384.

Answers to Self-Study Questions

A. The therapy of a missing single tooth has become a frequent and important indication in current dentistry. A variety of therapeutic options are available to restore a missing single tooth. These therapies range from resin-bonded bridges, to fixed dental prostheses (FDPs), up to the use of implant-supported [1–4].

The functional and biological advantages of implant-borne reconstructions compared with conventional reconstructive dentistry are for many clinical situations indisputable. Implant therapy can help minimize bone loss. In addition, the surrounding healthy, pristine teeth can be left unprepared [5,6]. Therefore, it can be estimated that a considerably increasing percentage of patients seeking dental care will present with implant-borne reconstructions in the future [7].

However, when it comes to the decision-making process between implant-supported single crowns (SCs) and a tooth-supported FDP, it is important to know the survival proportions and the determination of the incidence of biological and technical complications not only for the implants but also for the reconstructions. The related decision criteria should be essentially derived from systematic reviews of the available evidence [8,9] and objective surgically/prosthetically oriented risk assessments as well as patient-related factors, including cost effectiveness and quality of life [10].

When advising the patient on different treatment options, "long-term" survival rates and the incidence of biological and technical events should thus be based on mean follow-up periods of at least 5 years to supply the patient with reliable information [11,12].

If we class the "survival" observation period irrespective of its condition [13,14] and "success" as an FDP that remains unchanged and free of all complications over the entire follow-up period, then the systematic reviews conducted so far [12,15] indicate a 5-year survival of implant-supported SCs of 94.5%, and 5-year survival of conventional FDPs of 93.8%. The estimated 10-year survival was 89.4% for implant-supported SCs and 89.2% for conventional FDPs.

Complications with reconstructions can basically be grouped into technical ones (e.g., abutment tooth fracture, loss of retention, fractures of porcelain/framework/secondary parts, screw loosening) and into biological ones – which comprise peri-implant radiolucencies, signs of peri-implantitis (such as deepening of the peri-implant pocket probing depths) and radiographic signs of loss of osseointegration (i.e., horizontal bone loss and vertical defects for suprastructures on implants and caries, loss of pulp vitality, periodontal disease progression for tooth-borne FDPs).

For conventional tooth-supported FDPs, the most frequent complications are biological complications. However, the incidence of technical complications is significantly higher for implant-supported than for tooth-supported reconstructions [16].

Four studies [17–20] provided information on FDPs that remained intact over the observation period. In meta-analysis, the estimated 5-year complication rate of conventional FDPs was 15.7%. This value was 38.7% for implant-supported FDPs.

Comparing the success proportion of conventional tooth-supported and solely implant-supported FDPs, the tooth-supported FDPs have a significantly higher 5-year success proportion of 84.3% compared with 61.3% for the implant-supported FDPs. Hence, patients with implant-supported FDPs are at a higher risk of having complications than are patients with tooth-supported conventional FDPs.

The most frequent biological complication with tooth-supported reconstructions is loss of abutment vitality. One study [21] compared 255 abutment teeth with 417 non-abutment teeth and found a higher incidence of pulpal necrosis in abutment teeth (15% versus 3%). The 5-year rate of loss of abutment vitality for conventional FDPs is 6.1%. The second most common biological complication with tooth-supported prostheses is dental caries. Several studies reported the number of FDPs lost due to caries. The 5-year rate of conventional FDPs lost because of dental caries is 1.6%. The third most frequent biological complication with tooth-supported prostheses is their loss due to recurrent periodontitis, with a rate of 0.4%.

The most frequent biological complication with implant-supported reconstructions is peri-implant disease. Peri-implant mucosal lesions, soft tissue complications, and peri-implantitis are reported in various studies. Other studies reported signs of inflammation (pain, redness, swelling, and bleeding) or "soft tissue complications," defined as fistula, gingivitis, or hyperplasia. The annual rate of this complication is 9.7% for implant-supported SCs. For implant-supported SCs, 10 studies evaluated changes in marginal bone height, evaluated on radiographs, over the observation period. In a Poisson model analysis, the cumulative rate of implants with bone loss exceeding 2 mm after 5 years was 6.3%.

In the group of technical complications, the most frequent one by tooth-supported reconstructions is loss of retention, with a 5-year rate of 3.3% for conventional FDPs. This value is 5.5% for implant-supported SCs. The most common technical complication with implant-supported reconstructions is the fracture of a veneer material (acrylic, ceramic, or composite), with a 5-year rate of veneer fractures of 4.5% for implant-supported SCs. Tooth-supported FDPs have a significantly lower 5-year risk of ceramic fracture or chipping (2.9%). The second most common technical complication by implant-supported reconstructions is abutment or occlusal screw loosening. The 5-year rate of abutment or occlusal screw loosening for implant-supported SCs is 12.7%. Such a complication happens for conventional FDPs.

Fractures of components, such as implants, abutment, and occlusal screws, are other rare complications of implant-supported SCs. Some of these technical failures and complications today may seem to be irrelevant because of the continuous development of the implant components. Thus, by the introduction of controlled torque device and technical improvements of the abutment and transfer system, some risks might have been eliminated or heavily reduced [22].

On the other hand, more than 90% of the patients are completely satisfied with implant therapy, from both functional and esthetic points of view [23]. A dental implant is more expensive than a bridge, but, over a short observation period, the implant reconstruction demonstrates a more favorable cost/effectiveness ratio for single-tooth replacement compared with the conventional FPD. The implant reconstruction is to be recommended from an economical point of view especially in situations with either nonrestored or minimally restored teeth and sufficient bone [24].

B. There are different opinions regarding factors considered being of special relevance for the patient undergoing implant therapy. For example, patients with inadequate oral hygiene, microbial biofilm composition, history of periodontitis, radiation to the jaws, smoking habits, inadequate maintenance, and systemic diseases (such as uncontrolled diabetes, cancer, and cardiovascular diseases) are in a higher risk category for developing peri-implantitis and potential future implant loss [25].

Adequate bone density and quality are among the most important requirements for dental implant success. However, new advancements in implant designing now offer short and narrow implants, which can change the old criteria for hosting bone height/width. High success rates of bone grafting and expanding procedures make it possible to regenerate the resorbed bone to a certain level. The consensus is that enough bone must exist to achieve primary stability at the time of implant placement, and that the implant body should be at least 1.5 mm away from any anatomical landmark, such as adjacent tooth (root), mandibular nerve, floor of the maxillary sinus, or mental foramen, to prevent possible damage. A buccal bone crest thickness of at least 2 mm is recommended by many clinicians to minimize the risk for a biologic and/or esthetic complication as a result of normal crestal bone remodeling.

Any periodontal disease should be treated prior to implant placement, and the prospective implant sites must be free from any pathology, including residual endodontic lesions.

C. Cement-retained implants offer many advantages over their screw-retained alternatives. They offer flexibility, can aid in correcting misaligned implants, and improve esthetics – even when the alignment is not ideal – especially in anterior regions of the dentition. However, they are associated with a unique set of disadvantages as well. First, it is much more difficult to remove a cement-retained restoration than a screw-retained implant intact if, for some reason, it has broken or the abutment screw has loosened. The other disadvantage – and the one that tends to cause the most issues for restorative clinicians – is that the retention of cement below the mucosal margin can lead to catastrophic implant complications.

Excess cement could result in peri-implant disease under an cement-retained implant restoration, which is the reason dentists have returned to favoring screw-retained crowns these days. In addition, excess cement in subgingival spaces can be described as an "artificial calculus" and may have a similar irritating effect as a calcified calculus on periodontally involved teeth [26].

Peri-implant disease may affect the peri-implant mucosa only (peri-implant mucositis), which according to Present and Levine, this can "in esthetic areas in particular, this can severely disrupt implant treatment. Even if the implant remains osseointegrated, the resultant soft-tissue hyperplasia or recession can be an unacceptable outcome to both the patient and the clinician" [27]; or it may also involve the supporting bone (peri-implantitis). Peri-mucositis, by recent definition, is the presence of inflammation (bleeding upon probing) in the mucosa at an implant with no signs of associated bone loss, whereas peri-implantitis is inflammation not restricted to mucosa and is characterized by loss of bone around the implant [28–30].

In summary, the advantages of cement restorations are:
• simpler laboratory techniques;
• lesser risk for nonpassive fit;
• improved esthetics of the occlusal aspect of a restoration;
• facilitated design of the occlusal surface;
• elimination of occlusal screw loosening;
• lower cost of fabrication compared with screw retention.

In turn, the disadvantages are:
• inability to sufficiently remove excess cement, especially in the presence of submucosally located restorative implant or abutment margins;
• limited retrievability depending upon the type of cement utilized;
• unpredictable resistance and retention, depending upon the design and dimensions of an abutment;
• possibility of increased maintenance costs due to loss of retention [27].

D. A flapless surgical approach for implant placement can be chosen if the local bone volume in width and height is excellent (as identified via cross-sectional radiographs) and if a wide band of keratinized mucosa is present at the implant site. If the bone width diagnosed via a cross-sectional radiograph and diagnostic template is such that the maintenance of *at least* 1 mm of bone thickness buccally and/or lingually to the implant cannot be predicted, a flap elevation is necessary to facilitate a horizontal bone augmentation procedure. Furthermore, if the keratinized mucosa at the implant site is narrow and the risk exists that it is "punched away" in the process, a flapless surgery is contraindicated to avoid the risk of being left with a mobile peri-implant mucosa anywhere around the implant. Finally, the use of a precise and stably seated drill guide, which allows the reproduction of the radiographically planned implant position, is strongly recommended for a flapless implant surgery.

A flapless implant surgery makes the procedure quick and easy for the surgeon and the patient. It also reduces the level of postoperative discomfort for the patient substantially. Caution is required, however, to limit this surgical approach to those indications where the previously cited conditions are present.

Case 2

Anterior Implant Restoration

CASE STORY

A 61-year-old Caucasian male presented with a chief complaint of "my front tooth is moving and I am worried to lose it." The patient recalls having his central incisor (#8) fractured about 35 years ago during a rugby game and having it restored with a post and a crown. The patient has been seen regularly by his general dentist. His oral hygiene is fair even if his home care is questionable.

LEARNING GOALS AND OBJECTIVES

- To be able to understand the concept of immediate implant placement and implant provisionalization in the esthetic zone
- To understand the prosthetic procedures involved in the esthetic zone in order to achieve a proper soft tissue management
- To understand the importance of materials in the achievement of a proper esthetic result

Medical History

At the time of treatment, patient presented with no medical contraindications to any dental treatment. Patient has been a professional rugby player and now is in good health and does not take any medications.

Review of Systems

- Vital signs
  - Blood pressure: 128/78 mmHg
  - Pulse rate: 86 beats/min (regular)
  - Respiration: 16 breaths/min

Social History

The patient did not smoke or drink alcohol at the time of treatment.

Extraoral Examination

No significant findings were noted. The patient had no masses or swelling, and the temporomandibular joint was within normal limits. There was no facial asymmetry noted, and his lymph nodes were normal on palpation.

Intraoral Examination

- Oral cancer screening was negative.
- Soft tissue exam, including tongue and floor of the mouth, were within normal limits.
- Periodontal examination revealed pocket depths in the range of 2–3 mm except on tooth #8 (Figure 1).
- Generalized areas of gingival inflammation were noted.
- Several restorations in the form of single crowns and fixed partial dentures were present but nondefective.

Occlusion

There were no occlusal discrepancies or interferences noted. Patient had a class III tendency and anterior guidance.

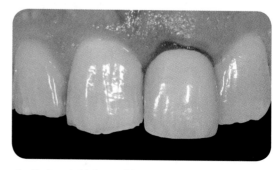

Figure 1: Patient initial condition, intraoral, frontal view.

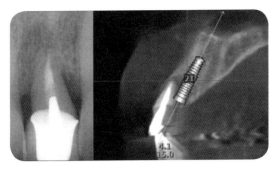

Figure 2: Patient initial condition, radiographic examinations.

Radiographic Examination

A full mouth radiographic series was ordered. A more detailed diagnostic radiograph (computed tomography scan) was taken for the central incisors (Figure 2).

Diagnosis

American Academy of Periodontology diagnosis of plaque-induced gingivitis with localized severe chronic periodontitis. Tooth #8 was also previously treated for a chronic apical abscess according to the classification of the American Association of Endodontists.

Treatment Plan

The treatment plan for this patient consisted of initial phase I therapy that included oral prophylaxis and oral hygiene instructions to address gingival inflammation. This was followed by extraction of tooth #8 and immediate implant placement with soft tissue graft. Immediately after the end of the surgical procedure a temporary Maryland bridge, with ovate pontic, was delivered. After 4 months of implant osseointegration, a screw-retained provisional restoration was inserted. Three months after soft tissue maturation a definitive abutment (titanium, gold hue) and a definitive crown (zirconia ceramic) were delivered.

Treatment

After the initial therapy, the patient presented for extraction of tooth #8 and implant placement. After obtaining profound anesthesia at the surgical site using local anesthetic, tooth #8 was extracted, paying attention to maintain the integrity of the buccal plate. Piezosurgery was utilized to create the implant osteotomy. The implant was then placed following the ideal prosthetic position; the gap between the implant and the buccal wall of the alveolus was filled with low rate resorbable material (xenograft). A rounded free gingival graft was utilized to seal the socket (Figures 3

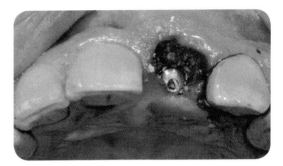

Figure 3: Immediate implant placement with bone-grafting procedure.

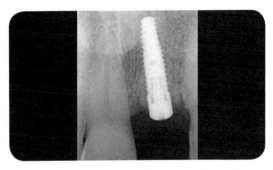

Figure 4: Postoperative periapical radiograph after implant placement.

and 4). Immediately after the surgical procedure a resin–metal temporary Maryland bridge was bonded to the palatal surfaces of the anterior teeth (Figure 5). The tissue surface of the Maryland bridge was ovate in shape, well polished, and was giving light pressure to the grafted soft tissue in order to mold it. Four months after implant placement, implant stage II took place (Figure 6). A pouch technique was utilized in order to minimize the surgical trauma and to maximize the soft tissue dimension on the buccal aspect of the implant (Figure 7). Immediately after the surgical procedure, an implant-level impression was taken and transferred

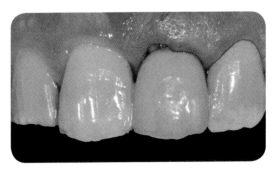

Figure 5: Delivery of acid-etched provisional fixed dental prosthesis with ovate pontic immediately after implant placement.

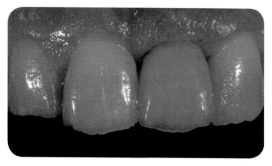

Figure 6: Acid-etched provisional fixed dental prosthesis at the end of the osseointegration period (4 months).

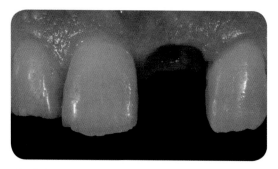

Figure 7: Soft tissue healing at the end of the osseointegration period (4 months).

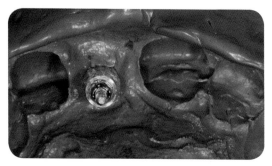

Figure 8: Implant-level impression without soft tissue profile customization.

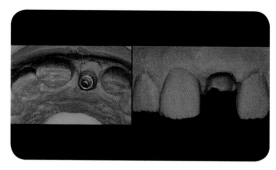

Figure 9: Determination of peri-implant soft tissue profile with modifications to the stone in the master cast.

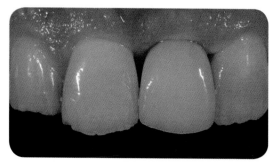

Figure 10: Implant-supported provisional crown, screw-retained, at delivery.

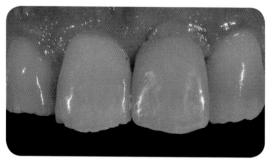

Figure 11: Implant-supported provisional crown, screw-retained, 3 months after insertion.

to the dental technician (Figure 8). In the stone model, the shape of the peri-implant soft tissue was molded in order to enable an adequate esthetic profile and soft tissue maturation with the screw-retained provisional restoration (Figure 9). The provisional restoration was inserted with light local anesthesia, giving pressure to the palatal and interproximal tissue, and torqued to 10 N cm (Figure 10). The soft tissues were conditioned for about 3 months prior to moving to the definitive steps; minimal modifications of the facial emergence profile were made (Figure 11).

About 7 months after implant placement the impressions for the definitive restorations were taken

with a customized impression coping and polyether material (Figures 12, 13, and 14). The definitive abutment was designed with the same shape principles adopted for the provisional restoration and fabricated in gold-hue titanium (Figure 15). After the abutment try-in, the definitive restoration was tried at the bisque stage and at the glazed stage. When both the patient and the dentist were satisfied, the definitive abutment was torqued down at 20 N cm and the definitive zirconia-ceramic crown was cemented with polycarboxylate provisional cement. Particular attention was addressed to the complete removal of the cement (Figures 16, 17, 18, and 19).

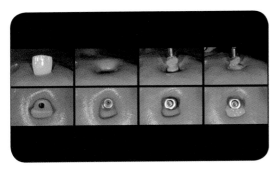

Figure 12: Customization of the implant impression coping.

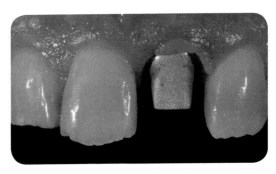

Figure 16: Definitive gold-hue titanium abutment at insertion.

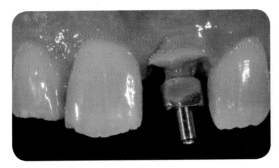

Figure 13: Implant-level final impression with customized impression coping; clinical view.

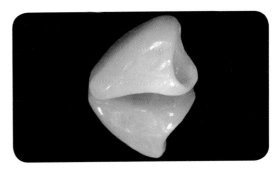

Figure 17: Definitive zirconia-ceramic crown.

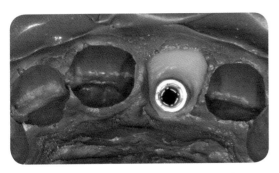

Figure 14: Implant-level definitive impression with customized impression coping, polyether material, and flowable composite.

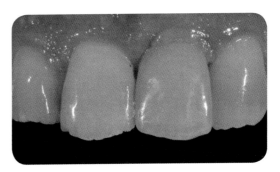

Figure 18: Definitive zirconia-ceramic crown 4 weeks after delivery.

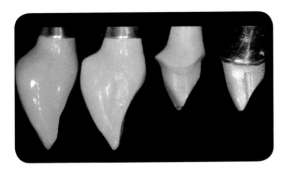

Figure 15: Customization of the peri-implant emergence profiles with initial screw-retained provisional restoration, modified screw-retained provisional restoration, definitive abutment wax-up, definitive gold-hue titanium abutment.

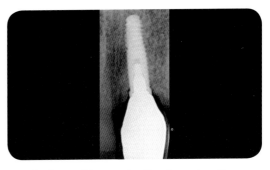

Figure 19: Radiographic examination 4 weeks after crown delivery.

Discussion

This case describes the treatment of a hopeless single tooth. The predictability of an anterior single implant tooth is related to a careful selection of the surgical and prosthetic steps.

The identification of the surrounding soft and hard tissue levels should be related to the planned or desired levels. A careful clinical and radiographic examination of some crucial anatomic landmarks should be performed. The success of the definitive restoration is strictly related to the presence of a good preextraction buccal plate and of interproximal bone peaks at an adequate level. If these structures are present, a good outcome is expected. The surgical procedure should include atraumatic extraction, minimal bone grafting procedure in the gap between the implant and the extraction socket, and soft tissue hypercorrection at implant stage I, and at implant stage II if thin tissue is present.

The prosthetic steps should follow the biologic timeline of the surgical procedures guiding the tissue maturation. Since soft tissue scalloping is determined by the prosthetic profiles, a proper shape of the prosthesis is crucial. The ovate pontic of the Maryland bridge molds the tissue in the healing phase and should never be removed in order to maintain the planned soft tissue contours.

When the implant is connected, either it is happening at stage I or II, the provisional and the definitive restorations should be modified the least possible number of times. Hence, the dentist should try to determine the exact prosthetic profile once and then, with minor modifications, transfer its shape to the definitive prosthesis. As described later, the market is nowadays filled with multiple offers in terms of materials, and the selection should focus on materials that combine esthetics, biology, and structural durability.

Self-Study Questions

(Answers located at the end of the case)

A. What are the initial radiographic requirements?

B. Is an immediate implant placement preferred to a delayed one in the esthetic zone?

C. Why is an ovate pontic selected for a temporary solution?

D. How should the peri-implant prosthetic profile be designed?

E. Why is a cemented type of restoration selected in the esthetic zone?

F. Does the material influence soft and hard tissue stability?

G. Does the material influence the final esthetic outcome?

H. Does the material influence the prognosis of the case?

References

1. Kois JC, Kan JY. Predictable peri-implant gingival aesthetics: surgical and prosthodontic rationales. Pract Proced Aesthet Dent 2001;13:691–698.
2. Kan JY, Roe P, Rungcharassaeng K, et al. Classification of sagittal root position in relation to the anterior maxillary osseous housing for immediate implant placement: a cone beam computed tomography study. Int J Oral Maxillofac Implants 2011;26(4):873–876.
3. Wohrle PS. Single-tooth replacement in the aesthetic zone with immediate provisionalization: fourteen consecutive case reports. Pract Periodontics Aesthet Dent 1998;10:1107–1114.
4. Kan JY, Rungcharassaeng K, Lozada J. Immediate placement and provisionalization of maxillary anterior

single implants: 1-year prospective study. Int J Oral Maxillofac Implants 2003;18:31–39.
5. Chen ST, Buser D. Clinical and esthetic outcomes of implants placed in postextraction sites. Int J Oral Maxillofac Implants 2009;24:186–217.
6. Stein RS. Pontic-residual ridge relationship: a research report. J Prosthet Dent 1966;16:251–285.
7. Zitzmann NU, Marinello CP, Berglundh T. The ovate pontic design: a histologic observation in humans. J Prosthet Dent 2002;88:375–380.
8. Orsini G, Murmura G, Artese L, et al. Tissue healing under provisional restorations with ovate pontics: a pilot human histological study. J Prosthet Dent 2006;96:252–257.

9. Gallucci GO, Belser UC, Bernard J, Magne P. Modeling and characterization of the CEJ for optimizing of Esthetic implant design. Int J Periodont Rest Dent 2004;24:19–29.

10. Rompen E, Raepsaet N, Domken O, et al. Soft tissue stability at the facial aspect of gingivally converging abutments in the esthetic zone. J Pros Dent 2007;97:119–125.

11. Su H, Gonzalez-Martin O, Weisgold A, Lee E. Considerations of implant abutment and crown contour: critical contour and subcritical contour. Int J Periodontics Restorative Dent 2010;30:335–343.

12. Chee W, Jivraj S. Screw versus cemented implant supported restorations. Br Dent J. 2006;201(8):501–507.

13. Hebel KS, Gajar RC. Cement-retained versus screw-retained implant restorations: achieving optimal occlusion and esthetics in implant dentistry. J Prosthet Dent 1997;77:28–35.

14. Michalakis KX, Hirayama H, Garefis PD. Cement-retained versus screw-retained implant restorations: a critical review. Int J Oral Maxillofac Implants 2003;18:719–728.

15. Wadhwani C, Rapoport D, La Rosa S, et al. Radiographic detection and characteristic patterns of residual excess cement associated with cement-retained implant restorations: a clinical report. J Prosthet Dent 2012;107(3):151–157.

16. Vigolo P, Givanu A, Majzoub Z, Cordioli G. A 4-year prospective study to assess peri-implant hard and soft tissues adjacent to titanium versus gold-alloy abutments in cemented single implant crowns. J Prosthodont 2006;15:250–256.

17. Welander M, Abrahamsson I, Berglundh T. The mucosal barrier at implant abutments of different materials. Clin Oral Implants Res 2008;19:635–641.

18. Jung RE, Holderegger C, Sailer I, et al. The effect of all-ceramic and porcelain-fused-to-metal restorations on marginal peri-implant soft tissue color: a randomized controlled clinical trial. Int J Periodontics Restorative Dent 2008;28:357–365.

19. Hefferman MJ, Aquilino SA, Diaz-Arnold AM, et al. Relative translucency of six all-ceramic systems. Part I: core and veneer materials. J Prosthet Dent 2002;88:4–9.

20. Bressan E, Paniz G, Lops D, et al. Influence of abutment material on the gingival color of implant-supported all-ceramic restorations: a prospective multicenter study. Clin Oral Implants Res 2011;22(6):631–637.

21. Paniz G, Bressan E, Stellini E, et al. Correlation between subjective and objective evaluation of peri-implant soft tissue color. Clin Oral Implants Res 2014;25(8):992–996.

22. Ishikawa-Nagai S, Da Silva JD, Weber HP, Par SE. Optical phenomenon of peri-implant soft tissue. Part II. Preferred implant neck color to improve soft tissue esthetics. Clin Oral Implants Res 2007;18:575–580.

23. Cho HW, Dong JK, Jin TH, et al. A study on the fracture strength of implant-supported restorations using milled ceramic abutments and all-ceramic crowns. Int J Prosthodont 2002;15(1):9–13.

24. Yildirim M, Fischer H, Marx R, Edelhoff D. In vivo fracture resistance of implant-supported all-ceramic restorations. J Prosthet Dent 2003;90(4):325–331.

25. Zembic A, Bösch A, Jung RE, et al. Five-year results of a randomized controlled clinical trial comparing zirconia and titanium abutments supporting single-implant crowns in canine and posterior regions. Clin Oral Implants Res 2013;24(4):384–390.

Answers to Self-Study Questions

A. To ensure successful immediate implant placement, in addition to the presence of an intact bony socket following extraction and the absence of active infection, primary implant stability must be achieved by engaging the implant with the palatal wall and the bone approximately 4–5 mm beyond the root apex [1]. Unfortunately, because the available bone around the failing tooth may not always be sufficient to achieve primary implant stability, alternative treatment options should be considered. Factors such as root length, sagittal root position, and the morphology of the osseous housing are important in determining the feasibility of the immediate placement and must be evaluated via the use of cone beam computed tomography. Understanding the importance of sagittal root position through the use of cone beam computed tomography will be a vital adjunct to treatment planning of immediate implant placement in the anterior maxilla [2].

B. Immediate implant placement of a single tooth in the esthetic zone was first advocated in the mid-1990s and has since been considered a predictable treatment option for replacing failing teeth [3]. In addition to reducing treatment time and providing the patient with the convenience of an immediate tooth replacement, the immediate implant placement procedures have also been documented with high success rates when established clinical guidelines are followed [4]. Evidence is lacking to demonstrate the superiority of one placement protocol over the other with respect to healing of peri-implant defects with postextraction implants. However, there is some evidence to show that regenerative outcomes are better with early placement (4–8 weeks) compared with immediate placement in the presence of dehiscence defects of the facial bone wall. The survival rates for postextraction implants are high, with the majority of studies reporting rates of over 95%. This shows that immediate and delayed (type 2) placement protocols have similar survival rates. Tissue alterations leading to recession of the facial mucosa and papillae are common with immediate placement. There is evidence that early placement (4–8 weeks) is associated with a lower frequency of mucosal recession compared with immediate placement. Risk indicators for recession with immediate placement include a thin tissue biotype, a facial malposition of the implant, and a thin or damaged facial bone wall [5]. Although patient-evaluated esthetic outcomes with postextraction implants are generally favorable, there are relatively few studies that evaluate esthetic outcomes using objective parameters.

C. In order to better control the implant osseointegration and the soft tissue scalloping and maturation, immediate provisionalization is not always recommended in the esthetic zone [1]. For this reason, excluding removable solutions, which are not well accepted by patients with high expectations, a fixed temporary solution like a Maryland bridge is suggested. In the esthetic zone, the Maryland bridge supports an ovate pontic and is inserted right after the surgical procedure, providing a natural gingival architecture and avoiding the postextraction soft tissue collapse [6]. The ovate pontic shape should extend about 1–2 mm inside the postextraction site, giving adequate support to the facial soft tissue (not excessive, avoiding recession), to the interproximal area (crucial, since the papillae act as a water bag), and to the palatal aspect (in order to give the patient adequate comfort, phonetics, and to avoid possible food impaction) [7]. It is crucial that nonconcavity is present underneath the pontic and that the surface is well polished [8].

D. The utilization of customized emergence profiles is critical in order to achieve a proper esthetic result with adequate shape and scalloping of the soft tissues. The peri-implant profile should be designed at the provisional stage and transferred to the definitive restorations through customized procedures [9]. A subcritical area, closer to the implant head, is characterized by a straight profile with reduced influences on the soft tissue. A concave emergence profile in this area might be useful to thicken the soft tissue and to favor its coronal migration [10]. A critical area, closer to the gingival margin, is responsible for the shape of the soft tissue and should be designed carefully: convexity determines tissue apicalization, concavity determines tissue coronalization [11].

E. In the finalization of a prosthetic case on implants, two different solutions could be selected: a cement-retained type or a screw-retained type [12]. Each has advantages and disadvantages. Considering single-unit cement-retained restorations in the esthetic zone, different advantages are present [13,14]:
• *Esthetics.* Since the prosthesis is cemented on abutments, in a similar manner to natural teeth, the screw access hole is not present and the esthetic appearance of the prosthesis is normally excellent, especially if the implant is slightly facially inclined.
• *Occlusion.* For the same reason, occlusion is not influenced by the presence of a screw access hole on the centric stops or on the excursive movements.
• *Porcelain stability.* Since no holes are present on the prosthesis, the integrity of the prosthesis porcelain is improved.
Nevertheless, particular attention should be given to possible disadvantages, such as retrievability (especially when screw loosening happens) and cement trapping in the peri-implant sulcus, which should be carefully avoided [15].

F. The stability of the peri-implant soft tissue is strictly related to surgical procedures that favor the presence of adequate buccal and interproximal hard and soft tissue. The selection of adequate materials contributes to improve this stability. Clinically, not many differences are present, but radiographically and histologically a few differences have been documented [16]. Materials such as titanium and zirconia are associated with less marginal bone loss, more coronal position of the barrier epithelium, higher amount of collagen, and fibroblast in the surrounding connective tissue [17]. Since clinical findings are less significant, this information should be considered but does not represent a crucial factor.

G. The selection of the definitive prosthesis material has a crucial role in the achievement of an adequate natural esthetic result, especially in restorations where natural teeth are still present and the comparison is easily made by the patient or by observers. The esthetic benefit of ceramic abutments over metal abutments has been well documented in recent clinical studies underlining an improved soft tissue color around implants [18]. On the other side, not many differences are present at the crown portion since, due to the increased thickness of the abutment, most of the materials present similar opacity [19]. More recent studies underlined the fact that, while the presence of gray titanium abutments creates an impairment of the soft tissue color, a

gold-hue metal abutment or gold-hue titanium abutments provide the same natural esthetic result of the soft tissue, and might be preferred for structural reasons [20–22].

H. The performance of white abutments (zirconia, lithium disilicate, alumina) has always been considered at a higher level of risk compared with a stronger abutment type, such as titanium and metal. Indeed, superior fracture strengths have been demonstrated for metal-ceramic crowns cemented on titanium abutments compared with all-ceramic crowns cemented on ceramic abutments [23]. Besides the esthetic considerations mentioned, several workers report a good prognosis for zirconia abutments, especially on anterior teeth, as the fracture resistance of implant-supported all-ceramic abutments (Al_2O_3 and ZrO_2) exceeds the maximum values for incisal load reported in the literature [24]. More recent systematic reviews report similar 5-year survival rates for ceramic and metal abutments as well as similar technical and biological complication rates also in posterior regions [25]. For these reasons all-ceramic abutments can be utilized with a good prognosis, but case-by-case selection is recommended.

Case 3

Full-Mouth Rehabilitation

CASE STORY

A 65-year-old Caucasian male presented with a chief complaint of: "I am tired of my lower denture, which is moving and interfering with my tongue. I want to improve my smile" (Figure 1). The patient has been wearing a removable complete maxillary denture for more than 30 years, with no significant problems. The patient has also been wearing a removable mandibular partial denture for the same amount of time. Twelve months before his appointment, teeth #28 and #29 had been extracted and the partial denture modified into a complete denture (Figures 2 and 3). The patient has an extremely positive attitude to his health and to the treatment of his mouth. He is thinking of a removable prosthesis in the maxilla and is

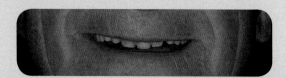

Figure 1: Patient's initial condition: extraoral, frontal view.

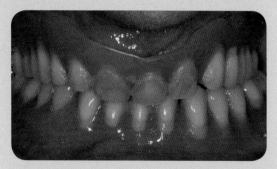

Figure 2: Patient's initial condition: intraoral, frontal view with existing dentures.

wondering if a fixed solution would be possible for his mandibular arch. The patient has financial limitations.

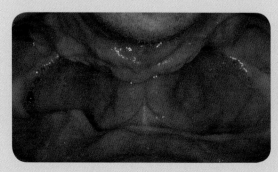

Figure 3: Patient's initial condition: intraoral, frontal view without existing dentures.

LEARNING GOALS AND OBJECTIVES

■ To be able to understand the possible treatment options for a completely edentulous patient

■ To understand the technique for immediate occlusal loading on a completely edentulous mandible

■ To understand the different types of prosthetic solutions for an implant-supported restoration, also in consideration of economic conditions

Medical History

At the time of treatment, the patient was in good health and presented no contraindication for any type of dental treatment.

Review of Systems

- Vital signs
  - Blood pressure: 130/85 mmHg
  - Pulse rate: 80 beats/min (regular)
  - Respiration: 14 breaths/min

Social History

The patient did not smoke; he drank one glass of wine at each meal.

Extraoral Examination

No significant findings were noted. The patient had neither masses nor swelling, and the temporomandibular joint was within normal limits. There was no significant facial asymmetry noted, and his lymph nodes were normal on palpation.

Intraoral Examination

- Oral cancer screening was negative.
- Soft tissue exam, including tongue and floor of the mouth, were within normal limits.
- The upper and the lower edentulous arches are V-shaped.

- Evaluation of the alveolar ridge in the areas #7–#10 (FDI #12–#22) presented reduced keratinized tissue.
- Horizontal and vertical resorption of bone was present in the posterior quadrants of the maxillary arch and the mandibular arches, with the exception of the area #27–#29 (FDI #43–#45).

Occlusion

The occlusal scheme of the existing denture was bilaterally balanced, but no occlusal morphology was present on the existing dentures due to advanced wear.

Radiographic Examination

Besides a panoramic radiograph for general screening, a computed tomography (CT) scan of the mandibular arch was taken to assess the possibility of a fixed prosthodontic reconstruction (Figures 4 and 5). A radiographic examination revealed significant horizontal and vertical bone resorption, but sufficient bone was present in the intraforaminal area from #21 to #28 (FDI #34–#44) for placement of four to five dental implants of standard diameter and height.

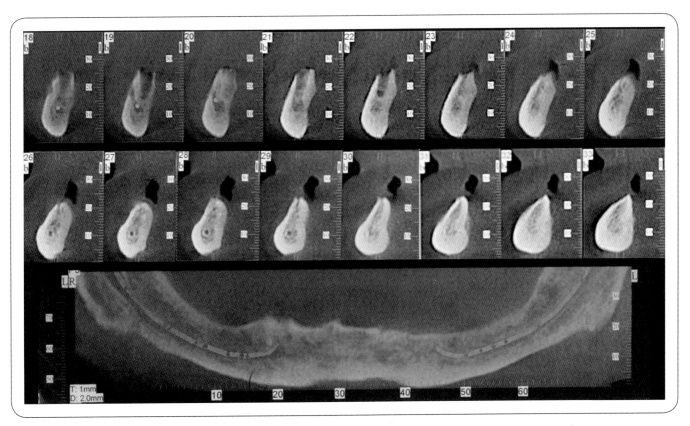

Figure 4: Patient's initial condition: mandibular radiographic examination with cross-sectional and panoramic views.

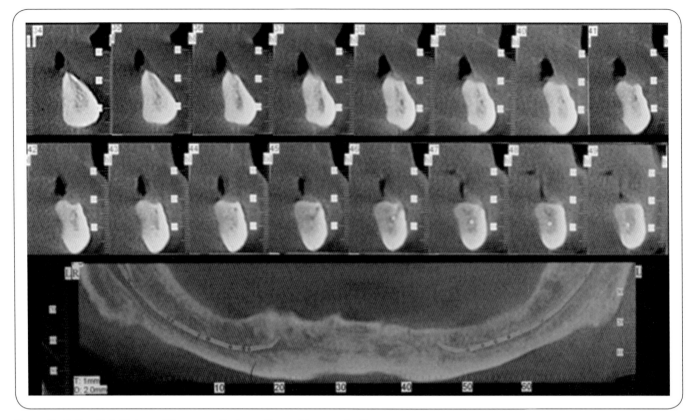

Figure 5: Patient's initial condition: mandibular radiographic examination.

Diagnosis

According to the Diagnostic Classification of Complete Edentulism of the American College of Prosthodontics, the patient was diagnosed as having a class IV condition. This means a severely compromised situation due to the mandibular bone height as measured at the least vertical height (≤10 mm is class IV). The maxillo-mandibular relationship was normal (class I), the residual maxillary ridge morphology well defined (class I), and the muscle attachments adequate in all regions except in the buccal vestibules (class II).

Treatment Plan

The treatment plan for this patient consisted of soft relining and tissue conditioning of the existing dentures prior to fabrication of a newly developed maxillary complete denture and mandibular implant-supported complete denture. Anterior vestibuloplasty was discussed with the patient for the maxillary arch, but not planned according to the patient's request. Four dental implants have been planned, placed and immediately loaded with a resin base complete denture. At the end of the osseointegration period and tissue stabilization period (3 months), a mandibular complete resin-veneered titanium prosthesis was to be fabricated and inserted.

Treatment

After a denture relining procedure with tissue conditioning material, a preliminary procedure for the fabrication of maxillary and mandibular complete dentures was performed. Irreversible hydrocolloid material was utilized with stock trays, and preliminary casts were fabricated with type III dental stone. In the maxillary arch a customized tray was fabricated and utilized for taking the impression for a definitive maxillary complete denture. Modeling plastic impression compound was utilized for border molding and polysulfide material for tissue impression (Figure 6). The definitive cast for the maxillary arch was fabricated with type IV dental stone. The interocclusal registration was obtained with the utilization of record bases with wax rims and aluminum-wax (Figure 7). A trial insertion was performed to visualize the final functional and esthetic outcome (Figure 8). A definitive complete denture was then fabricated for the maxillary arch, and

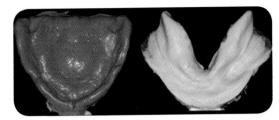

Figure 6: Final impressions for maxillary complete denture (polysulfide) and interim complete mandibular denture (irreversible hydrocolloid).

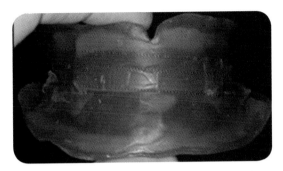

Figure 7: Interocclusal records with record base and wax rims.

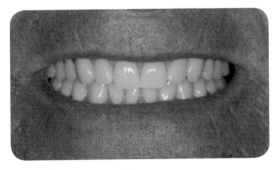

Figure 8: Tooth set-up at try-in.

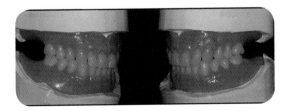

Figure 9: Lateral views of maxillary complete denture (definitive) and mandibular complete denture (interim for immediate loading).

an interim complete denture, prepared to be modified at the implant placement, was fabricated for the mandible (Figure 9). A duplication of the mandibular denture, in orthodontic resin, was utilized as a surgical stent.

On the day of the surgery, the patient was anesthetized. Then, a midline crestal incision was

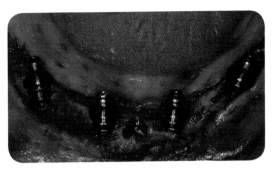

Figure 10: Implant placement in the mandibular arch (surgery by Andrea Chierico, DDS).

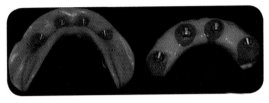

Figure 11: Immediate loading procedure, prior and after prosthesis finalization.

made, and a full-thickness mucoperiosteal flap was elevated. A reduction of the knife-edge residual bone was performed mainly in the right quadrant, and four dental implants were placed between the mental foramens. The two distal implant were inclined in the distal direction to increase the support polygon and reduce cantilever lengths (Figure 10; surgery by Andrea Chierico, DDS). All of the implants revealed an insertion torque higher than 50 N cm and an implant stability quotient (ISQ) higher than 70. Four straight conical abutments were inserted and torqued at 32 N cm, and the tissues were sutured. The resin complete denture was minimally reduced to accommodate the titanium temporary cylinders screwed on the conical abutment, and autopolymerizing acrylic resin was utilized to fix the cylinders to the denture. Once the acrylic resin was polymerized, the abutments were unscrewed and the prosthesis finalized with reduction of the distal cantilever and flanges (Figure 11). The interim implant-supported complete denture was then inserted, and the screws were torqued to 12 N cm. The occlusion was verified and adjusted to even contact in centric and light group function (Figure 12). The sutures were removed 1 week after prostheses insertion, and the occlusion was verified and minimally adjusted. The patient's progress was assessed at 3 weeks and at 2 months after the procedure. Three months after the implant placement, when osseointegration was considered completed and the tissues were remodeled,

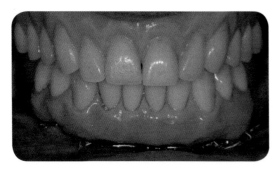

Figure 12: Maxillary definitive complete denture and mandibular temporary denture, implant-supported and immediately loaded.

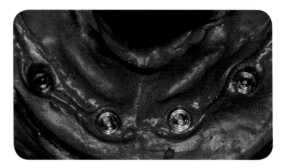

Figure 15: Final impression for mandibular prosthesis with polyether material.

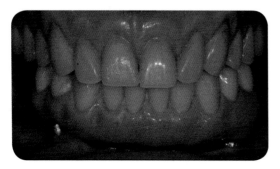

Figure 13: Four-month follow-up after prostheses insertion.

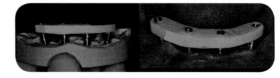

Figure 16: Stone index verification.

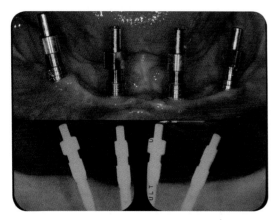

Figure 14: Impression copings for final impression placed and accurate seating verified with radiograph.

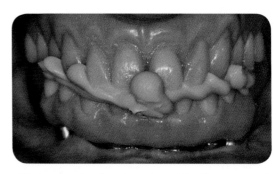

Figure 17: Interocclusal registration with silicone material.

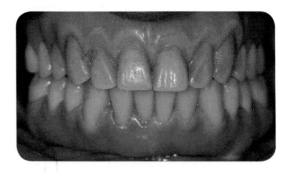

Figure 18: Teeth try-in for mandibular denture.

the definitive implant-supported complete denture was fabricated with computer-aided design (CAD)/computer-aided manufacturing (CAM) (Figure 13).

A definitive implant-level impression was taken with polyether impression material and verified with a stone index (Figures 14, 15, and 16). Interocclusal registration was performed utilizing the existing restoration with the interposition of silicone bite-registration material (Figure 17). A resin–wax try-in was made prior to

framework fabrication in order to design the titanium structure in the best possible way (Figures 18 and 19). The titanium–acrylic resin prosthesis was torqued to the implant heads at 32 N cm. The distal cantilever extensions were set to the first molar, and a lingualized occlusal scheme was followed (Figures 20 and 21). The patient has been observed for 3 years, and no complications have occurred (Figures 22 and 23).

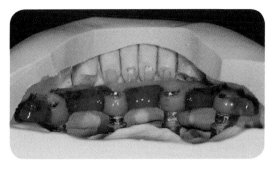

Figure 19: Resin mandibular framework prior to milling process.

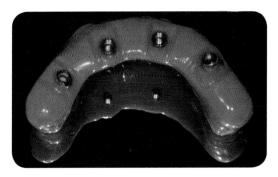

Figure 20: Implant-supported mandibular complete denture, tissue surface.

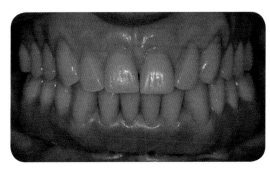

Figure 21: Maxillary complete denture (removable) and mandibular implant-supported complete denture (fixed).

Discussion

In this case, the treatment of a fully edentulous patient is described. In treating these types of patients, the evaluation of the residual ridges and the analysis of the existing dentures and the patient's comfort with them are crucial diagnostic steps prior to deciding which treatment to follow.

When a patient is satisfied with the existing dentures, especially in the maxillary arch, the

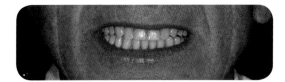

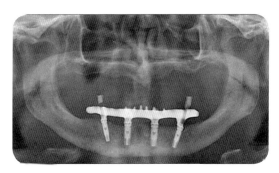

Figure 22: Patient's condition posttreatment, extraoral, frontal view.

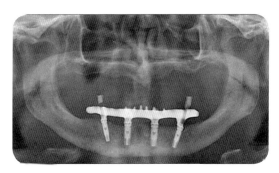

Figure 23: Patient's condition posttreatment, radiographic examination.

fabrication of a new denture should be considered prior to selecting more extensive treatment. Especially in the maxillary arch, like in this particular case, the achievement of good support, retention, and stability is predictable.

In the mandibular arch, the situation is often different from the maxillary arch as the morphology of the mandible is different, and anatomical components, like the tongue, play a significant role in the achievement of good retention and stability. For these reasons, the placement of implants, either for assisting or supporting a complete denture, should be considered as standard of care. Implant-assisted complete overdentures are characterized by improved stability and retention. This solution does not change the patient's ability to remove and insert the removable denture, significantly helping maintenance. Implant-supported complete dentures play an important role in improving patient comfort, but their applicability should be considered more carefully. In the mandibular arch, thanks to the extremely good quality of the bone between the alveolar foramens, implant-supported solutions are predictable and often easy to manage. Also, immediate occlusal loading is a predictable and common way to treat an edentulous mandible.

Self-Study Questions

(Answers located at the end of the case)

A. Which radiographic examinations are necessary for treating an edentulous patient with implants?

B. Should a fixed restorative solution be preferred over a removable one in a completely edentulous patient?

C. Is the immediate occlusal loading predictable and useful for a completely edentulous patient?

D. Which material should be utilized for a full-arch immediate occlusal loading?

E. How many implants should be placed on an edentulous mandible?

F. How should the implant position be transferred to the dental laboratory?

G. What are the advantages of a screw-retained prosthesis compared with a cemented type?

H. Can the utilization of CAD/CAM technology improve the quality of definitive restoration?

I. Is the utilization of resin veneering material advantageous compared with ceramic material?

References

1. Tyndall AA, Brooks SL. Selection criteria for dental implant site imaging: a position paper of the American Academy of Oral and Maxillofacial radiology. Oral Surg Oral Med Oral Pathol Oral Radiol Endodontol 2000;89(5):630–637.
2. Harris D, Buser D, Dula K, et al. E.A.O. guidelines for the use of diagnostic imaging in implant dentistry. A consensus workshop organized by the European Association for Osseointegration in Trinity College Dublin. Clin Oral Implants Res 2002;13(5):566–570.
3. Feine JS, Carlsson GE, Awad MA, et al. The McGill consensus statement on overdentures. Mandibular two-implant overdentures as first choice standard of car for edentulous patients. Gerodontology 2002;19(1):3–4.
4. Bressan E, Tomasi C, Stellini E, et al. Implant-supported mandibular overdentures: a cross-sectional study. Clin Oral Implants Res 2012;23(7):814–819.
5. Emami E, Heydecke G, Rompré PH, et al. Impact of implant support for mandibular dentures on satisfaction, oral and general health-related quality of life: a meta-analysis of randomized-controlled trials. Clin Oral Implants Res 2009;20(6):533–544.
6. Romanos G, Froum S, Hery C, et al. Survival rate of immediately vs delayed loaded implants: analysis of the current literature. J Oral Implantol 2010;36(4):315–324.
7. Raghavendra S, Taylor T. Early wound healing around implants: a review of the literature. Int J Oral Maxillofac Implants 2005;20(3):425–431.
8. Dierens M, Collaert B, Deschepper E, et al. Patient-centered outcome of immediately loaded implants in the rehabilitation of fully edentulous jaws. Clin Oral Implants Res 2009;20(10):1070–1077.
9. Misch CM. Immediate loading of definitive implants in the edentulous mandible using a fixed provisional prosthesis: the denture conversion technique. J Oral Maxillofac Surg 2004;62(9 Suppl 2):106–115.
10. Paniz G, Chierico A, Cuel S, Tomasi P. A technique for immediate occlusal loading of a complete edentulous mandible: a clinical report. J Prosthet Dent 2012;107(4):221–226.
11. Maló P, Rangert B, Nobre M. "All-on-Four" immediate function concept with Brånemark System implants for completely edentulous mandibles: a retrospective clinical study. Clin Implant Dent Relat Res 2003;5(Suppl 1):2–9.
12. Branemark PI, Svensson B, van Steenberghe D. Ten-year survival rates of fixed prostheses on four or six implants ad modum Brånemark in full edentulism. Clin Oral Implants Res 1995;6(4):227–231.
13. Heydecke G, Zwahlen M, Nicol A, et al. What is the optimal number of implants for fixed reconstructions: a systematic review. Clin Oral Implants Res 2012;23(6):217–228.
14. Lee H, So JS, Hochstedler JL, Ercoli C. The accuracy of implant impressions: a systematic review. J Prosthet Dent 2008;100(4):285–291.
15. Vigolo P, Fonzi F, Majzoub Z, Cordioli G. Evaluation of the accuracy of three techniques used for multiple implant abutment impressions. J Prosthet Dent 2003;89(2):186–192.
16. Hariharan R, Shankar C, Rajan M, et al. Evaluation of accuracy of multiple dental implant impressions using various splinting materials. Int J Oral Maxillofac Implants 2010;25(1):38–44.
17. Michalakis KX, Hirayama H, Garefis PD. Cement-retained versus screw-retained implant restorations: a critical review. Int J Oral Maxillofac Implants 2003;18(5):719–728.

18. Karl M, Graef F, Taylor TD, Heckmann SM. In vitro effect of load cycling on metal-ceramic cement- and screw-retained implant restorations. J Prosthet Dent 2007;97(3):137–140.

19. Keith SE, Miller BH, Woody RD, Higginbottom FL. Marginal discrepancies of screw-retained and cemented metal-ceramic crowns on implant abutments. Int J Oral Maxillofac Implants 1999;14(3):369–378.

20. Ortorp A, Jemt T. Clinical experience of CNC-milled titanium frameworks supported by implants in the edentulous jaw: a 3-year interim report. Clin Implant Dent Relat Res 2002;4(2):104–109.

21. Paniz G, Stellini E, Meneghello R, Cerardi A, Gobbato EA, Bressan E. The precision of fit of cast and milled full-arch implant-supported restorations. Int J Oral Maxillofac Implants 2013;28(3):687–693.

22. Papaspyridakos P, Chen CJ, Chuang SK, et al. A systematic review of biologic and technical complications with fixed implant rehabilitations for edentulous patients. Int J Oral Maxillofac Implants 2012;27(1):102–110.

23. Bozini T, Petridis H, Garefis K, Garefis P. A meta-analysis of prosthodontic complication rates of implant-supported fixed dental prostheses in edentulous patients after an observation period of at least 5 years. Int J Oral Maxillofac Implants 2011;26(2):304–318.

24. Nedir R, Bischof M, Szmukler-Moncler S, et al. Prosthetic complications with dental implants: from an up-to-8-year experience in private practice. Int J Oral Maxillofac Implants 2006;21(6):919–928.

Answers to Self-Study Questions

A. Assessment of available alveolar bone and bone morphology with clinical examination and palpation of the bone ridge at the implant site is essential in preoperative implant planning. Various presurgical imaging techniques, including conventional radiographs (intraoral and panoramic radiographs, tomography, cephalometry, etc.) and CT, are proposed to localize the mandibular canal [1].

Although the need for cross-sectional imaging has been strongly recommended, panoramic radiographs are considered to be the standard radiographic diagnostic examination for implant treatment as it imparts a low radiation dose [2].

B. Implant overdentures have been characterized as the best solution for an edentulous patient to achieve a good balance between costs and benefits [3]. On the other hand, if the diagnostic clinical solutions allow a fixed restoration, esthetics, phonetics, masticatory function, and psychological attitude are better achieved with a fixed restoration [4].

Nevertheless, in order to define whether a fixed or removable solution, such as an implant overdenture, is to be preferred for a specific patient, a few variables should be considered. First, the residual amount of bone in the mandible and especially in the maxilla should be considered to understand how many implants can be positioned in the specific arch and how the denture will integrate with the tissue profiles. Furthermore, the patient skeletal classification as well as the residual bone relation to anatomical extraoral structures (such as lip support and profile) should be considered, and a removable solution is preferred when increased discrepancies are present. Finally, patient compliance should be considered in regard to their ability and motivation to maintain an adequate oral hygiene with a fixed solution. Patients with limitations might not be able to adopt sufficient home care [5].

C. Immediate occlusal loading has been documented as a predictable option for restoring missing teeth when bone quantity and quality are favorable for adequate bone-to-implant contact. In order to be able to perform immediate loading, primary stability of the implant is required. Primary stability could be measured by the insertion torque (a minimal insertion torque of 25–30 N cm is recommended), predicted radiographically (Hounsefield units are a useful tool for measurements of bone quality), helped by a correct implant insertion protocol and assessed with resonance frequency analysis (ISQ value) [6]. When ISQ values are between 45 and 60, the implant stability is good, but not good enough for immediate occlusal loading. If ISQ values are higher than 60, immediate occlusal loading can be performed with good predictability. Its application in the completely edentulous mandible is well described in the literature, especially when implants are positioned between the alveolar foramens [7]. This procedure is useful to reduce treatment time (soft tissue maturation), patient discomfort (avoiding the utilization of an unstable and relined removable denture), especially in the first weeks after the surgical procedure, and postoperative care. In addition, immediate loading has been demonstrated to have a positive psychological effect on both partially and especially completely edentulous patients [8].

D. A full-arch implant-supported restoration delivered immediately after implant placement must be rigid. Cross-arch stabilization is important to increase the good prognosis of implant osseointegration. Moreover, the prosthesis must incorporate functional and esthetic properties, since it is not recommended to remove it from the patient's mouth during the osseointegration period. For this reason, an accurate case assessment and diagnostic wax-up or set-up should be made prior to the surgical procedure [9]. In this way, complications such as fracture of the structure and the teeth will be avoided. In the mandible, when prosthesis height is adequate, a good compromise can be achieved with the utilization of resin only [10]. In the maxilla, or in particular situations of the mandible, the height of the prosthesis could be reduced and the addition of reinforcements (metal or fiber) is recommended [11].

E. Even if there are many opinions on the number of implants needed for full-mouth rehabilitation, there is a lack of evidence to define the optimal number for a fixed rehabilitation of an edentulous arch. In the mandible, six implants have been defined as the required number since the beginning of osseointegration [12]. More recent studies and clinical reports confirmed good survival and success rates with the utilization of four implants for full-arch implant restorations of the mandible. When a reduced number of implants are selected, particular care should be addressed on implant distribution and angulation, especially if immediate loading is involved [13].

F. Marginal adaptation is a fundamental requirement of dental prosthesis and, due to the absence of the periodontal ligament, must be even more precise with implant-supported restorations to reduce biological and mechanical complications. The precision of fit is the result of multiple clinical and laboratory procedures, and implant-level impression is the first step. Most research concludes that the indirect impression technique, also called the closed-tray technique, creates higher distortions than the direct technique, also known as the open-tray technique [14]. Precise materials such as polyether and polyvinylsiloxane should be utilized in conjunction with custom trays, and adjunctive procedures should be used to verify the precision of the impression procedures with resin and stone indexing and improve accuracy by splinting the impression posts with acrylic material [15,16].

G. Implant-supported restorations can be classified as either screw-retained or cement-retained prostheses. The biggest advantage of a screw-retained prosthesis is that, at any time, the prosthesis can be easily unscrewed and removed by the dentist [17]. There is also no risk of leaving cement in the peri-implant sulcus, which has been documented as a hazard to optimal biologic integration and performance of the implant-supported prosthesis. Finally, a screw-retained prosthesis is a versatile solution, especially when occlusal limitations are present, and presents reduced fabrication costs [18]. Limitations should also be considered, since a cement-type prosthesis presents improved esthetics, occlusal stability, ceramic prognosis, and improved passive fit [19].

H. CAD and CAM have been introduced in the dental field to reduce the possible errors resulting from multiple technique-sensitive procedures. For these reasons, the utilization of digital technology can improve the quality of prosthesis, improving accurate fit of implant-supported restorations [20]. Compatible materials such as titanium or zirconia, or less expensive materials such as cobalt–chromium, can be utilized predictably. The development of technology significantly influenced the technical possibilities for the fabrication of full-arch implant-supported restorations with frameworks fabricated with milling techniques [21].

I. A layering procedure over implant frameworks can be done with ceramic material or with composite/resin material. Resins are often selected owing to their reduced cost and ease of handling and repair. On the other hand, plaque accumulates faster on resins than on ceramics, and the color of resins is less stable in the mid and long term [22]. Recent studies investigated biologic and technical complications over time, concluding that complications happen constantly over time as a result of fatigue and stress. These events may not lead to implant/prosthetic failures, but they are significant in relation to the amount of repair and maintenance needed and time and cost to both the clinician and patient. Resin layering is related to increased prosthodontic complications such as fracture and material wear after long-term function [23,24].

Case 4

Implant-Supported Mandibular Overdentures

A 62-year-old Caucasian female presented with an internal referral from Tufts University School of Dental Medicine Undergraduate Clinic, with a chief complaint of: "Both of my dentures are loose, my bottom denture constantly causes both pain and ulcers, I find it difficult to chew food with my lower denture in and often eat with it out. I would like to have a set that look clean and stay in" (Figure 1).

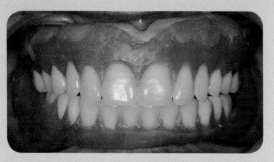

Figure 1: Existing maxillary and mandibular dentures.

LEARNING GOALS AND OBJECTIVES
- Proper diagnosis of an edentulous patient
- Understanding the role of implants in edentulous patients
- Utilizing implants in the xerostomia patient

Medical History

A review of the patient's medical history revealed that she has struggled with bouts of anorexia nervosa. She reports that this behavior is now in the past and no longer affects her. She also has hypothyroidism and suffers from anxiety and depression. The patient also reports migraines. She is taking levothyroxine for the hypothyroidism, Cymbalta (duloxetine) and lorazepam for anxiety, Prilosec (omeprazole) for gastroesophageal reflux disease, amitriptyline for depression, and Imitrex (sumatriptan) for migraines.

Review of Systems

- Vital statistics
  - Average blood pressure: 118/81 mmHg
  - Average respiration rate: 16 breaths/min
  - Average pulse rate: 65 beats/min

Social History

The patient has no history of smoking or use of tobacco-containing products. She does not consume alcohol owing to interactions with medications.

Extraoral Examination

The patient had no palpable lymph nodes in the head and neck region, no muscle tenderness, and no temporomandibular joint sounds or symptoms. Patient exhibits good facial symmetry. Mandibular range of motion was smooth and free of clicking, and there was no deviation of the mandible upon opening. The patient exhibited a straight soft tissue profile and an even, high upper lip line when smiling with existing dentures.

Intraoral Examination

Examination of the lips, tongue, floor of the mouth, oral mucosa, and pharyngeal tissues revealed no pathology. Maxillary residual ridge was ovoid shaped, and denture-bearing areas appeared firm and keratinized. Posterior left ridge was wider and slightly irregular from extraction sockets. Palatal form was classified as House class I form [1] (Figure 2).

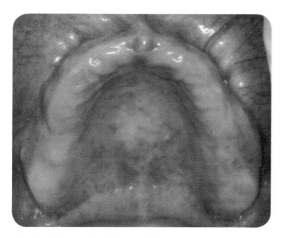

Figure 2: Maxillary edentulous ridge.

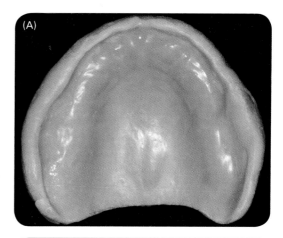

(A)

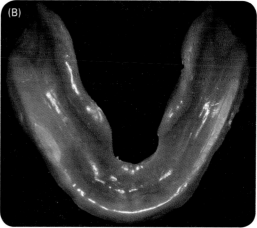

(B)

Figure 4: (A) Maxillary and (B) mandibular dentures.

The mandibular residual ridge was ovoid in shape, and denture-bearing tissue appeared firm and keratinized. However, the tissue is inflamed and several small, ulcerated lesions are present on the ridge. An amalgam tattoo is present near the ulcerated lesion. The patient suffers from severe xerostomia, which is evident in Figure 3. The retromylohyoid fossa was classified as Neil's class II lateral throat form [2]. The buccal shelf areas are adequate in size for denture support. However, the vertical height of mandibular ridge remaining is minimal, evident by the lack of buccal vestibule depth.

The patient had adequate interarch space at the approximate occlusal vertical dimension. Maxillary and mandibular residual ridges appear regular shape and in class 1 relationship.

Prosthetic Analysis

Regarding the immediate maxillary denture, the peripheral extensions of the denture are impinging the buccal frena. The soft liner material is hard, brittle,

and breaking. Underextension of denture flanges was seen in the retrozygomatic fossa area. The mandibular immediate denture was relined with a hard reline material that was not well trimmed and separating from the denture base. There was no retention due to lack of lingual vestibule extension in the retromylohyoid fossa (Figure 4).

Radiographic Examination

Maxillary residual ridge showed a minimal amount of horizontal resorption. The mandibular ridge has moderate resorption in the posterior areas. There appears to be no major sinus proximity. Both ridges show a normal trabecular bone pattern (Figure 5).

Diagnosis

- Maxillary and mandibular complete edentulism.
- Severe xerostomia.
- The patient was classified as prosthodontic diagnostic index class III completely edentulous patient [3].

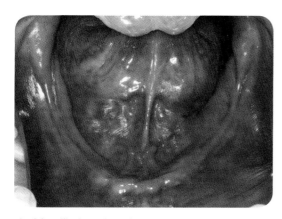

Figure 3: Mandibular edentulous ridge.

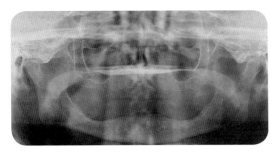

Figure 5: Pretreatment radiograph.

Treatment Plan

The treatment plan for this patient consisted of maxillary complete denture opposing an implant-retained mandibular overdenture. With the patient's permission, both dentures were relined for comfort and better stability. The mandibular denture was duplicated and converted to a radiographic stent. Both surgical and restorative assessments were performed using the SAC classification [4]. The surgical and restorative risk assessment was categorized as straightforward. Presurgical treatment planning included the use of a cone beam computed tomography (CBCT) scan with radiographic guide (Figure 6) for placement

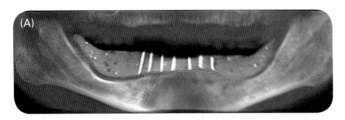

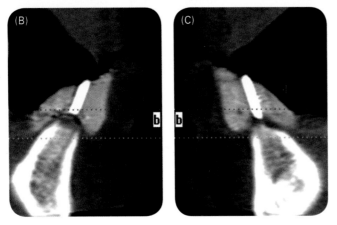

Figure 6: CBCT scans. (A) Panoramic view with diagnostic template in place. Note gutta-percha channels in diagnostic template to mark possible implant locations in anterior mandible. (B) Sagittal view of planned implant site #22 (FDI #33). (C) Sagittal view of planned implant site #27 (FDI #43). b: buccal.

of two tissue-level Roxolid SLActive regular-neck 4.1 mm × 12 mm implants (Straumann Implant System, Switzerland). These implants were selected owing to their improved strength and accelerated ossintegration [5,6]. A diameter of 4.1 mm was indicated given the width of the residual ridge. The radiographic guide was converted to a surgical stent and made ready for surgery.

Treatment

Surgical

Surgical risks were reviewed with the patient. At 1 h prior to implant surgery, 2 g amoxicillin was administered. The patient rinsed with chlorhexidine gluconate 0.12% for 1 min. Anesthesia of the site was achieved via local infiltration with 2% Xylocaine 1:100,000 epinephrine, a midcrestal incision was made from site #22 through #27. A vertical releasing incision was made facial to the area of #24 and #25 and the full-thickness flap was reflected. The surgical stent was used during the procedure. The osteotomy was created with a 2.2 mm diameter drill and incrementally enlarged by 2.8 and 3.5 mm diameter drills. Both implants were placed (4.1 mm diameter × 12 mm height) according to manufacturer's specifications. Confirmation of primary stability was assessed when a torque equal to 35 N cm was necessary to finalize the implant placement, radiography confirmed implant placement, and closure caps were placed. The site was then sutured with interrupted 5-0 Vicryl resorbable sutures until tension-free site closure was obtained.

Postoperative

The patient was prescribed a 5-day regimen of amoxicillin, ibuprofen for pain as needed, and a 7-day routine of 0.12% chlorhexidine gluconate. The patient was seen 1 week after surgery for a follow-up, and 2 weeks after surgery for remaining suture removal. The site was allowed to heal for an additional 2 weeks, and at this point the cover screws were replaced with locator abutments torqued to 35 N cm (Figures 7 and 8). There was no mobility detected. Following the early loading guidelines [7], the patient's immediate denture was engaged to the implants by picking up the locator attachments using the direct method. This allowed the patient to place some occlusal load on the implants, allowing the ulcers to heal.

Prosthetic Restoration

Preliminary impressions were made and custom impression trays fabricated. The custom tray was border

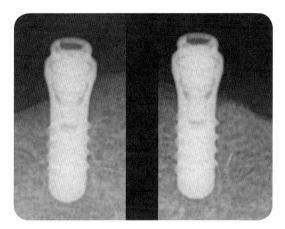

Figure 7: Periapical radiograph after locator abutments placed.

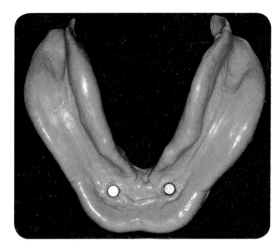

Figure 9: Mandibular final impression.

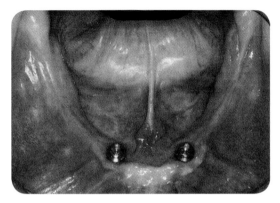

Figure 8: Locator abutment on mandibular arch.

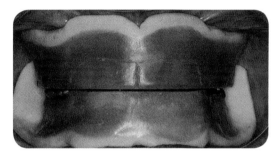

Figure 10: Maxillomandibular relationship.

molded to the muscles and soft tissue attachments of the mouth using modeling compound. The final impressions were made using a selective pressure technique [8] with medium-body polysulfide impression material. The postpalatal seal area was then marked on the palate and transferred to the maxillary impression and later to the definitive cast. Locator impression pickup copings were attached prior to impression making (Figure 9). Locator analogs were then attached to pickup copings in the mandibular impression. The impressions were boxed and poured.

Acrylic record bases and wax occlusal rims were fabricated. The maxillary occlusal rim was tried in the patient's mouth and adjusted for adequate occlusal plane based on patient's phonetics, esthetics, facial tissue support, and anatomical landmarks. The mandibular occlusal rim was then adjusted and aligned with the maxillary rim to gain the appropriate occlusal vertical dimension. Centric relation interocclusal record was made using aluwax added to the mandibular occlusal rim (Figure 10). Final casts were mounted on a whipmix articulator with the aid of an arbitrary ear-bow transfer.

Anterior teeth were selected, set on the articulator, and tried in the mouth. Occlusal plane and occlusal vertical dimension were reevaluated. The maxillomandibular relationship was verified intraorally. The tooth set-up was completed and the patient approved the appearance of the trial dentures (Figure 11).

The completed trial dentures were processed utilizing standard laboratory procedures. The locator attachments were processed with the denture. The

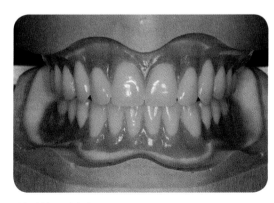

Figure 11: Wax trial dentures.

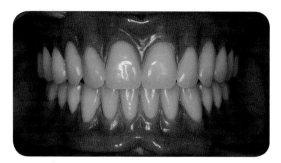

Figure 12: Complete final prosthesis

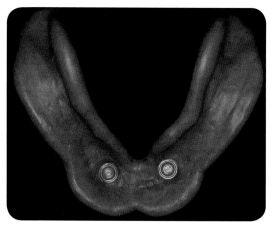

Figure 13: Mandibular denture intaglio view displaying retentive components.

completed dentures were polished and delivered to the patient (Figure 12). The dentures were inserted into the mouth. Denture base adaptation and border extensions were evaluated using pressure indicator paste. Lastly, the black processing caps were removed from the locator attachments and replaced with two Nylon 3.0 lbs (1.36 kg) retentive components (Figure 13).

Discussion

This case describes the rehabilitation of a completely edentulous patient. This case proved challenging in the management of soft tissue. The patient's severe xerostomia and minimal mandibular ridge height often led to many ulcerated lesions on the mandibular mucosa. It was recommended to restore the patient with a complete maxillary denture and implant-supported mandibular complete denture. Given the amount of remaining mandibular bone, it was determined to place two 4.1 mm × 12 mm tissue-level implants. The coronal portion would be restored with locator abutments. The implant-supported mandibular prosthesis is ideal for this patient; by helping transfer some occlusal forces from the tissue and being removable, this would give the patient's dry tissue the rest it needs to prevent ulcer formation.

A thorough examination and complete diagnosis is key before starting any surgical and restorative procedures. Utilizing a CBCT scan and a surgical guide helps to minimize any surgical complications and increases accurate placement of implants. Envisioning the restorative space and adhering to ideal prosthetic fabrication ensures a favorable outcome that will serve the patient well.

Self-Study Questions
(Answers located at the end of the case)

A. What is the primary cause of xerostomia in this patient? What are the side effects of xerostomia in the edentulous patient?

B. What are current treatment modalities for edentulous patients with xerostomia?

C. What are the indications for using a mandibular bar attachment instead of locator attachments?

D. Are there any potential benefits from utilizing TiZr implant versus traditional Ti(Cp) implants?

E. What are the effects of chemically treated surfaces on osseointegration?

F. Is immediate loading of mandibular implant-retained dentures recommended?

References

1. House M.M. The relationship of oral examination to oral diagnosis. J Prosthet Dent 1958;8(2):208–219.
2. Levin B. Impressions for Complete Dentures. Chicago, IL: Quintessence Publishing; 1984, pp 51–55.
3. McGarry TJ, Nimmo A, Skiba JF, et al. Classification system for the completely dentate patient. J Prosthodont 2004;13(2):73–82.
4. Dawson A, Martin W, Belser U. Edentulous mandible – removable prosthesis. In: DawsonA, ChenS (eds), The SAC Classification in Implant Dentistry. Berlin: Quintessence Publishing; 2009, pp 106–111.
5. Grandin HM, Berner S, Dard M. A review of titanium zirconium (TiZr) Alloys for use in endosseous dental implants. Materials 2012;5(8):1348–1360.
6. Ikarashi Y, Toyoda K, Kobayashi E, et al. Improved biocompatibility of titanium–zirconium (Ti–7r) alloy: tissue reaction and sensitization to Ti–Zr alloy compared with pure Ti and Zr in rat implantation study. Mater Trans 2005;46(10):2260–2267.
7. Buser D, Broggini N, Wieland M, et al. Enhanced bone apposition to a chemically modified SLA titanium surface. J Dent Res 2004;83(7):529–533.
8. Boucher CO, Hickey JC, Zarb GA (eds). Prosthodontic Treatment of Edentulous Patients, 7th edn. St Louis, MO: Mosby; 1975.
9. Turner M, Jahangiri L, Ship JA. Hyposalivation, xerostomia, and the complete denture wearer: a systematic review. J Am Dent Assoc 2008;139(2):146–150.
10. Ahuja S, Cagna DR. Classification and management of restorative space in edentulous implant overdenture patients. J Prosthet Dent 2011;105(5):332–337.
11. Lee CK, Agar J. Surgical and prosthetic planning for a two-implant-retained mandibular overdenture: a clinical report. J Prosthet Dent 2006;95(2):102–105.
12. Schimmel M, Srinivasan M, Herrmann FR, Müller F. Loading protocols for implant-supported overdentures in the edentulous jaw: a systematic review and meta-analysis. Int J Oral Maxillofac Implants 2014;29(Suppl):271–286.
13. Gallucci GO, Benic GI, Eckert SE, et al. Consensus statements and clinical recommendations for implant loading protocols. Int J Oral Maxillofac Implants 2014;29(Suppl):287–290.

Answers to Self-Study Questions

A. This patient's xerostomia is a direct result of her medications.

Xerostomia in a denture patient can cause the following side effects:

- lack of retention due to decrease in adhesion, cohesion, and surface tension;
- increase in incidence of *Candida albicans* infections;
- idiopathic dysesthesia (burning mouth syndrome);
- mucosal irritation.

B. The current treatment modalities for edentulous patients with xerostomia are [9]:

- properly constructed denture that is stable and not overextended;
- use of salivary substitutes and water to keep the mucosa moist;
- the use of an implant prosthesis to decrease the pressure put directly on the mucosa;
- communication with patient's physician to decrease, eliminate, or change medications to those that have less xerostomia side effects.

C. The indications for using a mandibular locator attachments instead of a bar attachment are as follows [10,11]. The main consideration is restorative arch space. The locator attachment system requires roughly 8.5 mm of restorative space. This includes 1.8 mm osseous level to implant platform, 1.5 mm for the shortest locator abutment, 3.2 mm for the locator attachment housing, and finally 2 mm of acrylic resin above the locator attachment. This, however, does not include the denture teeth, which, depending on position and size, can take an additional 3–7 mm of space. The bar attachment system requires additional minimum space for cleaning underneath the bar and bar thickness. This puts the bar attachment at a minimum of 13 mm from the bone crest to the acrylic resin base, not including denture teeth.

D. There are three benefits reported [5,6]:

- increased higher fatigue strength;
- increased resistance to corrosion;
- improved biocompatibility.

E. The effects of chemically treated SLA (sand blasted, large grit, acid etch) implant surface on osseointegration are as follows [7]. Chemical treatment of the SLA implants creates a hydrophilic surface. This improves initial wettability during placement, accelerating osseointegration and decreasing the amount of time needed to reach secondary stability. These improvements have increased the success in immediate and early loading of implant cases.

F. The recommendations for immediate loading of mandibular implant-retained dentures are as follows [12,13]. The proceedings from the fifth ITI Consensus Conference address this topic specifically, stating: "Although all three loading protocols provide high survival rates, early and conventional loading protocols are still better documented than immediate loading and seem to result in fewer early implant failures compared to immediate loading". The consensus further adds, "Splinting of implants and the type of attachment system had no effect on 1-year survival rate compared to freestanding implants."

Case 5

Immediate Provisionalization (Temporization)

CASE STORY

A 32-year-old Asian female presented for consultation. She had received a porcelain-fused-to-metal (PFM) crown on her upper right lateral incisor 5 years earlier. The crown was loose and had been recemented at a local dental clinic 2 weeks previously. A thorough clinical and radiographic examination revealed that tooth #7 had a root canal filling and a large cast post with a loose PFM crown (Figure 1). Insufficient tooth structure was noted after removal of large secondary caries, and tooth extraction was indicated.

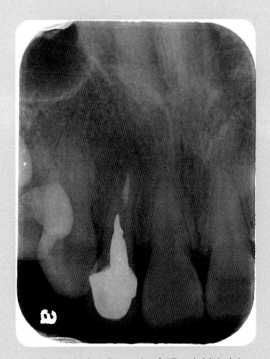

Figure 1: Periapical radiograph of #7 at initial visit.

LEARNING GOALS AND OBJECTIVES

- To identify diagnostic criteria for the application of immediate provisionalization
- To review risk factors and contraindications for the immediate provisionalization protocol
- To recognize the advantages and disadvantages of immediate provisionalization
- To highlight the importance of provisional restoration (shaping of soft tissue contours) and the role they play when dealing with implants in the esthetic zone

Medical History

The patient was in good general health, and the medical history was not contributory at the time of treatment. There was no history of food or drug allergies according to her statement.

Review of Systems

- Vital signs
  - Blood pressure: 127/67 mmHg
  - Pulse rate: 84 beats/min (regular)
  - Respiration: 16 breaths/min

Social History

The patient did not smoke or drink alcohol.

Extraoral Examination

No significant findings were noted. The patient had no masses or swelling, and the temporomandibular joint was within normal limits. There was no facial asymmetry noted, and her lymph nodes were normal on palpation. Average smile line was observed.

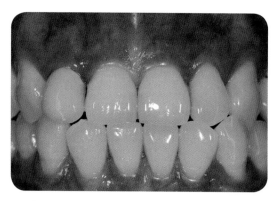

Figure 2: Secondary caries and local gingival inflammation at #7 were noted.

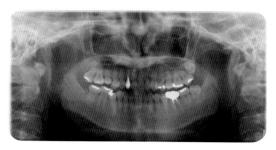

Figure 4: Initial panoramic radiograph showing normal crestal bone levels.

Intraoral Examination

- Local gingival inflammation around tooth #7 (Figure 2).
- PFM crown at #7.
- Large cast post with secondary caries at tooth #7.
- Periodontal examination revealed pocket depths in the range of 2–4 mm (Figure 3).
- Oral cancer screening was negative.
- Soft tissue exam, including her tongue and floor of the mouth, was within normal limits.

Occlusion

Mild crowding of lower anterior teeth and almost edge-to-edge contact relationship in the anterior region were noted. There were no occlusal discrepancies or interferences noted.

Radiographic Examination

Panoramic and periapical radiographs of upper anterior teeth were ordered (Figure 4). A radiographic

examination revealed normal crestal bone levels. Teeth #7 and #19 had previous root canal treatment, and posts and PFM crowns were noted. Impacted tooth #16 and amalgam restoration on #2, #3, #12, #14, #15, #18, #29, #30, and #31 were observed.

Diagnosis

Secondary caries at #7 with insufficient tooth structure.

Treatment Plan

An initial-phase therapy including oral prophylaxis and oral hygiene instructions to eliminate gingival inflammation and infection was scheduled. Restoration of the failing tooth with a dental implant or a three-unit fixed partial denture was recommended. However, she did not want to damage her natural teeth, and a removable interim prosthesis was not acceptable owing to her social activity. Immediate implant placement and provisionalization (temporization) were planned in this case.

Treatment

Before implant surgery, a thorough clinical and radiographic examination was performed (Figure 5).

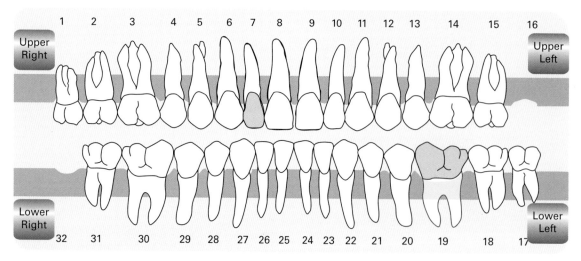

Figure 3: Probing pocket depth measurements during initial visit.

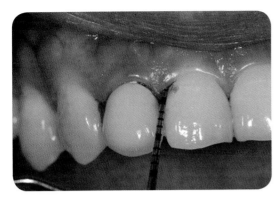

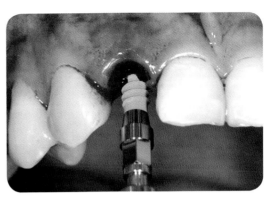

Figure 7: Immediate flapless implant placement in an ideal prosthetically driven position.

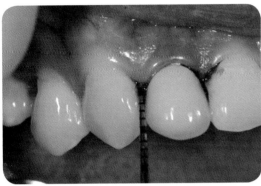

Figure 5: Pre-op bone sounding revealed normal attachment level of neighboring teeth.

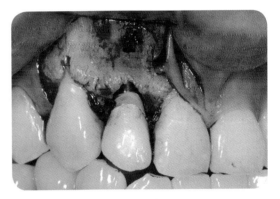

Figure 8: Temporary abutment and crown.

According to the result of SAC (simple/straightforward, advanced, complex) assessment, this case was classified as complex. Additional procedures such as simultaneous guided bone regeneration (GBR) and adjunctive soft tissue graft would be required.

After obtaining profound anesthesia at the surgical site using local anesthetic, tooth #7 was removed carefully and atraumatically with the aid of periotomes (Figure 6). A rough surface (SLA) narrow neck (3.3 mm diameter × 12 mm height; Straumann Dental Implant System) implant was placed flapless and palatally in relation to the extraction socket (Figure 7).

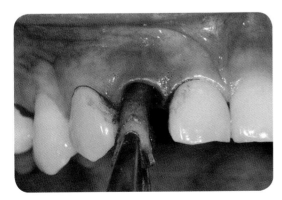

Figure 6: Atraumatic tooth extraction of #7 with the use of periotomes.

Full-thickness buccal and palatal flaps were reflected owing to an apical fenestration that was detected before implant placement. An interim (provisional) restoration was fabricated. The interim restoration was connected to the implant after finishing and polishing with flour of pumice (Figure 8).

Decortication of the labial bone using a small round bur was performed. Xenograft bone particles were placed on top of the buccal plate and packed into the gap between the inner surface of the buccal plate and implant surface (Figure 9). Subepithelium connective tissue was retrieved from the hard palate and secured on the inner surface of the labial flap. The flap was repositioned and primary closure made by 5-0 Nylon (Figures 10 and 11).

The sutures were removed 10 days later and the wound was healing uneventfully. After 3 months of healing and soft tissue conditioning with the provisional crown, the prosthodontic procedures for fabrication of the definitive restoration commenced. A customized impression coping technique was used for definitive impression (Figure 12).

On the definitive cast, a zirconia abutment was fabricated and tried-in intraorally. Once the abutment

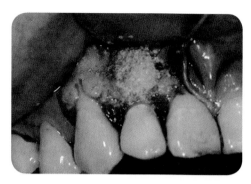

Figure 9: Xenograft and connective tissue graft were applied on the facial aspect of the implant. Intra-op presentation after flap elevation (facial view).

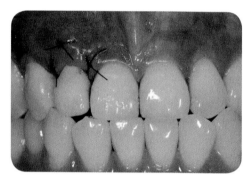

Figure 10: Post-op clinical view, with provisional crown out of occlusion.

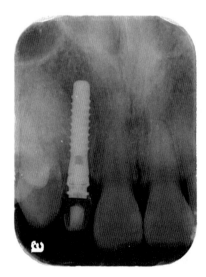

Figure 11: Post-op periapical radiograph confirming implant placement in an ideal position.

finishing line was confirmed clinically to be slightly subgingivally on the buccal side, the shade was selected and the abutment was sent to the laboratory for fabrication of an implant-supported all-ceramic single crown. At the next visit the definitive all-ceramic single crown was delivered (Figures 13, 14, and 15).

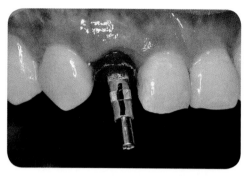

Figure 12: Customized impression coping in place to capture the conditioned soft tissue emergence profile.

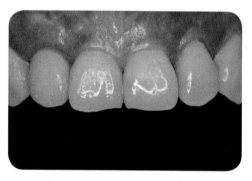

Figure 13: Definitive crown delivery (facial view).

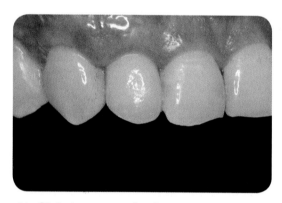

Figure 14: Clinical outcome after 3 years.

Discussion

Immediate provisionalization is the immediate loading of dental implants with a prosthesis within 1 week after implant placement. Immediate implant placement with implant provisionalization has gained popularity owing to the shortening of the treatment time and reduction of surgical interventions. Successful outcomes have been reported with immediate provisionalization of implants placed in fresh extraction sockets, especially in regard to interproximal papilla [1–6]. On the other hand, midfacial gingival recession is the most common encountered complication with

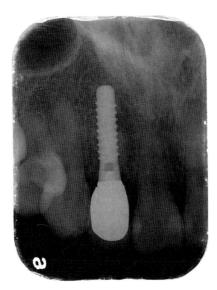

Figure 15: Stable crestal bone levels around the implant after 3 years.

this treatment approach [7–9]. Case selection and accurate three-dimensional (3-D) implant positioning are of outmost importance since there is a high risk for esthetic complications [9].

In the present case, immediate provisionalization was performed for an immediately placed implant. The esthetically pleasing final anterior implant crown relied heavily on correct 3-D implant placement and management of the soft tissue profile around the dental implant during the fixed provisionalization. A stable and esthetic outcome was maintained at the 3-year clinical follow-up with great patient satisfaction. Undercontouring the transmucosal part of the interim (provisional) crown during healing is crucial for soft tissue conditioning and may prevent gingival apical recession.

Specifically for immediate loading with implant-supported single crowns, the following prerequisites are necessary: (a) postdoctoral training, clinical skills, and experience, (b) proper patient selection, adequate bone volume and density, (c) primary stability, measured with insertion torque >20 N cm and resonance frequency analysis values >60 implant stability quotient (ISQ), (d) implant length >10 mm, and (e) absence of systemic or local contraindications (large bone defects in need of structural bone augmentation, poor bone volume and density, parafunctional activities, need for sinus floor elevation, systemic health) [8,10].

In general, there is a high level of short-term comparative evidence in terms of implant survival and marginal bone level stability that supports the use of both immediate and conventional loading [8].

Based on the scientific literature, the most common inclusion/exclusion criteria for immediate loading included minimal insertion torque in the range of 20–45 N cm, a minimal ISQ in the range of 60–65, and implant length >10 mm.

There is limited scientific data comparing immediate and conventional loading in terms of stability of the papilla height and the facial mucosal margin. Esthetics and patient satisfaction were measured only in a few trials that compared immediate and conventional loading, rendering insufficient data to draw conclusions [8].

Self-Study Questions

(Answers located at the end of the case)

A. What is immediate provisionalization?

B. What are the prerequisites for immediate provisionalization?

C. What are the differences between immediate and conventional provisionalization?

D. How predictable is immediate provisionalization?

E. What are the factors that influence the outcome of immediate provisionalization?

F. What are the differences between screw-retained and cement-retained provisionalization?

G. What are the alternatives to immediate provisionalization?

H. What are the recent advances and/or new techniques for immediate provisionalization?

References

1. Morton D, Chen ST, Martin WC, et al. Consensus statements and recommended clinical procedures regarding optimizing esthetic outcomes in implant dentistry. Int J Oral Maxillofac Implants 2014;29(Suppl):216–220.

2. Kan JY, Rungcharassaeng K, Lozada JL, Zimmerman G. Facial gingival tissue stability following immediate placement and provisionalization of maxillary anterior single implants: a 2- to 8-year follow-up. Int J Oral Maxillofac Implants 2011;26:179–187.

3. Botticelli D, Renzi A, Lindhe J, Berglundh T. Implants in fresh extraction sockets: a prospective 5-year follow-up clinical study. Clin Oral Implants Res 2008;19:1226–1232.

4. Chen ST, Buser D. Clinical and esthetic outcomes of implants placed in postextraction sites. Int J Oral Maxillofac Implants 2009;24(Suppl):186–217.

5. Roe P, Kan JY, Rungcharassaeng K, et al. Horizontal and vertical dimensional changes of peri-implant facial bone following immediate placement and provisionalization of maxillary anterior single implants: 1-year cone beam computed tomography study. Int J Oral Maxillofac Implants 2012;27:393–400.

6. Cosyn J, Eghbali A, Hanselaer L, et al. Four modalities of single implant treatment in the anterior maxilla: a clinical, radiographic, and aesthetic evaluation. Clin Implant Dent Relat Res 2013;15:517–530.

7. Lang NP, Pun L, Lau KY, et al. A systematic review on survival and success rates of implants placed immediately into fresh extraction sockets after at least 1 year. Clin Oral Implants Res 2012;23(Suppl 5):39–66.

8. Gallucci GO, Benic GI, Eckert SE, et al. Consensus statements and clinical recommendations for implant loading protocols. Int J Oral Maxillofac Implants 2014;29(Suppl):287–290.

9. Cosyn J, Sabzevar MM, De Bruyn H. Predictors of inter-proximal and midfacial recession following single implant treatment in the anterior maxilla: a multivariate analysis. J Clin Periodontol 2012;39:895–903.

10. Benic GI, Mir-Mari J, Hammerle CHF. Loading protocols for single implant crowns: a systematic review and meta-analysis. Int J Oral Maxillofac Implants 2014;29(Suppl):222–238.

11. Schrott A, Riggi-Heiniger M, Maruo K, Gallucci GO. Implant loading protocols for partially edentulous patients: a systematic review and meta-analysis. Int J Oral Maxillofac Implants 2014;29(Suppl):239–255.

12. Buser D, Chappuis V, Kuchler U, et al. Long term stability of early implant placement with contour augmentation. J Dent Res 2013;92(12 Suppl):176S–182S.

13. Buser D, Chappuis V, Bornstein MM, et al. Long-term stability of contour augmentation with early implant placement following single tooth extraction in the esthetic zone: a prospective, cross-sectional study in 41 patients with a 5- to 9-year follow-up. J Periodontol 2013;84:1517–1527.

14. Hürzeler MB, Zuhr O, Schupbach P, et al. The socket-shield technique: a proof-of-principle report. J Clin Periodontol 2010;37:855–862.

Answers to Self-Study Questions

A. Immediate provisionalization is the connection of a prosthesis to dental implants within 1 week following implant placement. The placement of the implant can be done at a healing and/or healed site or a postextraction socket [8].

B. The recommendations for immediate loading of implant-supported single crowns and implant-supported fixed dental prostheses are limited to situations fulfilling the following prerequisites:
- primary implant stability (insertion torque ≥20–45 N cm and/or ISQ ≥60–65);
- implant length >10 mm;
- absence of systemic or local contraindications (large bone defects in need of structural bone augmentation, poor bone volume and density, parafunctional activities, need for sinus floor elevation, systemic health);
- clinician experience and knowledge;
- when the clinical benefits exceed the risks;
- immediate implant placement postextraction is not a contraindication for immediate loading if primary stability is attained.

C. Conventional implant loading is the connection of a prosthesis to dental implants after 2 months or more following implant placement. Conventional loading is predictable in all clinical situations and is particularly recommended in the presence of treatment modifiers such as poor primary implant stability, substantial bone augmentation, reduced implant dimensions, and compromised host conditions [8].

On the other hand, immediate loading is the connection of the prosthesis within 1 week after implant placement. Where indicated, immediate loading has similar survival rates to conventional loading [8].

D. For the implant-supported single crowns in the *anterior and premolar regions*, immediate loading is a predictable procedure in terms of implant survival and stability of the marginal bone. However, data regarding soft tissue aspects are not conclusive enough to recommend immediate or early loading of single implant crowns in the esthetically demanding sites as a routine procedure. Immediate loading in such sites should be approached with caution and by experienced clinicians [8].

For the *mandibular molar region*, immediate loading of implant-supported single crowns is a predictable procedure and can generally be recommended in cases where clinical benefits are identified.

For the *maxillary molar region* there is a limited amount of data on immediate loading of implant-supported single crowns, and in these sites conventional loading should be the procedure of choice.

For partially edentulous patients with *multiple missing posterior adjacent teeth*, limited scientific evidence shows that immediate implant loading in patients with healed posterior multi-unit sites presents similar implant survival rates to early or conventional loading [11].

Insufficient evidence exists to support immediate loading in *anterior maxillary and mandibular multi-unit partially edentulous sites* [11]. Hence, it should be approached with caution and by experienced clinicians since there is a limited volume of evidence.

For *completely edentulous patients*, strong scientific evidence from the dental literature shows that immediate loading has the same effect on implant survival as conventional loading. In completely edentulous patients and when using dental implants with a microtextured surface, immediate, early, or conventional loading with a one-piece fixed interim prosthesis results in high implant and prosthesis survival rates in the mandible and maxilla [8].

E. Besides the previously mentioned prerequisites that are necessary for application of immediate loading, occlusal factors influence the outcome of immediate provisionalization. Clearance from interferences at all functional movements and centric stops are necessary to achieve osseointegration and prevent excessive overload on the implants with subsequent failures. Patient compliance with a soft diet regimen is incumbent in the first 6 weeks after immediate provisionalization.

Conventional loading is predictable in all clinical situations and is particularly recommended in the presence of treatment modifiers such as poor primary implant stability, substantial bone augmentation, reduced implant dimensions, and compromised host conditions.

F. Both retention methods present with their own advantages and limitations. Besides clinician preference, there are clinical issues that may dictate one retention type. These include 3-D positioning of implant placement (depth, buccolingual, mesiodistal), ease of fabrication, passive fit, retrievability and accessibility, esthetics, and ease of maintenance. There is no difference in patient preference toward one or the other.

G. As stated in the answer to self-study question E, conventional loading is predictable in all clinical situations and is particularly recommended in the presence of treatment modifiers such as poor primary implant stability, substantial bone augmentation, reduced implant dimensions, and compromised host conditions. In these cases, removable provisionalization or tooth-supported provisionalization is indicated [8].

In the absence of modifying factors, an early loading of 6–8 weeks in healed single-tooth gaps or extended edentulous sites of partially edentulous patients should be considered routine.

When part of the buccal bone is missing following extraction of the failing tooth, early implant placement after soft healing time of 6–8 weeks has been suggested [12]. The implant installation is performed with simultaneous GBR to restore facial contour. A submerged approach is performed followed by removable provisionalization during the osseointegration period. The long-term results of this facial contour augmentation have been encouraging clinically and esthetically after 5–9 years of follow-ups [13].

H. Computer-planned, template-guided implant surgery has gained increased popularity. It has been proposed that implant 3-D planning software should be used in every case whether or not it will be coupled with template-guided surgery. Planning and visualizing the implant surgery prior to performing the actual procedure has great advantages.

The "socket shield" technique has been recently introduced and includes the retention of a root segment facially or interproximally in order to maintain the facial contours or interproximal papilla heights respectively [14]. No long-term data exist with this technique. Immediate provisionalization can be done by using the patient's own extracted tooth instead of an acrylic crown, whenever it can be used. This can lead to an enhanced transmucosal emergence profile.

Conclusions

Conventional implant loading is predictable in all clinical situations and is particularly recommended in the presence of treatment modifiers such as poor primary implant stability, substantial bone augmentation, reduced implant dimensions, and compromised host conditions [8].

For the anterior maxillary and mandibular regions, immediate loading of implant-supported single crowns is a predictable procedure in terms of implant survival and stability of the marginal bone. Immediate loading in such sites should be approached with caution and by experienced clinicians [8,10]. This is due to the fact that data regarding soft tissue aspects is not conclusive enough to recommend immediate loading of single implant crowns in the esthetically demanding sites as a routine procedure.

For partially edentulous patients with multiple missing adjacent teeth, limited scientific evidence shows that immediate implant loading in patients with healed posterior multi-unit sites presents similar implant survival rates compared with early or conventional loading [11]. Insufficient evidence exists to support immediate loading in anterior maxillary and mandibular multi-unit partially edentulous sites [8,11]. Hence, it should be approached with caution and by experienced clinicians since there is a limited volume of evidence.

For completely edentulous patients, strong scientific evidence shows that immediate loading has the same effect on implant survival as conventional loading [8].

Acknowledgments

We would like to thank Dr. Lian-Ping Mau and Dr. Chih-Wen Cheng, Chi-Mei Medical Center, Tainan, Taiwan, for their contribution to the clinical care provided for the patient.

Case 6

Immediate Loading

CASE STORY

A 48-year-old Asian patient presented for consultation. His chief complaint was: "I want to fix my dentures because they are not working well. I also want to have teeth in my mouth all the time." This patient lost most of his molars several years ago. Some fixed partial dentures (FPDs) and a mandibular, ill-fitting removable partial denture were present. Upon clinical and radiographic examination, multiple caries lesions and gingival recession were observed (Figure 1). The patient reported that he did not visit his dentist regularly. He never used dental floss or an interdental brush and he brushed his teeth twice daily.

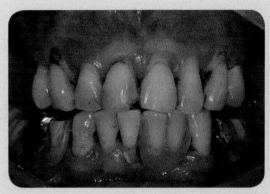

Figure 1: Pre-op presentation (facial view).

LEARNING GOALS AND OBJECTIVES

■ To indicate the most appropriate implant loading protocol for different clinical in dications
■ To understand the advantages of immediate loading
■ To highlight the contraindications for an immediate loading protocol
■ To describe the criteria for immediate loading
■ To review the scientific evidence leading to clinical recommendations for implant loading protocols

Medical History

At the time of treatment, this patient was healthy and the medical history was not contributory.

Review of Systems

• Vital signs
  ○ Blood pressure: 129/73 mmHg
  ○ Pulse rate: 84 beats/min (regular)
  ○ Respiration: 17 breaths/min

Social History

The patient did not drink alcohol but had smoked cigarettes (about one pack per day) for more than 10 years at the time of treatment.

Extraoral Examination

No significant findings were noted. The patient had no masses or swelling, and the temporomandibular joint was within normal limits. There was no facial asymmetry, and his lymph nodes were normal on palpation.

Intraoral Examination

• Oral cancer screening was negative.
• Soft tissue exam, including her tongue and floor of the mouth, were within normal limits.

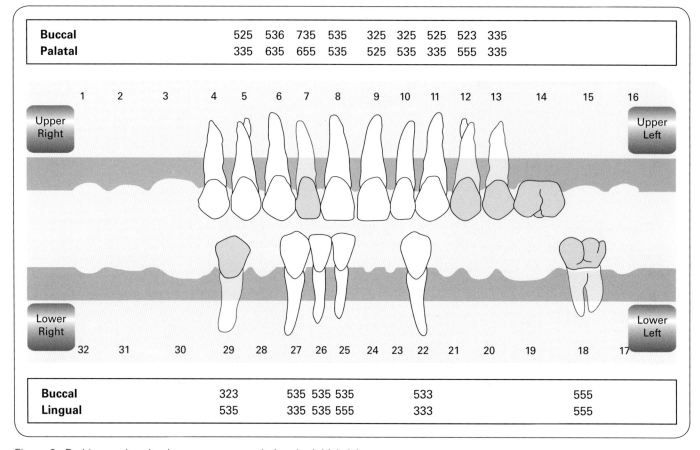

Buccal					525	536	735	535		325	325	525	523	335		
Palatal					335	635	655	535		525	535	335	555	335		

	1	2	3	4	5	6	7	8	9	10	11	12	13	14	15	16

Buccal			323		535	535	535		533			555			
Lingual			535		335	535	555		333			555			

Figure 2: Probing pocket depth measurements during the initial visit.

- Periodontal examination revealed pocket depths in the range of 2–3 mm (Figure 2).
- Localized areas of gingival inflammation noted.
- Evaluation of the alveolar ridge in the areas #4 and #5 revealed both horizontal and vertical resorption of bone.
- Extensive restorations in the form of single crowns and FPDs.

Occlusion

Facial midline was coincident with dental midline with 3 mm overjet and 2 mm overbite. Maximum mouth opening was 40 mm, and there were no occlusal discrepancies or interferences.

Radiographic Examination

A full mouth radiographic series was ordered (Figure 3). Radiographic finding including:
- Residual roots: #3, #4.
- Missing teeth: #1, #2, #14, #15, #16, #17, #19, #20, #21, #23, #24, #28, #30, #31, #32.
- Previous root canal treatment: #27.
- Caries: #6, #22, #25, #26, #27.

- Ill-fitting fixed prosthesis: #12 to #14, #18, #29.
- Angular bony defect: #18.
- Horizontal bony defect: #5, #6, #7, #8, #9, #10, #11, #25, #26.
- Furcation involvement: #18.

Diagnosis

According to the American Academy of Periodontology (AAP), the diagnosis was generalized chronic periodontitis. Secondary caries and partial edentulism were also diagnosed.

Definition of Loading Protocols

In accordance with published consensus statements, the following definitions of loading protocols are currently used [1]:
- *Immediate loading* – a prosthesis is connected to the dental implants within 1 week following implant placement.
- *Early loading* – a prosthesis is connected to the dental implants between 1 week to 2 months following implant placement.

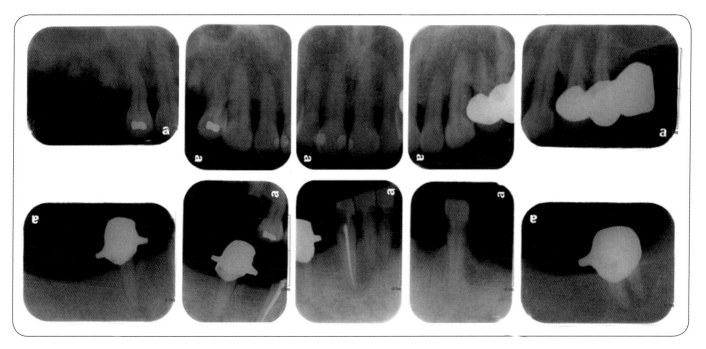

Figure 3: Pre-op full mouth series radiographs.

- *Conventional loading* – a prosthesis is connected to the dental implants after 2 months or more following implant placement.

Treatment Plan

The treatment plan for this patient consisted of initial phase I periodontal therapy that included oral prophylaxis with scaling, root planing, and oral hygiene instructions to eliminate all gingival inflammation and infection.

Extraction of all remaining teeth on the mandible followed by insertion of an immediate denture was recommended. Definitive rehabilitation would be carried out with an implant complete-arch fixed dental prosthesis. Tooth #4 would be restored by a single implant, and two crowns of #12 and #13 would be fabricated. A shortened dental arch concept of the maxilla was applied in the present case in order to avoid sinus elevation surgery.

Treatment

During the initial-phase therapy, nonsurgical periodontal treatment was performed. Residual roots of #3 and #4 were extracted and #12–#14 FPD was replaced by #12 and #13 provisional crowns. The definitive treatment included extraction of all remaining mandibular teeth and restoration by an immediate complete denture in order to maintain esthetic, phonetics, and occlusal

function. Six weeks postextraction, cone beam computed tomography scanning was performed for presurgical evaluation and three-dimensional (3-D) implant positioning for six implants was planned. Furthermore, immediate loading with the "pick-up technique" was planned.

A midcrestal incision was made from site #18 to #31 after obtaining profound local anesthesia of the mandible (Figure 4). Full-thickness buccal and lingual flaps were reflected after incision. Six implants were placed on #19, #21, #22, #27, #28, and #30 as planned (Figure 5). Implant stability was checked by resonance frequency analysis (Ostell), and the implant stability

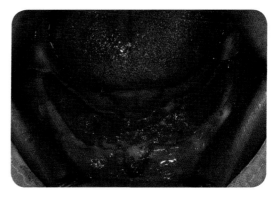

Figure 4: Intra-op presentation after flap elevation (facial view).

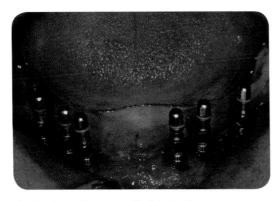

Figure 5: Implant placement (facial view).

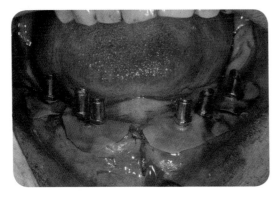

Figure 6: Temporary abutments placed intraorally with rubber dam after flap repositioning and suturing (facial view).

quotient (ISQ) was more than 65 for all of the implants. Temporary abutments were screwed on the implants and a rubber dam was used for isolation of the surgical field (Figure 6).

A prefabricated interim prosthesis was relieved to accommodate the temporary abutments and picked-up with the "conversion prosthesis" technique (Figure 7). Subsequently, the prosthesis was trimmed and polished in the laboratory. Even occlusal contact and group

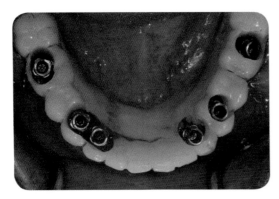

Figure 7: Conversion prosthesis placed intraorally with relief to accommodate the temporary abutments (occlusal view).

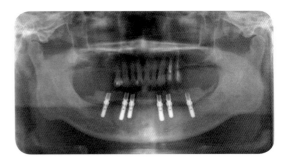

Figure 8: Post-op panoramic radiograph.

function were achieved after delivery of the screw-retained interim prosthesis (Figure 8).

All the sutures were removed 10 days later, and the wound healing was uneventful. One more implant at maxillary site #4 was placed 1 week later. Eight weeks later, definitive polyether impressions were made after splinting the impression copings with dental floss and acrylic resin [2]. After the interocclusal record appointment, the segmented zirconia frameworks were tried-in (Figures 9, 10, and 11). A new interocclusal record was taken and the prostheses were sent to the laboratory for porcelain veneering.

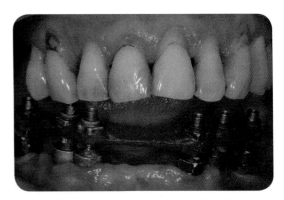

Figure 9: Impression copings splinted with acrylic resin (facial view).

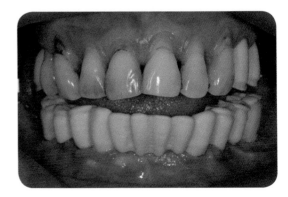

Figure 10: Modified monolithic zirconia frameworks placed intraorally (facial view).

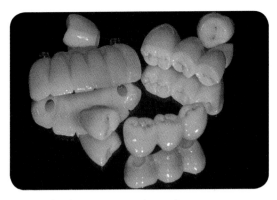

Figure 11: Definitive segmented prostheses.

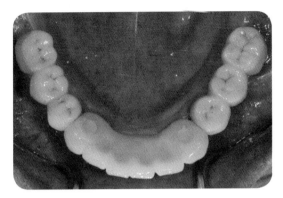

Figure 12: Definitive mandibular implant FPDs intraorally (occlusal view).

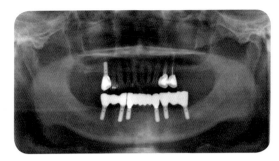

Figure 13: Panoramic radiograph after 1 year of clinical function.

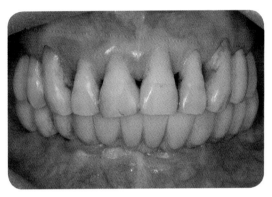

Figure 14: Definitive rehabilitation after 2 years of clinical function.

At the final insertion appointment, three segmented mandibular FPDs, a maxillary implant-supported crown, and two tooth-supported crowns were delivered (Figures 12 and 13). At the 2-year follow-up, the patient was still satisfied with the quality of his rehabilitation (Figure 14). No biologic or technical complications were observed.

Discussion

The advent of implant dentistry gave a reliable solution to the treatment of edentulism, and the longitudinal effectiveness of microtextured rough surface dental implants has been demonstrated for both partially and fully edentulous patients [3,4].

In the USA the percentage of edentulous patients is 10% of the total population, and this is expected to increase in the future as the life expectancy also increases [5]. Hence, it becomes clear that the need for prosthodontic treatment with dental implants for completely edentulous patients will increase. However, the extended healing time without loading of the implants using the conventional loading protocol is a disadvantage from the patient perspective. Hence,

reducing the healing period or time to loading is of great benefit to the patient. Rough implant surfaces and immediate loading protocols have led to faster healing times and immediate restoration of function and esthetics in carefully selected cases and represent scientifically and clinically validated treatment modalities [5,6]. Immediate loading can be applied in both partially and completely edentulous clinical situations and can be applied to implants placed in either healed sites (delayed placement) or in extraction sockets (immediate placement) [4].

The benefits of immediate loading have allowed for shortened treatment time and immediate function with fixed prostheses. Immediate loading also mitigates the psychological impact of edentulism on patients that are going to lose their teeth or have been wearing dentures for extended periods of time [5].

The treatment of complete edentulism with implant-supported fixed prostheses is complex. Hence, careful case selection and treatment planning as well as adequate knowledge, skill and experience of the clinician performing the procedures are key [1]. The existing literature provides strong scientific evidence that immediate loading of microtextured dental implants with a one-piece fixed interim prosthesis in both the edentulous mandible and maxilla is as predictable as early and conventional loading. Inclusion criteria, such as insertion torque ≥30 N cm, resonance frequency quotient (ISQ) ≥60, and minimal implant length ≥10 mm, have been used in the majority of the clinical studies [1,5,6].

Primary implant stability is critical for predictable osseointegration regardless of the loading protocol.

It is suggested that, prior to immediate loading in the edentulous arch, the primary stability of each implant must be confirmed. The number, size, and distribution of implants for a full-arch fixed prosthesis needs to be based on the implant–prosthodontic plan, arch form, and bone volume, regardless of the loading protocol. The need for simultaneous procedures such as bone augmentation or sinus floor elevation is considered a relative contraindication for immediate loading [1,5,6].

Self-Study Questions

(Answers located at the end of the case)

A. What is immediate loading?

B. What are the prerequisites for immediate loading?

C. What are the advantages of immediate loading?

D. What are the contraindications for immediate loading?

E. How predictable is immediate loading?

F. What are the differences between immediate and conventional loading?

G. What are the recent advances in immediate implant loading?

References

1. Gallucci GO, Benic GI, Eckert SE, et al. Consensus statements and clinical recommendations for implant loading protocols. Int J Oral Maxillofac Implants 2014;29(Suppl):287–290.
2. Papaspyridakos P, Lal K. Computer-assisted design/computer-assisted manufacturing zirconia implant fixed complete prostheses: clinical results and technical complications up to 4 years of function. Clin Oral Implants Res 2013;24:659–665.
3. Papaspyridakos P, Chen CJ, Chuang SK, et al. A systematic review of biologic and technical complications with fixed implant rehabilitations for edentulous patients. Int J Oral Maxillofac Implants 2012;27:102–110.
4. Morton D, Chen ST, Martin WC, et al. Consensus statements and recommended clinical procedures regarding optimizing esthetic outcomes in implant dentistry. Int J Oral Maxillofac Implants 2014;29(Suppl):216–220.
5. Papaspyridakos P, Chen CJ, Chuang SK, Weber HP. Implant loading protocols for edentulous patients with fixed prostheses: a systematic review and meta-analysis. Int J Oral Maxillofac Implants 2014;29(Suppl):256–270.
6. Schrott A, Riggi-Heiniger M, Maruo K, Gallucci GO. Implant loading protocols for partially edentulous patients: a systematic review and meta-analysis. Int J Oral Maxillofac Implants 2014;29(Suppl):239–255.
7. Papaspyridakos P, Mokti M, Chen CJ, et al. Implant and prosthodontic survival rates with implant fixed complete dental prostheses in the edentulous mandible after at least 5 years: a systematic review. Clin Implant Dent Relat Res 2014;16:705–717.
8. Bornstein MM, Al Nawas B, Kuchler U, Tahmaseb A. Consensus statements and recommended clinical procedures regarding contemporary surgical and radiographic techniques in implant dentistry. Int J Oral Maxillofac Implants 2014;29(Suppl):78–82.
9. Lal K, Eisig SB, Fine JB, Papaspyridakos P. Prosthetic outcomes and survival rates of implants placed with guided flapless surgery using stereolithographic templates: a retrospective study. Int J Periodontics Restorative Dent 2013;33:661–667.
10. Patzelt SB, Bahat O, Reynolds MA, Strub JR. The All-on-Four treatment concept: a systematic review. Clin Implant Dent Relat Res 2014;16:836–855.

Answers to Self-Study Questions

A. Immediate loading is the clinical modality of connecting a prosthesis to the dental implants within 1 week following implant placement.

B. In order to use an immediate loading protocol, there are several prerequisites. It is important to understand that any treatment of edentulism with fixed implant-supported prostheses is considered complex. Hence, careful case selection and adequate knowledge, skill, and experience of the clinician performing the procedures are key.
- Postdoctoral training, clinical skills and experience.
- Proper patient selection.
- Primary stability, measured with insertion torque >30 N cm and resonance frequency analysis values >60 ISQ.
- Cross-arch stabilization.
- Number of implants depends on implant-prosthodontic plan, arch shape, bone volume, bone density and other factors, minimum of four implants.
- Implant size and length >10 mm.
- Precise coordination of the treatment team (surgeon, prosthodontist, dental technician).

C.
- Immediate restoration of masticatory function.
- Shorten overall treatment times (fewer office visits for adjustments and overall treatment).
- Eliminate the need for interim removable prosthesis.
- Psychological and social aspect.
- Increased patient comfort throughout the healing period and reduction of postoperative discomfort caused by removable interim prostheses.
- Additionally, the patient can also evaluate the esthetics and phonetics of the future rehabilitation without the difficult adaptation to a complete denture during the transitional phase.
- Fixed provisionalization aids in proper soft tissue conditioning with ovate pontics and does not allow any deleterious pressure from complete dentures to the implants. It also facilitates an equal distribution of load, while with a removable prosthesis there is a danger of uneven occlusal

load on one or more implants and a need for frequent adjustment or relining procedures.
- Prosthodontic control is enhanced by the fixed interim restorations, and established landmarks are easy to transfer to the definitive restorations by cross-articulation, silicone key index, and the cutback technique.

D.
- Lack of appropriate postdoctoral training and clinical experience.
- Need for guided bone regeneration as treatment modifier.
- Bruxism is a relative risk factor (treatment modifier), not an absolute contraindication, and it applies to all loading protocols; additional implants may be recommended.
- Non-careful case selection, patient incompliance with soft diet.
- Systemic risk factors that may affect the outcome of treatment involving dental implants (e.g., uncontrolled diabetes, smoking, history of periodontal disease) apply to all loading protocols.

E. Strong scientific evidence from dental literature shows that immediate loading has the same effect on implant survival and failures as early and conventional loading. In edentulous patients and when using dental implants with a microtextured surface, immediate, early, or conventional loading with a one-piece fixed interim prosthesis results in high implant and prosthesis survival rates in the mandible and maxilla. The estimated 1-year implant survival is above 99% (95% confidence intervals) with all three loading protocols (immediate, early, and conventional) [1]. A recent meta-analysis of prospective studies with more than 500 patients showed that the implant treatment of mandibular edentulism yields high implant and prosthesis survival rates that exceed 96% after 10 years, irrespective of the loading protocol [7].

F. Conventional implant loading is the connection of a prosthesis to the dental implants after 2 months or more following implant placement. Conventional loading is predictable in all clinical situations and is particularly recommended in the presence of treatment modifiers such as poor primary implant stability, substantial bone augmentation, reduced implant dimensions, and compromised host conditions. On the other hand, immediate loading is the connection of the prosthesis within 1 week after implant placement. Where indicated, immediate loading has similar survival rates with conventional loading [1].

G. Computer-guided flapless surgery is currently gaining popularity. The flapless surgery can be efficiently combined with immediate loading with a prefabricated interim prosthesis or conversion prosthesis [8,9]. Implant survival rates are similar to the ones achieved with conventional surgical procedures in the medium term and for completely edentulous patients [5]. More long-term clinical studies are necessary as technology continues to improve.

In an attempt to avoid sinus elevation and extensive grafting procedures in the posterior maxilla and mandible, the inter-sinus or inter-foraminal placement of axial and tilted implants has been proposed. The use of tilted implants (All-on-Four concept) for immediate loading of completely edentulous jaws with fixed prosthesis shows good medium-term results, but long-term results are lacking [10].

Conclusions

Conventional implant loading is predictable in all clinical situations and is particularly recommended in the presence of treatment modifiers such as poor primary implant stability, substantial bone augmentation, reduced implant dimensions, and compromised host conditions. For immediate loading, minimal insertion torque of 30 N cm, implant length of minimum 10 mm, and careful case selection are clinically recommended. Clinical experience and postdoctoral training are necessary.

For completely edentulous patients, strong scientific evidence shows that estimated 1-year implant survival was above 99% (95% confidence intervals) with all three loading protocols (immediate, early, and conventional) [1,5]. When selecting cases carefully and using dental implants with a rough surface, immediate loading with fixed prostheses in edentulous patients results in similar implant and prosthesis survival and failure rates as with early and conventional loading.

For partially edentulous patients, limited scientific evidence shows that immediate implant loading in patients with healed posterior multi-unit sites presents similar implant survival rates to early or conventional loading [1,6]. Insufficient evidence exists to support immediate loading in anterior maxillary and mandibular multi-unit partially edentulous sites [1,5]. Hence, it should be approached with caution and by experienced clinicians, since there is a limited volume of evidence.

Acknowledgments

We would like to thank Dr. Chih-Wen Cheng, Chi-Mei Medical Center, Tainan, Taiwan, for his contribution to the clinical care provided for the patient.

9

Special Interdisciplinary Considerations

Case 1

Implants for Periodontally Compromised Patients

CASE STORY

A 53-year-old man presented with a chief complaint of pain, swelling, and bleeding that developed in the last few days. Half a year ago he had been informed that his teeth in the lower right had "hopeless prognoses." A hopeless prognosis was also given to #30 due to a perforation during post preparation, and #31 due to a fracture. The patient delayed seeking care, as there was no pain associated with these teeth. This dental neglect led to chronic periodontal disease and acute infections, including a periodontal abscess. In this case, we discuss the option of implant therapy in a site with previous periodontal disease and potential risk factors for peri-implantitis (Figure 1).

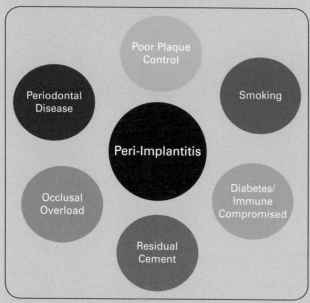

Figure 1: Risk factors for peri-implantitis.

LEARNING GOALS AND OBJECTIVES

■ To understand how to sequence periodontal and implant therapy
■ To understand common risk factors for periodontitis and peri-implantitis
■ To understand about implant success and survival in periodontitis patients

Medical History

The patient has high blood pressure and high cholesterol. Both conditions are controlled with medications (propranolol, Lipitor). The patient has no known allergies.

Review of Systems

- Vital signs
  ○ Blood pressure: 120/70 mmHg
  ○ Pulse rate: 76 beats/min

Social History

The patient denies drinking, smoking cigarettes, and recreational drug use.

Extraoral Examination

There are no significant findings. There are no masses or swelling, and the temporomandibular joint is within normal limits.

Intraoral Examination

- The oral cancer screening is negative.
- The patient's hard palate, soft palate, vestibule, and saliva are all within normal limits.
- The patient has a low smile line.
- Periodontal examination reveals localized severe periodontitis in the lower right quadrant (Figure 2).

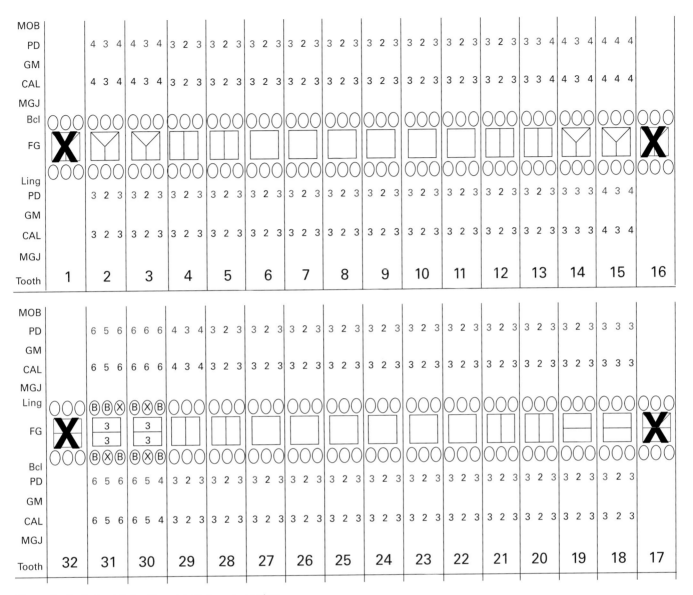

Maxillary arch (Teeth 1–16)

	1	2	3	4	5	6	7	8	9	10	11	12	13	14	15	16
PD (Buccal)	X	4 3 4	4 3 4	3 2 3	3 2 3	3 2 3	3 2 3	3 2 3	3 2 3	3 2 3	3 2 3	3 2 3	3 2 3	3 3 4	4 3 4	4 4 4
CAL (Buccal)	X	4 3 4	4 3 4	3 2 3	3 2 3	3 2 3	3 2 3	3 2 3	3 2 3	3 2 3	3 2 3	3 2 3	3 2 3	3 3 4	4 3 4	4 4 4
PD (Lingual)		3 2 3	3 2 3	3 2 3	3 2 3	3 2 3	3 2 3	3 2 3	3 2 3	3 2 3	3 2 3	3 2 3	3 2 3	3 3 3	4 3 4	
CAL (Lingual)		3 2 3	3 2 3	3 2 3	3 2 3	3 2 3	3 2 3	3 2 3	3 2 3	3 2 3	3 2 3	3 2 3	3 2 3	3 3 3	4 3 4	

Mandibular arch (Teeth 32–17)

	32	31	30	29	28	27	26	25	24	23	22	21	20	19	18	17
PD (Lingual)	X	6 5 6	6 6 6	4 3 4	3 2 3	3 2 3	3 2 3	3 2 3	3 2 3	3 2 3	3 2 3	3 2 3	3 2 3	3 2 3	3 3 3	
CAL (Lingual)	X	6 5 6	6 6 6	4 3 4	3 2 3	3 2 3	3 2 3	3 2 3	3 2 3	3 2 3	3 2 3	3 2 3	3 2 3	3 2 3	3 3 3	
PD (Buccal)		6 5 6	6 5 4	3 2 3	3 2 3	3 2 3	3 2 3	3 2 3	3 2 3	3 2 3	3 2 3	3 2 3	3 2 3	3 2 3	3 2 3	
CAL (Buccal)		6 5 6	6 5 4	3 2 3	3 2 3	3 2 3	3 2 3	3 2 3	3 2 3	3 2 3	3 2 3	3 2 3	3 2 3	3 2 3	3 2 3	

Figure 2: Periodontal charting at initial presentation.

- Patient has a number of gold restorations.
- Tooth #30 has a missing crown and moderate inflammation.
- Tooth #31 has a significant infection.

Occlusion

The patient presents with a normal molar and canine relationship on the right side. Anterior crossbite is present between #11 and #22.

Radiographic Examination

An examination of a full mouth series of radiographs reveals that there is moderate to severe bone loss localized to the lower right quadrant. Both #30 and #31 have significant furcation involvement apparent on the periapical film (Figure 3).

Diagnosis

The patient has a localized severe chronic periodontitis and a periodontal abscess.

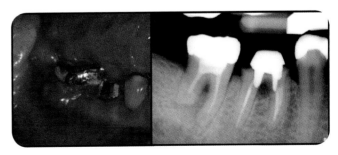

Figure 3: Clinical and radiographic presentation at initial presentation.

Treatment Plan

The treatment plan for this patient includes an initial phase of debridement along with systemic antibiotics and oral hygiene instructions. Consequently, as these teeth have hopeless prognosis, #30 and #31 will have to be extracted and replaced with dental implants.

Treatment

In the areas of #30 and #31, there was localized inflammation associated with the periodontal abscess (Figures 2 and 3). A Glickman grade 3 furcation involvement was noted and a diagnosis of localized severe periodontitis was made.. It was decided to first treat the abscess with debridement and a prescription of 675 mg of Augmentin PO TID for 7 days [1].

Seven days following the administration of the medication the patient presented to extract #30 and #31 and to preserve the ridge in preparation for implant placement. The swelling had significantly improved in the last week due to the debridement and the pharmacologic intervention. On the day of the surgery, two carpules of 2% Xylocaine were used and both teeth were sectioned and extracted atraumatically in order to preserve the buccal plate as much as possible (Figure 4A). Freeze-dried bone allograft (FDBA) was used to preserve both sockets (Figure 4B). Bio-guide membrane was employed to drape the area [2]. Expanded polytetrafluorethylene sutures were used

to gain primary closure (Figure 4C) in order for optimal healing and regeneration to take place [3]. Postoperative instructions were given along with medications (azithromycin 500 mg QD for 5 days). Two weeks later, the patient presented for suture removal. Other than a minor dehiscence measuring 2 mm × 2 mm, the site healed well.

Six months following the preservation procedure, the patient presented for his implants on #30 and #31. No sign of inflammation was present. Anesthesia was achieved with two carpules of 2% Xylocaine 1 : 100k epi – one via local infiltration and one via inferior alveolar nerve block. An incision was made slightly lingual to the midcrestal area with an intention to apically position the keratinized flap. The ridge was healthy and sound to bone sounding (Figure 5A). Two Straumann implants were placed: #30 (4.1 mm × 10 mm RN) and #31 (4.8 mm × 10 mm WN) (Figure 5C). Owing to a low insertion torque, both implants were submerged with primary closure for maximal healing (Figure 5B). The patient healed with no complications.

Four months following the implant placement, the implants were exposed and healing abutments were placed. At the same time, an Osstell device was used to measure implant stability [4]. Both #30 and #31 had values greater than 80 from all directions.

Two months following the second-stage procedure, the implants were restored with screw-retained implant crowns. The patient is committed to maintenance

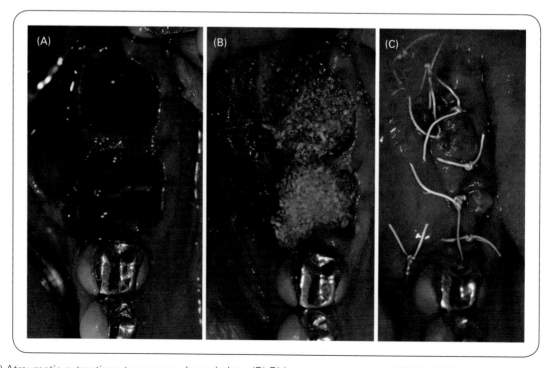

Figure 4: (A) Atraumatic extractions to preserve buccal plate. (B) Ridge preservation with FDBA. (C) Primary closure.

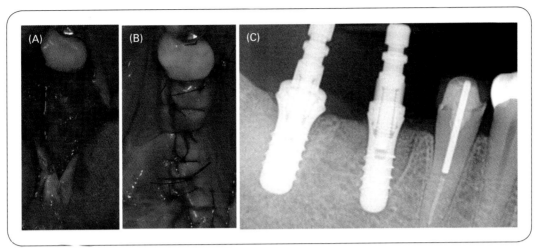

Figure 5: (A) Ridge is preserved 4 months following the preservation. (B) Primary closure is achieved. (C) Periapical radiograph at the time of the implant insertion.

every 4 months to protect his remaining dentition and implants. Bone levels around the implant are maintained 24 months after implant placement (Figure 6).

Discussion

Implants have been used for rehabilitation of complete or partially edentulous cases for over 30 years. They have successfully become the primary tooth replacement choice of most patients and clinicians, due to their high success rates and tooth-like qualities presented in their natural appearance, ease of maintenance, and lack of need to involve surrounding teeth for support. Success rates of implant therapies have been routinely reported to be above 90%. Implant failures, although relatively small, are not uncommon, and usually range between 1 and 8%. Failures of implants have been attributed to two main etiologies: either mechanical failures or biological failures, or the combination of both. The prevalence of periodontal disease has been reported by the US Centers for Disease Control and Prevention to be 47% in adults over the age

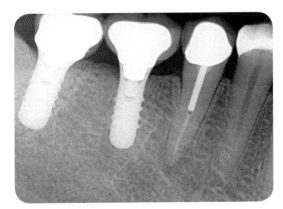

Figure 6: Periapical radiograph 24 months following implant placement.

of 30 and 70.1% in adults over the age of 60 [5]. As the demand on dental implants continues to grow, it is more common for patients with an active or treated periodontitis to be candidates for implant therapy. In this case study, we present and discuss the treatment of a patient with a history of periodontal disease with dental implants. The aim is to discuss the success and failure of dental implants in periodontally compromised versus healthy patients.

Microbiological evaluation of peri-implantitis [6] revealed high numbers of common periodontal pathogens, such as *Porphyromonas gingivalis*, *Aggregatibacter actinomycetemcomitans*, and *Prevotella intermedia*, suggesting that bacteria in periodontal pockets may cross infect and, furthermore, act as a reservoir for the colonization of subgingival areas around dental implants. Beyond the bacterial challenge, the host response appears to play a major role in the progression and amount of tissue destruction that occurs around dental implants. It is therefore not the mere presence of periodontal pathogens that likely contributes to the onset and progression of peri-implantitis, but rather the complex events resulting from the interaction and exchanges that occur between bacterial plaque and the immune system. Susceptible patients are thought to react more intensively to the infectious agent, leading to more tissue breakdown during the progression of periodontal disease [7].

The presence and extent of peri-implantitis were evaluated [8,9], the investigators concluding that patients with periodontal disease are at an increased risk for more tissue breakdown compared with healthy individuals. While this is true, the variance in the criteria for periodontal disease diagnosis was significant and served as a confounder. Furthermore, there are only a limited number of controlled studies available on the subject.

Careful examination, diagnosis, and successful treatment of periodontal disease is therefore strongly recommended before implant therapy is initiated. Furthermore, a tailored maintenance program after periodontal therapy and implant treatment have been completed is prudent to successfully maintain periodontal health and implant success.

Self-Study Questions

(Answers located at the end of the case)

A. Is periodontitis a risk factor for peri-implantitis?

B. What is the rationale of periodontal therapy prior implant surgery?

C. Describe peri-implantitis diagnosis.

D. What are the risk factors for peri-implantitis?

E. Describe the peri-implantitis classification system.

F. What are the survival rates of implants placed in healthy versus periodontally compromised patients?

G. What are treatment modalities for peri-implantitis?

References

1. Herrera D, Roldán S, O'Connor A, Sanz M. The periodontal abscess (II). Short-term clinical and microbiological efficacy of 2 systemic antibiotic regimes. J Clin Periodontol 2000;27:395–404.
2. Camelo M, Nevins ML, Schenk RK, et al. Clinical, radiographic, and histologic evaluation of human periodontal defects treated with Bio-Oss and Bio-Gide. Int J Periodontics Restorative Dent 1998;18(4):321–331.
3. Bowers GM, Chadroff B, Carnevale R, et al. Histologic evaluation of new attachment apparatus formation in humans. Part I. J Periodontol 1989;60(12):664–674.
4. Meredith N, Book K, Friberg B, et al. Resonance frequency measurements of implant stability in vivo. A cross-sectional and longitudinal study of resonance frequency measurements on implants in the edentulous and partially dentate maxilla. Clin Oral Implants Res 1997;8(3):226–233.
5. Eke PI, Dye B.A, Wei L, et al. Prevalence of periodontitis in adults in the United States: 2009 and 2010. J Dent Res 2012;91(10):914–920.
6. Mombelli A. Microbiology and antimicrobial therapy of peri-implantitis. Periodontol 2000 2002;28:177–189.
7. Page RC, Offenbacher S, Schroeder HE, et al. Advances in the pathogenesis of periodontitis: summary of developments, clinical implications and future directions. Periodontol 2000 1997;14:216–248.
8. Van der Weijden GA, van Bemmel KM, Renvert S. Implant therapy in partially edentulous peridoontally compromised patients: a review. J Clin Periodontol 2005;32:506–511.
9. Schou S, Holmstrup P, Worthington HV, Esposito M. Outcome of implant therapy in patients with previous tooth loss due to periodontitis. Clin Oral Implants Res 2006;17(Suppl 2):104–123.
10. Karoussis IK, Kotsovilis S, Fourmousis I. A comprehensive and critical review of dental implant prognosis in periodontally compromised partially edentulous patients. Clin Oral Implants Res 2007;18:669–679.
11. Peri-implant mucositis and peri-implantitis: a current understanding of their diagnoses and clinical implications. J Periodontol 2013;84(4):436–443.
12. Zheng H, Xu L, Wang Z, et al. Subgingival microbiome in patients with healthy and ailing dental implants. Sci Rep 2015;5:10948. doi: 10.1038/srep10948.
13. Albrektsson T, Zarb G, Worthington P, Eriksson AR. The long-term efficacy of currently used dental implants: a review and proposed criteria of success. Int J Oral Maxillofac Implants 1986;1(1):11–25.
14. Heitz-Mayfield LJ. Peri-implant diseases: diagnosis and risk indicators. J Clin Periodontol 2008;35(8 Suppl):292–304. doi: 10.1111/j.1600-051X.2008.01275.x.
15. Ferreira S, Silva G, Cortelli J, et al. Prevalence and risk variables for peri-implant disease in Brazilian subjects. J Clin Periodontol 2006;33:929–935.
16. Lindquist L, Carlsson G, Jemt T. Association between marginal bone loss around osseointegrated mandibular implants and smoking habits: a 10-year follow-up study. J Dent Res 1997;6:1667–1674.
17. Quirynen M, Abarca M, Van Assche N, et al. Impact of supportive periodontal therapy and implant surface roughness on implant out- come in patients with a history of periodontitis. J Clin Periodontol 2007;34:805–815.
18. Strietzel FP, Reichart PA, Kale A, et al. Smoking interferes with the prognosis of dental implant treatment: a systematic review and meta-analysis. J Clin Periodontol 2007;34:523–544.
19. Galindo-Moreno P, Fauri M, Avila-Ortiz G, et al. Influence of alcohol and tobacco habits on peri-implant marginal bone loss: a prospective study. Clin Oral Implants Res 2005;16:579–586.
20. Froum SJ, Rosen PS. A proposed classification for peri-implantitis. Int J Periodontics Restorative Dent 2012;32(5):533–540.
21. Etter TH, Håkanson I, Lang NP, et al. Healing after standardized clinical probing of the perlimplant soft tissue seal: a histomorphometric study in dogs. Clin Oral Implants Res 2002;13(6):571–580.

22. Baelum V, Ellegaard B. Implant survival in periodontally compromised patients. J Periodontol 2004;75(10):1404–1412.
23. Hardt CR, Gröndahl K, Lekholm U, Wennström JL. Outcome of implant therapy in relation to experienced loss of periodontal bone support: a retrospective 5- year study. Clin Oral Implants Res 2002;13(5):488–494.
24. Karoussis IK, Salvi GE, Heitz-Mayfield LJ, et al. Long-term implant prognosis in patients with and without a history of chronic periodontitis: a 10-year prospective cohort study of the ITI Dental Implant System. Clin Oral Implants Res 2003;14(3):329–339.
25. Mengel R, Schröder T, Flores-de-Jacoby LJ. Osseointegrated implants in patients treated for generalized chronic periodontitis and generalized aggressive periodontitis: 3- and 5-year results of a prospective long-term study. J Periodontol 2001;72(8):977–989.
26. Araújo MG, Sukekava F, Wennstrom JL, Lindhe J. Ridge alterations following implant placement in fresh extraction sockets: an experimental study in the dog. J Clin Periodontol 2005;32(6):645–652.
27. Lang NP, Pun L, Lau KY, et al. A systematic review on survival and success rates of implants placed immediately into fresh extraction sockets after at least 1 year. Clin Oral Implants Res 2012;23(Suppl 5):39–66.
28. Renvert S, Roos-Jansåker AM, Claffey N. Non-surgical treatment of peri-implant mucositis and peri-implantitis: a literature review. J Clin Periodontol 2008;35(8 Suppl):305–315.
29. Felo A, Shibly O, Ciancio SG, et al. Effects of subgingival chlorhexidine irrigation on peri-implant maintenance. Am J Dent 1997;10(2):107–110.
30. Karring ES, Stavropoulos A, Ellegaard B, Karring T. Treatment of peri-implantitis by the Vector system. Clin Oral Implants Res 2005;16(3):288–293.
31. Büchter A, Meyer U, Kruse-Lösler B, et al. Sustained release of doxycycline for the treatment of peri-implantitis: randomised controlled trial. Br J Oral Maxillofac Surg 2004;42(5):439–444.

Answers to Self-Study Questions

A. Although many studies explored periodontitis as a risk factor for peri-implantitis, significant variation in study design, length of follow-up, outcome measurement, and confounders such as smoking add challenges to drawing a clear conclusion, yet current evidence suggests this association.

Schou et al. [9] performed a meta-analysis comparing the outcomes of implant treatment in individuals with periodontitis-associated tooth loss and non-periodontitis-associated tooth loss. They concluded that there was a significantly increased incidence of peri-implantitis and increased marginal bone loss around implants in those with periodontitis-associated tooth loss.

On the other hand, Karoussis et al. [10] demonstrated through a systemic review that there was no statistically significant differences in both short- (<5 years) and long-term (>5 years) implant survival between patients with a history of chronic periodontitis and periodontally healthy individuals. However, it was noted that those with a history of chronic periodontitis may exhibit more probing pocket depth, more marginal bone loss, and incidence of peri-implantitis compared with periodontally healthy subjects.

Periodontal disease is one of several important risk factors that may lead to the establishment and progression of peri-implant mucositis and peri-implantitis (Figure 1) [11].

B. Periodontal pockets can act as reservoir for pathogenic bacteria. Samples taken from peri-implantitis sites have been shown to harbor a significantly higher number of periodontal pathogens [12]. Eliminating these reservoirs will not only decrease the possibility of cross-infection but will also decrease or eliminate the need to mount an immune response from potentially susceptible hosts, which contributes to the onset and progression of peri-implant tissue destruction. As a general principle in dentistry it is recommended to treat any active disease before the prosthetic rehabilitation is initiated. This is important in particular from an overall comprehensive treatment planning standpoint. Patients are best served with a comprehensive, long-term, and predictable treatment plan that will lead to a comfortable, stable, and easily maintainable dentition. The placement of implants in patients with active periodontal disease, who might experience future tooth loss, might lead to an unpredictable outcome and a treatment plan that constantly needs to be altered and updated to address continuous future tooth loss. The treatment and stabilization of the periodontal status will allow for more accurate assessment and prognostication of current and future need of implants, allowing the clinician to present the patient with an efficient and predictable treatment plan that best addresses their dental needs.

C.

- *Radiographic examination.* Periapical and bitewing radiographies are important tools to determine the extent of bone resorption and bone levels around implants. Successful implant therapy results in stable bone levels with minimal changes during the implant life. Initial stages of peri-implantitis might result in minimal bone level changes, which are difficult to detect on nonstandardized periapical radiographs. It was suggested by Albrektsson et al. [13] that 0.2 mm of annual bone loss around a dental implant fixture is acceptable; however, the ability to detect this change on periodic periapical radiographs is extremely difficult. Therefore, radiographic examination of dental implants should always be paired with a careful clinical examination.

- *Clinical examination.* Peri-implant probing is not only a method to measure peri-implant probing depths but also the presence or absence of bleeding, presence or absence of suppuration, as well as presence and extent of recession around the implant fixture. It is important to note that probing around an implant is in some cases challenging due to the implant macrotopography coupled with the crown anatomy and probe angulation. It is also important to note that the vertical level of implant placement might result in an increased probing depth if the implant is placed at a more apical level than ideal. In such a case, a deep probing depth measurement might be a result of a deep sulcus created by the apical position of the implant rather than the disease process. This highlights that implant probing depths should be interpreted in conjunction with multiple other parameters, including radiographic examination and presence or absence of inflammation before a diagnosis is determined.

- *Microbiologic examination.* The value of microbiological testing for the diagnosis or prediction of peri-implantitis has been a controversial topic. It could, however, be a valuable tool in the treatment phase of a peri-implantitis case, providing a biological guide for the selection of an appropriate and effective systemic antibiotic as an adjunctive therapy.

Based on the earlier examinations, the diagnosis of peri-implantitis should be made based on a thorough medical and dental history and a combination of thorough clinical and radiographic examination.

D. Because peri-implant diseases may take years to develop, as with periodontitis, long-term prospective studies are most valuable in identifying risk factors. The literature we have today varies significantly in study design, length of follow-up, definition of patient population in terms of periodontal status, and outcome measurement. However, in 2008, Heitz-Mayfield completed a comprehensive review and organized the risk factors for peri-implantitis with respect to the level of evidence [14]. Given the evidence we have so far, there is substantial evidence for the following risk factors: poor oral hygiene [15,16], history of periodontitis [8–10,17], and cigarette smoking [18]. There is limited evidence for the following risk factors for peri-implantitis: diabetes [15] and alcohol consumption [19].

E. According to Froum and Rosen [20], the lack of a standardized classification to differentiate the various degrees of peri-implantitis has resulted in confusion when interpreting the results of studies evaluating the prevalence, treatment, and outcomes of therapy. They authors have developed a classification system (Table 1).

According to the AAP position paper in 2013 [11], a number of risk factors have been identified that may lead to the establishment and progression of peri-implant mucositis and peri-implantitis, including previous periodontal disease, poor plaque control/inability to clean, residual cement, smoking, diabetes, occlusion and overload, and other

Table 1: Peri-implantitis Classification System

Stage	Classification system
Early	Probing depth ≥4 mm (bleeding and/or suppuration on probing) Bone loss <25% of the implant length
Moderate	Probing depth ≥6 mm (bleeding and/or suppuration on probing) Bone loss 25–50% of the implant length
Advanced	Probing depth ≥8 mm (bleeding and/or suppuration on probing) Bone loss >50% of the implant length

potential risk factors (rheumatoid arthritis, alcohol consumption).

A list of diagnostic considerations for the early detection of peri-implantitis has been proposed by AAP [11] that includes probing, bleeding, and suppuration. Initial probing of the implant should be done once the final restoration has been installed. According to Etter et al. [21], this can be done with a traditional periodontal probe using light force (0.25 N) because of the delicate and unique anatomy of the peri-implant mucosa. In addition, periapical radiographs of the implant following placement and then following the prosthesis installation should function as the baseline by which all future radiographs are to be compared. Secondary diagnostics, such as bacterial culturing, have been suggested; inflammatory markers and genetic diagnostics may further be useful in the diagnosis of peri-implant diseases.

F. Implant survival in periodontally compromised patients has been investigated and the 5-year survival rates were 97% and 94% for two- and one-stage implants respectively [22]. Clinical trials compared the success of implants in patients with a history of periodontitis and those without a history of periodontitis [23,24]. These studies demonstrated an increased survival of implants in healthy patients. The success rate of implant placement in chronic and aggressive periodontitis patients was evaluated longitudinally [25]. The authors concluded that the outcome of implant therapy in terms of loss of supporting bone and implant loss may be different in periodontitis patients compared with individuals without a history of the disease.

In prospective and retrospective cohort studies, Schou et al. [9] systematically reviewed at least 5-year studies with the outcome of implant treatment in individuals with periodontitis-associated and non-periodontitis-associated tooth loss. In a meta-analysis study, they concluded that there was a significantly increased incidence of peri-implantitis and increased peri-implant marginal bone loss in individuals with periodontitis-associated tooth loss.

In corroboration with many studies, Araújo et al. [26] have shown that ridge alterations following implant placement in dogs increase the risk for implant complications. Karoussis et al. [10] used a systematic approach to identify 15 prospective studies regarding the short-term (<5 years) and long-term (>5 years) prognosis of osseointegrated implants placed in periodontally compromised partially dentate patients. The authors found no statistically significant differences in both short- and long-term implant survival between patients with a history of chronic periodontitis and periodontally healthy individuals. However, they found that patients with a history of chronic periodontitis may exhibit significantly greater long-term probing pocket depth, peri-implant marginal bone loss, and incidence of peri-implantitis compared with periodontally healthy subjects.

G. The biggest obstacle of treating a peri-implantitis case appears to be surface decontamination. Almost all implants currently used have roughened titanium surfaces. Although a rough titanium surface offers a larger surface area for osseointegration to occur, decontaminating the complex microtopography of the roughened titanium surface in peri-implantitis cases is a very challenging task. However, novel tools continue to be developed in order to decontaminate the surface of the implants, including the use of the TiBrush, lasers, ultrasonics, and chemicals (citric acid, peroxide).

The treatment modalities for peri-implant mucositis and peri-implantitis have been divided into surgical and nonsurgical. Algorithms for treatment choices have been proposed [27]. According to Renvert [28], mechanical therapy is effective for peri-implant mucositis, and adjunctive use of antimicrobial uses are beneficial [29]. On the other hand, mechanical therapy alone was considered, in some cases, insufficient for peri-implantitis [30]. This was confirmed in both cases when antimicrobials were administered locally and systemically [6,31].

Case 2

Dental Implants in an Orthodontic Case

CASE STORY

An 11-year-old Caucasian female initially presented to our clinic in 2005 with missing lateral incisors. Congenitally missing lateral incisors were diagnosed and the patient decided to proceed with orthodontic treatment. This case report illustrates a multidisciplinary treatment planning integrating dental implants with orthodontic treatment. Management of potential complications was also implemented and discussed.

LEARNING GOALS AND OBJECTIVES

■ To be able to comprehensively treatment plan dental implants for orthodontic patients
■ To understand the concerns and to foresee potential complications
■ To be able to enhance orthodontic treatment with dental implants when indicated
■ To explore the possibility of accelerated orthodontics

Medical History

There were no contributing medical issues, and the patient was not taking any medications. There were no known drug allergies.

Review of Systems

- Vital signs
  - Blood pressure: 121/68 mmHg
  - Pulse rate: 74 beats/min
  - Respiration: 16 breaths/min

Social History

The patient denied any smoking habit, alcohol drinking, and use of recreational drug. She was a full-time student and worked part time at a fast-food restaurant later when she was 18 years old.

Extraoral Examination

There was no facial asymmetry, and no significant findings were noted during palpation of the lymph nodes. No lesions, masses, or swelling were found, and the temporomandibular joint was within normal limits.

Intraoral Examination

See Figure 1.
- Oral cancer screening was negative.
- Soft tissue examination, including her lips, tongue, floor of the mouth, hard and soft palate, and buccal mucosa, was all within normal limits.
- Periodontal examination revealed all probing depths were within normal limits.
- An adequate amount of attached gingiva was generally present around most teeth.
- Mild plaque accumulation and localized gingival inflammation were noted.
- Large diastema (about 3 mm) was noted between maxillary central incisors, and significant spacing was present over premaxilla region.
- Dental examination showed missing lateral incisors and partially erupted maxillary second molars.
- Saliva was of normal flow and consistency.

Occlusion

Angle's molar class I and canine class II occlusion were noted. Normal overjet and overbite were noted.

Radiographic Examination

Panoramic radiograph, periapical and bitewing radiographs were taken (Figure 2). Congenitally missing

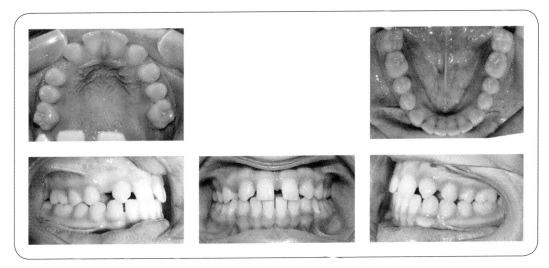

Figure 1: Initial intraoral examination at the age of 11 showed missing maxillary lateral incisors, prominent diastema, and spacing for the maxillary anterior teeth.

lateral incisors were noted. There was no evidence of periapical radiolucency or any other pathologic findings.

Diagnosis
- Congenitally missing lateral incisors.
- American Academy of Periodontology diagnosis of dental plaque-induced gingivitis.

Treatment Plan
The initial phase of therapy included full mouth prophylaxis and oral hygiene instruction to resolve the gingival inflammation. After reevaluation and observing an improvement in her plaque control ability, orthodontic treatment was planned in conjunction with 3-month periodontal maintenance visits. Dental implants were planned to be placed after the completion of the orthodontic treatment and skeletal growth to restore the missing lateral incisors. Additional hard and soft tissue augmentation may be implemented if needed. The final prosthesis would be fabricated after proper soft tissue contouring.

Treatment
The patient's oral hygiene improved after periodontal phase 1 therapy, which allowed the beginning of her orthodontic treatment. One and a half year after orthodontic treatment started, most spacing was closed and sufficient space was created for #7 and #10 implant

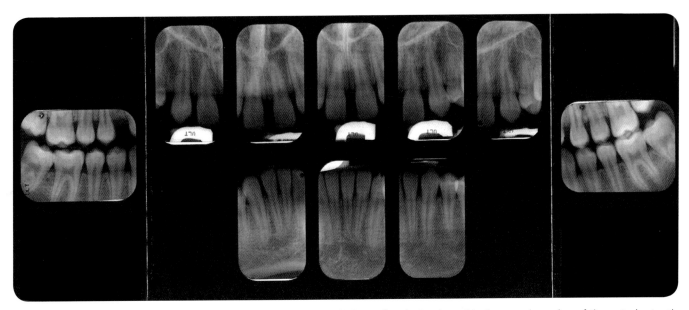

Figure 2: Initial radiographs at the first consultation visit revealed bilaterally missing lateral incisors and spacing of the anterior teeth.

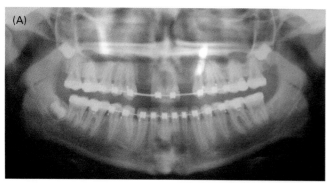

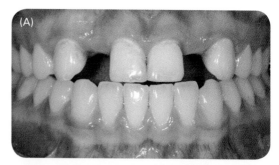

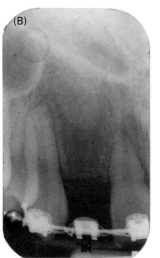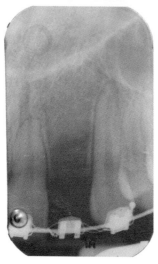

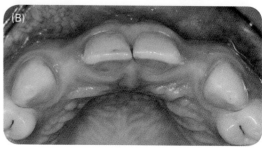

Figure 4: Patient presented at the age of 18 (3 years after the orthodontic treatment completion) with adequate space maintained for implant placement. However, clinical examination showed teeth cervical decalcification and anterior open bite (A). The occlusal view showed moderate deficiency over the facial contour of the ridge (B).

Figure 3: (A) After orthodontic treatment, space was created for proper implant site development. (B) However, significant external root resorption occurred, especially for two maxillary central incisors.

guidance, the anterior open bite was to be corrected with prosthetic treatment. Another concern was the progression of the external root resorption. The resorption of the roots for most of the teeth seemed to remain stable, but teeth #6 and #8 showed additional progression (Figure 5). Although there was no significant mobility, the compromised crown-to-root ratio (C/R) gave a questionable prognosis for tooth #8 (C/R < 1) and raised the possibility of changing the

sites (Figure 3A). However, significant root resorption was noted over teeth #6, #8, and #9 on the periapical radiographs (Figure 3B). Brackets were removed and it was decided to monitor the root resorption closely and maintain the central incisors since the mobility of the teeth were only grade 1. Although the patient requested to have dental implants as soon as possible, it was explained to the patient that dental implant placement should be deferred until the cessation of the puberty growth. She wore a vacuum-formed retainer (Essix) during the waiting period.

After confirming the completion of the skeletal growth, she was examined again to assess the current dental conditions before implant placement. Intraoral examination showed anterior open bite and cervical decalcification of the maxillary anterior teeth (Figure 4A). Adequate space was created and maintained with the retainer. It was suspected that the anterior open bite was developed due to a later mandibular growth. Given the presence of canine

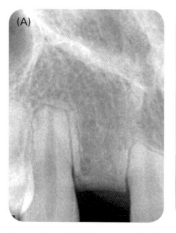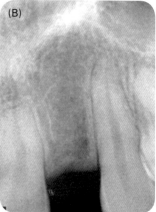

Figure 5: (A, B) Periapical radiographs reveal that significant root resorption is present and further progression of the resorption is suspected over #6 and #8 that may require revisiting the treatment plan.

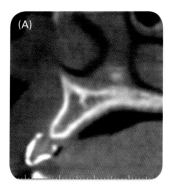 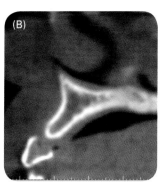

Figure 6: CBCT demonstrated the dimension of the ridge may be just enough for narrow-neck dental implants. (A) The #7 site showed a more favorable contour of the alveolar ridge with a 4.3 mm width. (B) The #10 site showed a more narrower ridge (3.5 mm in width) and pronounced labial concavity that might lead to dehiscence or fenestration-type defect around the dental implant after placement.

final prosthetic treatment plan to extract both central incisors and to have a two-implant-supported four-unit bridge from #7 to #10. The concern and alternative plan was discussed with the patient. As the patient expressed her strong will to save the teeth, the original plan was kept with the amendment of protective occlusion design and night guard fabrication. The patient also understood that, in the long term, the two single implant-supported crowns might eventually need to be replaced to support a four-unit prosthesis.

Clinical assessment before implant placement included hard and soft tissue examination. The frontal view of the intraoral examination showed a bilateral 6 mm edentulous space and symmetrical gingival margin with adequate keratinized attached tissue (Figure 4A). The occlusal view revealed a deficiency over the buccal contour of the edentulous ridge (Figure 4B), which suggested that contour augmentation procedure may be needed. Cone beam computed tomography (CBCT) was performed with a radiographic stent for better prosthetically driven implant planning (Figure 6). CBCT revealed the alveolar ridge underneath #7 had a 4.3 mm width and a 3.5 mm width over the #10 site with a rounded crest that may result in a dehiscence defect after placing a 3–4 mm diameter implant. More prominent facial concavity was also noted for the #10 site where a fenestration defect was anticipated. A resin-retained temporary bridge (Maryland bridge) was also fabricated for the healing phase of the implants (Figure 7).

After administering local anesthetics, a lingual–crestal incision was made, and a full-thickness flap was raised. The osteotomy for implant placement was performed using surgical stent and leaning against the

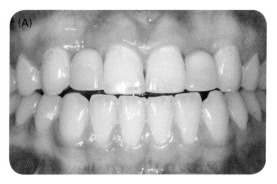

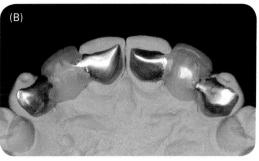

Figure 7: (A) The vacuum-formed (Essix) retainer was replaced by a Maryland bridge for better esthetic results and less interference during healing process. (B) Incisal guidance and occlusal interference was adjusted to minimal.

palatal wall. Two dental implants (3.3 mm × 12 mm) were then placed. No facial dehiscence-type defect was noted, but the remaining facial plate was only about 1–1.5 mm (Figure 8A). A palatal dehiscence defect was evident over the palatal side of #10 after implant

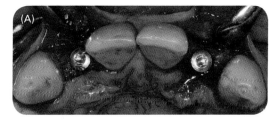

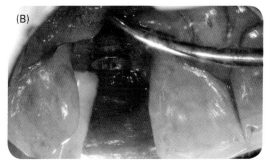

Figure 8: (A) After the implant placement leaning against the palatal wall, the buccal bone plate was intact yet thin. (B) A dehiscence-type defect over the palatal plate was noted over the #10 site.

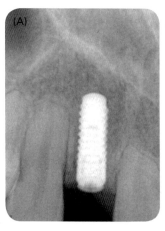 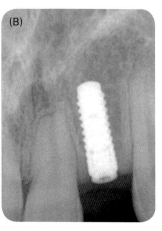

Figure 9: Periapical radiographs showed proper position and angulation of the dental implants. Proper long-axis alignment with a safe distance of 1.5 mm to the natural root was noted over (A) #7 and (B) #10.

placement (Figure 8B). Although palatal dehiscence-type defects may not contribute to an esthetic complication as critical as facial side defects, palatal ridge augmentation procedure was performed together with facial contour augmentation. Freezed-dried bone allograft with a cross-linked resorbable collagen membrane was placed over the facial side of implant #7 and around implant #10. Primary closure was achieved after periosteum fenestration releasing over the facial flap. A periapical radiographic film taken immediately after the implant placement showed proper position and angulation of the implants (Figure 9).

After 4 months of uneventful healing, a second-stage procedure was performed together with temporary crowns fabrication for soft tissue development. A minimal midcrestal incision was made under local anesthesia, and the flap was reflected carefully to insert an impression coping to maximize the amount of keratinized tissue (Figure 10). Cement-retained crowns were planned for the implants due to the angulation of the implants that was limited by the deficient alveolar

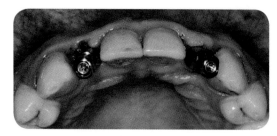

Figure 10: A minimal crestal incision was made to preserve the soft tissue for a second-stage procedure. An impression coping was placed to fabricate the fixed temporary prosthesis.

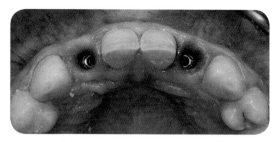

Figure 11: Healthy peri-implant soft tissue was developed with the augmented facial contour of the ridge. Minimal tooth preparation for veneers was also completed.

ridge. Veneers were also planned to address patient's high esthetic demand.

A proper soft tissue contour was achieved after 4 months of temporization phase with serial adjustments in its emergence profile. Successful facial contour augmentation could also be recognized compared with the preoperation status (Figure 11). The ideal esthetic outcome was achieved after delivery of the permanent prosthesis (Figure 12A). Limited overbite and overjet were designed in accordance with her present canine guidance to avoid excessive incisal guidance. A night guard was also fabricated for her as a protective device. A periapical radiograph was taken after 6 months' functional loading (Figure 12B). The patient was content about the outcome of the treatment and was aware of the precaution for long-term maintenance of the implants and the central incisors.

Discussion

Congenital missing of lateral incisors is a common agenesis of the permanent teeth. The prevalence varies between different ethnicities but is estimated to be about 1–2% [1]. The treatment options include removable partial dentures, conventional fixed bridges, resin-bonded bridges, autotransplantation, canine substitution, and single implant-supported crown. The advantages and disadvantages of these approaches have been widely discussed in the literature [2–4]. It has been a debate in the orthodontic literature whether to close the space with canine substitution or to create the space in conjunction with a fixed prosthesis to achieve the best clinical outcome [5,6]. With the integration of a dental implant into the treatment plan, implant-supported restoration with an interdisciplinary approach can provide a predictable and ideal esthetic outcome [7–9]. This case report presents a multidisciplinary approach for a patient with congenitally missing lateral incisors and the management of the complications.

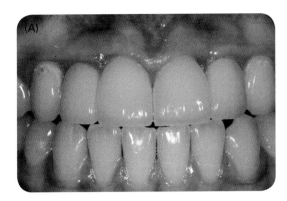

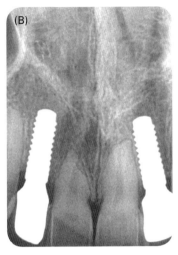

Figure 12: The desired esthetic outcome was achieved following the delivery of the final prosthesis. (A) Minimal overjet and overbite were designed together with an occlusal guard to control trauma from occlusion. (B) Radiographic film demonstrated stable crestal bone remodeling after functional loading.

Three major concerns in the treatment progress of the present case were:
1. timing of the implant placement;
2. insufficient space and hard tissue for implant site;
3. management of the complications related to the orthodontic treatment.

Dental implant placement in adolescence should be postponed until after the cessation of skeletal growth. One of the irreversible consequences of early placement is a nonfunctional infra-occluded implant-retained crown that would result in both functional and esthetic complications. (For more discussion, please refer to Chapter 9 Case 4.) Several observations showed that the patient in the present case had already passed the cessation of growth spurt at the time of implant placement.

Another concern for utilizing dental implants to replace missing lateral incisors is potentially the lack of sufficient alveolar bone. It has been shown that after distalizing the canines to create the space, the alveolar bone width decreased on average from 17% to 25% along the height of the ridge, resulting in an increased labial concavity [10]. A similar observation could be found in this case where the edentulous area had limited alveolar bone width and significant labial concavity after orthodontic treatment. Thus, simultaneous ridge augmentation was performed together with the implant placement to augment the deficient ridge. A CBCT study revealed that fenestration defect is common (about 20%) if dental implants are placed following the cingulum position of the restoration in the maxillary incisors [11]. In this case, no fenestration defect was detected clinically.

In this case, the complication resulting from the orthodontic treatment was the severe resorption of the roots, especially for both central incisors. Although clinical mobility did not linearly correlate with the poor C/R, the prognosis of the teeth was considered questionable. The alternative option may be to extract both central incisors and to have a two-implant-supported four-unit bridge for a more stable long-term outcome. A patient-centered final decision was obtained after a detailed consultation with the patient and her parents. The use of a night guard and a protective design of the occlusion was amended to the final treatment plan to avoid excessive occlusal force to the central incisors. It is critical to communicate with the patient regarding the potential complications beforehand, and an alternative treatment option will need to be presented to the patient should the complication occur. A case series of retaining maxillary incisors with severe root resorption with a long–term follow up was presented by Savage and Kokich [12]. In the case series, designing a protective occlusion, lingual wire splinting, and close monitoring seemed to be the key to success.

In summary, this case report enlightened several issues regarding integrating dental implants in patients with orthodontic treatment. A well-coordinated multidisciplinary team is necessary in managing such cases.

Self-Study Questions

(Answers located at the end of the case)

A. What are the general concerns to integrate dental implants in an orthodontic treatment plan?

B. How can we place dental implants during orthodontic treatment?

C. Can dental implants enhance orthodontic treatment? And vice versa?

D. What is the difference between implant therapy and orthodontic treatment in view of occlusion?

E. What are the complications in orthodontic treatment and implant therapy and how does it affect the treatment plan?

F. What is accelerated orthodontics?

References

1. Polder BJ, van't Hof MA, van der Linden FP, Kuijpers-Jagtman AM. A meta-analysis of the prevalence of dental agenesis of permanent teeth. Community Dent Oral Epidemiol 2004;32:217–226.

2. Kinzer GA, Kokich Jr VO. Managing congenitally missing lateral incisors. Part I: canine substitution. J Esthet Restor Dent 2005;17:5–10.

3. Kinzer GA, Kokich Jr VO. Managing congenitally missing lateral incisors. Part II: tooth-supported restorations. J Esthet Restor Dent 2005;17:76–84.

4. Kinzer GA, Kokich Jr VO. Managing congenitally missing lateral incisors. Part III: single-tooth implants. J Esthet Restor Dent 2005;17:202–210.

5. Zachrisson BU, Rosa M, Toreskog S. Congenitally missing maxillary lateral incisors: canine substitution. Point. Am J Orthod Dentofacial Orthop 2011;139:434, 436, 438.

6. Kokich Jr VO, Kinzer GA, Janakievski J. Congenitally missing maxillary lateral incisors: restorative replacement. Counterpoint. Am J Orthod Dentofacial Orthop 2011;139:435, 437, 439.

7. Kokich VG. Maxillary lateral incisor implants: planning with the aid of orthodontics. J Oral Maxillofac Surg 2004;62:48–56.

8. Spear FM, Kokich VG. A multidisciplinary approach to esthetic dentistry. Dent Clin North Am 2007;51(2):487–505.

9. De Avila ÉD, de Molon RS, de Assis Mollo Jr F, et al. Multidisciplinary approach for the aesthetic treatment of maxillary lateral incisors agenesis: thinking about implants? Oral Surg Oral Med Oral Pathol Oral Radiol 2012;114(5):e22–e28.

10. Uribe F, Padala S, Allareddy V, Nanda R. Cone-beam computed tomography evaluation of alveolar ridge width and height changes after orthodontic space opening in patients with congenitally missing maxillary lateral incisors. Am J Orthod Dentofacial Orthop 2013;144(6):848–859.

11. Chan HL, Garaicoa-Pazmino C, Suarez F, et al. Incidence of implant buccal plate fenestration in the esthetic zone: a cone beam computed tomography study. Int J Oral Maxillofac Implants 2014;29(1):171–177.

12. Savage RR, Kokich Sr VG. Restoration and retention of maxillary anteriors with severe root resorption. J Am Dent Assoc 2002;133(1):67–71.

13. Nikgoo A, Alavi K, Alavi K, Mirfazaelian A. Assessment of the golden ratio in pleasing smiles. World J Orthod 2009;10(3):224–228.

14. Gobbato L, Avila-Ortiz G, Sohrabi K, et al. The effect of keratinized mucosa width on peri-implant health: a systematic review. Int J Oral Maxillofac Implants 2013;28(6):1536–1545.

15. Leung MT, Lee TC, Rabie AB, Wong RW. Use of miniscrews and miniplates in orthodontics. J Oral Maxillofac Surg 2008;66(7):1461–1466.

16. Salama H, Salama M, Kelly J. The orthodontic–periodontal connection in implant site development. Pract Periodontics Aesthet Dent 1996;8:923–932.

17. Nordquist GC, McNeill RW. Orthodontic vs. restorative treatment of the congenitally absent lateral incisor – long term periodontal and occlusal evaluation. J Periodontol 1975;46:139–143.

18. Senty EL. The maxillary cuspid and missing lateral incisors: esthetics and occlusion. Angle Orthod 1976;46:365–371.

19. Droukas B, Lindée C, Carlsson GE. Relationship between occlusal factors and signs and symptoms of mandibular dysfunction. A clinical study of 48 dental students. Acta Odontol Scand 1984;42:277–283.

20. Harzer W, Reinhardt A. Limiting factors of functional adaptation to orthodontic space closure. Eur J Orthod 1990;12:354–357.

21. Pullinger AG, Seligman DA, Gornbein JA. A multiple logistic regression analysis of the risk and relative odds of temporomandibular disorders as a function of common occlusal features. J Dent Res 1993;72:968–979.

22. Telles D, Pegoraro LF, Pereira JC. Prevalence of noncarious cervical lesions and their relation to occlusal aspects: a clinical study. J Esthetic Dent 2000;12:10–15.

23. Robertsson S, Mohlin B. The congenitally missing lateral incisor. A retrospective study of orthodontic space closure versus restorative treatment. Eur J Orthod 2000;22:697–710.

24. Marchi LM, Pini NI, Hayacibara RM, et al. Congenitally missing maxillary lateral incisors: functional and

periodontal aspects in patients treated with implants or space closure and tooth re-contouring. Open Dent J 2012;6:248–254.

25. Travess H, Roberts-Harry D, Sandy J. Orthodontics. Part 6: Risks in orthodontic treatment. Br Dent J 2004;196(2):71–77.

26. Stenvik A, Mjor IA. Pulp and dentine reactions to experimental tooth intrusion. A histologic study of the initial changes. Am J Orthod 1970;57(4):370–385.

27. Harry MR, Sims MR. Root resorption in bicuspid intrusion. A scanning electron microscope study. Angle Orthod 1982;52(3):235–258.

28. Weltman B, Vig KW, Fields HW, et al. Root resorption associated with orthodontic tooth movement: a systematic review. Am J Orthod Dentofacial Orthop 2010;137(4):462–476.

29. Trossello VK, Gianelly AA. Orthodontic treatment and periodontal status. J Periodontol. 1979;50(12):665–671.

30. Ketcham AH. A progress report of an investigation of apical root resorption of vital permanent teeth. Int J Orthod Oral Surg Radiogr 1929;15(4):310–328.

31. Linge L, Linge BO. Patient characteristics and treatment variables associated with apical root resorption during orthodontic treatment. Am J Orthod Dentofacial Orthop 1991;99(1):35–43.

32. Sadowsky C, BeGole EA. Long-term effects of orthodontic treatment on periodontal health. Am J Orthod 1981;80(2):156–172.

33. Artun J, Osterberg SK. Periodontal status of teeth facing extraction sites long-term after orthodontic treatment. J Periodontol 1987;58(1):24–29.

34. Wennström JL, Stokland BL, Nyman S, Thilander B. Periodontal tissue response to orthodontic movement of teeth with infrabony pockets. Am J Orthod Dentofacial Orthop 1993;103(4):313–319.

35. Ferreira SD, Silva GL, Cortelli JR, et al. Prevalence and risk variables for peri-implant disease in Brazilian subjects. J Clin Periodontol 2006;33(12):929–935.

36. Frost HM. The regional acceleratory phenomena: a review. Henry Ford Hosp Med J 1983;31(1):3–9.

37. Yaffe A, Fine N, Binderman I. Regional accelerated phenomenon in the mandible following mucoperiosteal flap surgery. J Periodontol 1994;65(1):79–83.

38. Wilcko WM, Wilcko T, Bouquot JE, Ferguson DJ. Rapid orthodontics with alveolar reshaping: two case reports of decrowding. Int J Periodontics Restorative Dent 2001;21(1):9–19.

39. Kim SH, Kook YA, Jeong DM, et al. Clinical application of accelerated osteogenic orthodontics and partially osseointegrated mini-implants for minor tooth movement. Am J Orthod Dentofacial Orthop 2009;136(3):431–439.

40. Dibart S, Sebaoun JD, Surmenian J. Piezocision: a minimally invasive, periodontally accelerated orthodontic tooth movement procedure. Compend Contin Educ Dent 2009;30(6):342–344, 346, 348–350.

Answers to Self-Study Questions

A. The development of dental implants has dramatically revolutionized treatment planning in dentistry. A multidisciplinary approach is considered the highest standard of care, and orthodontists have embraced implant therapy to provide the best treatment options for different cases. The challenges for coordination and treatment planning are staging, implant-site development, and complication management.

The first question is whether we should place the implants before or after the orthodontic treatment. Conventionally, the sequence would be to place the dental implants after orthodontic treatment has been completed. Because the position of the dental implants is permanent after osseointegration with the bone, it cannot be adjusted as the natural tooth with orthodontic treatment. Therefore, it would be difficult to predict and plan the final position of the implant according to the dynamic tooth movement.

On the other hand, placing the dental implant after the orthodontic treatment would increase the overall treatment time; meanwhile, the orthodontist also loses the opportunity to utilize dental implants to enhance the orthodontic treatment by providing static anchorage. Developmental issues are another concern that affects the treatment plan. Adolescents after completion of the orthodontic treatment are eager to receive implant therapy if needed. However, dental implants should not be placed before skeletal growth cessation.

The second concern is the potential lack of space or hard and soft tissue defects at the implant site. It is critical for the restorative provider to communicate with the orthodontist to determine the space required for the prosthesis. The ideal space needed for different teeth varies between individuals. The remaining teeth could serve as a reference to determine the required space. For the anterior teeth, the golden proportion has been widely used as a guideline; however, it may not be a decisive factor for an attractive smile [13]. A diagnostic wax-up may be the most effective way to facilitate the agreement between different specialties and the patient during treatment planning. For posterior teeth, the contralateral tooth can serve as a reference; however, a smaller crown may favor occlusal loading for an implant-supported prosthesis. For severely resorbed alveolar ridges, extensive ridge augmentation procedures will be needed as a separate surgery before implant placement. Soft tissue augmentation should also be performed for the better maintenance of the dental implants if there is not enough keratinized attached tissue [14]. All procedures that are required to optimize the implant site should be presented to the patients as part of the comprehensive treatment plan. If proper planning is done, it is possible to proceed with these procedures during the orthodontic treatment.

The potential complications associated with orthodontic treatment and dental implants must be discussed with the patients before finalizing the treatment plan. The complication of an orthodontic treatment like external root resorption impacts the final treatment plan significantly. The potential risk of peri-implantitis should also be evaluated and discussed. These complications are further discussed in the answer to self-study question E.

In summary, the key to successful orthodontic and implant treatment is through a well-coordinated multidisciplinary team to develop a comprehensive plan and careful communication between all disciplines and patients.

B. If placement of the dental implants during the orthodontic treatment is the sequence of choice, careful interdisciplinary planning should be conducted. Conventionally, implants could be placed 3–4 months prior to completion of the orthodontic treatment as final restoration could be fabricated immediately after debonding of the bracket. However, in order to utilize the anchorage provided by the dental implants, earlier placement may be beneficial; yet, locating the final prosthetically driven position is a great challenge, and a full mouth wax-up should be made to provisionalize the case.

In most of the cases, dental implants should not be placed in the early phase of the orthodontic treatment. Midline shifting or significant spacing from the adjacent teeth would greatly affect the ideal position of the dental implants. The opposing arch should also be assessed to foresee a proper occlusion. In addition, implant site development may be required to precede implant placement. Maintaining the space, ensuring proper plaque control, and keeping the dental implants clean throughout the healing process are also important and often neglected.

C. Historically, the integration of dental implants in orthodontics may only be limited to facilitate tooth replacement. However, by proper multidisciplinary planning, dental implants and orthodontic treatment can work together and mutually benefit each other to enhance the overall treatment outcomes.

Temporary anchorage devices, like miniscrews, have been shown to successfully facilitate orthodontic treatment by providing additional anchorage [15]. Standard dental implants could also be planned and placed carefully to serve as a favorable anchorage for tooth movement. The incorporation of implants into the orthodontic treatment planning makes each decision pathway more predictable either to open or to close an edentulous space. Miniscrews could assist in the closure of the space, and dental implants could restore the space after opening. Dental implants with a temporary crown could act as an effective anchorage for the overall movement of the teeth. This gives the clinicians the confidence to provide different treatment options to the patients based on their interests.

Orthodontic treatment can also enhance the final outcome of dental implant-supported prostheses. For a narrow edentulous space, implant placement is not possible without the orthodontic treatment. Proper teeth alignment can eliminate unnecessary embrasure space and the discrepancy of the bone level, which would help with the patient's comfort and create a better environment for maintenance. For more advanced cases, orthodontic extrusion could increase the vertical dimension of the hard and soft tissue and provide a more harmonious profile for dental implants [16]. Therefore, orthodontic extrusion should be considered before extraction of any nonperiodontally involved tooth.

In conclusion, dental implants and orthodontics can mutually enhance each other in many ways. However, proper multidisciplinary treatment planning is required to avoid complications and to achieve the best treatment outcome.

D. Establishing a stable occlusion is critical for the long-term stability of the treatment outcome. The goal is the same for different disciplines, but each may have a different focus. For orthodontic treatment, the goal is to achieve an Angle class I molar and canine relationship with proper interincisal overlap. However, instead of focusing on the occlusion system, dental implants in orthodontic patients usually require individual attention where eccentric interference should be minimized to exert less lateral force to the implants. Therefore, the final restoration on the dental implant should be fabricated after orthodontic treatment and even after patient has adapted to the occlusion.

For patients with congenitally missing lateral incisors, there are several considerations for occlusion stability. From a functional standpoint, there is a controversy regarding whether or not to achieve an Angle class I molar relationship at the end of orthodontic treatment [17,18]. In cases treated with space closure from a canine substitute, the lack of canine protected occlusion may predispose the patient to cervical abfraction and temporomandibular disorder (TMD) [19–22]. On the other hand, the first premolar may be considered an ideal substitute for the canine as some clinical studies found no difference in occlusal function or signs and symptoms of TMD in these patients [17,18,23]. As for patients treated with dental implants, the occlusion may be able to be established with the "ideal" canine protected occlusion and minimal incisal guidance over the implant-supported crowns. One study showed that TMD is not influenced by different treatment options, and 44% of all patients presented mild TMD regardless of the different treatment group [24]. Although there is limited evidence regarding its effect, occlusion remains an important consideration for all specialties.

E. Orthodontic treatment can be associated with unfavorable side effects, such as enamel demineralization, increased caries risk, enamel trauma, enamel wear, pulpal reaction, allergy to orthodontic components, gingival hyperplasia, root resorption, and acceleration of periodontal tissue destruction [25].

One of the common complications of orthodontic treatment is external root resorption. Histologic studies have shown than more than 90% of orthodontically treated teeth were affected by some degree of root resorption [26–28]. However, clinical studies using radiographic diagnostic tools have reported an incidence rate of root resorption ranging from 8 to 16% of orthodontically treated teeth [29]. The etiology of root resorption in orthodontically treated teeth is considered to be complex and multifactorial. There are several conditions that appear to be risk factors, such as duration of applied force, type and magnitude of applied force, abnormal root morphology, hormonal deficiency, genetic factors, and previous history of root resorption [28]. It has been found that maxillary central incisors are the teeth that tend to be most affected [30]. Furthermore, it has been shown that the duration of the force is a more influential factor than the force magnitude [31]. Therefore, it is necessary for clinicians to identify and consider the risk factors for root resorption and discuss those risk factors with the patient. Moreover, the patient must be informed about the risks of orthodontic treatment, especially the risk of root resorption before initiation of the treatment. During orthodontic treatment, teeth should be monitored closely to detect any sign of root resorption. If root resorption is identified, the active phase of treatment should be stopped for 3 months. In the case of severe root resorption, the treatment plan should be revised and an alternative treatment option should be considered.

Proper orthodontic treatment in periodontally healthy patients who have good oral hygiene does not cause any periodontal destruction. However, in patients who have preexisting periodontal disease, orthodontic treatment may accelerate periodontal destruction [32–34]. Hence, orthodontic treatment of patients with active periodontal disease is not recommended. Furthermore, clinicians should monitor periodontal conditions closely to detect early signs of periodontal disease during orthodontic treatment in order to prevent periodontal destruction.

Proper oral hygiene during orthodontic treatment is crucial to maintain a healthy periodontium. Orthodontic treatment with fixed appliances is known to make oral hygiene difficult and increase the accumulation of dental plaque. Plaque control during orthodontic treatment is crucially important, especially when implant placement during the orthodontic treatment is planned, since poor oral hygiene is considered as the main risk factor for peri-implantitis. It is well documented that patients with poor oral hygiene are more likely to develop peri-implantitis with an odds ratio up to 14.3 [35]. Therefore, it is essential to educate patients on effective plaque control techniques and to reinforce oral hygiene instructions according to an individual's need at each visit.

F. Shortening the treatment time has always been the wish of the patient and the goal of the clinicians.

Incorporating implant site development and implant placement collaterally with orthodontic treatment could potentially reduce the overall treatment time. In addition, selective decortication of the alveolar bone may further accelerate the movement of the teeth. This observation was first called the regional accelerated phenomenon [36,37]. It was later incorporated with a bone grafting procedure by Dr. William M. Wilcko and termed periodontally accelerated osteogenic orthodontics [38]. The mechanism behind this technique may be the inflammation that increased the bone turnover rate. A case series was published using this technique with miniscrews to treat extremely difficult cases, such as intrusion of severely elongated molar and closure of large molar edentulous space [39]. The main issue for patients' acceptance is the invasive nature of such an approach. A minimally invasive approach with piezo-instruments is also proposed to minimize the morbidity [40]. The accelerated orthodontics techniques are gradually gaining popularity among clinicians and patients, and this approach could be a field of great potential in the near future.

Case 3

Patients with Systemic Disease (A Genetic Disorder)

CASE STORY

A 17-year-old female patient diagnosed with Papillon–Lefèvre syndrome (PLS) was referred to a prosthodontist for their expert opinion and management of the case. The chief complaint was generalized teeth mobility, which affected the patient's teeth function. She also reported bleeding with brushing, which affected her home oral care practice. The patient visited her dentist regularly for uninterrupted dental care.

LEARNING GOALS AND OBJECTIVES

■ To learn the oral manifestations of the PLS
■ To learn how to restore a case of PLS using dental implants

Medical History

At the time of treatment the patient was not aware of any medical conditions besides PLS.

Review of Systems

• Vital signs
  ○ Blood pressure: 122/76 mmHg
  ○ Pulse rate: 76 beats/min
  ○ Respiration: 15 breaths/min

Social History

The patient is a high school student who had never smoked before.

Extraoral Examination

No significant findings were noted on the face and lips. Hyperkeratosis of palms and soles of feet was noted (Figure 1).

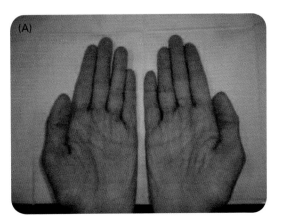

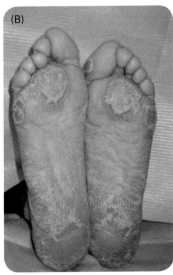

Figure 1: Hyperkeratosis of (A) the palm and (B) the feet.

Intraoral Examination

• Oral cancer screening was negative.
• Soft tissue exam, including her tongue and floor of the mouth, were within normal limits.
• Missing teeth: #1, #16, #17, #32.
• Restorations: there are several amalgam restorations in the posterior teeth.

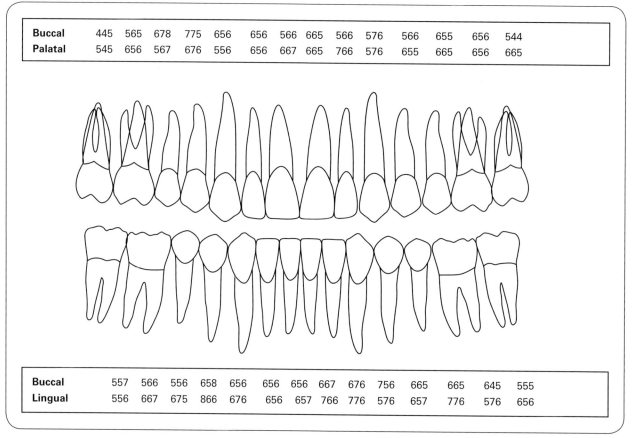

Buccal	445	565	678	775	656		656	566	665	566	576		566	655	656	544
Palatal	545	656	567	676	556		656	667	665	766	576		655	665	656	665

Buccal	557	566	556	658	656		656	656	667	676	756		665	665	645	555
Lingual	556	667	675	866	676		656	657	766	776	576		657	776	576	656

Figure 2: Periodontal charting.

- Periodontal examination revealed pocket depths in the range of 4–10 mm and spontaneous bleeding on probing (Figure 2).
- Generalized severe gingival inflammation (Figure 3).
- Generalized erythematous gingiva (Figure 3).
- Generalized recession (Miller class IV).

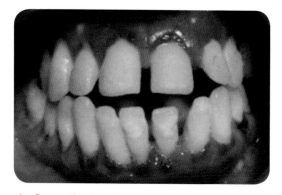

Figure 3: Generalized erythematous gingiva with plaque deposition and gingival recession.

Occlusion

It was difficult to determine whether there were any occlusal discrepancies or interferences owing to the severe teeth mobility the patient was experiencing.

Radiographic Examination

A full mouth radiographic series was ordered. Radiographic examination revealed generalized severe bone loss except in the second molar area, where the bone loss was mild/moderate (Figure 4).

Diagnosis

The diagnosis according to American Academy of Periodontology was generalized severe chronic periodontitis associated with genetic disorders (PLS).

Treatment Plan

Considering her age and the prognosis of the teeth, a decision was made to extract all the teeth except for the second molars of both upper and lower arches. To restore function and esthetics, implant-supported fixed

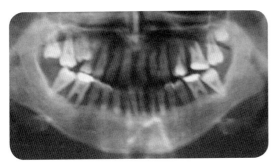

Figure 4: Pretreatment panoramic radiograph showing generalized bone loss giving a floating teeth appearance.

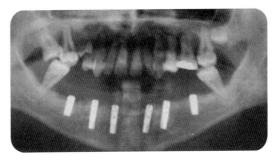

Figure 6: Panoramic radiograph after implant insertion in the mandibular arch.

prostheses was considered as the treatment option. This treatment plan consisted of a staged approach to prevent any long disturbance of the function or any psychological trauma to the patient, considering her age.

Treatment

After discussing the treatment plan with the patient and her parents, initial-phase therapy was performed on the first visit; during her second visit to the clinic, scaling and root planing was performed for the second molars. Atraumatic extraction was performed for all the teeth in the lower jaw except the second molars using a periotome and universal forceps after obtaining profound anesthesia at the surgical sites using local anesthetic; the erupting third molars were extracted as well. No flaps were reflected during the procedure. Sutures were placed to approximate the edges of the soft tissue (Figure 5). After soft tissue relining and occlusal adjustments, the lower immediate transitional removable partial denture was inserted. Two months after extraction of the lower teeth, six dental implants (OsseoSpeed™, Astratech Dental Implant System, Mölndal, Sweden) in the canino, first premolar, and first molar region were placed in the lower arch. Bone grafting (Bio-Oss®, Geistlich AG, Switzerland) was

carried out in the lower right first premolar and molar region. In the canine as well as premolar region, implants of size 3.5 mm diameter and 13 mm length (OsseoSpeed, Astratech Dental Implant System, Mölndal, Sweden) were used, whereas 4 mm × 9 mm implants (OsseoSpeed, Astratech Dental Implant System, Mölndal, Sweden) were used in the lower molar area (Figure 6).

Two months later the extraction of the upper teeth took place using a periotome and universal forceps after obtaining profound anesthesia at the surgical sites; an upper immediate transitional removable partial denture was inserted after extraction. Two month later, eight implants were placed in the upper central incisor, canine, second premolar, and first molar region on both sides (Figure 7). Implants (OsseoSpeed, Astratech Dental Implant System, Mölndal, Sweden) of size 5.0 mm diameter, 9 mm length, and 3.5 mm diameter, 11 mm length were used. Wider and shorter implants were used at the molar sites. Bone grafting (Bio-Oss, Geistlich AG, Switzerland, 0.5 g, 0.25–1 mm) was performed in the premolar and molar region.

After 4 months, all the implants were surgically exposed and impression procedures and jaw relation

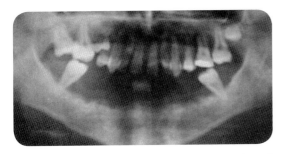

Figure 5: Panoramic radiograph taken after extraction of mandibular arch (except teeth #17 and #31).

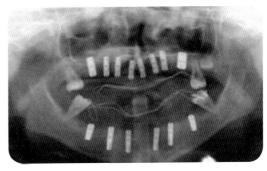

Figure 7: Panoramic radiograph, after the placement of implants in both arches.

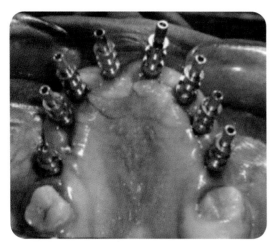

Figure 8: Fixture-level impression copings on the implants with the guide pins.

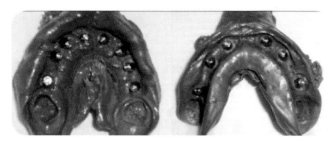

Figure 9: Definitive fixture-level impression for both maxillary and mandibular arches.

recording carried out (Figures 8 and 9). The transitional denture was converted to an interim fixed partial denture (Figure 10). After framework try-in it was then sent to the laboratory for porcelain application (Figures 11 and 12). Finally, esthetic and occlusion corrections were made on the prosthesis. The occlusion of the prosthesis was adjusted to achieve simultaneous centric relation contact and canine protected occlusion.

In the final visit, the abutments were torqued to 25 N cm and the screw holes were sealed with light polymerizing provisional resin (Fermit-N; IvoclarVivadent, GmbH, Bolzano, Italy) and composite resin (Tetric

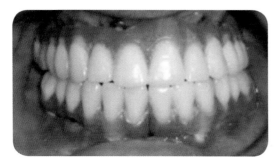

Figure 10: Interim fixed partial denture in occlusion.

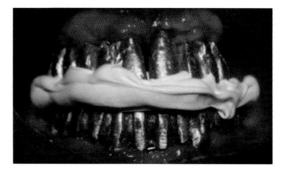

Figure 11: Try-in of metal framework and new centric relation record.

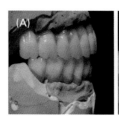 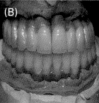 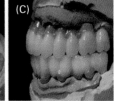

Figure 12: Ceramo-metal implant-supported fixed prosthesis mounted in semi-adjustable articulator with mutually protected occlusion: (A) right view; (B) front view; (C) left view.

Ceram HB; Ivoclar, Vivadent, GmbH, Bolzano, Italy). The final prosthesis was cemented using temporary cement (TempBond NE, Kerr/Sybron, Romulus, MI, USA) (Figures 13, 14, and 15). After the final insertion of the prosthesis, the interfaces were checked for accuracy radiographically. The occlusal vertical dimension, esthetics, phonetics, occlusion, and patient satisfaction were evaluated. Post-insertion instructions regarding maintenance of oral hygiene, use of water jet (Waterpik® Ultra Cordless Dental Water Jet, Surrey, UK), and dental floss were provided.

Periodic follow-up of the case was carried out up to 1 year (Figure 16). Oral hygiene maintenance and

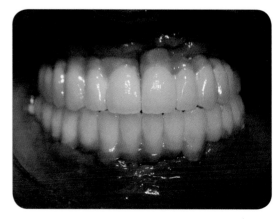

Figure 13: Post-insertion of the final prosthesis.

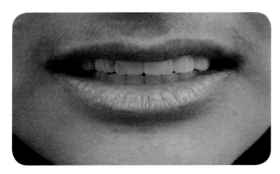

Figure 14: Extraoral frontal view of patient smile with final prosthesis cemented.

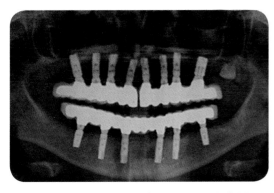

Figure 15: The panoramic view of completed definitive prosthesis.

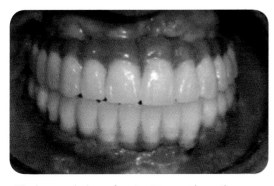

Figure 16: Intraoral view after 1 year post-insertion.

occlusion were evaluated during the recall visits. She was satisfied with the esthetics and functioning of the prosthesis.

Discussion

PLS is a devastating disease process characterized by rapid destruction of the dental alveolar complex affecting primary and permanent teeth. Early extraction of permanent dentition and prosthodontic rehabilitation has been suggested as a method of managing such cases [1,2]. Our patient had a poor dental prognosis as most of the teeth had grade III mobility. The second molars were retained to be used as abutments, and also to maintain the vertical dimension of occlusion.

There are not many case reports that have been published describing the placement and restoration of dental implants in PLS patients. Implants can act as an ankylosed tooth if placed before the growth of the alveolar process has stopped, and thus is a contraindication in young children [3]. Prosthetic rehabilitation becomes difficult in patients with atrophic mandibles and maxillae. This may call for various additional surgical techniques, such as distraction osteogenesis, bone augmentation procedures, and nerve lateralization to achieve adequate bone level in atrophic jaws before implant placement. Some studies have reported only implant placement for severely atrophic mandibles as the surgical procedures could lead to possible bone fracture [4]. Normal healing was observed postsurgery. After 1 year of follow-up, the clinical and radiological conditions of the osseointegrated implants and the denture were accessed and no signs of infection or unexpected bone loss around the implants were noticed.

Self-Study Questions

(Answers located at the end of the case)

A. What are the main characteristics of PLS?

B. What is PLS caused by?

C. Does PLS respond to conventional periodontal treatment?

D. Can we control PLS?

E. How do we manage a PLS patient to achieve successful dental treatment?

F. Can dental implants be used to treat an edentulous PLS patient?

References

1. Ullbro C, Crossner CG, Lundgren T, et al. Osseointegrated implants in a patient with Papillon–Lefèvre syndrome. A 4 1/2-year follow up. J Clin Periodontol 2000;27:951–954.

2. Woo I, Brunner DP, Yamashita DD, Le BT. Dental implants in a young patient with Papillon–Lefèvre syndrome: a case report. Implant Dent 2003;12:140–144.

3. Oesterle LJ, Cronin Jr RJ, Ranly DM. Maxillary implants and the growing patient. Int J Oral Maxillofac Implants 1993;8:377–387.

4. Etoz OA, Ulu M, Kesim B. Treatment of patient with Papillon–Lefèvre syndrome with short dental implants: a case report. Implant Dent 2010;19:394–399.

5. Gorlin RJ, Sedano H, Anderson VE. The syndrome of palmar–plantar hyperkeratosis and premature periodontal destruction of the teeth. A clinical and genetic analysis of the Papillon–Lefèvre syndrome. J Pediatr 1964;65:895–906.

6. Hart TC, Hart PS, Bowden DW, et al. Mutations of the cathepsin C gene are responsible for Papillon–Lefèvre syndrome. J Med Genet 1999;36:881–887.

7. Rao NV, Rao GV, Hoidal JR. Human dipeptidyl-peptidase I. Gene characterization, localization, and expression. J Biol Chem 1997;272:10260–10265.

8. Albandar JM, Khattab R, Monem F, et al. The subgingival microbiota of Papillon–Lefèvre syndrome. J Periodontol 2012;83:902–908.

9. De Vree H, Steenackers K, de Boever JA. Periodontal treatment of rapid progressive periodontitis in 2 siblings with Papillon–Lefèvre syndrome: 15-years follow-up. J Clin Periodontol 2000;27:354–360.

10. Ishikawa I, Umeda M, Laosrisin N. Clinical, bacteriological, and immunological examination and the treatment process of two Papillon–Lefèvre syndrome patients. J Periodontol 1994;65:364–371.

11. Nickles K, Schacher B, Schuster G, et al. Evaluation of two siblings with Papillon–Lefèvre syndrome 5 years after treatment of periodontitis in primary and mixed dentition. J Periodontol 2011;82:1536–1547.

12. Nickles K, Schacher B, Ratka-Kruger P, et al. Long-term results after treatment of periodontitis in patients with Papillon–Lefèvre syndrome: success and failure. J Clin Periodontol 2013;40:789–798.

Answers to Self-Study Questions

A. PLS is a rare hereditary disease, with a prevalence of 1–4 per million. The disease is characterized by palmoplantar hyperkeratosis (Figure 16) combined with severe periodontal destruction affecting both the deciduous and permanent dentitions [5].

B. PLS is caused by mutations in the cathepsin C gene [6], whose main functions are protein degradation and proenzyme activation [7]. Microbiological studies of plaque samples from PLS patients have shown the presence of Gram-negative anaerobic pathogens often but not always including *Aggregatibacter actinomycetemcomitans* [8].

C. Conventional periodontal therapy failed in PLS patients most of the times [9]. Conventional treatment leads to unsuccessful outcomes with eventual tooth loss leading to edentulism. Another approach that has been suggested is to extract all the erupted teeth at an early stage, followed by an edentulous period, to prevent subsequent infection of the nonerupted teeth [10]. This can result in successful outcomes, but is a drastic treatment, particularly in children or young adults, and has orthodontic, physiognomic, and potential psychological consequences. In general one should wait until skeletal development is completed.

D. There is some evidence that, in some patients with PLS, periodontal disease may be arrested by combined mechanical and antibiotic periodontal treatment, extraction of severely diseased teeth, oral hygiene instructions, intensive maintenance therapy and microbiological monitoring and treatment of the infection with *A. actinomycetemcomitans* [11].

E.
- Early diagnosis and anti-infective therapy (scaling and root planing with systemic amoxicillin metronidazole and the extraction of severely diseased teeth).
- Suppression of *A. actinomycetemcomitans* below detection limits.
- Intensive maintenance therapy [12].

F. Dental implants in PLS patients is a treatment option, but it should be kept in mind that they are at high risk of peri-implantitis and implant loss if they do not follow the prescribed regimen for maintenance care. Overall, dentists and PLS patients should bear in mind that treatment of PLS patients always has to be considered as high-risk cases. There are very few cases that have been documented, and therefore it is difficult to predict the long-term success of these cases. In this case the implants have been fully functional and maintained for more than five years.

Case 4

The Use of Dental Implants in the Child/Adolescent

CASE STORY

A 16-year-old Caucasian male was brought to the Emergency Department of Boston Children's Hospital (BCH). The day before, the patient was struck in the face with a baseball, resulting in injury to the maxilla and mandible. The initial emergency evaluation was completed by a local emergency department. It was determined that teeth #23, #25, and #26 had been avulsed. Tooth #25 was not recovered. Parental report noted tooth #23 had been reimplanted within 20 min of the accident, and tooth #26 had been reimplanted 1 h after the injury. The patient was then referred to BCH Department of Dentistry for further evaluations.

LEARNING GOALS AND OBJECTIVES

■ To understand the decision-making process for implant placement after traumatic injuries to the teeth in adolescents
■ To understand the sequence of treatment after dental traumatic injuries
■ To be able to consider suitable short-term and long-term management of such injuries

Medical History

This patient had a medical history significant for seasonal allergy and persistent cough, for which he was taking Flonase® nasal spray. Otherwise, no other significant medical problems were noted. He reported his overall health as excellent and had no known allergies to any medication, metal, or food.

Review of Systems

• Vital signs
  ○ Blood pressure: 122/80 mmHg
  ○ Pulse rate: 70 beats/min (regular)
  ○ Respiration: 15 breaths/min

Dental History

The patient brushed and flossed at least once a day. He had low caries risk with no history of decay.

Social History

He was a sophomore in high school and denied smoking, drinking alcohol, and use of recreational drugs.

Extraoral Examination

Extraoral examination revealed swelling of the lower lip. Otherwise, no lesions, masses, or swelling were noted, and the temporomandibular joint was within normal limits.

Intraoral Examination

A gross intraoral exam revealed the presence of gingival bleeding and swelling around the mandibular anterior teeth. An anterior mandibular alveolar fracture was observed from tooth #23 to #26, with the presence of a mobile segment. The fracture did not extended to the inferior border of the mandible. Teeth #23, #25, and #26 were avulsed. At the time of dental evaluation, teeth #23 and #26 had been reimplanted. One tooth had been reimplanted within 20 min of the injury, and the other over an hour later; however, the parents were unable to identify which was which. Tooth #25 had not been retrieved. Tooth #26 had been reimplanted in the socket of tooth #25. The reimplanted teeth were extruded by 3 mm with hyperocclusion against maxillary incisors. A bony and soft tissue defect was observed around tooth #26 due to the loss of buccal bone. Teeth #9 and #10 had uncomplicated enamel–dentin fractures without pulp exposure. All other soft tissues were healthy with the exception of mild plaque accumulation. No mobility, displacement, or fractures were noted to any other teeth.

Occlusion

Teeth #23 and #26 were in hyperocclusion as a result of incomplete reimplantation. No other occlusal discrepancies or interferences were detected. Overbite and overjet could not be assessed due to the presence of fractures on teeth #8 and #9.

Radiographic Examination

Panoramic and periapical radiographs were taken. Radiographic examination demonstrated fracture of the anterior mandibular segment. Periapical radiographs of anterior mandibular teeth demonstrated widened periodontal ligament spaces that are consistent with incomplete reimplantation of avulsed teeth (Figure 1). Furthermore, the panoramic radiograph showed no condylar fracture (Figure 2).

Radiographic examination of the other teeth showed no horizontal or vertical bone loss, and the crestal bone level appeared to be within normal limits. There was no evidence of periapical radiolucencies or any other pathologic findings.

Diagnosis

Mandibular fracture involving teeth #23–#26 with mobile segment. Avulsion of teeth #23, #25, and #26 with reimplantation of teeth #23 and #26. Avulsion of buccal bone tooth #26. Enamel–dentin fracture of teeth #8 and #9 noted.

Treatment

Treatment for this patient was completed over several visits. At the time of initial presentation (emergency visit), after achieving local anesthesia, tooth #23 was better repositioned into the socket and tooth #26 was reimplanted in its own socket. Then, teeth #21–#28 were splinted using a flexible wire–composite splint (Figure 3).

A 1 week follow-up appointment was performed to evaluate the health of the soft tissues, assess the stability of the splint, and initiate pulpal therapy for the avulsed teeth. Pulpectomies were initiated on teeth #23 and #26. Root canals were filled with calcium hydroxide paste, and the access cavity was adequately sealed with a resin-modified glass-ionomer. Subsequently, a pontic for the missing lower incisors was bonded to the mandibular splint. In addition, teeth #8 and #9 were restored for esthetics with dental composites.

In order to manage the severe gingival recession on tooth #26, a free gingival graft was done in the area 3 months after the incident.

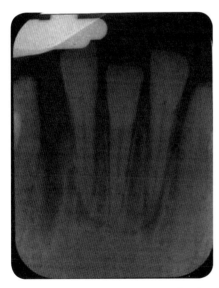

Figure 1: Periapical radiograph taken immediately after trauma.

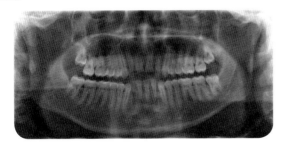

Figure 2: Panoramic radiograph taken immediately after trauma.

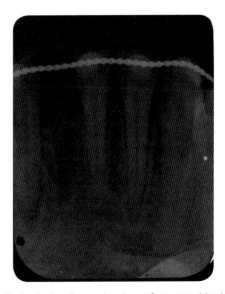

Figure 3: Periapical radiograph taken after repositioning teeth.

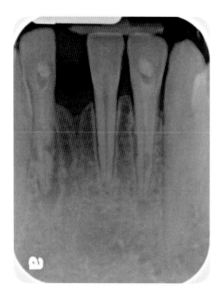

Figure 4: Periapical radiograph taken 6 months after trauma demonstrating internal and external root resorption on teeth #23, #24, and #26.

Completion of endodontic therapy was postponed to assess the stability of reattachment. Six months after the trauma, teeth #23, #24, and #26 were diagnosed as hopeless due to signs of internal and external root resorption (Figure 4). A hand–wrist radiograph was taken in order to determine the stage of skeletal maturity. The hand–wrist radiograph revealed the completion of skeletal growth. Consequently, extraction of those teeth and immediate implant placement at the position of teeth #23 and #26 was considered as the treatment of choice.

The patient was premedicated with diazepam 5 mg 1 h before the surgery. After administering local anesthesia, teeth #23, #24, and #26 were extracted atraumatically. Following the extractions, the sockets were examined and granulation tissue was removed. A large buccal bone dehiscence was evident. Implant bed sites were prepared using sequential drills according to the protocol recommended by the manufacturer. Osteotomies were extended to 2 mm beyond the apical portion of the extraction sockets. Two implant fixtures with a length of 13 mm and a diameter of 3.75 mm were then placed. A combination of bovine-derived xenograft and demineralized freeze-dried bone allograft was placed on the buccal aspect to cover the existing dehiscence. The bone particles were covered by a resorbable cross-linked collagen membrane, and the flap was sutured over the membrane. A temporary removable partial denture was delivered to replace teeth #23–#26 (Figure 5). Postsurgical instructions were given, and the patient received a prescription

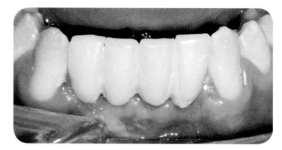

Figure 5: A temporary removable partial denture was delivered to replace teeth #23–#26.

for amoxicillin (500 mg tid. for 7 days), a nonsteroidal analgesic, and an oral rinse. Sutures were removed after 10 days, and healing was uneventful. Three months postoperatively, the second-stage surgery was performed and the implants were uncovered (Figure 6). Healing abutments were then connected to the implants. The final implant-supported screw-retained porcelain-fused-to-metal (PFM) fixed partial denture was delivered after 4 weeks (Figures 7 and 8).

Discussion

This case illustrates failure of reattachment of reimplanted permanent incisors. In the present case, the reimplanted avulsed teeth had a hopeless prognosis and were extracted primarily due to presence of

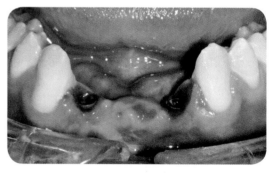

Figure 6: Uncovered implants before placement of healing abutments.

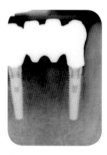

Figure 7: Periapical radiograph taken after delivery of final prosthesis.

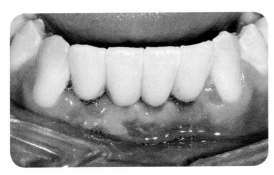

Figure 8: The final implant-supported screw-retained PFM fixed partial denture was delivered.

external root resorption. Once external resorption is discovered in reimplanted teeth, the extent of resorption should be assessed clinically and radiographically. One of the most important factors influencing treatment decision-making is the location of resorption. When the resorption is coronal to the bone crest, a dental restoration can be placed in the external resorption cavity. The restoration might arrest the resorption, or at least postpone the need for tooth extraction until completion of skeletal growth. In these cases, special consideration should be taken into account to prevent violation of the biologic width. If the external resorption occurs at the lateral root surface and apical to the bone crest, extraction of the tooth is indicated [1]. However, when the replacement external root resorption occurs

at the apical end of the root surface, it is recommended to wait as long as possible for root resorption and its replacement by bone in order to have sufficient bone volume for future implant placement.

For patients with complete skeletal growth, once the avulsed teeth are diagnosed as hopeless, the implant can be placed either immediately after extraction or with a delayed approach after ridge preservation. Several factors influence this decision-making process, including, but not limited to, clinician experience, the presence or absence and thickness of the buccal bone wall, presence of active infection, the dimensions of extraction socket, the esthetic demands, the anatomy of the site, and the quality and quantity of bone. In order to achieve optimal outcome, it is crucial to assess the need for soft tissue or bone augmentation, consider the esthetic demands of the patient, and coordinate the treatment sequence accordingly.

For the cases that there would be a long delay between tooth extraction and implant placement due to incomplete skeletal growth, tooth decoronation and preservation of roots in the alveolar bone is recommended in order to maintain bone volume for future implant treatment. However, when the roots are infected, preservation of roots is not indicated. In these cases, it is necessary to perform a ridge preservation procedure at the time of tooth extraction in order to maintain the ridge dimensions.

Self-Study Questions

(Answers located at the end of the case)

A. What are the treatment options for avulsed teeth in adolescents?

B. What are the complications after reimplantation of avulsed teeth?

C. What is the earliest age for implant placement in children and adolescents?

D. What indicators can be used to determine the completion of skeletal growth?

E. What are the consequences of implant placement when skeletal growth is not completed?

References

1. Block MS, Casadaban MC. Implant restoration of external resorption teeth in the esthetic zone. J Oral Maxillofac Surg 2005;63(11):1653–1661.
2. Andersson L, Andreasen JO, Day P, et al. International Association of Dental Traumatology guidelines for the management of traumatic dental injuries: 2. Avulsion of permanent teeth. Dent Traumatol 2012;28(2):88–96.
3. Heithersay GS. Replantation of avulsed teeth. A review. Aust Dent J 1975;20(2):63–72.
4. Andreasen JO, Borum MK, Jacobsen HL, Andreasen FM. Replantation of 400 avulsed permanent incisors. 2. Factors related to pulpal healing. Endod Dent Traumatol 1995;11(2):59–68.
5. Flores MT, Andersson L, Andreasen JO, et al. Guidelines for the management of traumatic dental injuries. II. Avulsion of permanent teeth. Dent Traumatol 2007;23(3):130–136.

6. Nasjleti CE, Castelli WA, Caffesse RG. The effects of different splinting times on replantation of teeth in monkeys. Oral Surg Oral Med Oral Pathol 1982;53(6):557–566.

7. Kahler B, Heithersay GS. An evidence-based appraisal of splinting luxated, avulsed and root-fractured teeth. Dent Traumatol 2008;24(1):2–10.

8. Andreasen JO, Hjorting-Hansen E. Replantation of teeth. I. Radiographic and clinical study of 110 human teeth replanted after accidental loss. Acta Odontol Scand 1966;24(3):263–286.

9. Hammarström L, Pierce A, Blomlöf L, et al. Tooth avulsion and replantation – a review. Endod Dent Traumatol 1986;2(1):1–8.

10. Fuss Z, Tsesis I, Lin S. Root resorption – diagnosis, classification and treatment choices based on stimulation factors. Dent Traumatol 2003;19(4):175–182.

11. Thilander B, Odman J, Grondahl K, Friberg B. Osseointegrated implants in adolescents. An alternative in replacing missing teeth? Eur J Orthod 1994;16(2):84–95.

12. Iseri H, Solow B. Continued eruption of maxillary incisors and first molars in girls from 9 to 25 years, studied by the implant method. Eur J Orthod 1996;18(3):245–256.

13. Carmichael RP, Sandor GK. Dental implants, growth of the jaws, and determination of skeletal maturity. Atlas Oral Maxillofac Surg Clin North Am 2008;16(1):1–9.

14. Heij DG, Opdebeeck H, van Steenberghe D, et al. Facial development, continuous tooth eruption, and mesial drift as compromising factors for implant placement. Int J Oral Maxillofac Implants 2006;21(6):867–878.

Answers to Self-Study Questions

A. The treatment of choice for avulsed teeth is immediate dental reimplantation. The prognosis of avulsed teeth is directly affected by time of extraoral storage, type of storage, stage of root development, and age of patient [2]. The prognosis is negatively influenced by a delay of more than 5 min in replantation and by presence of mature apex [3–5].

In an adolescent patient presenting with avulsed teeth with closed apex, reimplantation of the avulsed teeth is indicated when extraoral dry time is less than 60 min and teeth were kept in Hank's balanced salt solution, milk, saline, or saliva. In order to decrease the chance of ankylosis, it is recommended that the avulsed tooth be splinted to the adjacent unaffected teeth for no more than 2 weeks [6,7]. Initial root canal therapy should be initiated within 7–10 days following replantation and before removal of splint [2]. Calcium hydroxide should be placed in the root canal to provide an alkaline environment that could inhibit bacterial growth and reduce chance of root resorption.

When extraoral dry time is more than 60 min, the reimplantation is usually not indicated. In those cases, implant-supported crown is the treatment of choice when skeletal growth is completed. However, in children and adolescents, the delayed reimplantation can be done to maintain the space and preserve ridge dimensions for later implant treatment.

B. Following the reimplantation of an avulsed tooth, several phenomena can occur. Generally, avulsed teeth have poor long-term prognosis if they are not immediately replanted. It has been shown that root resorption occurred in 95% of the cases when there was a delay of more than 2 h in reimplantation [8]. The root resorption after reimplantation can be categorized as inflammatory external root resorption and replacement external root resorption (also known as ankylosis).

The inflammatory external root resorption is usually detected radiographically within 6 months following the replantation. Inflammatory root resorption is the result of injury to cementum following the trauma. It is caused by an inflammatory process in the periradicular tissues in response to the passage of bacteria and toxic products from the infected necrotic pulp to the root surface [9]. This inflammatory process can lead to progressive root resorption if not resolved. Inflammatory external root resorption can be arrested by removal of bacterial stimulation from the dentinal tubules and application of calcium hydroxide for 6–24 months in the root canal [10].

Replacement external root resorption causes the tooth structure to be gradually replaced by bone. Teeth with this type of resorption usually can be clinically diagnosed by the absence of mobility and metallic percussion sound [1]. It occurs as the result of severe injury to periodontal ligament. In these cases, the cells from the alveolar bone repopulate the exposed root surfaces and replace periodontal ligament by bone tissue causing dento-alveolar ankylosis. Replacement root resorption in growing children is problematic because of decreased alveolar growth and noticeable defects.

Although in many cases teeth can be saved by successful implantation, there are some cases where posttraumatic complications eventually necessitate tooth extraction or tooth decoronation and preservation of roots in the alveolar bone in order to maintain bone volume for future implant treatment.

C. Placement of dental implants should be postponed until after completion of skeletal growth. It has been shown that osseointegrated implants behave similar to ankylosed teeth. Dental implants, unlike adjacent natural teeth, do not displace in the sagittal and transversal dimensions during the growth of maxilla and mandible, and they do not follow the changes of alveolar process during growth [11,12]. Therefore, in order to avoid future complications, dental implants should not be placed in growing adolescents.

D. The pattern of skeletal development varies widely between individuals. Therefore, analyzing an individual's growth curve is recommended in estimating skeletal growth cessation. Furthermore, hand–wrist radiographic assessment and

superimposition of serial lateral cephalograms, taken at least 6 months apart, are of great value to determine skeletal maturation.

Neither chronological age nor dental age can be used as the guidance for implant placement in young individuals since they do not closely represent the stage of skeletal growth. This statement is supported by the study of Thilander et al., who evaluated the vertical relation between the implant crown and adjacent teeth in adolescents. They reported that patients who were at the same chronological age and same dental stage at the time of implant placement showed different degrees of infraocclusion of the implant crowns, which is the result of continuous growth of the jaw after implant placement [11].

E. Since dental implants behave similar to ankylosed teeth, early implantation in young individuals could lead not only to unfavorable esthetic outcomes but also to a discrepancy in occlusal plan and submergence of the implant-supported restoration [11]. This submergence of implant crown can result in overeruption of opposing teeth and tipping of adjacent teeth [13]. Furthermore, it can cause alveolar height reduction and periodontal destruction around the teeth adjacent to the implant. Early implantation in a growing child leads to even greater complications, since it may affect the normal development of the jawbones [14].

10

Peri-implantitis: Diagnosis, Treatment, and Prevention

Case 1

Ailing and Failing Implants

AILING IMPLANT

CASE STORY

A 49-year-old Caucasian female presented on 12/17/2001 with a chief complaint of: "I have pain around the implants in the left side of my upper jaw." She described the pain as a mild discomfort.

The patient had congenital absence of tooth #12 and 6 years ago had lost teeth #13–#15 due to periodontal disease (Figure 1). Two machined surface implants were placed in the area of # 12 and #13 at 9 months after the extraction (Figure 2). Nine months afterwards, the implants were restored with implant-supported single crowns (Figure 3). At the

time of her presentation with the chief complaint, the implants had been loaded for almost 4 years.

The patient brushed and flossed at least once a day. The patient has high caries risk, and she had received a significant number of dental procedures, such as crowns, inlays, amalgam restorations, and root canal therapy. Furthermore, there was a history of bruxism, and a night guard had been delivered with some occlusal adjustment. The patient had received nonsurgical and surgical periodontal treatment 10 years ago. Since then, she had been on a regular maintenance program.

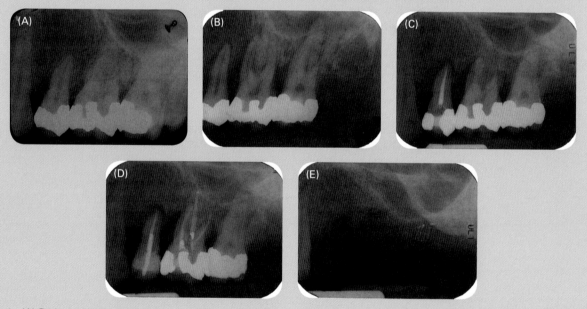

Figure 1: (A) Periapical radiograph taken 14 years before teeth extraction demonstrating relatively normal bone level around teeth #13–#15. (B) Radiograph taken 8 years before teeth extraction depicting intrabony defects surrounding teeth #13–#15. (C) Radiograph taken 4 years before teeth extraction showing progression of bone loss around the teeth. (D) Radiograph taken before teeth extraction showing severe bone loss and lack of supporting bone around teeth #13–#15. (E) Radiograph taken after extraction of teeth #13–#15.

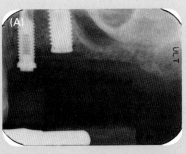
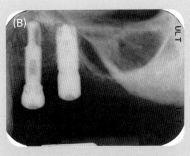

Figure 2: (A) Periapical radiograph taken after implant placement in sites #13 and #14. (B) Radiograph taken after the second-stage surgery and placement of healing abutments.

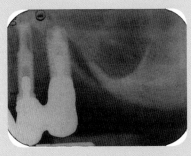

Figure 3: Periapical radiograph taken after restoring implants #12 and #13 with implant-supported single crowns.

LEARNING GOALS AND OBJECTIVES
- To identify factors that are used for determining the prognosis of teeth versus implants
- To be able to determine if an implant is ailing but might still be maintained
- To be able to determine if an implant is failing or failed

Medical History
There were no significant medical problems, and she was not taking any medication. The patient reported allergy to sulfa drugs. She reported her overall health as good.

Review of Systems
- Vital signs
  - Blood pressure: 120/71 mmHg
  - Pulse rate: 93 beats/min (regular)
  - Respiration: 15 breaths/min

Social History
The patient had been smoking around 10 cigarettes daily for the last 17 years. Although she had been well informed about the adverse impact of smoking on periodontal health and general health, she was not interested in stopping smoking. She denies any alcohol dependency or use of recreational drugs.

Extraoral Examination
No lesions, masses, or swelling were found in extraoral examination, and the temporomandibular joint (TMJ) was within normal limits.

Intraoral Examination
Oral cancer screening was negative. Soft tissues, including lips, tongue, floor of the mouth, hard and soft palate, and buccal mucosa, appeared normal. There was an adequate amount of attached gingiva present. A hard tissue examination was completed. Mild plaque accumulation with slight supra- and subgingival calculus was present. Saliva was of normal flow and consistency.

Probing depths of 7 and 8 mm were detected on the distobuccal surface and mesiobuccal surface of implants #12 and #13 respectively. Bleeding upon probing was also present. However, no suppuration was detected, and no clinical mobility was evident.

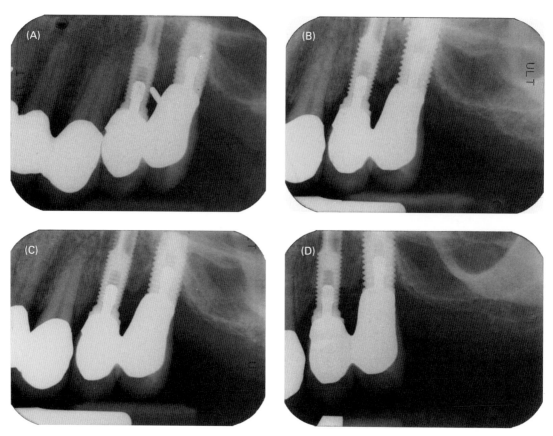

Figure 4: Periapical radiographs depicting the bone level around implants #12 and #13: (A) after 1 month of loading; (B) after 1 year of loading; (C) after 2 years of loading; (D) after 4 years of loading.

Radiographic Examination

A periapical radiograph of implants #12 and #13 was taken (Figure 4D). The radiograph showed both vertical and horizontal bony defects around implants #12 and #13. The marginal bone level was noted to be at the level of the third thread on the mesial and the fifth thread on the distal of implant #12 and at the level of the third thread on the mesial of implant #13. Comparing this radiograph with the baseline radiograph taken almost 5 years prior to the presentation (11/4/1996), it was apparent that a significant amount of bone loss occurred around implants #12 and #13 after implant placement (Figures 2 and 4).

Diagnosis

Based on the presence of bleeding on probing and deep pockets associated with bone loss around implants #12 and #13, a diagnosis of peri-implantitis and acute periodontal abscess was made.

Treatment Plan

The treatment plan for this patient included open flap debridement and surface decontamination for implants #12 and #13 after initial scaling and root planing, with antibiotic administration to treat the acute abscess.

Treatment

The surgical intervention was done on 2/1/2002. Anesthesia was obtained using buccal and palatal local infiltration of 2% lidocaine with 1 : 100,000 of epinephrine. A sulcular incision was made from mesial of tooth #11 to the distal of implant #13, and a vertical releasing incision was then made buccally on the mesial of the incision. Buccal and palatal full-thickness flaps were elevated. A thorough debridement was done using titanium scalers, and the implants' surfaces decontaminated with Arestin® (minocycline hydrochloride). The bony defects were completely degranulated, and all granulation tissues were removed. Then, the flap was repositioned and sutured with 4-0 silk sutures. Postoperative instructions were given, and the patient was seen 2, 4, and 6 weeks postoperatively to monitor the healing.

Reevaluation and Maintenance Care

Six weeks after the surgical intervention, clinical signs and symptoms were improved. The patient was then placed on a supportive maintenance care program including every 3 months recall for regular prophylaxis and clinical, radiographic, and hygiene controls. The patient was followed for 10 years. Implants remained stable over time. A chronologic sequence of the case is presented in Figure 5.

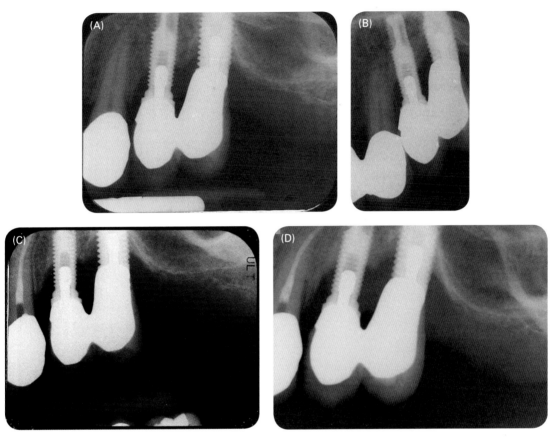

Figure 5: Periapical radiographs demonstrating stable bone level around implants #12 and #13 over time: (A) 1 year after the treatment; (B) 4 years after the treatment; (C) 9 years after the treatment; (D) 10 years after the treatment.

FAILED IMPLANT

CASE STORY

The same patient presented 10 years later (11/17/2011) with a chief complaint of pain around the right mandibular implants.

Teeth #29 and #30 were lost 15 years ago as a result of periodontal disease (Figure 6). At 6 months after the extraction, two machined-surface implants with a length of 10 mm and diameter of 3.75 mm were placed in the area of #29 and #30, which were placed in 11/4/1996 (Figure 7). Nine months after implant placement, the final single implant-supported porcelain-fused-to-metal crowns were delivered.

Tooth #31 was extracted 5 years ago due to insufficient tooth structure available after crown facture and being diagnosed as nonrestorable (Figure 8). Three months after extraction, a 5 mm × 10 mm rough-surface implant with tapered design and wide neck platform was inserted (Figure 9). The implant was then loaded after 3 months (Figure 10). The patient had been receiving maintenance therapy on an irregular basis afterwards.

At the time of this appointment, the implants #29 and #30 had been loaded for almost 14 years, and the implant #31 had been in function for 4 years.

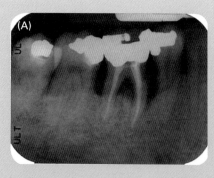
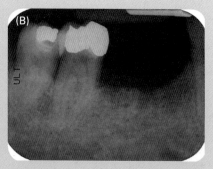

Figure 6: (A) Periapical radiograph taken before teeth extraction showing severe vertical and horizontal bone loss and intrabony defects around teeth #29 and #30. (B) Radiograph taken after extraction of teeth #29 and #30.

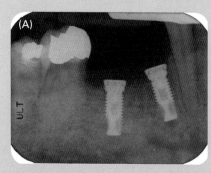
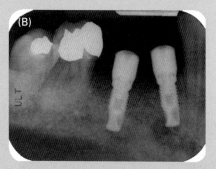

Figure 7: (A) Radiograph taken after implant placement in sites #29 and #30. (B) Radiograph taken after the second-stage surgery and placement of healing abutments.

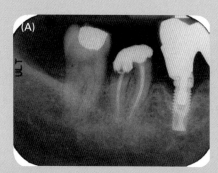
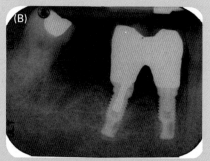

Figure 8: (A) Periapical radiograph of tooth #31 before the extraction. (B) Radiograph taken after extraction of tooth #31.

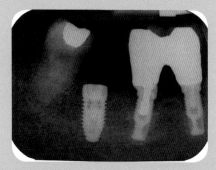
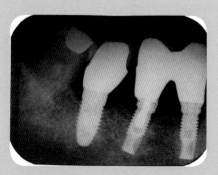

Figure 9: Radiograph taken after implant placement in site #31 at 3 months after the extraction.

Figure 10: Periapical radiograph taken after restoring implant #31.

Medical History

There was no significant change in the patient's medical history.

Social History

The patient was still smoking around 10 cigarettes a day. She denies any alcohol dependency or use of recreational drugs.

Extraoral Examination

There were no detectable lesions, masses, or swelling, and the TMJ was within normal limits.

Intraoral Examination

On the day the patient presented (11/17/2011), implant #29 was found to be clinically mobile. The peri-implant mucosa of implant #29 was swollen and bled on probing. A probing depth of 5 mm was noted on both mesial and distal aspects of implant #29. Furthermore, there were probing depths of 6 mm and 7 mm with bleeding on probing on the mesial and distal surfaces of implant #30 respectively.

No suppuration was evident.

In general, soft tissues of the mouth appeared normal, and oral cancer screening was negative. Slight supra- and subgingival calculus was seen. Saliva was of normal flow and consistency.

Radiographic Examination

After removal of the crowns of implants #29 and #30, a periapical radiograph of the area was taken. The radiograph showed a horizontal fracture in the implant #29 (Figure 11A).

Vertical and horizontal bony defects were evident around implant #30. Comparing this radiograph with the one taken at the time of implant placement showed that a significant amount of bone loss had occurred around implant #30 (Figure 7A). However, comparing this radiograph with the radiograph taken 9 years ago, after 5 years of loading, revealed that the bone level had remained stable since then (Figure 11).

Diagnosis

Implant #29 was considered to have failed due to the mobility and fracture. Implant #30 was considered as an ailing implant since deep probing depth and bone loss was evident but the condition was stable over the time.

Treatment Plan

The treatment plan included the explantation of implant #29 and placement of an implant in #29 position.

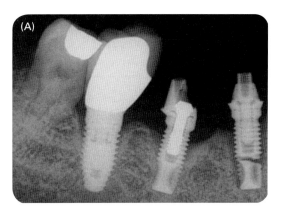

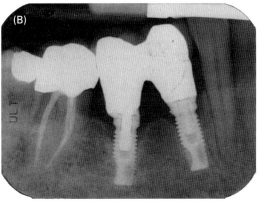

Figure 11: (A) Periapical radiograph depicting a horizontal fracture in the implant #29. Also, note the vertical bone loss around implant #30 after 14 years of loading. (B) Periapical radiograph taken 9 years prior to the radiograph in (A). Notice relatively stable bone level around implant #30 during the last 9 years.

Furthermore, open-flap debridement and administration of a locally delivered antibiotic was considered for implant #30.

Treatment

Following the administration of local anesthesia, a sulcular incision was performed from mesial of tooth #28 to distal of implant #31 with a vertical releasing incision at the mesiobuccal line angle of tooth #28. Full-thickness flaps were then elevated bucally and lingually. Implant #29 was removed using a trephine (Figure 12).

After removal of implant #29, mesial and distal surfaces of implant #30 were thoroughly debrided using carbon scalers. Complete degranulation of the bony defects was then done, and all granulation tissues were removed. Afterwards, minocycline HCl microspheres were locally administrated into bony defects. The flap was repositioned and primary closure was achieved. Postoperative instructions, including oral hygiene instructions, were provided. The patient was seen for postoperative appointments 2 and 4 weeks afterwards.

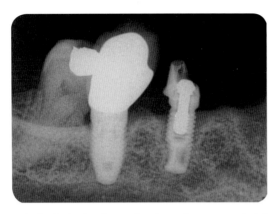

Figure 12: Periapical radiograph taken after removal of the fractured implant.

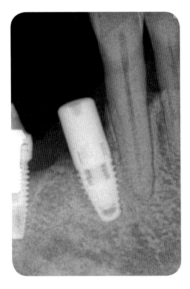

Figure 13: Periapical radiograph taken after placement of a wider implant in the site #29.

Healing was uneventful thereafter. Three months later, a rough-surfaced, threaded, tapered implant with a length of 8 mm and diameter of 4.3 mm was placed in the site #29 (Figure 13).

The patient was again placed on a regular maintenance care program and has been seen every 3 months for periodontal maintenance therapy. Implants have been stable since then without any further complications.

Discussion

In the present case, implants #12 and #13 have been in function for more than 15 years. Although there were some biological complications, these implants were considered as ailing implants since they had been stable over time after receiving treatment. It is noteworthy to

mention that there is a distinction between irreversible failing implants and ailing implants. Failing implants are those with bleeding on probing, deep pockets, purulence, and evidence of continuing bone loss that does not respond to the treatment. On the other hand, ailing implants refer to those with deep pockets and bone loss but stable at the maintenance visits [1].

It is important to note that almost all implants placed for this patient were affected by peri-implantitis. This susceptibility to peri-implantitis can be related to the fact that the patient is a heavy smoker. Furthermore, her history of periodontal disease can be another contributing factor. A history of periodontitis and smoking are risk factors that have been shown to increase the incidence of peri-implantitis. There is substantial evidence that indicates peri-implantitis is more frequent in individuals with a history of periodontitis [2–6]. It has also been shown that smoker patients are at higher risk for peri-implantitis, with the odds ratio ranging from 3.6 to 4.6 [7,8]. Furthermore, a practice-based cross-sectional study reported that 80% of smoker patients with a history of periodontitis develop peri-implantitis [9]. Therefore, clinicians should identify the risk factors associated with peri-implantitis in their patients and inform the patients about the possible consequences. Moreover, maintenance visits with shorter intervals are strongly recommended for patients at a higher risk for peri-implantitis.

Implant #29 was considered as a failed implant. In this case, the failure was due implant fracture, which is one of the technical complications that can lead to the failure. In general, implant fracture is a rare complication. A systematic review by Berglundh et al. [10] reported that fracture of implant occurred only in 0.08–0.74% of cases. Another study by Eckert et al. [11] reported an incidence of 1.5% for implant fracture in partially edentulous arches. They found that fracture of implants mostly occurred in the posterior mandible. They also reported all fractured implants had 3.75 mm diameter [11]. Interestingly, the fractured implant in our case had exactly the same diameter (3.75 mm) as of fractured implants in that study. Owing to the proximity of posterior teeth to the TMJ, a higher magnitude of masticatory force is applied on them. Placing a narrow-diameter implant where a high magnitude of force is applied might be the reason for the implant fracture in this case. Furthermore, the history of bruxism of the patient could be another contributing factor for this implant fracture. The other factors that can result in implant fracture are framework misfit, excessive occlusal load, poor prosthetic design, and unfavorable leverage [11].

Self-Study Questions

(Answers located at the end of the case)

A. What are determinants of implant success and implant failure?

B. What are the risk factors for an implant to ail/fail

C. What are the biological reasons for an ailing/failing implant?

D. What are the restorative/physical reasons for implant failure?

References

1. Meffert RM. How to treat ailing and failing implants. Implant Dent 1992;1(1):25–33.
2. Van der Weijden GA, van Bemmel KM, Renvert S. Implant therapy in partially edentulous, periodontally compromised patients: a review. J Clin Periodontol 2005;32(5):506–511.
3. Schou S, Holmstrup P, Worthington HV, Esposito M. Outcome of implant therapy in patients with previous tooth loss due to periodontitis. Clin Oral Implants Res 2006;17(Suppl 2):104–123.
4. Karoussis IK, Kotsovilis S, Fourmousis I. A comprehensive and critical review of dental implant prognosis in periodontally compromised partially edentulous patients. Clin Oral Implants Res 2007;18(6):669–679.
5. Lindhe J, Meyle J. Peri-implant diseases: Consensus Report of the Sixth European Workshop on Periodontology. J Clin Periodontol 2008;35(8 Suppl):282–285.
6. Task Force on Peri-Implantitis. Peri-implant mucositis and peri-implantitis: a current understanding of their diagnoses and clinical implications. J Periodontol 2013;84(4):436–443.
7. Strietzel FP, Reichart PA, Kale A, et al. Smoking interferes with the prognosis of dental implant treatment: a systematic review and meta-analysis. J Clin Periodontol 2007;34(6):523–544.
8. Heitz-Mayfield LJ, Huynh-Ba G. History of treated periodontitis and smoking as risks for implant therapy. Int J Oral Maxillofac Implants 2009;24(Suppl):39–68.
9. Rinke S, Ohl S, Ziebolz D, et al. Prevalence of periimplant disease in partially edentulous patients: a practice-based cross-sectional study. Clin Oral Implants Res 2011;22(8):826–833.
10. Berglundh T, Persson L, Klinge B. A systematic review of the incidence of biological and technical complications in implant dentistry reported in prospective longitudinal studies of at least 5 years. J Clin Periodontol 2002;29(Suppl 3):197–212; discussion 232–233.
11. Eckert SE, Meraw SJ, Cal E, Ow RK. Analysis of incidence and associated factors with fractured implants: a retrospective study. Int J Oral Maxillofac Implants 2000;15(5):662–667.
12. Buser D, Weber HP, Lang NP. Tissue integration of non-submerged implants. 1-year results of a prospective study with 100 ITI hollow-cylinder and hollow-screw implants. Clin Oral Implants Res 1990;1(1):33–40.
13. El Askary AS, Meffert RM, Griffin T. Why do dental implants fail? Part I. Implant Dent 1999;8(2):173–185.
14. Esposito M, Hirsch JM, Lekholm U, Thomsen P. Biological factors contributing to failures of osseointegrated oral implants. (II). Etiopathogenesis. Eur J Oral Sci 1998;106(3):721–764.
15. Weyant RJ. Characteristics associated with the loss and peri-implant tissue health of endosseous dental implants. Int J Oral Maxillofac Implants 1994;9(1):95–102.
16. Karoussis IK, Salvi GE, Heitz-Mayfield LJ, et al. Long-term implant prognosis in patients with and without a history of chronic periodontitis: a 10-year prospective cohort study of the ITI Dental Implant System. Clin Oral Implants Res 2003;14(3):329–339.
17. Vervaeke S, Collaert B, Cosyn J, et al. A multifactorial analysis to identify predictors of implant failure and peri-implant bone loss. Clin Implant Dent Relat Res 2015;17(Suppl 1):e298–e307.
18. Drago CJ. Rates of osseointegration of dental implants with regard to anatomical location. J Prosthodont 1992;1(1):29–31.
19. Buser D, Mericske-Stern R, Bernard JP, et al. Long-term evaluation of non-submerged ITI implants. Part 1: 8-year life table analysis of a prospective multi-center study with 2359 implants. Clin Oral Implants Res 1997;8(3):161–172.
20. Esposito M, Hirsch JM, Lekholm U, Thomsen P. Biological factors contributing to failures of osseointegrated oral implants. (I). Success criteria and epidemiology. Eur J Oral Sci 1998;106(1):527–551.
21. Lambert PM, Morris HF, Ochi S. Positive effect of surgical experience with implants on second-stage implant survival. J Oral Maxillofac Surg 1997;55(12 Suppl 5):12–18.
22. Sakka S, Baroudi K, Nassani MZ. Factors associated with early and late failure of dental implants. J Investig Clin Dent 2012;3(4):258–261.
23. Han HJ, Kim S, Han DH. Multifactorial evaluation of implant failure: a 19-year retrospective study. Int J Oral Maxillofac Implants 2014;29(2):303–310.
24. Lambert PM, Morris HF, Ochi S. The influence of 0.12% chlorhexidine digluconate rinses on the incidence of infectious complications and implant success. J Oral Maxillofac Surg 1997;55(12 Suppl 5):25–30.

25. Esposito M, Grusovin MG, Worthington HV. Interventions for replacing missing teeth: antibiotics at dental implant placement to prevent complications. Cochrane Database Syst Rev 2013;(7):CD004152.

26. Sanz-Sánchez I, Sanz-Martín I, Figuero E, Sanz M. Clinical efficacy of immediate implant loading protocols compared to conventional loading depending on the type of the restoration: a systematic review. Clin Oral Implants Res 2015;26(8):964–982.

27. Gunne J, Jemt T, Linden B. Implant treatment in partially edentulous patients: a report on prostheses after 3 years. Int J Prosthodont 1994;7(2):143–148.

28. Ferreira SD, Silva GL, Cortelli JR, et al. Prevalence and risk variables for peri-implant disease in Brazilian subjects. J Clin Periodontol 2006;33(12):929–935.

29. Marcelo CG, Filie Haddad M, Gennari Filho H, et al. Dental Implant fractures – aetiology, treatment and case report. J Clin Diagn Res 2014;8(3):300–304.

30. Hsu YT, Fu JH, Al-Hezaimi K, Wang HL. Biomechanical implant treatment complications: a systematic review of clinical studies of implants with at least 1 year of functional loading. Int J Oral Maxillofac Implants 2012;27(4):894–904.

31. Jung RE, Zembic A, Pjetursson BE, et al. Systematic review of the survival rate and the incidence of biological, technical, and aesthetic complications of single crowns on implants reported in longitudinal studies with a mean follow-up of 5 years. Clin Oral Implants Res 2012;23(Suppl 6):2–21.

Answers to Self-Study Questions

A. Based on the Buser criteria for success [12], an implant is considered clinically successful when the following conditions are fulfilled:

- lack of persistent subjective complaints, including pain, foreign body sensation, and/or dysesthesia;
- lack of mobility;
- lack of recurrent peri-implant infection with suppuration;
- lack of a continuous radiolucency around the implant.

On the other hand, implant failure is a term used to describe implants that failed to fulfill functional, esthetic, and phonetic purposes, which can be due to biological or technical complications [13].

B. There are several factors that can affect the outcome of implant treatment. These factors in general can be divided in two categories of patient-related factors and procedure-related factors.

A variety of local and systemic patient-related conditions can interfere with bone healing, osseointegration, or maintenance of successful osseointegration. It has been suggested that systemic conditions such as irradiation therapy, bone metabolic disorders, hormonal diseases, rheumatic disorders, deficiency of neutrophil granulocytes, lichen planus, malabsorption syndromes, and immunological disorders are associated with higher implant failure rates [14]. Furthermore, patients with compromised medical status are more likely to have implant failure

[15]. Smoking and history of periodontal disease are other conditions that are considered as risk factors for implant failure [2,6–8,16,17]. Poor bone quality and quantity and location of implant are among the local patient-related factors that might influence implant failure. The implant failure has been reported to be higher in the maxilla than in the mandible and in the posterior sites compared with the anterior sites, which can be due to the differences in bone quality and quantity [18–20]. Parafunctions habits are other patient-related factors that seem to negatively affect the implant outcomes [14,20].

In addition to the patient-related factors, there are several procedure-related factors that may increase the risk of implant failure, such as insufficient clinician experience [21], bone overheating and excessive surgical trauma [22], lack of primary implant stability [22,23], bacterial contamination [24], lack of prophylactic antibiotics [25], immediate loading protocol [26], insufficient number of supporting implants [24,27], and nonoptimal surface properties and implant design [14].

Therefore, it is necessary for clinicians to identify and consider the patient-related risk factors and discuss those risk factors with the patient. Moreover, the patient presenting with risk factors should be informed about the increased chance of implant failure before initiation of the treatment. Furthermore, clinicians should try to eliminate procedure-related risk factors by employing appropriate surgical techniques, clinical guidelines, and prostheses.

C. Biological complications and failures refer to those affecting soft and hard tissues surrounding the implant. Biological implant failures can be classified into early and late failures. Early biological failures are the result of lack of osseointegration in the early stages prior to implant loading, which can be due to infection, lack of stability, or impaired wound healing. Late biological failures are caused by failure to maintain osseointegration due to bone loss following implant loading, which can occur for several reasons, including implant overload and peri-implantitis.

Overloading can result from poor prosthetic designs or a patient's parafunctional habits. In order to prevent implant overload, occlusion must be evaluated, and heavy or premature contacts and occlusal interferences should be eliminated. Furthermore, patients with parafunctional habits require an increased number of implants to bear the occlusal forces.

Peri-implant diseases are inflammatory lesions and are strongly associated with poor oral hygiene [28]. From the clinical perspective, it is crucial for clinicians to detect early signs of peri-implant diseases. Therefore, probing depths around the implant should be recorded annually in order to monitor the peri-implant conditions. It is important to mention that probing using a conventional periodontal probe does not cause damage to the

implant surface or soft tissue attachments [5]. Furthermore, patients should be informed about the necessity of long-term and regular maintenance care.

D. Technical complications and failures refer to mechanical damage of the implant, implant components, and prostheses, such as abutment screw loosening or fracture, prosthesis fracture, and implant fracture. These technical complications may or may not lead to implant failure, but they may lead to an increased need for repair.

Implant fractures are one of the technical complications that are considered as clear implant failures. Several factors such as peri-implant bone loss, overload, bruxism, small-diameter implants, and cantilevers have been suggested to be associated with implant fractures [29]. In the case of implant fracture, the removal of the fractured implants and the placement of new implants is the treatment of the choice.

Abutment- or screw-loosening are the most frequent technical complications [30,31]. The main etiologies for abutment or screw loosening are overloading and lack of passive fit of the superstructures. A retrospective study of fractured implants has reported that abutment or screw loosening preceded implant fracture in the majority of the cases [11]. Therefore, these minor complications should not be ignored, since unaddressed etiologies can lead to more invasive and irreversible damage, such as implant fracture.

Case 2

Patient's Plaque Control Around Implants

Medical History

The patient denies any present and past illnesses and conditions, and she does not consume any medications, other than over-the-counter multivitamin, calcium, and fish oil.

Review of Systems

- Vital signs
  - Blood pressure: 130/87 mmHg
  - Pulse: 80 beats/min
  - Respiration: 16 breaths/min

Social History

The patient has never smoked and does not drink alcohol.

Extraoral Examination

The extraoral examination revealed no significant findings. The patient presented with no suspicious masses or swellings. An assessment of the temporomandibular joints showed no alteration of the anatomical structures as well as mandibular excursions and function. Her face was symmetric, and there were no swollen lymph nodes noted on palpation and direct observation. Her eyes were of normal dimension, with the interpupillary line parallel to the occlusal plane. The patient's skin was of normal color.

Intraoral Examination

The oral cancer screening was negative. The soft tissues exam, including her tongue, floor of the mouth, and the throat, appeared to be normal in color, shape, and dimension.

The patient was missing natural teeth #1, #3, #14, #15, #16, and #32. No caries and no defective restorations were detected on the remaining teeth. The patient did not present with any open interproximal contacts; however, her teeth had moderate to severe wear facets.

The following clinical records were obtained:
- intra- and extraoral photographs (Figure 1);
- complete series of periapical and bitewing radiographs (Figure 2);

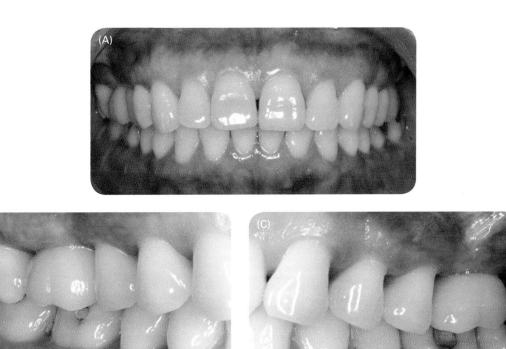

Figure 1: (A) Frontal and (B, C) lateral views of the clinical situation.

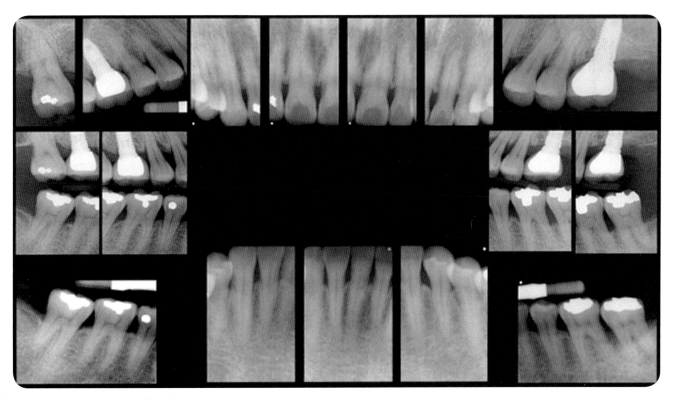

Figure 2: Complete series of radiographs.

- periodontal charting (including probing depth, bleeding on probing (BOP), clinical attachment loss, mobility, suppuration, furcation, mucogingival defects, recessions);
- study casts.

Periodontal Charting

The periodontal examination (Figure 3) revealed probing depths of:
- 4–6 mm for #2, #3, #4, #13, #18, #20, #28, and #31
- 7–9 mm for #5 and #12.

The gingival tissue exhibited a thick morphotype. The gingiva was of normal size, a flat shape and a firm consistency. Also, slight generalized marginal erythema was observed.

The patient presented with class I (oral hygiene index) BOP on teeth #3, #4, #5, #12, #13, #14, #20, #28, and #29, with no evidence of suppuration.

Localized presence of subgingival plaque and slight subgingival calculus accumulation was noted on teeth #4, #5, #12, #13, #18, #19, and #31.

The patient exhibited gingival recession on teeth #4, #5, #11–#13, #19–#21, and #28–#30 and an absence of attached gingiva associated with #4 and #13.

Occlusion

The patient has a class I Angle canine and molar occlusion. The evaluation of functional occlusion revealed a bilateral canine guidance as well as an incisor-guided anterior guidance with no discrepancies and interferences. There was evidence of parafunctional habits with attrition noted on the incisal edge of the cuspids.

Radiographic Examination

A complete mouth radiographic series was exposed (Figure 2). The radiographic examination revealed a generalized mild horizontal bone loss pattern with crestal lamina dura well defined. The exam also revealed a localized severe bone loss associated with teeth #2, #5, #18, and #19.

There was no sign of bone loss around the dental implants.

Diagnosis

- Generalized mild chronic periodontitis with localized severe chronic periodontitis associated with teeth #2, #5, #18, and #19 [1].
- Peri-implant mucositis #3 and #14.
- Developmental or acquired deformities and conditions around teeth.
- Acquired deformities and conditions around teeth [1]:
  ○ soft tissue recession #4, #5, #11, #12, #13, #19, #20, #21, #28, #29, and #30;
  ○ lack of attached gingiva #4 and #13.
- Partial edentulism.
- Generalized attrition.

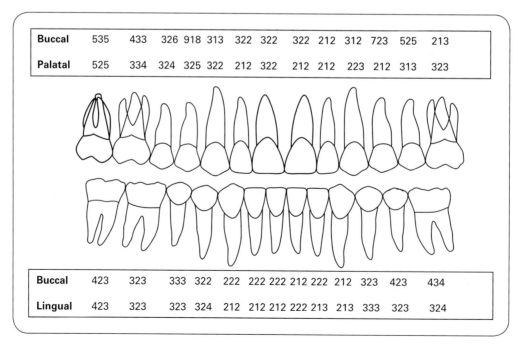

Buccal	535	433	326	918	313	322	322	322	212	312	723	525	213
Palatal	525	334	324	325	322	212	322	212	212	223	212	313	323

Buccal	423	323	333	322	222	222	222	212	222	212	323	423	434
Lingual	423	323	323	324	212	212	212	222	213	213	333	323	324

Figure 3: Periodontal charting.

Treatment Plan

The treatment plan for this patient consisted of initial phase I therapy. which included:

- patient motivation;
- oral hygiene technique instructions;
- complete mouth debridement (prophylaxis and scaling and root planing of dentition as well as implant debridement);
- reevaluation of initial phase (4–6 weeks).

Treatment

The most important step before initiating mechanical periodontal treatment is patient motivation for their personal oral hygiene. Without patient cooperation the teeth/implants will likely not have a favorable prognosis and the treatment outcome will also not be successful. At the outset of therapy, the patient's plaque removal habits were observed and the techniques modified in order to achieve better subgingival control of the biofilm. As an important part of this first phase, the patient demonstrated the recommended plaque control techniques for the clinician in front of a mirror. It is critical to observe the patient perform the suggested methods in order to assure its effectiveness and to help correct improper and ineffective techniques. The patient was introduced to the modified Bass technique as well as a thorough flossing technique. When implants present with increased interdental spaces, the patients can utilize Superfloss® and interproximal brushes for effective interdental plaque removal. Other aids that were utilized for this patient included a rubber tip, which compresses the soft tissue against the implant or its prosthesis to help dislodge interproximal plaque when there is no access for dental floss. This patient was shown how to use the rubber tip in the proximal areas next to the dental implants. She was instructed in the use of all recommended plaque removal aids, and she was asked to demonstrate the aforementioned devices to ensure that she understood the techniques and their applications.

Following her plaque control technique instruction, the natural teeth were scaled and root planed and the implants were debrided in two sessions (right side and left side of the mouth) 1 week apart utilizing local anesthesia.

The oral hygiene techniques were again reviewed, during the second session of root planing and debridement, in order to assess the patient's technical abilities. Following the assessment the remaining half of the mouth was debrided as before.

Four weeks following the initial hygiene therapy, a comprehensive periodontal charting and evaluation was completed.

Discussion

Once a diagnosis of peri-implant mucositis is established, the clinician must plan for two important treatment steps. The first task should be patient education to assist the patient in understanding why proficient plaque removal is necessary. If the patient understands the benefits of self-plaque removal they will likely be motivated to be consistent and thorough with performing the necessary techniques for plaque removal. This is called "concordance" versus "compliance." Compliance is doing plaque removal techniques because someone said to do it, whereas concordance is doing the techniques because the patient believes it is beneficial to their well-being and thus wants to do it. A concordant patient is likely to maintain the consistency indefinitely. The second task is to assist the patient with the techniques for plaque removal that best address the specific needs. In general, a sulcular technique of brushing is indicated, and there are a variety of techniques and devices for cleaning interproximally, which need to be individualized for each patient depending on the design of the implant prosthesis.

This patient presents with two implants that demonstrated clinical bone stability after 2 years in function. In order to debride the peri-implant area, the patient needs to be meticulous with plaque removal.

As in most cases of cleaning implant-supported prostheses, the implant surface itself is not accessible for debridement. In the cases of bone-level implants, the implant is surrounded by bone; however, the abutment is often exposed to bacterial contamination and will require debridement by the patient. In the case of a tissue-level implant, there is often an approximate 1.8 mm polished collar. In many instances the epithelial attachment is attached to this collar and the patient or clinician only needs to access the implant crown for debridement. In some instances of soft tissue and bone recession, the polished collar will be exposed to bacterial contamination and will need to be accessed by the patient for debridement. Additionally, it is important to understand the character of the surrounding soft tissue. If it is masticatory mucosa, then a sulcular brushing technique is advised. If it is alveolar mucosal tissue a more gentle technique of brushing might be advocated, such as a Stillman technique [2]. Also, it is advised to identify the material of the abutment (i.e., titanium, zirconia) before choosing the devices and abrasiveness of the toothpaste that the patient should use for mechanical hygiene therapy. It is also important to evaluate the three-dimensional position of every implant, as it is known that different angulations and apico-coronal depths require different strategies for plaque removal. In a situation where there is apical placement of the implant below the surrounding crest of bone, the implant will have increased probing depths, and thus the patients will not be efficient in their plaque removal procedures. Those implants many times have a chronic state of inflammation, and strict monitoring and short professional hygiene intervals are indicated.

Self-Study Questions

(Answers located at the end of the case)

A. Should implants be cleaned similarly as natural teeth?

B. Is there a contraindication to using toothpaste when cleaning implants?

C. What brushing technique(s) should be used?

D. What is the optimum stiffness of the bristles of a toothbrush and why?

E. Is there a special design of a toothbrush for implants?

F. Should a power brush be used and does it have any advantage over manual brushing? If so, is there a power brush that is best for implants?

G. Does the width of masticatory mucosa around an implant affect the brushing technique?

H. What interproximal oral hygiene aids are available to remove the biofilm from implants?

I. What other aids can be used in addition to a toothbrush or interproximal aids?

J. How should the patient clean a single implant restoration, a multiunit splinted implant restoration, or a hybrid appliance?

References

1. Armitage GC. Development of a classification system for periodontal diseases and conditions. Ann Periodontol 1999;4:1–6.
2. Berglundh T, Lindhe J, Marinello C, et al. Soft tissue reaction to de novo plaque formation on implants and teeth. An experimental study in the dog. Clin Oral Implants Res 1992;3:1–8.
3. Lang NP, Bragger U, Walther D, et al. Ligature-induced peri-implant infection in cynomolgus monkeys. I. Clinical and radiographic findings. Clin Oral Implants Res 1993;4:2–11.
4. Mombelli A. Etiology, diagnosis, and treatment considerations in peri-implantitis. Curr Opin Periodontol 1997;4:127–136.
5. Pinto TM, de Freitas GC, Dutra DA, et al. Frequency of mechanical removal of plaque as it relates to gingival inflammation: a randomized clinical trial. J Clin Periodontol 2013;40:948–954.
6. Axelsson P, Kocher T, Vivien N. Adverse effects of toothpastes on teeth, gingiva and bucal mucosa. In: Proceedings of the 2nd European Workshop on Periodontology. Chemicals in Periodontics. Quintessence; 1997, pp 259–261.

7. Meyers IA, McQueen MJ, Harbrow D, Seymour GJ. The surface effect of dentifrices. Aust Dent J 2000;45:118–124.
8. Van der Weijden F, Echeverría JJ, Sanz M, Lindhe J. Mechanical supragingival plaque control. In: Lindhe J, Lang NP, Karring T (eds), Clinical Periodontology and Implant Dentistry, 5th edn. Wiley-Blackwell; 2008, p 705.
9. Leonard HJ. Conservative treatment of periodontoclasia. J Am Dent Assoc 1939;26:1308–1318.
10. Fones AC (ed.). Mouth Hygiene, 4th edn. Philadelphia, PA: Lea & Febiger; 1934.
11. Bass CC. The optimum characteristics of toothbrushes for personal oral hygiene. Dent Items Interest 1948;70:697–718.
12. Stillman PR. A philosophy of treatment of periodontal disease. Dent Dig 1932;38:315–332.
13. Cagna DR, Massad JJ, Daher T. Use of a powered toothbrush for hygiene of edentulous implant-supported prostheses. Compend Contin Educ Dent 2011;32:84–88.
14. Truhlar RS, Morris HF, Ochi S. The efficacy of a counter-rotational powered toothbrush in the maintenance of endosseous dental implants. J Am Dent Assoc 2000;131:101–107.

15. Vandekerckhove B, Quirynen M, Warren PR, et al. The safety and efficacy of a powered toothbrush on soft tissues in patients with implant-supported fixed prostheses. Clin Oral Investig 2004;8:206–210.

16. Newman MG, Takei H, Klokkevold PR, Carranza FA. Plaque control for the periodontal patient. In: Perry AD (ed.), Clinical Periodontology, 10th edn. Elsevier; p 728.

17. Grender J, Williams K, Walters P, et al. Plaque removal efficacy of oscillating-rotating power toothbrushes: review of six comparative clinical trials. Am J Dent 2013;26:68–74.

18. Costa MR, Marcantonio RA, Cirelli JA. Comparison of manual versus sonic and ultrasonic toothbrushes: a review. Int J Dent Hyg 2007;5:75–81.

19. Wilson S, Levine D, Dequincey G, Killoy WJ. Effects of two toothbrushes on plaque, gingivitis, gingival abrasion, and recession: a 1-year longitudinal study. Compend Suppl 1993;(16):S569–S579; quiz S612–S614.

20. Rasperini G, Pellegrini G, Cortella A, et al. The safety and acceptability of an electric toothbrush on peri-implant mucosa in patients with oral implants in aesthetic areas: a prospective cohort study. Eur J Oral Implantol 2008;1:221–228.

21. Wolff L, Kim A, Nunn M, et al. Effectiveness of a sonic toothbrush in maintenance of dental implants. A prospective study. J Clin Periodontol 1998;25:821–828.

22. Esposito M, Worthington HV, Thomsen P, Coulthard P. Interventions for replacing missing teeth: maintaining health around dental implants. Cochrane Database Syst Rev 2004;(3):CD003069.

23. Gobbato L, Avila-Ortiz G, Sohrabi K, et al. The effect of keratinized mucosa width on peri-implant health: a systematic review. Int J Oral Maxillofac Implants 2013;28:1536–1545.

24. O'Leary TJ. Plaque control. In: ShanleyD (ed.), Efficacy of Treatment Procedures in Periodontology, vol 38. Chicago: Quintessence; 1980, pp 41–52.

25. ADA. Accepted dental therapeutics. Council of Dental Therapeutics 1994;40:222.

26. Christou V, Timmerman MF, Van der Velden U, Van der Weijden FA. Comparison of different approaches of interdental oral hygiene: interdental brushes versus dental floss. J Periodontol 1998;69:759–764.

27. Bergenholtz A, Olsson A. Efficacy of plaque-removal using interdental brushes and waxed dental floss. Scand J Dent Res 1984;92:198–203.

28. Waerhaug J. The interdental brush and its place in operative and crown and bridge dentistry. J Oral Rehabil 1976;3:107–113.

29. Barton J, Abelson D. The clinical efficacy of wooden interdental cleaners in gingivitis reduction. Clin Prev Dent 1987;9:17–20.

30. John CA. The dental water jet: a historical review of the literature. J Dent Hyg 2010;84:114–120.

31. Barnes CM, Russell CM, Reinhardt RA, et al. Comparison of irrigation to floss as an adjunct to tooth brushing: effect on bleeding, gingivitis, and supragingival plaque. J Clin Dent 2005;16:71–77.

32. Gorur A, Lyle DM, Schaudinn C, Costerton JW. Biofilm removal with a dental water jet. Compend Contin Educ Dent 2009;30(Spec No 1):1–6.

33. Goyal CR, Lyle DM, Qaqish JG, Schuller R. Evaluation of the plaque removal efficacy of a water flosser compared to string floss in adults after a single use. J Clin Dent 2013;24:37–42.

34. De Araujo Nobre M, Cintra N, Malo P. Peri-implant maintenance of immediate function implants: a pilot study comparing hyaluronic acid and chlorhexidine. Int J Dent Hyg 2007;5:87–94.

35. Felo A, Shibly O, Ciancio SG, et al. Effects of subgingival chlorhexidine irrigation on peri-implant maintenance. Am J Dent 1997;10:107–110.

36. Simon H, Yanase RT. Terminology for implant prostheses. Int J Oral Maxillofac Implants 2003;18:539–543.

Answers to Self-Study Questions

A. Plaque accumulation and indices of inflammation on dental implants occur in a similar pattern to natural teeth [2–4]. Studies demonstrated that an effective and accurate oral hygiene technique prevents an increase in the severity of gingival inflammation if performed at least once every 24 h [5]. Nonetheless, it appears that often patients have not been taught accurate plaque removal techniques, and some have difficulties with manual dexterity. It is usually recommended that a patient with implants performs oral hygiene based on their individual needs two times a day. Performing oral hygiene using incorrect techniques does not improve the results even if it is repeated two or more times a day. There are mainly three aspects in a patient's plaque control that need to be evaluated. First, patients have to be motivated to perform regular oral hygiene procedures. Second, they have to concentrate on their techniques in order to be thorough. This means they need to have a logical and repeatable sequence each time they are doing their plaque removal that will effectively clean all tooth surfaces exposed to oral fluids. Third, they need to acquire dexterity and knowledge in order to reach this goal. The latter aspect needs to be taught by a knowledgeable clinician. Evidence suggests that plaque control is as critically important for the maintenance of dental implants as it is for natural dentition. Devices that are effective in removing plaque from a crown on a natural tooth will also be effective in removing plaque on an implant crown. However, there are differences found in the morphologies of implant crowns and their relation to proximal crowns or natural teeth and to the surrounding soft tissues when compared with a natural tooth. Although plaque control techniques for dental implant-supported restorations are generally similar to traditional oral hygiene procedures on natural teeth, modifications are advised dependent on the prosthetic design (discussed in more detail in answer to self-study question J).

B. Different studies analyzed toothpaste usage during personal oral hygiene and its effect on plaque control [6,7]. There are many different brands and formulations of dentifrices. The agents contained in these pastes are multiple and they offer different functions (i.e., detergents, abrasives, polishing agents, binders, humectants, water, flavoring, coloring agents, active ingredients such as fluoride, antiplaque, anticalculus, desensitizing). The number and variation of chemical agents evaluated are quite large, and most have antiseptic or antimicrobial activity. It has been noted that the abrasives in the dentifrice mainly cause hard tissue damage when a scrub brushing technique is practiced. However, there has been no evidence

suggesting contraindication of toothpaste for patients with dental implant prosthesis.

C. Various studies demonstrated that different brushing techniques are almost similar in plaque removal efficacy [8]. Furthermore, all those methods were found to be inefficient in removing the plaque from interproximal areas. To be completely effective, these techniques must be customized according to the patient's needs. There are several techniques reported in the literature. In the vertical brushing technique [9], the movement is applied in vertical direction using up and down strokes. The circular brushing introduced by Fones in 1934 [10] is a combination of fast circular motions from the maxillary gingiva to the mandibular gingiva using light pressure. The sulcular brushing technique [11] (Bass technique 1948) can be the most efficacious when performing plaque control around implants. Generally speaking, implants have deeper crevices than natural teeth, and thus a sulcular technique of brushing should be more effective in cleaning an implant below the mucosa than a scrub or sweep technique. The Bass method emphasizes plaque removal of the area directly under the gingival margin by inclining the brush towards the apex of the tooth/implant. The bristles are directed into the sulcus at approximately 45° with respect to the long axis of the tooth (Figure 4). The brush is moved in a horizontal fashion with short strokes always maintaining the bristles stationary inside the sulcus against the tooth. For this reason, the Bass technique is considered an effective technique for plaque removal subgingivally in addition to

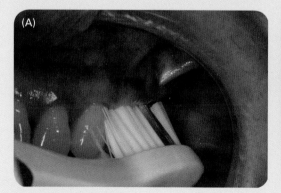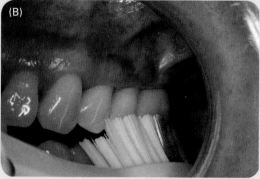

Figure 4: (A, B) Images showing the inclination of 45° angle used in the Bass brushing technique. The bristles are positioned in the area corresponding to the gingival sulcus.

the gingival margin. Some other techniques are considered "vibratory methods." One of these is the Stillman method [12] that was applied for massaging and stimulating the gingiva. The "roll or sweep technique" is based on rolling movements of the brush over the gingiva and tooth in an occlusal/incisal direction. Finally the modified Bass technique adds to the classic methods a rolling stroke.

In most cases with implants, adapting the toothbrush bristle tips to the junction of the tooth/implant crown and gingival margin and concentrating on working the bristle tips on the implant crown beneath the soft tissue margin is helpful in achieving biofilm removal. Some studies have suggested that powered toothbrushes might be more effective in removing bacterial biofilm than the manual brushes; however, the most important factor is the technique used, not whether the brush is powered with a battery or by hand [13–15]. An improper toothbrushing technique, such as scrubbing, may cause injury of the mucosal tissue, especially in patients with alveolar mucosa surrounding the implant rather than keratinized masticatory mucosa.

D. Toothbrushes were originally made of natural bristles using animal hair, and although at that time they were relatively effective they had some disadvantages. Animal hair toothbrushes lacked sufficient hygienic level, as bacteria colonizes on their surfaces, and they dry more slowly than the synthetic materials such as nylon used commonly today. Contemporary toothbrushes typically consist of either Nylon or a Nylon–polyester blend bristle. Nylon-bristled brushes exist in a variety of shapes, sizes, textures, and densities. Some companies claim that natural bristle can provide the patient with more degrees of softness, since animal hair can have a stiffness ranging from extra soft to hard (Fuchs®); artificial surfaces like Nylon allow less bacterial accumulation. Natural bristles fray, deteriorate, soften, and lose their elasticity quickly [16]. Nylon bristles dry significantly faster and are also more resistant to breakdown than natural bristle brushes.

The stiffness of a toothbrush relates to the diameter of the bristles and the length and the number of bristles in a tuft. A stiff bristle might be shorter in length or wider in diameter than a soft bristle. The stiffer the bristle the less the patient is able to access the surface of the crown beneath the mucosal crevice. A soft bristle is more flexible than a stiff bristle and is usually of a smaller diameter; thus, it is more likely to access the mucosal sulcus and do less damage to the soft tissue than a hard bristle will. If a stiff bristle brush were to be forced into the gingival crevice, it could lead to recession and/or create peri-implant dehiscence. Additionally, as alveolar mucosa has no keratinized surface, it is more sensitive to a toothbrush bristle, and thus a patient might not clean the cervical area thoroughly, therefore leaving plaque on the implant in the mucosal crevice. In 1948 Bass [11] advocated the use of soft, Nylon bristle brushes with an intrasulcular technique, stating that the plaque (biofilm) does not require abrasion to be dislodged from a tooth.

Most of the studies on toothbrush bristles take into consideration only the tooth structure damage; there are no studies with regard to implant crown surfaces. However, it is generally recommended to prescribe soft bristle toothbrushes to avoid traumatizing of the gingival tissue around teeth and implants and to better access the mucosal sulcus.

E. Some brands have proposed an exclusive design. For instance, the brand TePe® manufactured Implant Care™ (Figure 5), a special implant brush with a unique design for easy access. The neck has an angle that provides easier access to the implant surfaces where it is difficult to reach with the normal brush. The shape of the brush head is slim and facilitates cleaning even in very narrow areas. Another product from the same manufacturer is called TePe Compact Tuft™, which is characterized by soft, end-rounded filaments that can remove plaque around attachments for overdentures. To date, there is no comparative research showing that an implant brush is more effective than a regular hand toothbrush.

F. Studies seem to agree on the efficacy of power brushes for implant maintenance. A review paper [17] demonstrated that power brushes were more efficient in plaque reduction compared with regular manual brushes. The extent of the reduction was

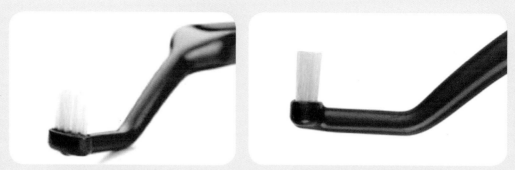

Figure 5: TePe manufactured Implant Care. This special implant brush has an angle that provides easier access to the implant surfaces where it is difficult to reach with the normal brush. The shape of the brush facilitates cleaning even in very narrow areas.

superior for the oscillating–rotating compared with either the sonic power or manual brush control in interproximal regions. When sonic brushes were tested in dental implant patients there was a more significant decrease in gingival and plaque indices [18]. The most important factor with the power brush is the application of a correct technique, so the bristles are activated and thus the handle of the brush does not require motion. The bristles should be placed against the implant prosthesis and guided into the mucosal sulcus. The action of the bristles of the power brush should be adequate to remove the biofilm. When manual and electric toothbrushes were compared in terms of their damaging potential, it seems that the latter tend to be less deleterious on soft tissues [19]. It is also important to consider that most studies involved a population of motivated participants (dental students) that clearly do not represent the general population. The effectiveness of both oscillating–rotating electric toothbrushes and sonic toothbrushes has been studied on patients with implants. Studies [15,20] reported a reduction in bleeding (up to 50% at 12 months) and probing depth (0.3 mm) and no adverse events. Although there was no control group in the study, the positive outcomes were patient acceptance and clinical changes even if only statistically and not clinically significant. Another study showed a sonic brush was better than a manual brush for plaque and bleeding reductions over time, but there was no difference in gingivitis scores after 6 months [21].

A systematic review reported no statistically significant difference between powered and sonic toothbrushes when compared with a manual technique [22].

G. There is still a controversy as to the width of masticatory mucosa necessary to facilitate maintenance of natural dentition and peri-implant health [23]. Some studies reported an association between reduced keratinized tissue and peri-implant inflammation. This might be due to the sensitivity of mucosal tissue, which might prevent the patient from removing plaque from the prosthesis at and/or beneath the mucosal sulcus, thus allowing for inflammation. Intrasulcular brushing techniques such as the Bass method have been associated with gingival recession [24] due to the action and pressure of the bristle tips against the margin of the sulcular soft tissue. An intrasulcular method of brushing would not be recommended in individuals with a narrow width of peri-implant masticatory mucosa, as it could contribute to recession of the soft tissue. (Also, reviewed in answer to self-study question K in Chapter 10 Case 3.)

H. The oral hygiene aids for proper plaque removal around implant-supported restorations are the same as those commonly used for natural teeth. Dental floss, interdental brushes, and rubber tips can be used safely around dental implants, and just as with the natural dentition, it should be customized on an individual basis. The patient's manual dexterity, the design of the prosthesis, and the type of prosthetic component must be taken into consideration when customizing interproximal hygiene techniques.

- *Dental floss.* The American Dental Association (ADA) reports that up to 80% of plaque biofilm may be removed by only flossing [25]. It has been demonstrated that a toothbrush is not successful in removing interproximal plaque effectively [26]. It is generally recommended to use floss around implant restorations for each individual unit, once or twice daily, doing plaque control techniques the same as for natural teeth. The number of times per day to use floss depends upon the patient's susceptibility to peri-implant inflammation (Figure 6).

- *Mechanical power flosser.* Studies reported minimal significant difference observed in plaque index of study subjects after 30 days of trial comparing a mechanical flosser and a manual flossing technique. Although there was no apparent clinical impact on gingival health, some patients seemed to markedly approve the use of the automatic flosser, which probably led to better compliance. For this reason an automatic device can be recommended.

- *Pre-threaded floss picks.* Although not as effective as regular floss due to the lack of proper adaptation to the tooth/implant surface, they are commonly used by people that cannot reach the posterior sextant of the mouth with regular floss mainly because of inadequate manual dexterity or desire to learn the proper technique. Regardless, the handle of the floss pick allows the patient to floss using only one hand and the arms of the picks can maintain the floss in tension without damaging the peri-implant soft tissues.

- *Superfloss.* It is known that the use of regular dental floss can be extremely difficult when attempting to remove plaque deposits in implant-supported fixed partial dentures. The great advantage of Superfloss is its stiff end that can be introduced between the abutment and the pontic area of the fixed prosthesis, which is not possible with the limp nature of regular floss. Another advantage of the Superfloss is the spongy portion that may facilitate the elimination of biofilm from the undersurface of a pontic area and also interproximally due to the increased surface area of the prosthesis, which is covered by the floss (Figure 7). Note that the "spongy" part of the Superfloss when wrapped tightly in a "C" around an implant loses its sponginess and becomes much thinner than when not stretched tightly against the implant or natural tooth.

  Reach DentoTAPE® (Johnson & Johnson) a waxed ribbon floss, is wider than regular floss and can accomplish plaque removal similarly as Superfloss.

- *Interproximal brush.* Also known as an interdental or proxy brush, was introduced in the 1960s as an alternative to wood picks. They are used as an effective device in plaque removal in the interproximal tooth surfaces [27]. These brushes consist of Nylon filaments attached to a stainless

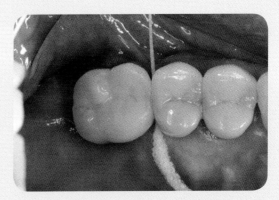

Figure 7: Image of Superfloss inserted under the implant-supported crown. Its stiff end can be introduced between the abutment and the pontic area of the fixed prosthesis, which is not possible with the limp nature of regular floss. The spongy portion facilitates the elimination of biofilm from the undersurface of a pontic area and also interproximally.

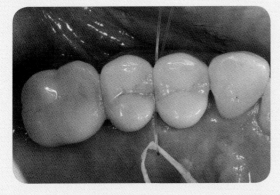

Figure 6: Regular dental floss used in conjunction with a floss threader in order to facilitate its insertion under the crowns.

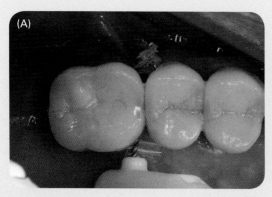
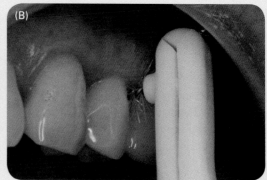

Figure 8: (A) Interproximal brush showed from an occlusal view. (B) Buccal view of interproximal brush inserted under the contact point of an implant-supported crown.

steel wire. This part can cause root sensitivity if not used properly (Figure 8). If the interproximal space is limited, the facial–lingual motion can create abrasions due to contact between the metal wire and root surface. Some brands have the metal wire coated with plastic to help reduce the abrasion. It is important to select the brush head of an appropriate size to fit into the interproximal area without creating damage to the soft tissue and to the root surface. In order to minimize the risk of hard tissue abrasion it is also advised to avoid the use of dentifrice with an interproximal brush and be replaced whenever the filaments appear to be deformed. Some studies demonstrated the individuals that routinely used an interproximal brush were able to maintain an adequate supragingival interproximal plaque control [28].

- *Rubber tip.* Another aid that can be utilized for plaque control around implants is a rubber tip; this device compresses the soft tissue against

the implant or its prosthesis to help dislodge interproximal plaque when there is no access for dental floss (Figure 9).

Another interproximal device available is Stim-U-Dent® (The Natural Dentist). This balsawood toothpick is triangular in section and it is designed for interproximal areas. The ADA Council on Scientific Affairs' acceptance of Stim-U-Dent plaque removers is based on "its finding that the product is effective for removing plaque between teeth and helping to prevent and reduce gingivitis, when used as directed" [25]. Studies demonstrated the efficacy of a toothpick as a supplement to brushing in reducing gingival inflammation [29].

I.
- *Water irrigation.* A water irrigator, also known by dental water jet or Waterpik®, is an oral hygiene

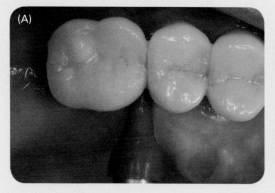
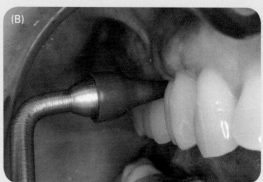

Figure 9: (A) Occlusal and (B) buccal views of rubber tip that is used to stimulate the interproximal papilla in between two crowns.

device that uses a stream of pulsating water to remove plaque and food debris between teeth and subgingivally. It has showed efficacy on patients under periodontal maintenance, and those with gingivitis, orthodontic appliances, crowns, and implants [30].

It has been demonstrated that the water irrigator is superior to dental floss in reducing bleeding and as effective in reducing plaque [31].

Another study found that a 3 s treatment of pulsating water at medium pressure removed almost 100% of plaque biofilm from treated sites [32].

The Waterpik water flosser was found to be more effective than string floss in interproximal plaque removal and had the added benefit of removing more plaque in areas such as the gingival margin and facial and lingual surfaces [33].

- *Mouthwash.* There is evidence that an antimicrobial mouthwash such as chlorhexidine can be a valid adjunct for maintaining peri-implant health [34].

In a cohort study [35], self-administration of subgingival irrigation with chlorhexidine compared with only rinsing with it in individuals with moderate signs of inflammation and shallow probing depths showed the group with subgingival irrigation demonstrated significant improvement in reducing signs of inflammation, in addition to less calculus and staining, compared with the rinsing group.

- *Toothpick.* The Perio-Aid® is a device that holds a toothpick at an angle and length which allows access to interproximal spaces. The Perio-Aid is used to remove plaque from the gingival margin interproximally. The Perio-Aid is available in two different versions (#2 and #3). The Perio-Aid #2 is double-ended with an adjustable nut on each end that fixes the toothpick in place. Each end gives the toothpick a different angle to access interproximal space. The Perio-Aid #3 does the same, but it has only one end.

J.

- *Single implant crown.* Despite anatomical differences on the supporting apparatus, a single dental implant crown needs to be considered like a single natural tooth in regard to plaque control. Healthy and successful implants should be enclosed in bone and covered by thick gingiva and not directly exposed to plaque biofilm and subject to oral environmental stresses. The tools and aids used for proper plaque removal for a single implant restoration are the same as that of natural teeth that were mentioned earlier. Nonetheless, the shape of an implant prosthesis differs from the natural tooth in most instances because the diameter of the implant head is significantly less than the diameter of a natural tooth by ~1–2 mm apical to the cemento-enamel junction. As a result of this, the emergence profile of the crown of a natural tooth emanating from the dental root is a gradual transition where the soft tissue dental papilla fills the interproximal space. In order to create this effect using an implant, the implant crown has to be made wide enough to allow the interproximal soft tissue to fill the space, and thus the transition from the implant head and the abutment is an abrupt widening creating a shelf-like contour, which makes this area more difficult to clean. One exception to this is the mandibular incisors, where the diameter of the implant might be equal to or greater than the incisor that it is replacing.

- *Splinted implant crowns.* Adequate removal of bacterial biofilm is even more of a challenge when implant restorations are splinted, as the patient must thread the floss through the interproximal space along with the bulky design of the suprastructure. Most of the time the interproximal spaces have limited access or the pontic design makes the access difficult when the design of the prosthesis results in a narrow embrasure for esthetics and to help prevent food entrapment. Flexible and soft instruments (i.e., Superfloss, interproximal toothbrushes) as well as irrigation devices are usually beneficial to get to these areas. The peri-implant mucosa and the pontic area should be free of plaque and food residues to avoid inflammation; the patient and the restorative dentist share this responsibility.

- *Hybrid appliances.* As with the splinted implants, hybrid dentures (or metal-resin implant fixed complete dentures) [36] represent a challenge to the patient's plaque removal ability. Therefore, proper design and adequate space to allow oral hygiene aids access to the abutments or the base of the denture are of crucial importance. Several tools ranging from regular toothbrushes to interdental toothbrushes and water pressure devices are useful. However, care has to be taken not to use any hard material that would damage the implant connections.

In summary, patients having implant restoration need to have regular maintenance appointments for professional hygiene therapy every 3 months. For patients with implant-supported hybrid dentures it is recommended to have the prosthetic portion removed in the office and cleaned properly at least once every 6 months, and we feel that every 3 months would provide a greater level of cleanliness than every 6 months.

Conclusion

The efficacy of toothbrushing, flossing, interproximal toothbrushes, Waterpik, rubber tips, and mouthwashes in maintaining health for the natural dentition is well established, and the same can be extrapolated to prevent inflammation of peri-implant mucosa.

The number of patients with dental implants is increasing exponentially as implant restorations are becoming standard of care to replace a missing tooth/teeth and prevent irreversible damage to healthy teeth or avoid removable prostheses. However, there is still no standard of care regarding their maintenance. The traditional methods of toothbrushing and flossing in control of inflammation is prudent; however, there are several differences between a natural tooth and an implant and their respective prosthetic restorations.

Every clinical case is different, as are patients' attitudes and capabilities in performing plaque control procedures. Many factors need to be taken into consideration in order to provide the patient with effective plaque control instructions (i.e., patient motivation and instruction, elimination of sources of risks, prosthetic evaluation and correction). In addition to handing a toothbrush to a patient and telling them to floss, adjunctive devices are often needed to complement their efforts in order to achieve an optimal plaque control. Thorough instruction by the clinician and consistent review in the use of all devices during maintenance visits, every 3–4 months, are essential.

It is recommended that the clinician modifies the patient's treatment and plaque control regimen on a case-by-case basis and customize the implant maintenance to the individual's needs. Plaque control around implants requires commitment, dexterity, and different techniques based on the position, angulation, type, and prosthetic component.

The message for the patient is that oral hygiene around implants is necessary since biofilm will form with the same processes that occur in a natural dentition, and although the implant will not decay, the bone holding it in will.

Case 3

Professional Plaque Control Around Implants

CASE STORY

A 37-year-old Caucasian man presented to the clinic with the chief complaint of "my dentist referred me here, because he said the gums around my implants were inflamed." Teeth #10, #19, #23, #26, #30, and #31 were lost 6 years ago, due to periodontitis. The missing teeth were replaced with dental implants restored with single porcelain-fused-to-metal crowns (Figure 1). The implants in the areas of teeth #23 and #26 were abutments for a four-unit fixed prosthesis (Figure 2). Following a comprehensive examination,

the implants in the areas of teeth #10, #19, #23, and #26 were diagnosed as having peri-implant mucositis (Figures 1, 2, 3, and 4). The patient stated his last professional debridement or prophylaxis was more than 18 months ago, and he reported brushing with a manual toothbrush twice a day and flossing once a day. It became apparent that the techniques the patient was using were inadequate to remove subgingival and submucosal plaque on the natural teeth and the implants.

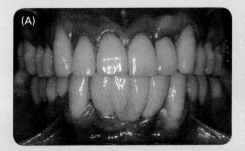 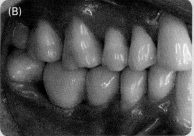 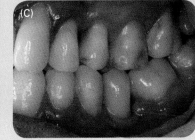

Figure 1: (A) Frontal and (B, C) lateral views.

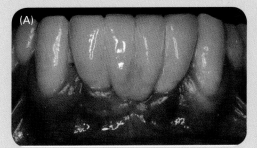 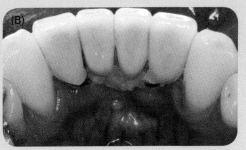

Figure 2: (A) Buccal and (B) lingual views of the mandibular anterior sextant.

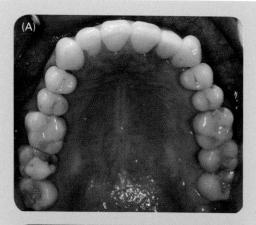

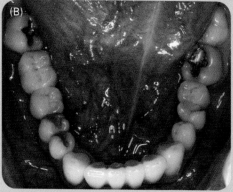

Figure 3: (A) Maxillary and (B) mandibular occlusal views.

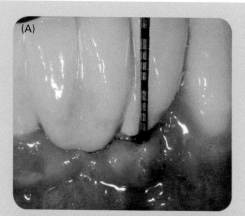

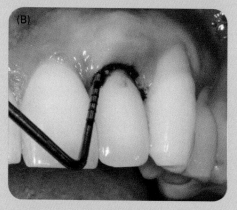

Figure 4: Probing depth of (A) implant #22 and (B) implant #10.

LEARNING GOALS AND OBJECTIVES

■ To be able to diagnose and treat peri-implant mucositis and monitor the health of the implants

■ To be able to know what instruments should be used to debride implants and the peri-implant tissues

■ To know what is the appropriate recall interval for each of our implant patients

Medical History

At the time of the initial visit the patient presented with a history of epilepsy. His most recent seizure was approximately 5–6 months ago. His condition is controlled with the anticonvulsant lamotrigine (Lamictal®) 200 mg/day. This medication does not cause any gingival overgrowth. He did not report any drug allergy.

Review of Systems

• Vital signs
  ○ Blood pressure: 122/67 mmHg
  ○ Pulse: 71 beats/min
  ○ Respiration: 15 breaths/min

Social History

The patient has never smoked and does not consume alcohol.

Extraoral Examination

No significant findings were noted. The patient exhibited no masses or swelling, and the temporomandibular joint was within normal limits, with no clicking, popping, or deviation of the mandible on opening. There was no facial asymmetry noted, and his lymph nodes felt normal on palpation.

Intraoral Examination

The oral cancer screening was negative. The soft tissue exam, including the tongue, cheeks, throat, and the floor of the mouth, were within normal limits.

The following information was collected as a part of the initial examination:

- full mouth periapical and bitewing series, and panoramic radiographs;
- study casts;
- intra- and extraoral photographs;
- periodontal charting (bleeding on probing, probing depths, clinical attachment loss, recession, mucogingival defects, mobility, suppuration, caries, and worn or defective restorations);
- occlusal and dental examination evaluating fremitus, centric relation prematurities and evaluation of working and nonworking side contacts, evaluation of occlusal wear, open interproximal contacts, and of caries.

The periodontal examination revealed the following probing depths (see Figure 5):

- 4–6 mm for #3, #5, #6, #11, #14, #15, #16, #17, #18, #19 (implant), #23 (implant), #26 (implant), #30 (implant), #31 (implant);
- 7–8 mm for #1, #2, #10 (implant), #32.

The gingiva surrounding the natural teeth and the peri-implant mucosa exhibited marginal erythema with moderate to severe bleeding on probing (see Figures 1, 2, 3, and 4).

There was generalized plaque and localized severe calculus accumulation in the lingual area of bridge #23–#26 (see Figure 2B).

There was caries on tooth #15 as well as defective restorations on teeth #2 and #15 (see Figures 3 and 6).

Occlusion

There were no occlusal discrepancies or interferences noted on clinical exam and on examination of the study casts. However, there was evidence of bruxism with generalized slight attrition.

Radiographic Examination

A full mouth series of periapical radiographs with bitewings was exposed (see Figure 6). The radiographic examination revealed a generalized horizontal bone loss pattern with an absence of crestal lamina dura. There was no radiographic evidence of bone loss beyond adaptive/physiologic remodeling around the dental implants.

The apico-coronal position of the implant in the area of tooth #10 with respect to the adjacent natural teeth #9 and #11 was due to preexisting horizontal bone loss prior to implant placement (Figures 4B, 6, and 7).

Diagnoses

Restorative

- Caries on tooth #15
- Defective restorations on teeth #2 and 15.

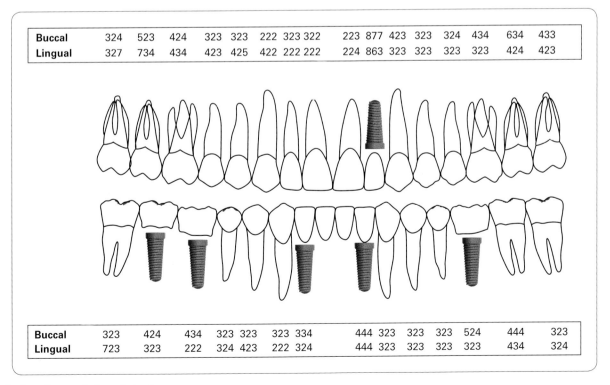

Buccal	324	523	424	323	323	222	323	322		223	877	423	323	324	434	634	433
Lingual	327	734	434	423	425	422	222	222		224	863	323	323	323	323	424	423

Buccal	323	424	434	323	323	323	334		444	323	323	323	524	444	323
Lingual	723	323	222	324	423	222	324		444	323	323	323	323	434	324

Figure 5: Baseline periodontal chart.

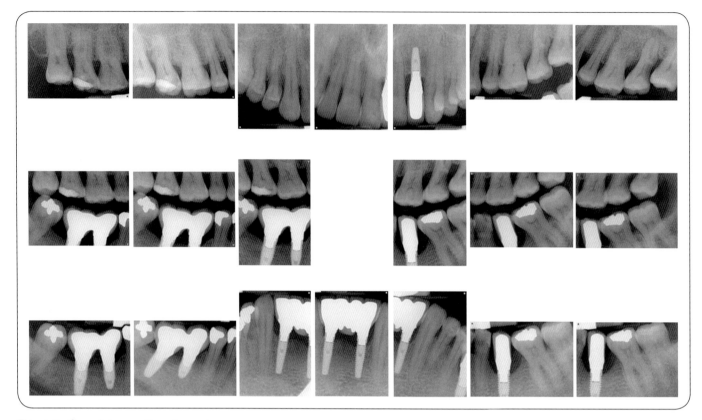

Figure 6: Complete mouth radiographs.

Periodontal

- According to Armitage [1]:
  - generalized moderate chronic periodontitis
  - developmental or acquired deformities and conditions around teeth
    - soft tissue recession
    - lack of attached gingiva associated with teeth #3, #6, #11, #12, #21, #22, and #27
    - primary and secondary occlusal trauma.
- According to Zitzmann and Berglundh [2]:
  - peri-implant mucositis associated with implants in the areas of teeth #10, #19, #23, and #26.

Treatment Plan

The treatment plan for this patient consisted of phase I or initial phase therapy (inflammatory control phase), which included:

- oral hygiene techniques instruction and patient motivation
- full mouth debridement
  - scaling, root planing, and polishing of the natural teeth

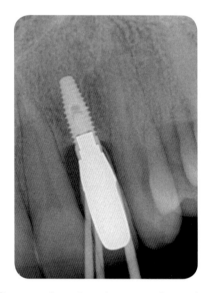

Figure 7: Gutta-percha points demonstrating no bone loss around the implant #10.

  - implant debridement
    - scaling with hand instruments and power scalers
    - air polishing
  - caries control
  - evaluation for endodontic therapy #15
  - reevaluation of initial phase (4–6 weeks).

Treatment

The importance of an adequate periodontal supportive therapy to ensure the best long-term prognosis of the patient's teeth and implants was discussed with him. Oral hygiene technique instruction was provided. With the help of a face mirror, the patient executed his normal brushing and flossing procedures for the clinician. After that, corrections were made to ensure an adequate brushing technique (modified Bass technique; see answer to self-study question C in Chapter 10, Case 2), as well as adequate flossing interdentally and under the fixed prosthesis using Superfloss®. Following his plaque removal technique instructions, the patient was asked to demonstrate those techniques to ensure he understood them. The review of his hygiene techniques was repeated frequently during the therapy, as there is a tendency for patients to continue with previous techniques, which were not effective.

The next step was to perform a complete mouth debridement in two sessions with scaling and root planing using local anesthesia for the natural teeth along with implant debridement. The right side of the mouth was treated in the first session. The left side of the mouth was treated the following week. Before this second session, oral hygiene techniques were observed to ensure that the patient was using the correct methods.

The instruments used to debride the implants were plastic and Teflon® scalers and curettes, plastic-protected ultrasonic tips, titanium curettes, and rubber cups with polishing paste (see Figures 8, 9, and 10). Regular hand and ultrasonic scalers were used to debride the crown portion of the implant-supported prosthesis.

Four weeks following therapy, new periodontal records were obtained, which included complete mouth periodontal charting. Oral hygiene techniques were again observed and modified where necessary. Thoroughness and consistency were emphasized to the patient.

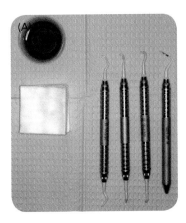
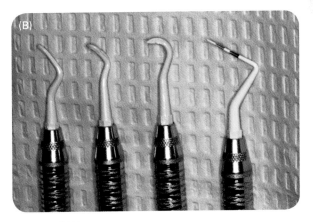

Figure 8: (A) Nonmetallic instruments used. (B) Magnified view of (A).

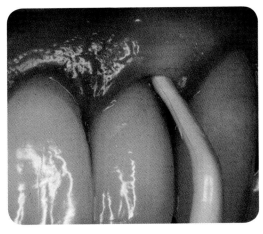
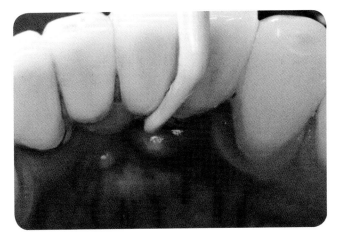

Figure 9: Plastic scalers used to debride peri-implant area.

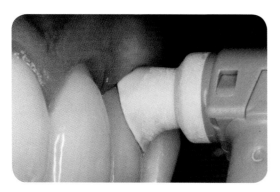

Figure 10: Polishing of implant #10 with rubber cup.

Discussion

With a diagnosis of peri-implant mucositis, therapy should be directed toward correcting or eliminating the etiologic factors producing the disease. Bacterial plaque (dental biofilm) is established as the primary etiologic factor for peri-implant mucositis [3]; thus, strong efforts should be focused toward its elimination.

Care must be taken when debriding the peri-implant area to use appropriate implant cleaning instruments in order not to scratch the implant or the restorative abutment's smooth surface. A rougher surface might lead to more plaque accumulation in the future. Thus, all efforts will be directed to debride with as little trauma as possible to the peri-implant tissues, to the implant abutment, and to the implant surface if it was exposed. For this, instruments equally as hard as or softer than titanium are recommended. However, the fabricated crown seated on the abutment is the same as a crown for a natural tooth and thus can be cleaned similarly.

In most of the cases of mucositis the implant surface itself will not be exposed to oral biofilm, as it is likely surrounded by bone, especially with bone-level implants; however, the restorative abutment or a polished collar might be exposed. It is therefore important to identify the areas that require debridement in order to determine what instruments should or should not be used to clean.

The apico-coronal implant position is a concept of concern, as we might find an implant placed subcrestally or in an area where there is excessive thickness of soft tissues (as in case of implant #10) (see Figures 4B, 6, and 7). In those situations, the implant will often have increased probing depths, and the patient will not be able to clean the area with daily plaque control efforts. Those implants usually exhibit a chronic state of inflammation or peri-implant mucositis, and those patients should be seen at least every 3 months for professional debridement. Those areas are considered as high-risk areas.

Self-Study Questions

(Answers located at the end of the case)

A. Should a clinician probe around implants? What type of probe should be used: metal or plastic?

B. How often should clinical periodontal records and radiographs be taken?

C. What is the goal of plaque control and supportive periodontal therapy (SPT) around implants?

D. What instruments should be used to debride implants?

E. Will peri-implant mucositis always resolve with adequate plaque control and SPT?

F. Should air polishing be used? If so, what is the most effective abrasive that should be used with it?

G. Should a rubber cup with polishing paste be used when cleaning an implant?

H. What is the efficacy of lasers, photodynamic therapy, and ozone (O_3) in treating peri-implant mucositis?

I. How should the clinician assess the results of therapy in the short term and long term?

J. What is the most appropriate interval between SPT appointments for implant patients?

K. Is masticatory mucosa around an implant important to assist in maintaining health?

References

1. Armitage GC. Development of a classification system for periodontal diseases and conditions. Ann Periodontol 1999;4(1):1–6.
2. Zitzmann NU, Berglundh T. Definition and prevalence of peri-implant diseases. J Clin Periodontol 2008;35(8 Suppl):286–291.
3. Lekholm U, Adell R, Lindhe J, et al. Marginal tissue reactions at osseointegrated titanium fixtures. (II) A cross-sectional retrospective study. Int J Oral Maxillofac Surg 1986;15(1):53–61.
4. Etter TH, Håkanson I, Lang NP, et al. Healing after standardized clinical probing of the perlimplant soft tissue seal: a histomorphometric study in dogs. Clin Oral Implants Res 2002;13(6):571–580.
5. Abrahamsson I, Soldini C. Probe penetration in periodontal and peri-implant tissues. An experimental study in the beagle dog. Clin Oral Implants Res 2006;17(6):601–605.
6. Schou S, Holmstrup P, Stoltze K, et al. Probing around implants and teeth with healthy or inflamed peri-implant mucosa/gingiva. A histologic comparison in cynomolgus monkeys (Macaca fascicularis). Clin Oral Implants Res 2002;13(2):113–126.
7. Fakhravar B, Khocht A, Jefferies SR, Suzuki JB. Probing and scaling instrumentation on implant abutment surfaces: an in vitro study. Implant Dent 2012;21(4):311–316.
8. Lindhe J, Lang NP, Karring T (eds). Clinical Periodontology and Implant Dentistry, 5th edn. Wiley Blackwell; 2008.
9. Humphrey S. Implant maintenance. Dent Clin North Am 2006;50(3):463–478, viii.
10. Lang NP, Wetzel AC, Stich H, Caffesse RG. Histologic probe penetration in healthy and inflamed peri-implant tissues. Clin Oral Implants Res 1994;5(4):191–201.
11. Albrektsson T, Zarb G, Worthington P, Eriksson AR. The long-term efficacy of currently used dental implants: a review and proposed criteria of success. Int J Oral Maxillofac Implants 1986;1(1):11–25.
12. Smith DE, Zarb GA. Criteria for success of osseointegrated endosseous implants. J Prosthet Dent 1989;62(5):567–572.
13. Buser D, Weber HP, Lang NP. Tissue integration of non-submerged implants. 1-year results of a prospective study with 100 ITI hollow-cylinder and hollow-screw implants. Clin Oral Implants Res 1990;1(1):33–40.
14. Papaspyridakos P, Chen CJ, Singh M, et al. Success criteria in implant dentistry: a systematic review. J Dent Res, 2012;91(3):242–248.
15. Misch CE, Perel ML, Wang HL, et al. Implant success, survival, and failure: the International Congress of Oral Implantologists (ICOI) Pisa Consensus Conference. Implant Dent 2008;17(1):5–15.
16. Lindhe J, Lang NP, Karring T. Clinical Periodontology and Implant Dentistry, 5th edn. Wiley Blackwell; 2003.
17. Cohen RE. Position paper: periodontal maintenance. J Periodontol 2003;74(9):1395–1401.
18. Newman MG, Takei HH, Klokkevold PR, Carranza FA. Carranza's Clinical Periodontology, 10th edn. Elsevier Health Sciences; 2006.
19. Louropoulou A, Slot DE, van der Weijden FA. Titanium surface alterations following the use of different mechanical instruments: a systematic review. Clin Oral Implants Res 2012;23(6):643–658.
20. McCollum J, O'Neal RB, Brennan WA, et al. The effect of titanium implant abutment surface irregularities on plaque accumulation in vivo. J Periodontol 1992;63(10):802–805.
21. Matarasso S, Quaremba G, Coraggio F, et al. Maintenance of implants: an in vitro study of titanium implant surface modifications subsequent to the application of different prophylaxis procedures. Clin Oral Implants Res 1996;7(1):64–72.
22. Grusovin MG, Coulthard P, Worthington HV, et al. Interventions for replacing missing teeth: maintaining and recovering soft tissue health around dental implants. Cochrane Database Syst Rev 2010;(8):CD003069.
23. Cochis A, Fini M, Carrassi A, et al. Effect of air polishing with glycine powder on titanium abutment surfaces. Clin Oral Implants Res 2013;24(8):904–909.
24. Marconcini S, Genovesi AM, Marchisio O, et al. In vivo study of titanium healing screws surface modifications after different debridment procedure. Minerva Stomatol 2016; in press.
25. Rapley JW, Swan RH, Hallmon WW, et al. The surface characteristics produced by various oral hygiene instruments and materials on titanium implant abutments. Int J Oral Maxillofac Implants 1990;5(1):47–52.
26. Todescan S, Lavigne S, Kelekis-Cholakis A. Guidance for the maintenance care of dental implants: clinical review. J Can Dent Assoc 2012;78:c107.
27. Renvert S, Roos-Jansaker AM, Claffey N. Non-surgical treatment of peri-implant mucositis and peri-implantitis: a literature review. J Clin Periodontol 2008;35(8 Suppl):305–315.
28. Bombeccari GP, Guzzi G, Gualini F, et al. Photodynamic therapy to treat periimplantitis. Implant Dent 2013;22(6):631–638.
29. Esposito M, Grusovin MG, De Angelis N, et al. The adjunctive use of light-activated disinfection (LAD) with FotoSan is ineffective in the treatment of peri-implantitis: 1-year results from a multicentre pragmatic randomised controlled trial. Eur J Oral Implantol 2013;6(2):109–119.
30. Renvert S, Polyzois I, Persson GR. Treatment modalities for peri-implant mucositis and peri-implantitis. Am J Dent 2013;26(6):313–318.
31. McKenna DF, Borzabadi-Farahani A, Lynch E. The effect of subgingival ozone and/or hydrogen peroxide on the development of peri-implant mucositis: a double-blind randomized controlled trial. Int J Oral Maxillofac Implants 2013;28(6):1483–1489.
32. Schwarz F, Bieling K, Bonsmann M, et al. Nonsurgical treatment of moderate and advanced periimplantitis lesions: a controlled clinical study. Clin Oral Investig 2006;10(4):279–288.
33. Peri-implant mucositis and peri-implantitis: a current understanding of their diagnoses and clinical implications. J Periodontol 2013;84(4):436–443.

34. Esposito M, Hirsch J, Lekholm U, Thomsen P. Differential diagnosis and treatment strategies for biologic complications and failing oral implants: a review of the literature. Int J Oral Maxillofac Implants 1999;14(4):473–490.

35. Hultin M, Komiyama A, Klinge B. Supportive therapy and the longevity of dental implants: a systematic review of the literature. Clin Oral Implants Res 2007;18(Suppl 3):50–62.

36. Adibrad M, Shahabuei M, Sahabi M. Significance of the width of keratinized mucosa on the health status of the supporting tissue around implants supporting overdentures. J Oral Implantol 2009;35(5):232–237.

37. Brito C, Tenenbaum HC, Wong BK, et al. Is keratinized mucosa indispensable to maintain peri-implant health? A systematic review of the literature. J Biomed Mater Res B Appl Biomater 2014;102(3):643–650.

38. Wennström JL, Derks J. Is there a need for keratinized mucosa around implants to maintain health and tissue stability? Clin Oral Implants Res 2012;23(Suppl 6):136–146.

39. Schrott AR, Jimenez M, Hwang JW, et al. Five-year evaluation of the influence of keratinized mucosa on peri-implant soft-tissue health and stability around implants supporting full-arch mandibular fixed prostheses. Clin Oral Implants Res 2009;20(10):1170–1177.

Answers to Self-Study Questions

A. Clinical probing is a reliable and important diagnostic parameter in the continuous monitoring of peri-implant tissues. When a light pressure (0.2 N) is applied during probing, the healing of the epithelial attachment seems to be complete at 5 days after clinical probing [4]. Probing around implants can be performed without causing permanent damage to the epithelial attachment.

Clinical probing and probe penetration at healthy implant sites is comparable to healthy natural tooth sites [5]. In cases where there is peri-implant mucositis or peri-implantitis, the probe tip will be closer to the bone when compared with gingivitis and/or periodontitis [6]. Peri-implant probing has to be interpreted according to implant positioning in the apico-coronal dimension, because this will influence the probing depth measurements. Therefore, it is crucial to establish a baseline probing depth at the time of prosthesis delivery that will allow a comparison with future probing depth measurements.

It has been suggested that metallic probes can alter or damage the implant surface. In most cases, the probe tip will not touch the implant surface, but at most only the abutment's surface. If that is the case, the surface alteration caused by the tip of a metallic probe against an abutment is minimal, and appears to be less than if probed with a plastic probe [7]. The clinician should not have any concern in probing with a conventional metallic probe; however, plastic probes are available and can be equally effective in measuring probing depth.

B. At each maintenance visit, a medical history update and the use of any new medications should be reviewed and changes recorded. An extraoral and intraoral examination, including oral cancer screening, should be performed for detection of any possible abnormalities. Next, an examination of the tooth or implant-related risk factors should be completed that includes: the patient's plaque levels and oral hygiene techniques and frequency, probing depths, clinical attachment levels, bleeding on probing or suppuration, mobility, presence of defective restorations or caries lesions, and the history of periodontitis [8].

The aforementioned examination is very important in assisting the patient to maintain peri-implant health, and the clinician should individualize how much information is needed for each patient based on the subject's oral hygiene, the local and systemic risk factors, and the frequency of maintenance visits [9].

Considering the supracrestal soft tissue healing will occur 5 days after clinical probing; implants can and should be probed at each maintenance visit [9,10], as mentioned previously in this chapter.

Radiographs are a useful method to monitor peri-implant bone level. Different annual marginal bone loss rates have been proposed by several researchers [11–15].

Baseline radiographs are very important at the time of implant placement and following crown–bridge installation. As most clinical changes occur during the first year of function, control radiographs should be taken at 6 and 12 months following prosthesis installation. In the absence of signs and symptoms of disease, radiographs should be obtained thereafter at intervals of 2–3 years, depending on the implant system used and the success rate obtained [16].

Radiographic interpretation should be done with caution, and should not be the only parameter to estimate implant success, as only mesial and distal bone levels are visible. Additionally, with the new implant designs and surfaces, minimal or no bone loss should be expected in a well-maintained patient population.

The consensus is that radiographs should be combined with a thorough clinical examination of the area in order to have adequate information and make the correct diagnosis.

C. Elevated plaque scores are correlated with increasing probing depth and peri-implant mucositis [3]. Therefore, the objective of plaque control and supportive periodontal therapy must be the continuous preservation of gingival and peri-implant health.

Regular and adequate supragingival plaque removal performed by the patient is the most important and challenging prerequisite to obtain a good long-term prognosis on the patients' teeth and implants. To achieve these results, not only is a thorough and frequent maintenance therapy needed, but continued reinforcement of the brushing and flossing techniques as well as patient motivation are also required.

D. Instrumentation around an implant-supported restoration is generally performed in a similar way as performed around teeth or teeth-supported restorations [17]. The main goal of instrumentation is to eliminate the bacterial biofilm. It is recommended [18] when debriding around dental implants to:
- utilize special instrumentation that will not scratch the implant or abutment when used for calculus removal;
- avoid acid fluoride prophylactic agents;
- apply nonabrasive prophy pastes.

Metal hand instruments and metal ultrasonic and sonic tips should be avoided owing to the risk of abrading the titanium surface [19]. Special instruments that would not scratch the implant or

abutment surface include Teflon, titanium, gold, or plastic tips.

Rubber cups with pumice, tin oxide, or special implant polishing pastes could be used with light and intermittent pressure on titanium surfaces [20].

Matarasso et al. [21] compared different prophylaxis procedures in vitro, including ultrasonic scalers, plastic-tip ultrasonic scalers, stainless steel curettes, titanium curettes, Teflon curettes, air-powered systems, abrasive rubber cups, polishing rubber cups, and a brush. They concluded that the instruments used could be divided in three groups in relation to surface alterations (see Table 1).

According to Cohen [17], there are no studies that have linked mechanical implant surface alterations to an increased incidence of mucositis or peri-implantitis.

In a systematic review, Grusovin et al. [22] found little evidence regarding the most effective interventions for maintaining and recovering health around peri-implant tissues long term.

E. In the great majority of the cases mucositis will resolve with adequate interproximal and toothbrushing habits, combined with professional maintenance debridement. Nevertheless, there are some specific cases where the implant will have a chronic inflammation that will not be resolved

Table 1: Surface Roughness Following Different Prophylaxis Methods

1. Methods that altered the implant neck surface producing increased roughness:
   - ultrasonic scalers
   - stainless steel curettes
   - titanium curettes
   - air jet polishing

2. Methods that left the implant neck surface unaltered:
   - rubber cup polishing
   - brush polishing
   - Teflon curette
   - plastic curette
   - plastic tip scaler

3. Methods resulting in a smoothening of the implant neck surface:
   - abrasive rubber cups

Modified from Matarasso et al. [21].

despite all the efforts of the patient and the clinician. These situations are often due to inadequate access to the peri-implant sulcus/pocket; for example, when implants are placed too apically or when the prosthetic components make the access impossible for any oral hygiene device. Those areas will be considered high-risk sites, and frequent maintenance visits should be recommended.

F. Presently, there is no implant polishing treatment able to completely clean the implant surface and at the same time preserve its properties [23].

When comparing air polishing with glycine powder or with sodium bicarbonate powder, it has been shown that the former material might be a better method to remove plaque from dental implants, because it is less abrasive. Moreover, the use of glycine powder seems to play an active role on the inhibition of bacterial recolonization of implants in the first 24 h after applications [23].

In comparison with laser and curettes, air polishing seems to be more efficient in debris removal [24]. However, there are conflicting reports in the literature, as some studies have shown that this method may alter the surface of the abutment, and powder deposits could be left on the surface [19,25]. More research is needed to determine the benefits of air polishing in the treatment of or the prevention of peri-implant mucositis as a part of professional hygiene therapy for implants.

G. Polishing with a fine paste does not appear to scratch the implant surface [26]. Moreover, Rapley et al. [25], in an in vitro study, demonstrated that using a rubber cup with flour of pumice on an implant abutment left the surface smoother compared with nontreated machined abutments.

As long as the preservation of the implant surface integrity is the primary goal, rubber cups and plastic curettes appear to be the instrument of choice [19].

A rubber cup with polishing paste might be recommended to decrease roughness of the implant/abutment surface if an aggressive debridement method has been performed previously. To our knowledge, Hawe Implant Paste, Kerr® is the only specific polishing paste available in the market for implants.

H. Studies treating peri-implant mucositis with the aforementioned techniques are scarce or nonexistent. Most of the evidence in application of these therapies relates to treating peri-implantitis [27–30]. To the best of our knowledge, there are no definitive studies that look at treating peri-implant mucositis with laser or photodynamic therapy.

However there was one study by McKenna et al. [31] regarding the use of O_3 therapy. O_3 is a powerful antimicrobial and oxidizing agent. The study compared the use of air (O_2) versus O_3 in 80 implants, dividing them into four different therapy groups:
- O_2 + saline
- O_2 + H_2O_2
- O_3 + saline
- O_3 + H_2O_2

O_3 therapies showed greater improvement in terms of plaque, gingival, and bleeding indices at 21 days compared with the use of O_2 therapies.

Despite the current lack of data in the literature, it is clear that as long as we mechanically remove the primary etiologic factor, bacterial plaque, resolution of peri-implant mucositis will occur. Future new approaches have the potential of enhancing the outcomes. Nevertheless, the results in the literature are probably not clinically significant and need to be further investigated to get the most adequate and significant therapy for each patient.

I. The early detection of both peri-implant mucositis and peri-implantitis is essential, as the treatment of peri-implantitis is not predictable. Once peri-implantitis is established, the therapy could be complex, difficult to perform, and in most of the cases noneffective or less effective when only nonsurgical therapy is performed [32]. A baseline radiograph is recommended at the time of both implant placement and prosthesis installation to facilitate comparison. To assess the results of therapy, the clinician should use a combination of probing data over time, "bleeding on light probing," inflammatory status of the mucosa, radiographic changes in bone levels over time, and, if possible, bacterial and/or peri-implant crevicular fluid sample data to arrive at an accurate diagnosis of peri-implantitis [33]. The short-term assessment of a successful result after treating peri-implant mucositis would be the elimination of inflammation, which would be determined by the absence of bleeding on light probing and purulence and the appearance of clinical health. On a long-term basis, the criteria for success would be the same as for the short term, in addition to the absence of progressing bone loss.

J. Evidence suggests that plaque control is as important around dental implants as it is around teeth. Periodontal maintenance should be performed at intervals no greater than 4 months if the reason for the implant placement is due to past caries or periodontitis. The determination of a hygiene maintenance interval should be decided on two factors: the present health and plaque levels of the patient and the susceptibility that patient has towards dental disease.

Patients with a history of periodontitis or at high risk of bone loss should obtain periodontal maintenance at least four times a year [17]. There is a lack of consensus in order to suggest frequency of recall intervals or to propose specific implant hygiene treatments [34,35]. The clinician should individualize each patient and tailor the adequate maintenance interval.

K. The literature reports contradictory results regarding the necessity of keratinized mucosa around dental implants. It is important to establish a differentiation on what type of prostheses is applied to each specific case, as a single-unit crown or an implant-supported overdenture might not present the same risk.

Adibrad et al. [36] showed that the absence of keratinized mucosa around implants supporting overdentures was associated with higher plaque accumulation, bleeding on probing, mucosal recession and gingival inflammation.

A recent systematic review [37] concluded that an adequate zone of keratinized tissue (or masticatory mucosa) might be necessary, as it is shown to be related to better peri-implant tissue health. On the other hand, Wennström and Derks [38] mentioned in their review that there is limited evidence to support the need of keratinized tissue around implants to maintain health and tissue stability.

Based on the existing literature, it is desired as far as possible to have an adequate ($\geq$2 mm [39]) band of keratinized mucosa in order to prevent or minimize possible gingival inflammation, plaque accumulation, mucosal recession, and bleeding on probing.

Moreover, the clinician should individualize each patient and each implant and assess the necessity of having keratinized mucosa, and the necessity of making a soft tissue graft for that purpose.

Plaque control is crucial, and if the implant can be maintained healthy and free of plaque, the presence or absence of keratinized mucosa might not affect the implant long-term stability. Today, no studies have been done to show the effect of brushing trauma on implants without masticatory mucosa.

Conclusions

Dental implants are a common replacement for lost teeth. Meticulous plaque control is essential in long-term success of dental implants.

Both the patient and the clinician have the responsibility of eliminating the plaque biofilm, as it has been proven to be the source of the inflammatory cascade. Patients have to maintain impeccable oral hygiene technique for plaque control. The clinician's responsibilities are to provide a properly designed prosthesis that is cleansable by the patient, to observe the patient's techniques and coach them as needed, and to see the patient regularly for hygiene maintenance therapy depending on the patient's susceptibility to dental/implant disease, their dental/implant hygiene, and the accessibility of the prosthesis for cleaning. The patient needs to be motivated and correctly instructed to be able to perform adequate techniques to remove plaque and to achieve and maintain peri-implant health. This teamwork should be enhanced at each maintenance appointment, preferably at a 3–4 months interval.

Case 4

Locally Delivered Drug Agents

CASE STORY

A 62-year-old Caucasian woman was referred by her dental hygienist with a chief complaint of: "My front implant (#9) bleeds." The patient claimed to brush her teeth three times per day and to floss once per day. The implant in the area of tooth #9 was placed by a general dentist 21 years ago (Figures 1, 2, 3, and 4).

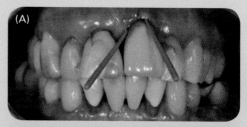

Figure 1: Pretreatment intraoral clinical picture.

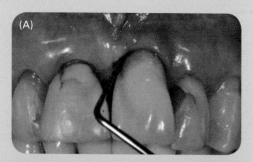

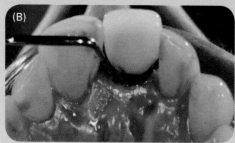

Figure 2: Clinical pictures demonstrating (A) bleeding on probing and 6 mm PD on the mesiobuccal and (B) 8 mm PD on the mesiopalatal of implant #9.

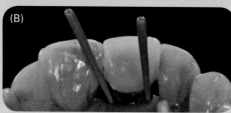

Figure 3: Clinical pictures demonstrating location of gutta percha points on (A) the mesiobuccal, distobuccal and (B) the mesiopalatal, distopalatal aspect of implant #9.

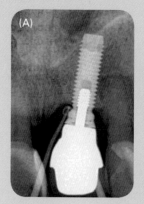
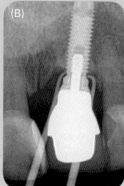

Figure 4: Radiographic pictures demonstrating the location of gutta percha points on (A) the mesiobuccal, distobuccal and (B) the mesiopalatal, distopalatal aspect of implant #9.

Medical History

The patient was diagnosed with osteopenia 3 years ago, and since then she had been taking Fosamax® (alendronate sodium) per oris 5–10 mg daily. She had no known allergies toward medications. There were no other systemic conditions.

Review of Symptoms

- Vital signs
  - ○ Blood pressure: 110/70 mmHg
  - ○ Pulse rate: 64 beats/min (regular)
  - ○ Respiration: 16 breaths/min

Social History

The patient stated that she quit smoking 10 years ago, that she drinks socially, and she denied alcoholism.

Extraoral Exam

No significant findings were noted. There were no areas of facial swelling or any facial asymmetry. The lymph nodes were non palpable. Skin, head, neck, temporomandibular joint and muscles were within normal limits.

Intraoral Examination

- An exam of the intraoral soft tissues, including the tongue and the floor of the mouth, was performed and was within normal limits. The oral cancer screening was negative.
- The patient's oral hygiene techniques were observed and found to be inadequate to thoroughly remove subgingival plaque.
- Teeth #1, #2, #3, #15, #16, #17, #18, #20, #24, #25, and #32 were missing.
- Implant-supported crowns were present in areas of teeth #4, #5, and #9.

- A four-unit fixed prosthesis was present from teeth #23 to #26.
- The periodontal charting revealed probing depth (PD) ranging from 1 to 3 mm (Figure 5).
- The implant in the area of tooth #9 presented with bleeding on probing and PD of 6, 4, and 4 mm buccally mesial to distal and 3, 9, and 8 mm palatally distal to mesial.

Occlusion

There was fremitus on tooth #8; however, there was no centric relation prematurity or slide. Tooth #8 had grade 1 mobility; there was no significant mobility on the other teeth. The patient denied any symptoms, and there were no signs associated with her temporomandibular joint such as crepitus, clicking, or pain.

Radiographic Examination

The complete periapical series of radiographs revealed generalized slight horizontal bone loss (Figure 6). Three implant-supported restorations were evident in the areas of teeth #4, #5, and #9.

Diagnosis

After careful review of the patient's medical and dental history, the clinical, and radiographic examinations, a periodontal diagnosis (according to Armitage classification 1999) was localized slight chronic periodontitis. Moreover, considering the bleeding on probing and the concomitant radiographic evidence of no bone loss, a diagnosis of peri-implant mucositis was made for the implant in the area of #9.

Treatment Plan

The treatment was as follows:
- delivery of oral hygiene instructions to the patient;
- periodontal prophylaxis with supra- and subgingival scaling and polishing of all teeth surfaces;
- nonsurgical debridement of implant #9 by means of curettes and air polishing, and administration of a locally delivered antibiotic (minocycline HCL 1 mg, Arestin®);
- 4–6 weeks reevaluation to assess the need for further therapy.

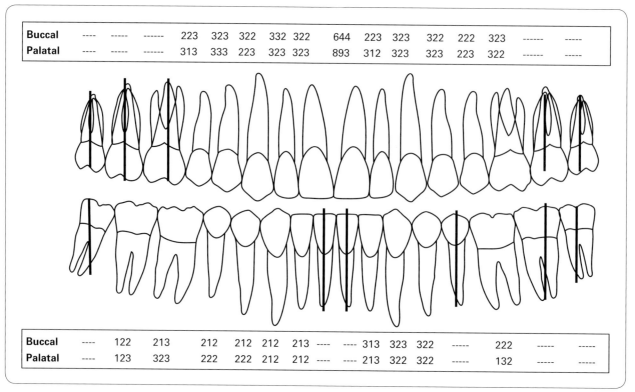

Buccal	----	-----	------	223	323	322	332	322	644	223	323	322	222	323	------	-----
Palatal	----	-----	------	313	333	223	323	323	893	312	323	323	223	322	------	-----

Buccal	----	122	213	212	212	212	213	----	----	313	323	322	-----	222	-----	-----
Palatal	----	123	323	222	222	212	212	----	----	213	322	322	-----	132	-----	-----

Figure 5: Periodontal chart.

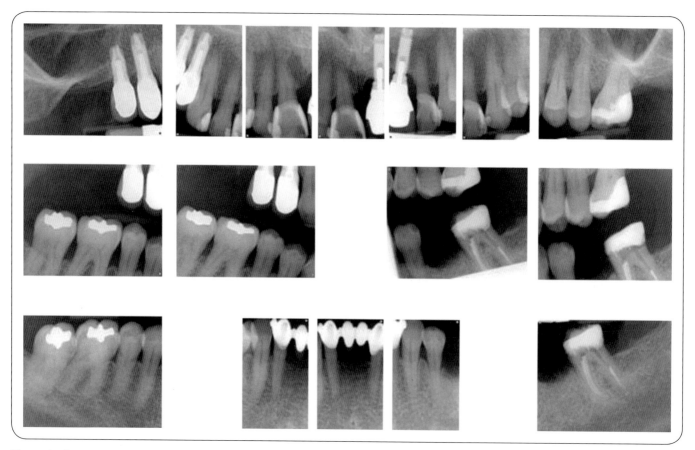

Figure 6: Complete series of periapical radiographs.

Discussion

The patient presented with bleeding upon probing around the implant in the area of tooth #9. As there was no evidence of bone loss, the diagnosis of peri-implant mucositis was made. A periodontal prophylaxis with supra- and subgingival scaling and polishing of all natural tooth surfaces was provided. Nonsurgical debridement of the implant #9 was completed using curettes and air polishing (Figure 7). The administration of a locally delivered antibiotic (minocycline HCL, Arestin) was placed on the mesial and on the palatal aspects (Figure 8). Two months following the therapy the patient presented for a follow-up visit and there was no bleeding upon probing associated with the implant in the area of #9 (Figure 9). The patient's brushing and flossing techniques are now excellent. The patient is presently on periodontal hygiene maintenance every 3 months. Research shows that regular hygiene visits to review the patient's plaque control techniques are fundamental for a good, long-term prognosis [1,2].

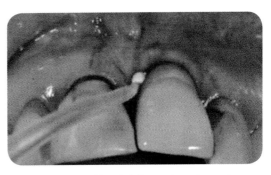

Figure 8: Application of local delivery Arestin on the mesiobuccal pocket on implant #9 immediately after nonsurgical debridement.

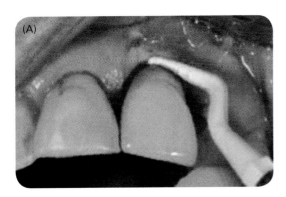

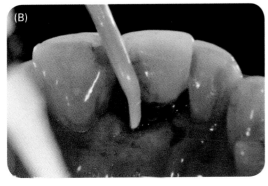

Figure 7: (A, B) Nonsurgical debridement of implant #9 using plastic curettes.

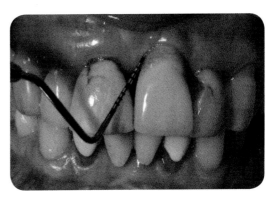

Figure 9: Two months follow-up after topical application of Arestin demonstrating no bleeding on probing.

Self-Study Questions

(Answers located at the end of the case)

A. What locally delivered drug agents (LDDAs) are vailable now?

B. Are there LDDAs that have been used in the past and are not available presently?

C. When should LDDAs be used around implants?

D. What are the methods of application of LDDAs?

E. Should LDDAs be used alone or only as an adjunctive treatment?

F. Are LDDAs indicated for use in pockets that do not exhibit bleeding?

G. When during therapy should LDDAs be administered: during or after phase I therapy?

H. Should LDDAs use be repeated? If so, at what interval, and is there a limit of their usage?

I. What are the instructions for the patient to observe after receiving LDDAs?

J. What time period after therapy of LDDAs should the outcome be assessed?

K. What are the advantages or benefits of using LDDAs?

L. What are the complications and contraindications to LDDAs?

References

1. Axelsson P, Nystrom B, Lindhe J. The long-term effect of a plaque control program on tooth mortality, caries and periodontal disease in adults. Results after 30 years of maintenance. J Clin Periodontol 2004;31(9):749–757.

2. Lindhe J, Axelsson P, Tollskog G. Effect of proper oral hygiene on gingivitis and dental caries in Swedish schoolchildren. Community Dent Oral Epidemiol 1975;3(4):150–155.

3. Schenk G, Flemmig TF, Betz T, et al. Controlled local delivery of tetracycline HCl in the treatment of periimplant mucosal hyperplasia and mucositis. A controlled case series. Clin Oral Implants Res 1997;8(5):427–433.

4. Mombelli A, Feloutzis A, Brägger U, Lang NP. Treatment of peri-implantitis by local delivery of tetracycline. Clinical, microbiological and radiological results. Clin Oral Implants Res 2001;12(4):287–294.

5. Lang NP, Berglundh T; Working Group 4 of Seventh European Workshop on Periodontology. Periimplant diseases: where are we now? – Consensus of the Seventh European Workshop on Periodontology. J Clin Periodontol 2011;38(Suppl 11):178–181.

6. Lindhe J, Meyle J; Group D of European Workshop on Periodontology. Peri-implant diseases: Consensus Report of the Sixth European Workshop on Periodontology. J Clin Periodontol. 2008;35(8 Suppl):282–285.

7. Javed F, Alghamdi AS, Ahmed A, et al. Clinical efficacy of antibiotics in the treatment of peri-implantitis. Int Dent J 2013;63(4):169–176.

8. Van Winkelhoff AJ. Antibiotics in the treatment of peri-implantitis. Eur J Oral Implantol 2012;(5 Suppl):S43–S50.

9. Heitz-Mayfield LJ, Salvi GE, Botticelli D, et al. Anti-infective treatment of peri-implant mucositis: a randomised controlled clinical trial. Clin Oral Implants Res 2011;22(3):237–241.

10. Renvert S, Lessem J, Dahlén G, et al. Topical minocycline microspheres versus topical chlorhexidine gel as an adjunct to mechanical debridement of incipient peri-implant infections: a randomized clinical trial. J Clin Periodontol 2006;33(5):362–369.

11. Roccuzzo M, Bonino F, Bonino L, Dalmasso P. Surgical therapy of peri-implantitis lesions by means of a bovine-derived xenograft: comparative results of a prospective study on two different implant surfaces. J Clin Periodontol 2011;38(8):738–745.

12. Bassetti M, Schär D, Wicki B, et al. Anti-infective therapy of peri-implantitis with adjunctive local drug delivery or photodynamic therapy: 12-month outcomes of a randomized controlled clinical trial. Clin Oral Implants Res 2014;25(3):279–287.

13. Renvert S, Lessem J, Dahlén G, et al. Mechanical and repeated antimicrobial therapy using a local drug delivery system in the treatment of peri-implantitis: a randomized clinical trial. J Periodontol 2008;79(5):836–844.

14. Wu PA, Anadkat MJ. Fever, eosinophilia, and death: a case of minocycline hypersensitivity. Cutis 2014;93(2):107–110.

15. Kanno K, Sakai H, Yamada Y, Iizuka H. Drug-induced hypersensitivity syndrome due to minocycline complicated by severe myocarditis. J Dermatol 2014;41(2):160–162.

Answers to Self-Study Questions

A. Arestin (minocycline HCL) microsphere 1 mg (Figure 12), Elyzol® (metronidazole 25%), and Atridox® (doxycycline hyclate 10%) are the locally delivered antibiotics indicated for treatment of periodontitis. The use of minocycline and doxycycline for peri-implant disease is considered by the US Food and Drug Administration (FDA) "off-label"; however, they can be safely used for implants, considering that Gram-negative anaerobic bacteria have been found in sites with peri-implant disease. Minocycline and doxycycline are broad-spectrum tetracycline, and therefore effective against both Gram-positive and Gram-negative bacteria; however, the concentration of the local drug is usually higher than those used systemically. Metronidazole is a nitroimidazole and targets anaerobic bacteria; Elyzol is not an FDA approved drug; therefore, its use is not considered safe and effective and is not marketed in the USA. Chlorhexidine, although not an antibiotic, is also indicated for the treatment of peri-implant mucositis. It is a bisbiguanide antiseptic/antimicrobial agent that is active against broad-spectrum microorganisms. In the USA it is available as a 0.12% solution or as biodegradable chips, which contain 2.5 mg of chlorhexidine and are marketed as Periochip®. In Europe it is also marketed as a 1% gel.

B. Actisite® periodontal fiber previously was marketed as an extended-release local antibiotic for treatment of periodontal sites; however, it is no longer available in the USA. It consisted of a monofilament of ethylene/vinyl acetate copolymer containing 25% tetracycline hydrochloride. The fiber was packed in the periodontal pocket, secured with adhesive, and left in place for 7–12 days, for continuous delivery of tetracycline. Actisite periodontal fiber in conjunction with supra- and subgingival scaling was found to decrease bleeding around implants with peri-implant mucositis in the short term [3]. In addition, there is some evidence suggesting that it can decrease the PD around implants with peri-implantitis [4]. The material is being modified and may in the future be marketed again (personal communication, Dr. Stephen Halem, Boston, MA).

C. Patients with implants that are diagnosed with peri-implant disease might be good candidates for LDDA therapy. Peri-implant disease is caused by a bacterial biofilm attached to the implant crown or abutment, and therefore the combination of mechanical debridement and locally delivered antibiotic or antimicrobial agents is indicated for its treatment. The current reference to help the clinician formulate the proper diagnosis is based on the VI and VII European Workshop on Periodontology consensus reports [5,6]. There are two types of peri-implant disease: peri-implant mucositis and peri-implantitis. The key parameter to diagnose peri-implant mucositis is inflammation of the sulcular mucosa with bleeding on gentle probing (<0.25 N) and without evidence of radiographic bone loss. Peri-implantitis is diagnosed when there is a diminished level of crestal bone around the implant, presence of bleeding on probing, and/or suppuration, with or without concomitant deepening of peri-implant pockets. Two recent reviews have pointed out that although indicated for sites with peri-implant mucositis, the clinical efficacy of LDDAs in the treatment of peri-implantitis remains unknown [7,8].

D. Locally delivered antibiotics are injected directly into the peri-implant pocket. Arestin is packaged in a specially designed unit-dose small blunt plastic needle that is inserted into the delivery metal syringe. Elyzol is packed in a carton containing a single-use applicator and a blunt needle. Arestin and Elyzol do not require to be mixed. Atridox is made with two different syringes, and their contents need to be mixed and then injected into the periodontal pocket through a blunt cannula. Chlorhexidine is available as a solution or gel that can irrigate the subgingival pocket through a plastic syringe, or as a small membrane (Periochip®) that is inserted into the pocket by means of cotton pliers. All the aforementioned LDDAs do not need to be removed because they are completely bioresorbable.

E. LDDAs are used as an adjunctive treatment to enhance the effect of mechanical debridement of the implant surfaces that are contaminated by bacteria.

They cannot be used alone since the oral biofilm acts as a barrier for the penetration of the active (antimicrobial) agent in the infected site. The aim of the application of LDDAs combined with mechanical debridement of the supra- and subgingival biofilm is to reduce the bacterial burden, decontaminate the implant surface, and reduce the peri-implant PD and bleeding [9,10]. LDAAs may be a successful means of treatment for peri-implant mucositis in conjunction with mechanical debridement since these lesions are well demarcated and controlled-delivery devices can release a sustained high dose of antimicrobial agent precisely into the affected site for several days.

F. The diagnosis of peri-implant disease is limited to the presence of bleeding on probing and/or suppuration [5]. This means that the use of LDDAs in pockets that do not bleed is indicated only if there is suppuration, since the presence of deep pockets without signs of bleeding and/or suppuration is not indicative of peri-implant disease. This is true especially for dental implants in esthetic areas, which are often placed subcrestally for esthetic concerns, and are often associated with PD deeper than 4 mm. (For this case, the term "deep pocket" refers to a PD around an implant that is inaccessible to the patient for daily biofilm removal.)

G. The optimum time of the administration of the LDDAs is during supra- and subgingival debridement. Locally delivered antibiotics are sometimes administered as part of the nonsurgical treatment in phase I therapy. Subgingival irrigation of chlorhexidine may also be part of the surgical protocol for decontaminating the surface of the implant diagnosed with peri-implantitis [11].

H. Evidence does not exist to support the concept that multiple applications of minocycline microspheres or chlorhexidine gel as an adjunctive therapy are indicated as an alternative for surgical therapy in peri-implant sites. The LDDAs may be administered after at least 1 month for up to three times in sites with bleeding and/or purulence on probing after active therapy [12,13]. No-one has investigated whether multiple applications versus a single one are more beneficial in reducing PD or

bleeding on probing. Surgical therapy, however, should always be considered for sites diagnosed with peri-implantitis that do not demonstrate clinical improvement after a nonsurgical approach. Similarly, if sites with peri-implant mucositis do not improve following three repeated applications of LDDAs over a period of 6 months or more, surgical therapy should be considered. Esthetics might modify the use of surgery.

I. After administering Atridox, it is necessary to instruct the patient not to brush and floss the treated area for 7 days. Similarly, after treating a site with Arestin, the patient should wait 12 h before brushing around the implant and should also postpone the use of any interproximal devices for at least 10 days. It is recommended to avoid eating hard, crunchy, or sticky foods for 1 week. If treated with Elyzol, the patient may eat and drink normally, as well as brush the teeth, but should avoid flossing and interdental brushing for 1 day following the procedure. Finally, patients should avoid flossing at the site of Periochip insertion for 10 days. The use of interproximal devices could dislodge the LDDAs from inside the pocket.

J. LDDAs differ from systemically delivered antibiotics since immediately after their application a high concentration of the active molecule is present at the site. The question is whether the antimicrobial effect can be maintained over the long term. Most of the studies include short-term follow-ups that report decreased PD and bleeding on probing several months after treatment with LDAAs, without providing longer term data.

K. The rationale for using LDAAs for treating peri-implant disease is to decrease the bacterial biofilm formation, which is the etiological factor for the disease. A theoretical advantage of LDDAs in comparison with systemically delivered antibiotics is that in the site a high concentration can be achieved, and therefore the risks of complications and side effects are minimized. Similarly, there is no risk of interactions with other antimicrobials or systemic medications and a minimal risk of emergence of antibiotic-resistant bacteria. Finally, since all the LDAAs are professionally delivered, compliance of the patient cannot affect the treatment outcome [8].

L. The administration of LDDAs to patients that are allergic to the antibiotic can lead to hypersensitivity reactions. Rash and fever can occur, and in very rare cases death is reported [14,15]. The clinician must do a thorough examination and collect a detailed medical history of the patient with particular attention to any drug allergy that the patient may have. Therefore, LDDAs are contraindicated in patients that are allergic to the antibiotic contained in them and having a history of predisposition to oral candidiasis.

Conclusions

Arestin (minocycline HCL) microsphere 1 mg, Elyzol (metronidazole 25%), Atridox (doxycycline hyclate 10%), Periochip (chlorhexidine gluconate) 2.5 mg, and chlorhexidine gluconate (0.12% solution and 1% gel) are the LDDAs indicated for the treatment of peri-implant mucositis and peri-implantitis. They are administered as an adjunctive treatment to supra- and subgingival scaling to reduce the bacterial biofilm and decontaminate the implant surface.

However, most of the studies include short-term follow-ups that report decreased PD and bleeding on probing several months after treatment with LDAAs without providing longer term data.

All studies agree that, in sites diagnosed with peri-implantitis that do not demonstrate clinical improvement, surgical therapy might be recommended.

Case 5

Systemic Antibiotics

CASE STORY

A 38-year-old Caucasian woman presented with a chief complaint of, "I want my broken tooth replaced." Tooth #9 had fractured at the gingival margin 3 months previously due to trauma. The patient claimed to brush her teeth two to three times daily and uses dental floss once per day. She also used mouth rinse once daily. On observing her plaque control techniques during her initial examination, she was using a scrub technique, and her flossing technique appeared adequate.

LEARNING GOALS AND OBJECTIVES

■ To review the history of systemic antibiotic use during implant treatment
■ To identify the indications for using systemic antibiotics during implant treatment
■ To better understand which antibiotic to use and the dosing schedule

Medical History

The patient was diagnosed with type I diabetes when she was 9 years old. She was taking regular insulin 8 U subcutaneously after lunch and Lantus® (insulin glargine) 16 U subcutaneously at bedtime. She maintains her health well; however, recently she has developed foot ulcers. She reported no allergies to any medications.

Review of Systems

- Vital signs
  - Blood pressure: 136/88 mmHg
  - Pulse rate: 81 beats/min
  - Respiration: 14 breaths/min
  - HbA1c: 6.8%
  - Fasting blood sugar: 122 mg/dL (high normal for diabetic based on Joslin Diabetic Center)

Social History

The patient reported that she never used tobacco or consumed alcohol.

Extraoral Examination

No significant findings were noted. The patient had no masses or swelling, and the temporomandibular joint was within normal limits. Facial asymmetry was noted, and her lymph nodes were normal on palpation.

Intraoral Examination

- The oral cancer screening was negative.
- The soft tissue examination, including the tongue and floor of the mouth, were within normal limits.
- The periodontal examination revealed probing depth measurements that were in the range of 2–3 mm (Figure 1).
- Localized areas of gingival inflammation were noted in area #9 (see Figures 2 and 3).
- There are extensive restorations in the form of single crowns.

Occlusion

The patient presented with an Angle class I molar relationship and no interference on extrusive movements. There were no premature contacts in centric relation position, and there was no fremitus. Tooth mobility was normal.

Radiographic Examination

A complete mouth periapical radiographic series (Figure 4) revealed normal bone levels from the

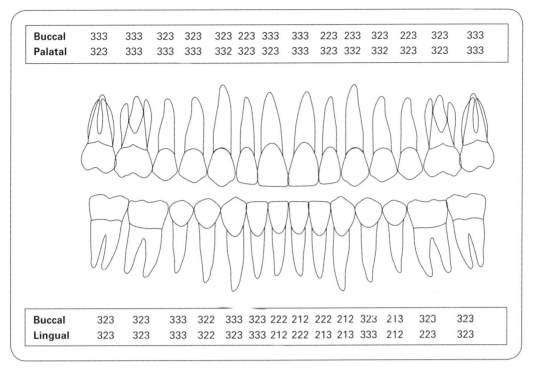

Buccal	333	333	323	323	323	223	333	333	223	233	323	223	323	333
Palatal	323	333	333	333	332	323	323	333	323	332	332	323	323	333

Buccal	323	323	333	322	333	323	222	212	222	212	323	213	323	323
Lingual	323	323	333	322	323	333	212	222	213	213	333	212	223	323

Figure 1: Probing pocket depth measurements during the initial visit.

cemento-enamel junction. A radiolucent lesion was noted at the apical region of tooth #9, which had been endodontically treated 3 months prior to this visit (Figure 5).

Diagnosis

After reviewing the dental history and the clinical and radiographic examinations, the diagnosis (Armitage 1999) was localized plaque induced gingivitis associated with #9. In addition, a tooth fracture and periapical lesion was noted on #9.

Prognosis

Tooth #9 was classified as nontreatable.

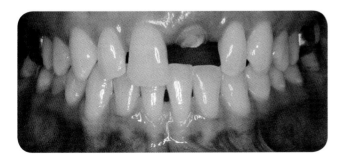

Figure 2: Pre-op presentation (facial view).

Treatment Plan

The plan was to have an initial consultation with the patient's physician regarding her diabetic status and its implications regarding possible periodontal surgery (extraction of tooth #9, ridge preservation, and implant placement). Following the medical consultation, oral hygiene therapy was done, which included a review of oral hygiene techniques and scaling and polishing. For the therapy to replace #9, several options were presented, including a fixed partial denture, a removable partial denture, or an implant. The patient opted for extraction of tooth #9 with ridge preservation, and following approximately 4 months of healing, an implant would be placed in the grafted area. Following an osseointegration period (4–6 months), an implant crown would be fabricated.

Treatment

After the initial therapy and the consultation with the patient's physician, tooth #9 was extracted atraumatically under local anesthesia (lidocaine 2% with epinephrine 1:100,000). A periotome and a universal forceps were used to extract tooth #9. However, owing to the subcrestal horizontal fracture, the root was retrieved in segments with the manipulation of small root elevators, which preserved the integrity of the

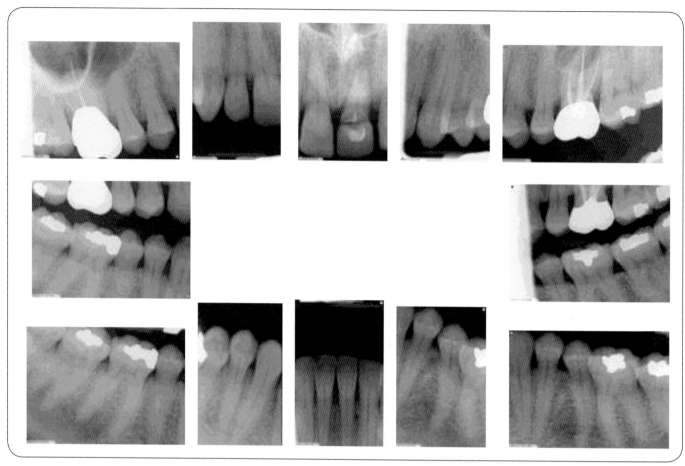

Figure 3: Full mouth series radiographs.

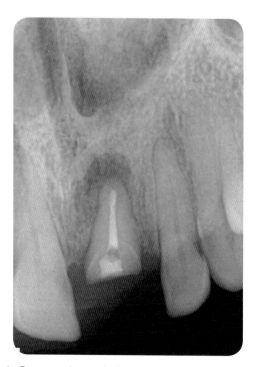

Figure 4: Preoperative periapical radiograph.

labial plate. Once the extraction socket was curretted to remove all granulation tissue, the site was irrigated with saline. Then, 0.5 cm^3 of freeze-dried mineralized bone allograft was hydrated with saline and placed in the socket up to the crestal level. A resorbable collagen membrane (Bio-Gide®, GeitlishPharma, Wolhusen, Switzerland) was placed over the augmented site and the flap was reapproximated. The flap was sutured over

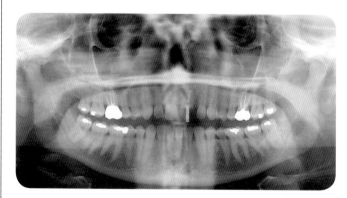

Figure 5: Pre-op presentation panoramic radiograph.

the membrane using Vicryl®. Primary closure was not attempted nor achieved. In addition to providing the patient with medication (600 mg ibuprofen) to treat any discomfort/pain, amoxicillin 500 mg tid was prescribed to the patient for 7 days. The patient was seen in 2 weeks. Sutures were removed and she reported completing the antibiotic regimen without any adverse reaction (Figure 6).

Six months postextraction, a bone-level Straumann implant was placed. On the day of the procedure, the patient's blood pressure was measured at 120/80 mmHg, which was within normal limits. Blood sugar was 126 mg/dL, which was on the high side of normal limits for a diabetic.

Lidocaine 2% (epinephrine 1:100,000) was given in the surgical area via labial and palatal infiltration. A midcrestal incision was made, and a full-thickness flap was raised. A surgical template was used to guide the sequential drilling with the copious irrigation to prepare the site for implant placement. A two-stage implant approach was utilized in this case. The implant used was a bone-level Roxolid® Straumann implant, size 4.1 mm by 12 mm. The implant was clinically stable, and a cover screw was used. A periapical radiograph confirmed angulation and safe distance from adjacent teeth (this radiograph will serve as a baseline for future

reference). The flap was sutured over the implant with primary closure. For management of discomfort and inflammation, 600 mg ibuprofen was given immediately postsurgery, and an ice pack was placed on the area.

Postoperative instructions were reviewed. The patient received prescriptions for amoxicillin 500 mg tid for 7 days, pain medication (600 mg ibuprofen) and chlorhexidine gluconate (0.12%) oral rinse. No bleeding was observed from the surgical site before the patient left the clinic.

At the 1 week follow-up appointment, the patient reported completing the antibiotic regimen without any adverse events. Minimal postoperative discomfort was reported. The patient had a provisional restoration during healing for esthetic reasons.

Six weeks postimplant, second-stage surgery was completed utilizing a punch technique to expose the implant, and the cover screw was removed and replaced with a 3 mm healing abutment. No antibiotic therapy or analgesics were needed.

The final prosthetic phase for the patient was initiated 1 month after the second stage. This phase began with a final impression, and all ceramic implant crowns were completed 4 weeks later. Oral hygiene instructions were reinforced, and the patient was scheduled for a re-care visit.

The patient was evaluated 1 year postoperatively, and the implant was found to be stable, functioning well, and esthetically pleasing to the patient.

Discussion

The use of systemic antibiotics with implant therapy remains controversial. The purpose of this chapter is to describe how the use of antibiotics in the placement of implants is for prophylactic reasons rather than to treat ongoing infection. Although the original Brånemark protocol advised the utiliziation of systemic antibiotics (penicillin V) as an adjunct to help prevent implant failure, not all cases require antibiotics. Systemic antibiotics should only be used when patient's treatment outcome can be improved [1]. If the patient's medical history includes recurrent infections or patient has high susceptibility for infection, antibiotics should be strongly considered. A medical consult is prudent in making that decision. The factors that should be taken into an account include the general condition of the patient, the surgical site and the extent of the treatment, the preoperative diagnosis, and the surgeon's preference [2]. It is imperative to minimize the use of antibiotics due to the risk of developing bacterial resistance.

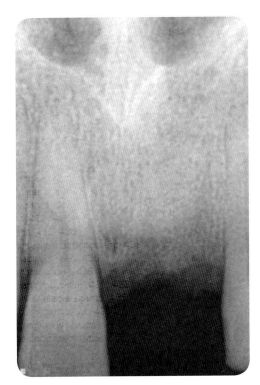

Figure 6: Postoperative periapical radiograph after extraction and bone graft.

If an antibiotic is indicated, a decision needs to be made as to whether it is administered prophylactically prior to or following the procedure. Similarly, the main considerations for this decision should be how high a risk the patient is for postsurgical infection. Currently, it is not clear whether a presurgical prophylactic regimen is superior to a postsurgical regimen in high-risk patients. Nonetheless, Resnik and Misch in 2008 developed recommendations for both presurgical and postsurgical antibiotic regimens in implant surgery. For presurgical use, they categorized procedures into risk levels for infection, and recommended specific antibiotic regimens for each [3]. For postsurgical antibiotic regimens, they reviewed the characteristics of each option and made recommendations as to which types of patients and indications are the most appropriate.

In the present case study, this patient had type I diabetes that had led to her foot ulcers, so she was considered a high risk for infection. However, the risk level was not high enough to consider a presurgical regimen. Also, since it was unclear if a presurgical regimen would have affected the outcome, postoperative antibiotic administration was selected. As reviewed by Resnick and Misch, amoxicillin is the preferred choice in the nonallergic patient, thus amoxicillin was prescribed [3]. Other considerations associated with choice of antibiotic include whether resistant strains are involved.

As the patient was compliant with antibiotic regimens and other instructions and tolerated treatment well, her dental implant was successful. Correct use of antibiotics in the appropriate patients will increase the likelihood of long-term implant success [1].

Self-Study Questions

(Answers located at the end of the case)

A. What is the history behind the use of antibiotics for implant therapy?

B. Why should systemic antibiotics be used during implant placement?

C. What systemic antibiotics are available for use, and for which conditions do they work the best?

D. When should systemic antibiotics be administered: before or after the treatment?

E. What are the side effects of antibiotics used in implant therapy?

F. How should systemic antibiotics be used so as to minimize the risk of bacterial resistance?

G. Which is better: a single dose of antibiotic or extended use?

H. Should a medical consult be done before prescribing antibiotics?

References

1. Esposito M, Grusovin MG, Talati M, et al. Interventions for replacing missing teeth: antibiotics at dental implant placement to prevent complications. Cochrane Database Syst Rev 2008;(3):CD004152.
2. Tan SK, Lo J, Zwahlen RA. Perioperative antibiotic prophylaxis in orthognathic surgery: a systematic review and meta-analysis of clinical trials. Oral Surg Oral Med Oral Pathol Oral Radiol Endod 2011;112:19–27.
3. Resnik RR, Misch C. Prophylactic antibiotic regimens in oral implantology: rationale and protocol. Implant Dent 2008;17:142–150.
4. Adell R, Lekholm U, Rockler B, Brånemark PI. A 15-year study of osseointegrated implants in the treatment of the edentulous jaw. Int J Oral Surg 1981;10:387–416.
5. Laskin DM, Dent CD, Morris HF, et al. The influence of preoperative antibiotics on success of endosseous implants at 36 months. Ann Periodontol Am Acad Periodontol 2000;5:166–174.
6. Dent CD, Olson JW, Farish SE, et al. The influence of preoperative antibiotics on success of endosseous implants up to and including stage II surgery: a study of 2,641 implants. J Oral Maxillofac Surg 1997;55:19–24.
7. Esposito M, Cannizzaro G, Bozzoli P, et al. Effectiveness of prophylactic antibiotics at placement of dental implants: a pragmatic multicentre placebo-controlled randomised clinical trial. Eur J Oral Implantol 2010;3:135–143.
8. Esposito M, Cannizzaro G, Bozzoli P, et al. Efficacy of prophylactic antibiotics for dental implants: a multicentre placebo-controlled randomised clinical trial. Eur J Oral Implantol 2008;1:23–31.

9. Morris HF, Ochi S, Plezia R, et al. AICRG, part III: the influence of antibiotic use on the survival of a new implant design. J Oral Implantol 2004;30:144–151.
10. Ata-Ali J, Ata-Ali F, Ata-Ali F. Do antibiotics decrease implant failure and postoperative infections? A systematic review and meta-analysis. Int J Oral Maxillofac Surg 2014;43:68–74.
11. Kashani H, Hossein K, Dahlin C, et al. Influence of different prophylactic antibiotic regimens on implant survival rate: a retrospective clinical study. Clin Implant Dent Relat Res 2005;7:32–35.
12. Wynn RL, Meiller TF, Crossley HL. Drug Information Handbook for Dentistry, 9th edn. Hudson, OH: Lexi Comp; 2003.
13. Lin RY. A perspective on penicillin allergy. Arch Intern Med 1992;152:930–937.
14. Grill MF, Maganti RK. Neurotoxic effects associated with antibiotic use: management considerations. Br J Clin Pharmacol 2011;72:381–393.
15. Heim-Duthoy KL, Caperton EM, Pollock R, et al. Apparent biliary pseudolithiasis during ceftriaxone therapy. Antimicrob Agents Chemother 1990;34:1146–1149.
16. Tedesco FJ, Barton RW, Alpers DH. Clindamycin-associated colitis: a prospective study. Ann Intern Med 1974;81:429–433.
17. Joshi N, Miller DQ. Doxycycline revisited. Arch Intern Med 1997;157:1421–1428.
18. Appel GB. Aminoglycoside nephrotoxicity. Am J Med 1990;88:S16–S20.
19. Hopkins S. Clinical toleration and safety of azithromycin. Am J Med 1991;91:S40–S45.
20. Binahmed A, Stoykewych A, Peterson L. Single preoperative dose versus long-term prophylactic antibiotic regimens in dental implant surgery. Int J Oral Maxillofac Implants 2005;20:115–117.
21. US Department of Health and Human Services. Guideline on antibiotic prophylaxis for dental patients at risk for infection. 2011.
22. Armitage GC. Commentary: evolution and application of classification systems for periodontal diseases – a retrospective commentary. J Periodontol 2014;85:369–371.

Answers to Self-Study Questions

A. The use of preoperative V-penicillin had been postulated by Brånemark for dental implant surgery in order to reduce bacteremia in his original protocol [4]. Several others suggested that antibiotic therapy might be important in implant therapy to prevent infections and to promote the osteointegration process [5,6]. A Cochrane review in 2013 suggests that, in general, antibiotics are beneficial for reducing failure of dental implants. Specifically, 2 or 3 g of amoxicillin given orally, as a single administration, 1 h preoperatively, significantly reduces failure rates [1]. However, there is no consensus about prescribing antibiotics with oral implants [1].

B. It is still debated whether early dental implant failure and postoperative infection can be reduced by antibiotic prophylaxis [5–10]. The mouth being an innately "septic medium," with a multitude of flora, the incidence of bacteremia is considered high. Conceptually, the goal of using prophylactic antibiotics is to prevent the onset of infection in the surgical wound by achieving an antibiotic concentration in the blood that should prevent bacterial proliferation [11]. While it is important

to minimize implant failure, there are concerns associated with the widespread use of antibiotics, since adverse events may occur [7]. The adverse effects of penicillin include the possibility of an allergic reaction, which affects 3–10% of the population and could lead to anaphylactic shock. Penicillin also cross-reacts with cephalosporins in 3–5% of the population [12]. The adverse effects of clindamycin include pseudomembranous colitis caused by a toxin produced by *Clostridium difficile* [12]. Side effects of metronidazole include an increased anticoagulant effect and disulfiram like reaction. The side effects of erythromycin include gastrointestinal upset and nausea [12].

A Cochrane review published in 2013 reviewed six studies including a total of 1162 participants [1]. Each study compared participants receiving systemic antibiotics with implant placement with ones who did not receive systemic antibiotics. It was found that implants were on average 67% less likely to be lost in the group that received systemic antibiotics, and this association was statistically significant [1].

The decision to administer prophylactic antibiotics, pre- or postsurgery, is based on various factors, including the general physical health of the patient, the surgical site and extension, the preoperative diagnosis, and surgeon preferences. Patients have different levels of risk for infection. A low-risk patient would be described as "young, healthy adults without significant co-morbidities" [2]; however, if a patient has significant co-morbidities (such as a patient with type I diabetes), this would constitute a moderate risk. A patient with an active infection or a compromised immune system (such as an HIV patient) would be considered a high-risk patient. Therefore, the level of risk of the patient should be considered strongly as a factor for the use of systemic prophylactic antibiotic therapy.

C. In 2008, Resnik and Misch described all the possible options for antibiotic use and associated considerations when selecting antibiotics as the following. However, they did not describe a particular dosage frequency [3].

- *Penicillin V.* This is well absorbed within 30 min. The main disadvantage is the frequent dosing needed to maintain blood levels and thereby prevent development of resistant bacteria. Penicillin is effective in streptococcus species and oral anaerobes and therefore is especially useful in implant therapy [4]. It has been found to be effective at eliminating pathogens red and orange complex, which are the main ones implicated in periodontal disease [5].
- *Amoxicillin.* This is the preferred antibiotic in the nonallergic patient, because it has better absorption and bioavailability than penicillin V. Those properties also make amoxicillin particularly useful in implants. Amoxicillin is preferred to penicillin (see answer to self-study question E) [12].
- *Augmentin®.* Augmentin is recommended for sinus augmentation as it inactivates resistant bacteria in cases where penicillinases are thought to be present.
- *Cephalexin.* This is a member of the first-generation cephalosporins, which are used in penicillin-allergic patients, and they are less prone to beta-lactamase destruction than penicillin.
- *Cefuroxime axetil (Ceftin®).* This has lower cross-reactivity, broader spectrum, and an improved resistance to beta-lactamase destruction. It will help in cases of implants associated with

acute bacterial maxillary sinusitis caused by *Streptococcus pneumoniae* or *Haemophilus influenzae* (non-beta-lactamase-producing strains only).
- *Erythromycin (a macrolide).* A narrow-spectrum antibiotic. This therapeutic is well absorbed and has a low toxicity, but it has a high incidence of nausea. It is usually used in penicillin-allergic patients.
- *Clindamycin.* This is an effective narrow spectrum against anaerobic bacteria, but also targets aerobic pathogens, especially *Bacteroides*. Its disadvantages include high toxicity, a high prevalence of diarrhea (20–30%), and pseudomembranous colitis (if taken over a long period).
- *Ciprofloxacin (first-generation quinolone).* A broad-spectrum bactericidal antibiotic used orally or parenterally. It will help in acute sinusitis caused by *H. influenzae*, penicillin-susceptible *S. pneumoniae*, or *Moraxella catarrhalis*. It can effectively treat rare oral infections caused by the Enterobacteriaceae group of bacteria.
- *Levaquin (third- or fourth-generation quinolone).* Useful against resistant and anaerobic bacteria and mainly used in sinus augmentation procedures.

The preferred order of antibiotic use in dental implant/bone graft proceures is amoxicillin, cephalexin, and then clindamycin [3]. In sinus augmentation procedures, Augmentin is the first option, followed by Ceftin and Levaquin [3].

Amoxicillin is preferred to be used over penicillin because (1) amoxicillin is better absorbed than penicillin (95% absorption versus 56%), (2) it has a longer serum half-life, and (3) it may be taken with food [12].

D. There is no difference whether systemic antibiotics are administered before or after implant placement [3]. The main concept is to use antibiotics to prevent infections, and to preserve the osseointegration process. Laskin et al. stated that "the results showed a significantly higher survival rate at each stage of treatment in patients who had received preoperative antibiotics" [5]. However, in a clinical trial [5] comparing four interventions – (1) 2 g of amoxicillin given 1 h preoperatively; (2) 2 g of preoperative amoxicillin plus 1 g twice a day for 7 days; (3) 1 g of postoperative amoxicillin twice a day for 7 days; and (4) no antibiotics (considered the control group) – at 3 months no implant failures were observed in the test groups (before or after), while there were two implant failures in the no antibiotic group [5]. However, there were no statistically significant differences reported between the experimental groups.

Resnik and Misch in 2008 developed the Misch prophylactic protocol [3]. They classified the categories with respect to the level of risk the procedure carries for infection. Their protocol is as follows.

Category 1: low risk of infection. This applies to simple extractions without grafting and second-stage surgery in healthy patients. No antibiotics are required. Chlorhexidine rinse (0.12%) is recommended pre- and postoperatively. There is no implant placement in this category.

Category 2: moderate risk of infection. This applies to traumatic extractions, socket grafting procedures, and immediate implant placements. Here, a preoperative loading dose of antibiotics and a single postoperative dose along with a 0.12% chlorhexidine rinse twice a day until suture removal is recommended.

Category 3: moderate to high risk of infection. This applies to multiple implants with extensive soft-tissue reflection or multiple immediate implants and bone grafts requiring membranes. A preoperative loading dose of antibiotics followed by three postoperative doses per day for 3 days and rinsing with 0.12% chlorhexidine twice daily until suture removal is also recommended.

Category 4: high risk of infection. This applies to implant placements with sinus floor lifts, autogenous block bone grafts and the same procedures as categories 2 and 3, but on medically compromised patients. The suggested regime is as category 3, but postoperative antibiotics should be continued for 5 days.

Category 5: also high risk of infection. This applies to all sinus augmentation procedures. Loading dose of antibiotics a day before the procedure (ensuring adequate levels in sinus tissues before surgery) and a beta-lactamase (Augmentin) antibiotic continued for 5 days. This is due to the high incidence of beta-

lactamase pathogens in maxillary sinus infections. Chlorhexidine rinse (0.12%) twice a day is also recommended, until suture removal.

E. The penicillin family has been associated with a wide range of hypersensitivity reactions, including fever, rash (maculopapular and urticarial), anaphylaxis, exfoliative dermatitis, erythema multiforme, serum sickness, and hemolytic anemia [13], in addition to central nervous system toxicity when administered intravenously in high doses, particularly to patients with renal impairment [14].

The cephalosporins can cause diarrhea, pseudomembranous colitis, and, rarely, hypersensitivity reactions, including drug fever, rash, interstitial nephritis, or immediate life-threatening events [15].

The most notorious side effect of clindamycin is diarrhea and *C. difficile*-related colitis [16]. This drug has rarely caused drug fever, rash, blood dyscrasias, and hepatotoxicity. Doxycycline has also been associated with diarrhea and, infrequently, photosensitivity, rash, hepatitis, and, particularly in elderly patients, esophageal ulcerations or strictures [17]. Concerns regarding administration of the aminoglycosides include nephrotoxicity, specifically nonoliguric acute renal failure, ototoxicity, both the auditory and vestibular components, and neuromuscular blockade, a rare event that has developed in patients with myasthenia gravis, renal disease, hypocalcemia, or hypermagnesemia [18].

Adverse events attributed to the macrolides have included nausea, vomiting, abdominal pain, diarrhea, and, rarely, antibiotic-associated colitis, pancreatitis, cholestatic jaundice, acute hepatitis, abnormal taste (clarithromycin), and reversible ototoxicity [19]. Clarithromycin and azithromycin cause fewer gastrointestinal adverse events than does erythromycin.

F. The prudent use of systemic antibiotics aims to minimize the risk of bacterial resistance [1,3]: (1) use antibiotics only when the patient's outcome can be improved; (2) use narrow-spectrum antibiotics whenever possible; (3) save the last-generation antibiotics for serious life-threatening infections; and (4) stop antibiotic therapy as soon as possible. When used prophylactically, a short course of antibiotics should be prescribed, typically only enough to last the duration of the surgical procedure, and the administration should begin prior to the surgery (about 2 h before the procedure), so that adequate systemic levels of antibiotic (two to eight times above minimum inhibitory concentration) are present at the time of surgical incision [1,3].

Amoxicillin has been commonly used as the antibiotic of choice (see answer to self-study question C); however, as noted in the answer to self-study question A, Brånemark used a narrow-spectrum antibiotic. The protocol for placing implants is to consider placement in a mouth free of periodontal disease. Thus, the use of narrow-spectrum antibiotics given prior to therapy is preferred when implants are placed under healthy conditions.

G. There appears to be no specific benefit based on two studies to use an extended course of antibiotics. Binahmed et al. compared the efficacy of prophylactic antibiotic regimens commonly used in dental implant surgery in single-dose and long-term regimens [20]. They included 215 patients.

In the first group, patients were administered a single preoperative dose with no postoperative antibiotics. In the second group, patients received a preoperative dose of antibiotics and were instructed to continue postoperatively for 7 days. They concluded that long-term prophylactic antibiotic was of no advantage or benefit over a single-dose preoperative antibiotic regimen in the study population [20]. This is because the outcome in terms of implant failure in the different groups was the same. In another study, Kashani et al. recommended a stricter regimen of a 1-day dose of prophylactic antibiotics compared with a full-week prescription [11].

H. Consultation with the patient's physician is always necessary to determine susceptibility to bacteremia-induced infections and to assess the patient's current medical situation [21]. Also, it is important to know the patient's current medication regimen to avoid cross-reaction with medications prescribed as part of the dental procedure.

Conclusion

A general rule about classifications of patients who should receive antibiotics prophylactically either pre-or postsurgically should be avoided. Information obtained through the medical consult should be weighed with other clinical information, and judgments should be made on a case-by-case basis.

It appears from the literature cited in this case report that the use of systemic antibiotic therapy is warranted to help prevent early implant failure. This brings to the table the question of the "overuse" of systemic antibiotics and the development of resistant organisms. Clearly, there is no easy answer. Assuming the literature is correct and that there is a significant chance for early implant failure without antibiotic prophylaxis, their use is justified from a dental perspective. It is important that a discussion of the facts presented in this case report is done with the patient and all the clinicians involved with the patient's therapy in order that a rational decision is made for and by the patient.

For the patient in this case report, with respect to their specific systemic concern of type I diabetes and considering the medical consultation, presurgical amoxicillin was not recommended; however, the postsurgical administration of systemic antibiotics was prescribed. Although previously the overuse of antibiotics has resulted in drug-resistant strains [22], their use in specific medical conditions and under the advice of a physician is warranted. The judicious use of prophylactic antibiotics with implant therapy is the current standard of care.

Case 6

Surgical Management of Peri-implantitis

Medical History
The patient presented with hypertension, controlled with medication (40 mg of lisinopril once a day). At the time of treatment, he was taking supplements, which included fish oil, green tea, and raspberry.

Review of Systems
- Vital signs
  - Blood pressure: 135/78 mmHg
  - Pulse rate: 69 beats/min
  - Respiration: 15 breaths/min

Social History
According to the patient, he did not smoke or drink alcohol. He did drink a few beers occasionally.

Extraoral Examination
No significant findings were noted. The patient had no masses or swellings. The temporomandibular joint was within normal limits. There was no facial asymmetry noted and his lymph nodes were normal on palpation.

Intraoral Examination
- Oral cancer screening was negative.
- The tongue, floor of mouth, and buccal mucosa were within normal limits.
- Periodontal examination revealed generalized probing depth in the range of 2–3 mm in most of the teeth. There were >5 mm probing depths around #23 (tooth), #19, #28, #29, and #30 (implants) (see Figure 1).
- Localized areas of gingival inflammation noted.
- Suppuration from #29 was observed.
- Evaluation of the alveolar ridge revealed generalized moderate horizontal resorption.
- Extensive restorations were present in the forms of single crowns and fixed partial dentures.

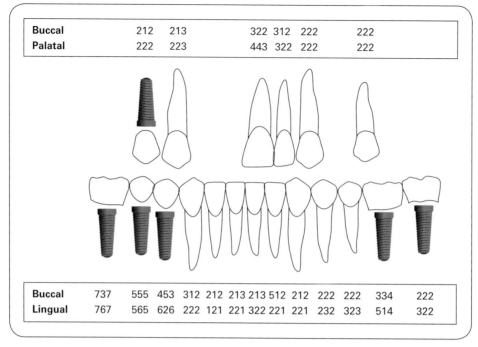

Buccal	212	213		322	312	222		222	
Palatal	222	223		443	322	222		222	

Buccal	737	555	453	312	212	213	213	512	212	222	222	334	222
Lingual	767	565	626	222	121	221	322	221	221	232	323	514	322

Figure 1: Probing pocket depth measurements during the initial visit. Note the implant restoration #6, two-unit fixed implant restoration #18–#19, and three-unit fixed implant restoration #28–#29–#30.

Occlusion

- There were no occlusal discrepancies or interferences noted.
- Overjet: 3 mm.
- Overbite: 3 mm.
- Crossbite: none.
- Angle's classification: canine class I for the right and left sides.

Radiographic Examination

A full mouth radiographic series and a panoramic radiograph were taken (Figures 2 and 3). Radiographic examination revealed mild to moderate horizontal bone loss. There was an angular bone loss noted in the mesial of #22. Circumferential peri-implant bone defect and crestal irregularities were observed around implant #30.

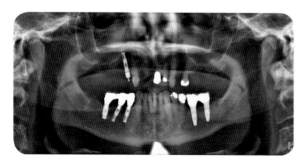

Figure 2: Preoperative presentation panoramic radiograph.

Diagnosis

- Generalized slight to moderate with localized severe chronic periodontitis.
- Peri-implantitis #19, #28, #29, and #30.
- Partial edentulism on the maxillary posterior.

Treatment Plan

The treatment plan for this patient consisted of initial-phase therapy of oral hygiene instructions, oral prophylaxis, and scaling and root planing to address gingival inflammation. Open-flap debridement with resective surgery on #28, #29, and #30 implants and guided tissue regeneration (GTR) on #23 were performed.

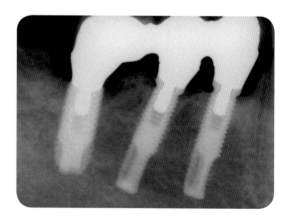

Figure 3: Preoperative periapical radiograph.

Treatment

After the initial-phase therapy, the clinical findings revealed a probing depth of 4–7 mm and bleeding on probing (BOP) around implants #28, #29, and #30. The preoperative view of the implant site is illustrated in Figures 4 and 5. Profound local anesthesia was obtained at the surgical site using two carpules of 2% lidocaine with 1:100,000 epinephrine. An intrasulcular incision was made from #28 to #30 with a vertical incision at the mesiofacial line angle of #28. Full-thickness buccal and lingual flaps were reflected

(Figures 6 and 7). The implant surfaces were thoroughly scaled. After all granulation tissues were removed, the bone defect morphologies around the implants were evaluated (Figure 7). Chemical decontamination of the implant surface was performed using 0.12% chlorhexidine, then thoroughly rinsed with sterile saline solution. Resective surgery was performed to eliminate a shallow but wide 2 mm intrabony defect on the lingual aspect of implants #28 and #29 (Figures 7 and 8). Osteoplasty was performed using a round diamond bur. The flaps were approximated and then sutured. External

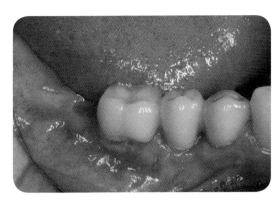

Figure 4: Preoperative presentation (facial view).

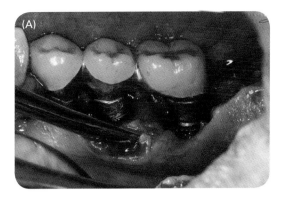

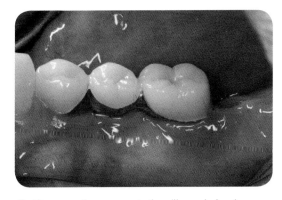

Figure 5: Preoperative presentation (lingual view).

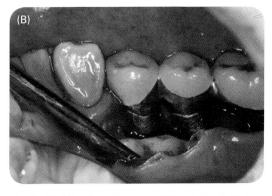

Figure 7: (A, B) After flap elevation (lingual view). Note intrabony defects on lingual #28 and #29.

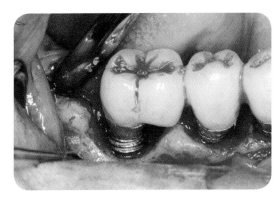

Figure 6: After flap elevation (facial view).

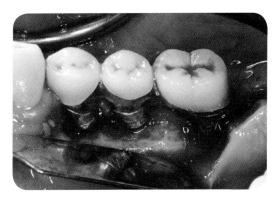

Figure 8: Post-osseous surgery (lingual view). Intrabony defect was removed with resective therapy.

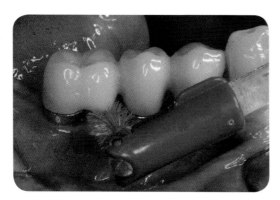

Figure 9: The patient is able to use an interdental brush after healing.

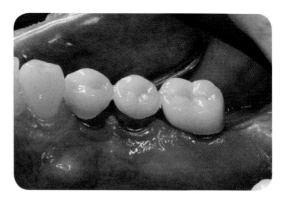

Figure 11: Follow-up at 2.5 years (lingual view).

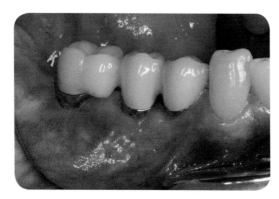

Figure 10: Follow-up at 2.5 years (facial view).

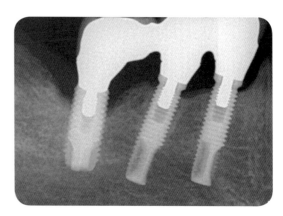

Figure 12: Periapical radiograph of the surgical area at 2.5 years follow-up.

vertical mattress sutures were placed to position the flaps apically. The patient was given systemic antibiotics (amoxicillin 500 mg TID) for 7 days postoperatively. Three months after the surgery, the treatment created spaces between implants that allowed for the use of an interproximal brush (Figure 9). The inflammation was reduced when compared with the preoperative status. Two and a half years after the surgery, peri-implant tissue was clinically stable (all probing depths were ≤3 mm and no BOP) (Figures 10, 11, and 12). At his regular checkups every 3 months, the patient was instructed to use the interproximal brush and maintain oral hygiene.

Discussion

In this case, the nonsurgical therapy was performed prior to the resective surgery. Owing to the presence of residual deep probing depths (>5 mm) and BOP, surgical therapy was performed for the defect debridement and decontamination of the infected implant surface. The goal of surgical treatment is the removal of biofilm from the implant surface, which is considered the primary etiology of peri-implantitis [1]. Elimination of toxins from the implant surface potentially may promote re-osseointegration, as shown in animal studies [2,3]. A recent study concluded that, "Cleansing of a previously plaque-contaminated implant is sufficient for re-osseointegration to occur, and rough surfaces can allow re-osseointegration" [1].

Several factors can contribute to the success of surface decontamination. Visualization of the implant surface is one of these factors [4]. Oftentimes, remnants of cement lead to peri-implantitis because it may not be detectable upon radiographic examination. In this case, there was clear access for all surfaces of the implants during the treatment [4].

Configuration and size of the defect is another factor. The defect morphology can be classified as follows: intrabony defects (one to four walls), dehiscence, or horizontal defect [5].

In this case, the defect was a combination of horizontal and intrabony defect (Figures 6 and 7). Open-flap debridement was the choice of treatment because horizontal bone loss was observed in most of the areas (#28, #29, and #30 implants) with a partial intrabony defect on the lingual aspect of #28 and #29 implants. The intrabony defect was wide and shallow (2 mm), which was not indicated for regenerative therapy. Therefore, the defect was removed by resective surgery. Additionally, resective surgery was performed to achieve better flap adaptation.

Prosthetic design can impact the patient's and therapist's ability to maintain the area. The patient was not able to use an interproximal brush nor Superfloss before surgical therapy due to the overcontoured prosthetic superstructure. After surgery, adequate space was created to allow for the patient to perform oral hygiene with an interproximal brush (Figure 9).

Similar to any other periodontal surgical procedures, the patient's systemic conditions, such as smoking or uncontrolled diabetes, negatively influence the clinical outcome. The patient's history in this case was noncontributory. The patient's oral hygiene improved after phase I and throughout the treatment. He was seeing the dentist regularly for periodontal recall, which is also a critical factor in the long-term success of treatment.

Self-Study Questions

(Answers located at the end of the case)

A. What are the goals of the surgical treatment?

B. Which option is better: surgical or nonsurgical treatment?

C. Which case is suitable for the surgical therapy?

D. What surgical modalities are available for surgical treatment?

E. What are the methods to decontaminate an infected implant surface?

F. What is the evidence for using a laser for surgical therapy?

G. If surgical therapy is selected, what is the treatment decision-making process between resective and regenerative therapy?

H. What are the factors that affect the surgical outcome?

I. How predictable is the surgical therapy for peri-implantitis?

J. With regenerative therapy, is reosseointegration possible or just bone fill?

References

1. Parlar A, Bosshardt DD, Cetiner D, et al. Effects of decontamination and implant surface characteristics on re-osseointegration following treatment of peri-implantitis. Clin Oral Implants Res 2009;20:391–399.

2. Claffey N, Clarke E, Polyzois I, Renvert S. Surgical treatment of peri-implantitis. J Clin Periodontol 2008;35:316–332.

3. Lindhe J, Meyle J; Group D of European Workshop on Periodontology. Peri-implant diseases: Consensus Report of the Sixth European Workshop on Periodontology. J Clin Periodontol 2008;35:282–285.

4. Wadhwani C, Hess T, Faber T, et al. A descriptive study of the radiographic density of implant restorative cements. J Prosthet Dent 2010;103:295–302.

5. Schwarz F, Herten M, Sager M, et al. Comparison of naturally occurring and ligature-induced peri-implantitis bone defects in humans and dogs. Clin Oral Implants Res 2007;18:161–170.

6. Schou S, Berglundh T, Lang NP. Surgical treatment of peri-implantitis. Int J Oral Maxillofac Implants 2004;19:140–149.

7. Renvert S, Roos-Jansåker AM, Claffey N. Non-surgical treatment of peri-implant mucositis and peri-implantitis: a literature review. J Clin Periodontol 2008;35(8 Suppl):305–315.

8. Klinge B, Meyle J; Working Group 2. Peri-implant tissue destruction. The Third EAO Consensus Conference 2012. Clin Oral Implants Res 2012;23:108–110.

9. Mombelli A, Lang NP. The diagnosis and treatment of periimplantitis. Periodontol 2000 1998;17:63–76.

10. Heitz-Mayfield LJA, Lang NP. Antimicrobial treatment of peri-implant diseases. Int J Oral Maxillofac Implants 2004;19:128–139.

11. Jovanoic SA. The management of peri-implant breakdown around functioning osseointegrated dental implants. J Periodontol 1993;64:1176–1183.

12. Gupta HK, Garg A, Bedi NK. Peri-implantitis: a risk factor in implant failure. J Clin Diagn Res 2011;5:138–141.

13. Leonhardt A, Dahlén G, Renvert S. Five-year clinical, microbiological, and radiological outcome following treatment of peri-implantitis in man. J Periodontol 2003;74:1415–1422.

14. Chen S, Darby I. Dental implants: maintenance, care and treatment of peri-implant infection. Aust Dent J 2003;48:212–220.

15. Romeo E, Lops D, Chiapasco M, et al. Therapy of peri-implantitis with resective surgery. A 3-year clinical trial on rough screw-shaped oral implants. Part II: radiographic outcome. Clin Oral Implants Res 2007;18:179–187.

16. Froum SJ, Froum SH, Rosen PS. Successful management of peri-implantitis with a regenerative approach: a consecutive series of 51 treated implants with 3- to 7.5-year follow-up. Int J Periodontics Restorative Dent 2012;32:11–20.

17. Dörtbudak O, Haas R, Bernhart T, Mailath-Pokorny G. Lethal photosensitization for decontamination of implant surfaces in the treatment of peri-implantitis. Clin Oral Implants Res 2001;12:104–108.

18. Schwarz F, Sahm N, Iglhaut G, Becker J. Impact of the method of surface debridement and decontamination on the clinical outcome following combined surgical therapy of peri-implantitis: a randomized controlled clinical study. J Clin Periodontol 2011;38(3):276–284.

19. Schwarz F, Hegewald A, John G, et al. Four-year follow-up of combined surgical therapy of advanced peri-implantitis evaluating two methods of surface decontamination. J Clin Periodontol 2013;40:962–967.

20. Mailoa J, Lin GH, Chan HL, et al. Clinical outcomes of using lasers for peri-implantitis surface detoxification: a systematic review and meta-analysis. J Periodontol 2014;85(9):1194–1202.

21. Romeo E, Ghisolfi M, Murgolo N, et al. Therapy of peri-implantitis with resective surgery. A 3-year clinical trial on rough screw-shaped oral implants. Part I: clinical outcome. Clin Oral Implants Res 2005;16:9–18.

22. Wetzel AC, Vlassis J, Caffesse RG, et al. Attempts to obtain re-osseointegration following experimental peri-implantitis in dogs. Clin Oral Implants Res 1999;10:111–119.

23. Yeung SC. Biological basis for soft tissue management in implant dentistry. Aust Dent J 2008;53:S39–S42.

24. Frisch E, Ziebolz D, Vach K, Ratka-Krüger P. The effect of keratinized mucosa width on peri-implant outcome under supportive postimplant therapy. Clin Implant Dent Relat Res 2015;17(Suppl 1):e236–e244.

25. Brito C, Tenenbaum HC, Wong BK, et al. Is keratinized mucosa indispensable to maintain peri-implant health? A systematic review of the literature. J Biomed Mater Res B Appl Biomater 2014;102(3):643–650.

26. Gobbato L, Avila-Ortiz G, Sohrabi K, et al. The effect of keratinized mucosa width on peri-implant health: a systematic review. Int J Oral Maxillofac Implants 2013;28(6):1536–1545.

27. Lin GH, Chan HL, Wang HL. The significance of keratinized mucosa on implant health: a systematic review. J Periodontol 2013;84(12):1755–1767.

28. Charalampakis G, Rabe P, Leonhardt A, Dahlén G. A follow-up study of peri-implantitis cases after treatment. J Clin Periodontol 2011;38:864–871.

Answers to Self-Study Questions

A. The primary goal of the surgical treatment of peri-implantitis is to get access to the implant surface for debridement and decontamination in order to achieve resolution of the inflammatory lesion around the implant, stop the disease progression, and maintain the implant in function with healthy peri-implant tissues [3,6]. Additionally, it may promote bone fill and could result in re-osseointegration [2].

B. Peri-implant mucositis can be treated successfully with mechanical debridement as nonsurgical therapy with the reduction of the level of microorganisms and inflammation [7]. In contrast, nonsurgical mechanical debridement alone has limited efficacy for the treatment of peri-implantitis [8]. Surgical therapy of peri-implantitis is considered to be superior to nonsurgical instrumentation, because it provides better access to perform a complete removal of all granulation tissue from the defect area and decontamination of the exposed implant surfaces [7]. However, in all cases, nonsurgical therapy is to be performed prior to surgical therapy to assess the healing response, patient compliance, and oral hygiene.

C. The indication for surgical therapy is the presence of considerable pocket formation (greater than 5 mm probing depth) and bone loss [9]. Acute infection must also be resolved, and the patient should follow proper oral hygiene instructions before proceeding to any surgical therapy [10].

The type of osseous defects should be identified before deciding on the surgical treatment modality. If the vertical (<3 mm) or one- to two-wall defects are found, then resective surgery can be used to reduce the pockets and correct the osseous architecture [11]. When three-wall or circumferential defects are present, regenerative therapy with various bone grafting techniques can be used for the regeneration of lost bone [12].

D.
- *Open-flap debridement.* Several animal studies showed that open-flap debridement including

surface decontamination was more effective in the treatment of peri-implantitis than closed debridement [2]. The long-term outcome of access surgery was evaluated in a case series. A complete healing of the peri-implant disease was found in 58% of the implants treated [13]. However, seven of 26 implants were lost, and disease progression occurred in an additional four implants [13].
- *Resective therapy.* This consists of ostectomy and/or osteoplasty with an apically positioned flap. The objectives of resective surgery are reducing probing depth and creating a soft tissue morphology that enhances good self-performed oral hygiene and peri-implant health. Resective therapy is generally confined to implants placed in nonesthetic sites [14].
- *Regenerative therapy.* This is an attempt to rebuild or regenerate lost peri-implant tissue. In intrabony defects such as crater defects, regenerative therapy is indicated. Autogenous bone, allograft, and xenograft materials in combination with nonresorbable or resorbable membranes are commonly used [2]. Better results have been reported with these methods when compared with surgical debridement and surface decontamination alone [2]. In human studies, regenerative procedures such as bone graft techniques with or without the use of barrier membranes resulted in various degrees of success [2]. However, the optimal treatment protocol is yet to be determined.

E.
- *Mechanical decontamination.* The following instruments are available for the mechanical decontamination of an implant surface.
  - Specially designed curettes made of pure titanium, plastic, or ceramic.
  - Ultrasonic instrument using tips with plastic or Teflon coatings.
  - Abrasive devices.
  - Titanium rotary instrument (TiBrush) (Figure 13A).
  - Erbium-doped yttrium aluminium garnet (Er:YAG) laser.

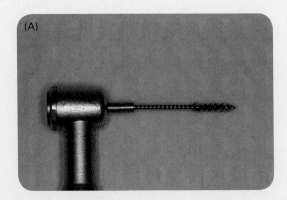

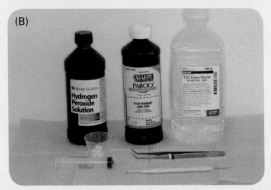

Figure 13: Implant surface decontamination: (A) a titanium brush for mechanical decontamination; (B) chemical agents (e.g., hydrogen peroxide, chlorhexidine gluconate) for chemical decontamination, sterile saline solution for irrigation.

○ Implantoplasty (surface modification) can be performed on the exposed threads of rough surface implants during surgery. In a radiographic study, the efficacy of implantoplasty was examined by comparing resective surgery with implantoplasty versus resective surgery only. The result suggested that implantoplasty seems to be effective and positively influences the implant survival rate [15].

• *Chemical decontamination.* After mechanical decontamination, chemical decontamination is suggested. Chlorhexidine gluconate, hydrogen peroxide, citric acid, and tetracycline hydrochloride have been used for chemical decontamination followed by thorough rinsing with sterile saline solution (Figure 13B).

There are several methods, but one of the well-known protocols is "the Froum protocol," which consisted of six steps [16]:

1. Application of fine bicarbonate powder.
2. Irrigation with sterile saline.

3. Application of tetracycline with cotton pellets or a brush.
4. A second exposure of the implant's surface to bicarbonate air abrasion.
5. Application of 0.12% chlorhexidine gluconate.
6. Second irrigation with sterile saline.

F. A laser can be used for the decontamination of implant surfaces. A clinical study evaluated the effectiveness of laser therapy for peri-implantitis by measuring the levels of periodontal pathogens (*Aggregatibacter actinomycetemcomitans*, *Porphyromonas gingivalis*, and *Prevotella intermedia*). The results indicated that the laser therapy resulted in a significant reduction in bacteria counts [17]. Among the lasers applied for surface decontamination, the Er:YAG laser is widely used by clinicians because it is considered to possess good properties for calculus removal, degranulation, and surface decontamination. A randomized controlled trial compared the effectiveness of an Er:YAG laser versus "plastic curettes + cotton pellets + sterile saline" for the surgical therapy of peri-implantitis; the study failed to demonstrate an impact of the method of surface decontamination on the clinical outcomes at 6-month follow-up [18]. A 4-year follow-up study also failed to show the differences between these methods on the long-term clinical outcomes [19]. A recent systematic review concluded that lasers resulted in similar probing depth reduction when compared with conventional implant surface decontamination methods in a short-term follow-up [20].

G. Resective or regenerative surgical approaches are proposed for the treatment of peri-implantitis depending on the morphology and the shape of bone defects [21]. In cases of particular clinical conditions, such as peri-implantitis with suprabony defects or one-wall intrabony defects in nonesthetic regions, the use of resective surgery with an apically repositioned flap and implantoplasty was suggested [21]. Regenerative therapy is indicated for well-defined crater defects, which are capable of retaining bone or bone substitute materials (Figure 14) [5].

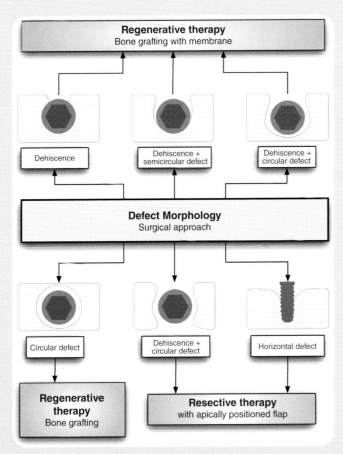

Figure 14: Diagram of decision-making tree based on the bony defect morphology.

H. There are several factors that may affect the outcome: the configuration of the defect and the surface composition of the implant. Various animal studies using artificially created peri-implant defects demonstrated that the width of the defect negatively affects the histological outcome [2]. The use of bone graft material also could be beneficial in terms of treatment outcome. It has also been shown that the deep, narrow peri-implant intrabony defect has greater clinical improvement following treatment compared with the wide, shallow defect [2]. In addition, the greater number of bony walls (e.g., three-wall defect versus one-wall defect) around the defect correlated to more success after the regenerative treatment [2].

Different implant surfaces could potentially lead to different defect characteristics [2]. Some studies showed no difference in the size of the defect created around titanium plasma-sprayed,

sand-blasted large-grit acid-etched, and commercially pure titanium machined surfaces [22]. In contrast, one study did show a greater defect associated with hydroxyapatite-coated implants following ligature-induced peri-implantitis [2].

Another factor to consider when comparing the healing around previously contaminated implants is the presence or absence of keratinized mucosa (KM). Although none of the studies described the amount of surrounding KM pre- and post-treatment [2], maintaining good oral hygiene around the implant is very difficult if no KM is present [23]. Whether a minimal width of KM is necessary to maintain peri-implant tissue health has been controversial [24]. However, recent systematic reviews concluded that a lack of adequate KM around implants appears to be associated with clinical parameters indicative of inflammation and poor oral hygiene [25–27]. The presence of an adequate zone of KM may be necessary, but the evidence is scarce due to the limited numbers of studies and heterogeneity among the studies included.

I. Degrees of success are varied. Success rates range from 3 years to 7.5 years [16], but there are no data for long-term observation. The success of surgical treatment after 6 years of follow-up can reach 45.3%, with the remainder being associated with either failure or the inability to arrest the progression of peri-implantitis [28]. Regarding procedures, an access flap alone with antibiotics was shown to be associated with failure, and regenerative surgery with antibiotics was associated with success, but both findings were not statistically significant [28]. Only an apically positioned flap with bone recontouring and antibiotics was associated with success [28].

J. Re-osseointegration is defined as the formation of new bone around the dental implant surfaces, which were previously lost to bacterial contamination. The consensus report of the Sixth European Workshop on Periodontology claimed, "open debridement including surface decontamination and regenerative procedure resolved peri-implantitis, promoted bone fill and could result in re-osseointegration" [3]. However, some studies found a significant difference in terms of both bone fill and re-osseointegration between different implant surfaces [16]. Re-osseointegration was reported in animal histological studies, but there are no clinical studies in humans that demonstrated re-osseointegration. In many human clinical cases, the postoperative radiographs indicate bone fill after regenerative procedures (Figure 15). Re-osseointegration can only be determined by histological means.

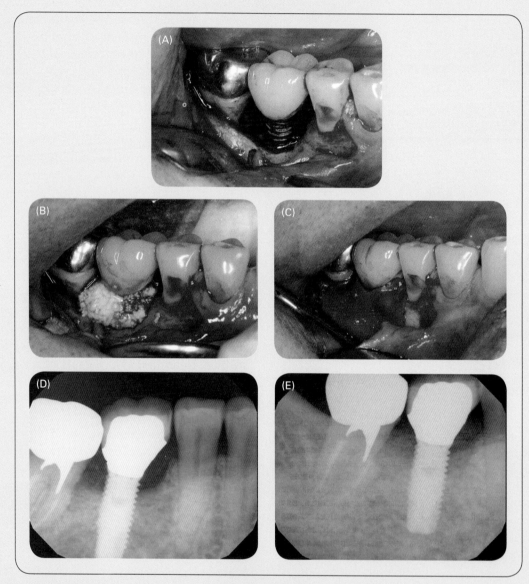

Figure 15: An example of regenerative therapy. (A) After flap elevation (facial view). A combination (horizontal and vertical) defect was observed. (B) Enamel matrix derivative and Xynograft (deproteinized bovine bone mineral) were applied in the defect. (C) The graft is covered with a collagen membrane. (D) Preoperative periapical radiograph. (E) Postoperative periapical radiograph.

Case 7

Removal/Replacement of Failed Implants

CASE STORY

A 58-year-old female patient had a chief complaint of pain and discomfort located in #2 and #3 areas. A review of medical history shows sinus problem, tinnitus, and vertigo in the past and implants placed 24 years ago.

On radiographic examination there were implants with no threads in #2, #3, #14, and #15 areas. There was a blade implant in #13 and bilateral blade implants in mandible.

The plan was for removal of the implants in #2 and #3 areas with the use of an implant removal kit in the least invasive way.

Figures 1 and 2 illustrate part of the initial clinical examination.

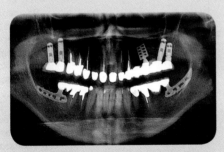

Figure 1: Notice different types of implants and radiolucent area in apical portion in #3.

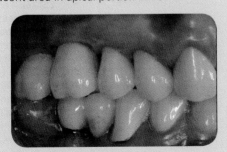

Figure 2: Lateral view of #2 and #3 area.

LEARNING GOALS AND OBJECTIVES

- To understand the factors that may cause an implant failure
- To understand different techniques that can be used for minimally invasive implant removal
- To be able to compare different techniques to remove the implant fixture

Medical History

The patient is in good health. She does report an allergy to dust.

Review of Systems

- Vital signs
  - Blood pressure: 155/93 mmHg
  - Pulse rate: 78 beats/min
  - Respiration: 16 breaths/min

Social History

The patient occasionally smokes. Occasional drinking.

Extraoral Examination

The patient has no masses or swelling, and no trismus. There were no masses felt on palpation of the lymph nodes. The temporomandibular joint evaluation showed mild deflection/deviation.

Intraoral Examination

- The soft tissues of the mouth, including the tongue, appear normal. The oral cancer screening was within normal limit.
- The gingival examination reveals generalized marginal erythema.

A periodontal charting was completed (Figure 3).

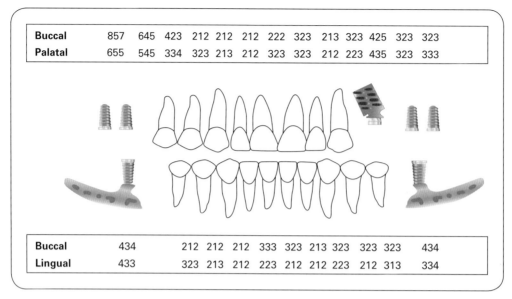

Buccal	857	645	423	212 212 212	222 323	213 323	425 323	323
Palatal	655	545	334	323 213 212	323 323	212 223	435 323	333

Buccal	434		212 212 212	333 323	213 323	323 323		434
Lingual	433		323 213 212	223 212	212 223	212 313		334

Figure 3: Probing pocket depth measurements during the consultation.

Occlusion

Group function was noted on lateral movement; patient presents flat curve of Spee, and class I occlusion (Figure 2).

Radiographic Examination

The #3 implant site was close to the sinus floor and presents a radiopaque mass in the right maxillary sinus (Figure 1).

Diagnosis

Periodontal status is II-chronic periodontitis, localized, moderate severity (Figure 3). The ridge is Seibert class III (horizontal and vertical bone loss) with lack of keratinized tissue, and low vestibular depth. Chronic maxillary sinusitis and failing dental implants on #2 and #3.

Treatment

The patient was premedicated with amoxicillin 875 mg 2 days before due to infection around dental implants #2 and #3 as well as in the right maxillary sinus. The implant fixtures were removed in #2 and #3 due to peri-implantitis and active infection. This was done atraumatically by using a specialized implant removal kit. Bone graft, a collagen resorbable membrane, and a titanium-reinforced expanded polytetrafluoroethylene (PTFE) membrane were used to cover the socket.

Preoperative Consultation

The medical history was reviewed. Consent for the procedure addressing benefits and risks was obtained.

After discussing all the relevant issues, the patient decided to remove the implants.

Implant Removal Procedure

Under intravenous sedation with 4 mg midazolam, topical anesthetic was applied and local anesthesia was given by infiltration: three carpules of 4% septocaine (Articaine) with epinephrine 1 : 100,000. The referring prosthodontist sectioned the implants for removal of the implants #2 and 3 (Figure 4). The prosthetic crowns were removed individually (Figure 5), then a #15 blade was used to make an incision in the buccal side of #2 and #3 area and a molt was used to release the flap to improve visibility (Figure 6).

Then we proceeded to use an implant removal kit. We connected the fixture remover (Figure 7) to the fixture with hex driver at 35 N cm (Figure 8); after that we connected the fixture remover (Figure 9) to a

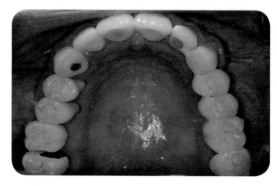

Figure 4: Occlusal view of the treated area.

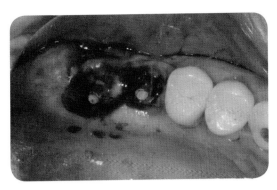

Figure 5: Treated area with crowns removed.

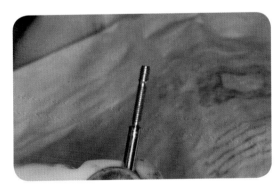

Figure 6: Buccal incision and flap release.

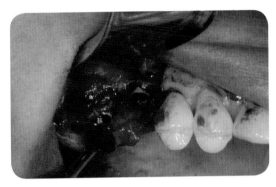

Figure 7: Fixture remover screw.

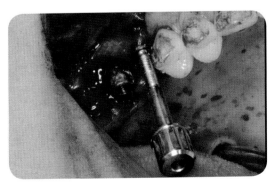

Figure 8: Connection of the fixture remover to the hex driver to 35 N cm.

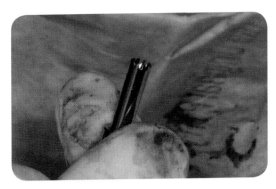

Figure 9: Fixture remover.

"fixture remover screw" by turning anticlockwise up to 300 N cm (Figures 10 and 11).

After the two implant removals (Figures 12, 13, and 14), infection distal of the implant in area #2 was found (Figure 15). All granulation tissues were removed with hemostatic forceps and we did lavage with Peridex and metronidazole. All irrigant and debris were suctioned from the wound site. The bone edges were smoothed with a bone file (Figure 16).

Freeze-dried bone allograft (FDBA) was mixed with metronidazole 250 mg/mL for 15 mins (Figure 17),

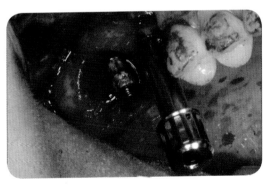

Figure 10: Connection of the fixture remover to the fixture remover screws.

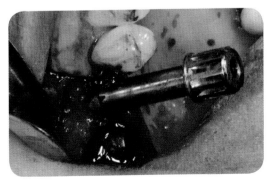

Figure 11: Turning fixture remover anticlockwise with torque wrench to 300 N cm.

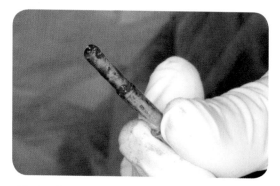

Figure 12: Implant removed atraumatically.

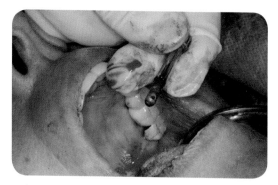

Figure 13: Implant #3 area removed.

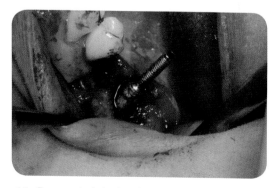

Figure 14: Removal of the implant in #2 area.

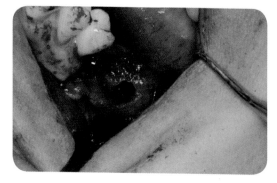

Figure 15: Granulation tissues in #2 area.

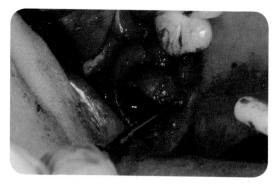

Figure 16: Granulation tissues removed.

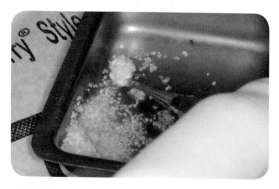

Figure 17: FDBA mixed with metronidazole 250 mg/mL solution.

and then we grafted it in the area (Figure 18). An open membrane technique was used with a Cytoplast collagen membrane (Figure 19) and a nonresorbable Cytoplast titanium reinforced membrane (Figures 20 and 21).

We sutured with a continuous suture technique with expanded PTFE Cytoplast suture (Figure 22). Three weeks later we removed the sutures and the nonresorbable membrane (Figure 23). Three months later the healing was normal (Figure 24).

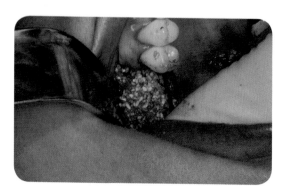

Figure 18: Placement of the FDBA in #2 and #3 area.

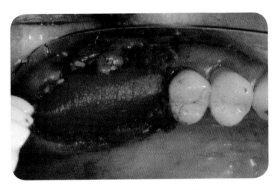

Figure 19: Colocation of Cytoplast resorbable collagen membrane.

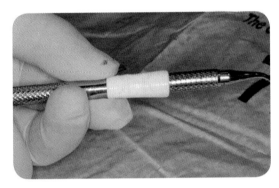

Figure 20: Molding the Cytoplast titanium-reinforced membrane before colocation.

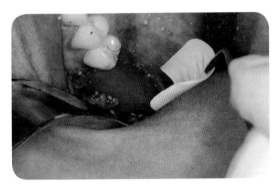

Figure 21: Colocation of Cytoplast titanium-reinforced membrane.

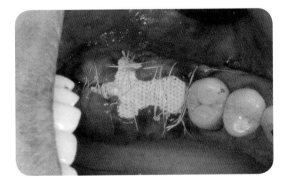

Figure 22: Open-membrane technique with Cytoplast PTFE continuous suture.

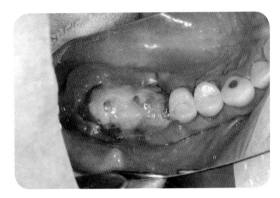

Figure 23: Reinforced membrane removal. Notice the resorbable collagen membrane still in the area.

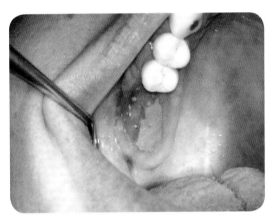

Figure 24: Four-week postoperative view.

Discussion

This case report discusses implants placed 24 years ago. Unfortunately, these had peri-implantitis. The treatment plan was for atraumatic removal and grafting process.

Burs, trephines, elevators, forceps, and piezoelectric instruments have been used for the removal of failing dental implants. Oftentimes these instruments and techniques remove too much alveolar bone, thus compromising the future implant site. However, when removal of an implant is necessary, the least invasive method should be the first option, in order to preserve the site for the possible future treatment and allow for an esthetic replacement, whether an implant restoration or pontic [1].

Many clinicians feel that implant placement is a success if the implant is not falling out or if there is no mobility. Nonetheless, the term "implant success" is commonly interchanged with "implant survival." This is a mistake, as implant survival is not necessarily implant success. Implant survival is defined as the continuation of the implant within the oral cavity regardless of the biological/technical complications that occur. Implant success is defined as an acceptable long-term (>10 years) nonmobile implant, without any evidence of radiographic radiolucency in the peri-implantar area, vertical bone loss (<0.2 mm) in the first year of service and annually subsequently, and absence of peri-implantitis, pain, and paresthesia [2–4].

Implant success is very susceptible to bacteria infiltration [1]. Therefore, it is very important to perform excellent phase 1 therapy, such as dental cleaning, periodontal treatment, and endodontic treatments if required. This will allow better postoperative healing.

Implant failures can be categorized as early and late. Late dental implant failure is mostly related to peri-implantitis, implant fracture, overloading before time of an adequate osseointegration, and occlusal trauma. Implants that fail due to peri-implantitis show many clinical signs similar to those found in periodontitis. These signs usually include bleeding on probing, pain, increased probing depth (>4 mm), suppuration, and bone loss [2,5,6]. The literature suggests that there are less late implant failures and that most implants fail in the early stages of healing [6].

Peri-implantitis can be treated nonsurgically or surgically in order to decontaminate implant surfaces with antibiotics and cleaning methods [7]. Nevertheless, when the maxillary sinus floor is involved in the infection, this approach might succeed due to the high risk of developing a new or aggravating sinusitis if the patient already presents it [8,9]. Literature suggests that one of the causes for an implant migration onto the sinus is the inflammatory reaction around the implant [10].

It was suggested that the use of a counter-torque ratchet is the least invasive method regarding damage to the surrounding structures when implant removal is needed [2]. However, counter-torquing cannot be achieved if part of the implant is still osseointegrated due to the internal connection being weaker than force required for removal.

Self-Study Questions

(Answers located at the end of the case)

A. What are some methods for implant removal?

B. What implant removal method is the least invasive option?

C. What three options have been reported in literature for the management of dental implant fracture?

References

1. Porter JA, von Fraunhofer JA. Success or failure of dental implants? A literature review with treatment considerations. J Acad Gen Dent 2005;53(6):423–432.
2. Froum S, Yamanaka T, Cho SC, et al. Techniques to remove a failed integrated implant. Compendium 2011;32(7):2–50.
3. Simonis P, Dufour T, Tenebaun H. Long-term implant survival and success: a 10–16 year follow-up of non-submerged dental implants. Clin Oral Implants Res 2010;21(7):772–777.
4. Albrektsson T, Zarb G, Worthington P, Eriksson AR. The long-term efficacy of currently used dental implants: a review and proposed criteria of success. Int J Oral Maxillofac Implants 1986;1(1):11–25.
5. Kim J-E, Shim J-S, Huh J-B, et al. Altered sensation caused by peri-implantitis: a case report. Oral Maxillofac Surg 2013;116(1):9–13.
6. Palma-Carrió C, Maestre-Ferrín L, Peñarocha-Oltra D, et al. Risk factors associated with early failure of dental implants. A literature review. Med Oral Patol Cir Bucal 2011;16(4):e514–e517.
7. Mombelli A, Moëne R, Décaillet F. Surgical treatments of peri-implantitis. Eur J Oral Implantol 2012;5(Suppl):S61–S70.
8. Prathapachandran J, Suresh N. Management of peri-implantitis. Dent Res J. 2012;9(5):516–521.
9. Viña-Almunia J, Peñarocha-Diago MA, Peñarocha-Diago M. Influence of perforation of the sinus membrane on the survival rate of implants placed after direct sinus lift. Literature update. Med Oral Patol Oral Cir Bucal 2009;14(3):E133–E136.
10. Fusari P, Doto M, Chiapasco M. Removal of a dental implant displaced into the maxillary sinus by means of the bone lid technique. Case Rep Dent 2013;2013:260707.

Answers to Self-Study Questions

A.

1. Counter-ratchet technique (reverse screw technique).
2. Use of piezotips or high-speed burs.
3. Use of trephine burs.
4. Use of electrosurgery to heat the implant (causing osteonecrosis around the fixture).

B. The use of a counter-torque ratchet is the least invasive option for implant removal. Other techniques involve damage to residual periodontium when removing bone around the implant.

C.

1. Removal of the coronal portion of the fractured implant, leaving the remaining apical part integrated in bone, complete removal of the fractured implant using explanation trephines, removal of the coronal portion of fractured implant with the purpose of placing a new prosthetic post.
2. Complete removal of the fractured implant using explanation trephines, removal of the coronal portion of the fractured implant, leaving the remaining apical part integrated in bone, removal of the apical portion of fractured implant with the purpose of placing a new prosthetic post.
3. Partial removal of the fractured implant using explanation trephines, removal of the coronal portion of the fractured implant, leaving the remaining apical part integrated in bone, removal of the apical portion of fractured implant with the purpose of placing a new prosthetic post.

Conclusion

The use of a nontraumatic technique for implant removal is preferred to preserve the peri-implant tissues compared with conventional use of trephine, bur, or piezo. This allows an easy minimally invasive approach and the future placement of implant and restoration. In this case report we have demonstrated a clever technique of grabbing the implant to overcome the required counter-torque to remove an implant atraumatically.

INDEX

Notes: Page numbers in *italics* indicate figures and those in **bold** denote tables and boxes

Clinical Cases in Implant Dentistry, First Edition. Edited by Nadeem Karimbux and Hans-Peter Weber.
© 2017 John Wiley & Sons, Inc. Published 2017 by John Wiley & Sons, Inc.